Diagnostic Imaging of Lung Cancers

Song Zhang
Editor

Ming-qi Zhang
Translator

Diagnostic Imaging of Lung Cancers

Science Press
Beijing

Springer

Editor
Song Zhang
Department of Respiratory and Critical Care Medicine
Shandong Provincial Hospital Affiliated to Shandong First Medical University
Jinan, Shandong
China

ISBN 978-981-99-6814-5 ISBN 978-981-99-6815-2 (eBook)
https://doi.org/10.1007/978-981-99-6815-2

Jointly published with Science Press
The print edition is not for sale in China (Mainland). Customers from China (Mainland) please order the print book from: Science Press.

This Springer imprint is published by the registered company Springer Nature Singapore Pte Ltd.
The registered company address is: 152 Beach Road, #21-01/04 Gateway East, Singapore 189721, Singapore

Paper in this product is recyclable.

Preface

When I Feel Sad

Written by Song Zhang

When I feel sad,
I miss the river in my memory—
The reddish brown water that flows
With all the trials and tribulations
And the sands of time that tell
The tales of speechless silence.

When I feel sad,
I miss the low hill, the pavilion,
The tall pines and cypresses
That watched me passing by time and again,
And the laughter of my childhood
That contrasts with the anguish of a wanderer.

When I feel sad,
I miss that afternoon in my childhood,
When the sunlight streamed through the window,
Bringing warmth to a puzzled boy,
And turning that moment
Into a lifetime of happiness.

When I feel sad,
I long for the vast expanse of wilderness,
Where the windswept grass
Brushes away many a difficult moment.
Then I'll be my old self again,
Living a free life like a dandelion.

Contents

Part II Mesenchymal Tumors

Part III Haematolymphoid Tumors

Contributors

Editor

Song Zhang Department of Respiratory and Critical Care Medicine, Shandong Provincial Hospital Affiliated to Shandong First Medical University, Jinan, Shandong, China

Translator

Ming-qi Zhang McGil University, Montreal, Quebec, Canada

Associate Editors

Xue-Peng Huang Department of Respiratory and Critical Care Medicine, People's Hospital of Rizhao Lanshan, Rizhao, Shandong, China

Jing Liu Department of Radiation Oncology, Shandong Cancer Hospital and Institute, Shandong First Medical University and Shandong Academy of Medical Sciences, Jinan, Shandong, China

Part I

Epithelial Tumors

Lung cancer is the most common cause of incidence and mortality of major cancers worldwide. Lung cancer incidence was estimated at 2,093,876 cases globally in 2018, accounting for 11.6% of the total cases. Estimated mortality for lung cancer in 2018 was 1,761,007 deaths globally, constituting around 18.4% of the total cancer deaths. The incidence varies according to geographic area, with Europe and Asia having the highest incidence rates. The global distribution for lung cancer incidence in 2018 was Asia (58.5%), Europe (22.4%), North America (12.1%), Latin American (4.3%), Africa (1.9%), and Oceania (0.81%). About 58% of lung cancer cases occur in underdeveloped countries. Compared to other highly incident malignancies (breast, colorectal, prostate, skin, and stomach cancer), lung cancer displays the lowest 5 years survival rate (10%– 20%) in most countries among those diagnosed during 2010 through 2014.

Classification

Lung cancer is divided into small cell lung cancer (SCLC) and non-small cell lung cancer (NSCLC). Small cell lung cancer is significantly more aggressive and is treated differently from other cell types. NSCLC accounts for about 85% of all lung cancer malignancies and is divided into a variety of histological subtypes, including adenocarcinoma, squamous cell carcinoma (SCC), and large cell carcinoma.

Although NSCLC and SCLC are commonly defined as different diseases because of their distinct biology and genomic abnormalities, the idea that these malignant tumors might share common cells of origin has been proved. A subset of NSCLCs with mutated EGFR return as SCLC when resistance to EGFR tyrosine kinase inhibitors develops this idea. Additionally, the coexistence of NSCLC and SCLC in some reports further challenges the commonly accepted view of their distinct lineages.

Etiology

Some environmental and lifestyle factors are related to the subsequent development of lung cancer. Smoking is the most important risk factor, accounting for approximately 90% of lung cancer cases in men and 80% of lung cancer cases in women. Among male smokers, SCC is the most common subtype. Tobacco smoke is also closely related to SCLC. Adenocarcinoma is the predominant subtype in never smokers and women, with increasing incidence rates over time. All histological types are strongly related to smoking, though the relative risks are considerably lower for adenocarcinoma than for SCC and SCLC. Toh et al. [1] found that smoking was associated with a worse prognosis in NSCLC. Sun et al. [2] also suggested that never smokers were increasingly prevalent and had a better prognosis than smokers with SCLC in Korea.

Given that about two-thirds of lung cancer deaths globally are attributed to smoking, the disease can be largely prevented through effective tobacco-control policies and regulations. Screening high-risk groups (current and former heavy smokers) with low-dose computed tomography (CT) can help diagnose cancer early. A Dutch-Belgian lung cancer screening trial involving high-risk persons reported that lung cancer mortality was significantly lower among those who underwent volume CT screening than among those who underwent no screening. The mortality reduction at 10 years of follow-up of 24% in men and 33% in women compared with no screening [3].

Other risk factors include age, family history, ionizing radiation, exposure to second-hand smoke, mineral and metal particles (arsenic, chromium, and nickel), polycyclic aromatic hydrocarbons, or asbestos. History of pulmonary fibrosis, human immunodeficiency virus infection, and alcohol consumption have also been confirmed as risk factors for lung cancer.

Because of reductions in smoking and improvements in early detection and treatment, the cancer death rate has fallen continuously from its peak in 1991 through 2018, for a total decline of 31%. The declines in mortality of lung cancer accounted for almost one-half of the total mortality decline from 2014 to 2018. The survival for SCLC remained at 14%–15%, but rapid gains in survival for NSCLC. For example, the 2-year relative survival for NSCLC increased from 34% for persons diagnosed during 2009 through 2010 to 42% during 2015 through 2016, including absolute increases of 5%–6% for every stage of diagnosis. Improved treatment has contributed to improved lung cancer-survival rates and drove a record drop in overall cancer mortality [4].

References

1. Toh CK, Gao F, Lim WT, et al. Never-smokers with lung cancer: epidemiologic evidence of a distinct disease entity. J Clin Oncol. 2006;24:2245–51.
2. Sun JM, Choi YL, Ji JH, et al. Small-cell lung cancer detection in never-smokers: clinical characteristics and multigene mutation profiling using targeted next-generation sequencing. Ann Oncol. 2015;26:161–6.
3. de Koning HJ, van der Aalst CM, de Jong PA, et al. Reduced lung-cancer mortality with volume CT screening in a randomized trial. N Engl J Med. 2020;382:503–13.
4. Siegel RL, Miller KD, Fuchs HE, et al. Cancer statistics, 2021. CA Cancer J Clin. 2021;71:7–33.

Adenocarcinoma

Song Zhang

Adenocarcinoma represents the most common histological type of lung cancer especially in non-smokers in most countries, accounting for almost half of all lung cancers. Adenocarcinoma originates from alveolar cells located in the smaller airway epithelium and tends to express immunohistochemical markers such as TTF-1 and Napsin A.

1 Classification

The classifications of lung tumors, published by the World Health Organization (WHO) in 1967, 1981, and 1999, were written primarily by pathologists for pathologists [1–3]. Histopathology is the basis of this classification, but lung cancer diagnosis is a multidisciplinary process that needs to be correlated with clinical, radiologic, molecular, and surgical information. Only in the 2004 revision, relevant genetics and clinical information were introduced [4].

Historically, pulmonary adenocarcinomas with lepidic growth have been termed bronchioloalveolar carcinoma (BAC), which was proposed by Dr. Averill Liebow in 1960 [5]. He introduced the term as bronchioloalveolar carcinoma, but it had lost its hyphen by the 1970s. Lepidic growth refers to neoplastic cells growing along pre-existing alveolar structures in a flat manner, without forming papillary or micropapillary structures. In the 1981 WHO histologic classification of lung tumors, lung adenocarcinoma was divided into 4 histologic subtypes: acinar adenocarcinoma, papillary adenocarcinoma, BAC, and solid adenocarcinoma with mucin. Noguchi et al. [6] in 1995 described patterns of non-mucinous BAC, some of which had "central collapse." These patients had 100% 5-year survival [7]. In the 1999 WHO classification of lung and pleural tumors, adenocarcinoma with mixed subtype was added as fifth major subtype. After 1999, the WHO classification narrowed the definition of BAC to include tumors with pure alveolar growth without invasion. Even after publication of the 1999 and 2004 WHO classifications, the term BAC is still used for a broad spectrum of tumors. According to the 2004 WHO histologic classification of lung tumors, lung adenocarcinoma is categorized into 5 main histologic subtypes: lepidic (formerly known as BAC), acinar, papillary, solid, and mixed subtype. Most cases of lung adenocarcinoma have been categorized as the mixed subtype. In 2011, based on advances in clinical, oncological, surgical, radiological, pathological, and molecular techniques, the International Association for the Study of

S. Zhang (✉)
Department of Respiratory and Critical Care Medicine, Shandong Provincial Hospital Affiliated to Shandong First Medical University, Jinan, Shandong, China

S. Zhang (ed.), *Diagnostic Imaging of Lung Cancers*, https://doi.org/10.1007/978-981-99-6815-2_1

Lung Cancer (IASLC), American Thoracic Society (ATS), and European Respiratory Society (ERS) proposed a new classification for lung adenocarcinoma that included a number of changes to previous classifications. The terms BAC and mixed subtype adenocarcinoma are no longer to be used. To clarify the nomenclature, the term BAC is referred to as "former BAC" in the new classification, and the concept is applicable to multiple categories in the new classification. For resected specimens, new terms of adenocarcinoma in situ (AIS) and microinvasive adenocarcinoma (MIA) are introduced to show pure lepidic growth and predominantly lepidic growth, with invasion ≤5 mm, respectively. The term "invasive mucinous adenocarcinoma" is introduced for adenocarcinomas formerly classified as mucinous BAC, excluding tumors that meet criteria for AIS or MIA. Invasive adenocarcinoma is classified as lepidic, acinar, papillary, and solid according to their predominant pattern; a micropapillary pattern is newly added. In the new classification, invasive mucinous adenocarcinoma, colloid, fetal and enteric adenocarcinoma are regarded as variants of invasive adenocarcinoma. Enteric adenocarcinoma is added to the variants based on histological and immunohistochemical features shared with colorectal cancer. For the diagnosis of enteric adenocarcinoma, the primary gastrointestinal origin should be excluded. This classification clearly emphasizes the significance of histological subtypes for prognosis and also provides guidance for small biopsies and cytology specimens.

Based on the 2011 IASLC/ATS/ERS classification [7], lung adenocarcinoma is classified as AIS, MIA, and invasive adenocarcinoma (IAC) in the WHO classification fourth edition in 2015 [8]. Tumors formerly known as large cell carcinomas that have pneumocyte marker expression (i.e., TTF-1 and/or Napsin A) are classified as solid adenocarcinomas. The expression of TTF-1 and/or Napsin A is sufficient not only to diagnose solid adenocarcinoma, but also to separate it from squamous cell carcinoma.

2 Molecular Pathology

Lung adenocarcinomas have relatively unique oncogenic driver mutations, such as EGFR exon 19 deletions and exon 21 point mutations, and EML4-ALK translocations, and matching these genotypes with associated targeted therapeutic agents becomes the basis for personalized therapy. Other driver mutations in oncogenes include ROS1, BRAF, RET, MEK1, NTRK, ERBB2, MET, and KRAS.

EGFR (epidermal growth factor receptor) is a transmembrane cell-surface receptor that is activated in around 10%–15% of Caucasian patients and 50% of Asian patients with NSCLC and is more common in Asians and non-smokers. EGFR exon 19 deletions or exon 18 (G719X, G719A, G719S, G719C, G719D), exon 20 (S768I), or exon 21 (L858R, L861Q, L861R) mutations are sensitive to EGFR-TKI therapy. Acquired resistance associated with EGFR-TKI therapy includes EGFR-dependent resistance(S768I, L861Q, G719X), MET and HER2 amplifications, small cell lung cancer, squamous cell carcinoma transformation, etc.

ALK (anaplastic lymphoma kinase) is a tyrosine kinase receptor encoded by the ALK gene and typically fusions with other genes, most commonly echinoderm microtubule-associated protein-like 4 (EML4). ALK gene rearrangement is largely independent of EGFR alterations and presents in approximately 2%–7% of patients with NSCLC. ALK-rearranged patients tend to be younger and have a limited history of smoking. Acquired ALK mutation (1151Tins, L1152R, C1156Y, F1174V/L, G1269A, and others) is the most common resistance mechanism. ALK translocation and EGFR mutation preclude first-line therapy with immune checkpoint inhibitors.

ROS1 (ROS proto-oncogene 1, receptor tyrosine kinase) rearrangements have been reported in 1%–2% of NSCLC patients and 2.4%–2.9% adenocarcinoma patients. ROS1 rearrangements are more prevalent in female sand smoker with a younger age. ROS1 rearrangements do not cor-

relate with worse prognosis. The homology between the tyrosine kinase domains of ROS1 and ALK determines the high sensitivity of ROS1 and ALK-positive NSCLC patients to targeted tyrosine kinase inhibitors (TKIs). Crizotinib treatment significantly improved outcomes in ROS1- and ALK-positive NSCLC patients.

BRAF (v-raf murine sarcoma viral oncogene homolog B) is a serine-threonine kinase belonging to the RAF kinase family lying downstream of KRAS and directly interacts with the MEK-ERK signaling cascade. BRAF mutations occur in 7% of NSCLC and 4% of lung adenocarcinoma cases and are more commonly found in current or former smokers and female patients. Half of them harbor the V600E mutation, and other mutations occur within exons 11 and 15.

RET (rearranged during transfection) rearrangements occur in approximately 1%–2% of NSCLC patients, with relatively high frequencies in young, non- or former light smokers. Activation of RET results in downstream pathway signaling including MAPK, AK/STAT, and PI3K/AKT, inducing cell proliferation and migration. The most common fusion variant is KIF5B-RET.

MEK1 (mitogen-activated protein kinase 1) encodes a serine-threonine kinase and is mutated in around 1% of NSCLC, mainly adenocarcinoma.

NTRK (neurotrophic tyrosine kinase receptor) genes (NTRK1, NTRK2, and NTRK3) encode three TRK proteins (TRKA, TRKB, and TRKC). NTRK1 and NTRK2 rearrangements occur in around 3% of lung adenocarcinomas.

MET (mesenchymal epidermal transition factor) is a receptor tyrosine kinase (RTK) that binds to hepatocyte growth factor (HGF). MET alterations or HGF activation promote the activation of signal pathways, including the RAS-RAF-mitogen-activated protein kinase (MAPK) and PI3K-AKT-mTOR (mammalian target of rapamycin) pathways. MET amplification is found in 3%–5% of newly diagnosed NSCLC patients, predominantly in adenocarcinoma. MET exon 14 skipping mutations have also been identified as oncogenic drivers and have been found in 4% of lung cancers.

KRAS (Kirsten Rat Sarcoma viral oncogene homolog) mutations account for approximately 25%–32% of lung adenocarcinomas and 4% of lung squamous cell carcinomas, most often in codons 12 or 13. They are usually found in non-Asians and smokers and associated with intrinsic EGFR-TKI resistance. The KRAS p.G12C mutation occurs in 13% of NSCLCs and in 1%–3% of colorectal cancers and other cancers. Sotorasib is a small molecule that selectively and irreversibly targets KRAS G12C. Hong et al. [9] conducted a phase 1 trial of sotorasib in patients with advanced solid tumors harboring the KRAS p.G12C mutation. In the NSCLC subgroup, 32.2% (19 patients) received a confirmed objective response and 88.1% (52 patients) achieved disease control. Sotorasib showed encouraging anticancer activity in patients with heavily pretreated advanced solid tumors harboring the KRAS p.G12C mutation.

In 2017, the College of American Pathologists (CAP), the International Association for the Study of Lung Cancer (IASLC), and the Association for Molecular Pathology (AMP) updated their recommendations for molecular testing for the selection of patients with lung cancer for treatment with targeted tyrosine kinase inhibitors. It strongly recommends against evaluating EGFR expression by immunohistochemistry for selection of patients for EGFR-targeted therapy. New for 2017 are recommendations for stand-alone ROS1 testing with additional confirmation testing in all patients with advanced lung adenocarcinoma, and RET, ERBB2 (HER2), KRAS, and MET testing as part of larger panels. ASCO also recommends stand-alone BRAF testing in patients with advanced lung adenocarcinoma [10].

3 Case Analysis

3.1 Case 1

A 46-year-old woman found a lung lesion for 4 days on physical examination.

Chest CT: A quasi-circular pure ground-glass nodule in the right upper lung lobe, with a diameter of approximately 5.0 mm (Fig. 1).

[Diagnosis] Atypical adenomatous hyperplasia.

[Diagnosis Basis] The transverse CT scan shows a 5.0 mm well-defined round nodule with pure ground-glass opacity in the apical segment of the upper right lung lobe. The pulmonary vessel penetrates the ground-glass opacity lesion without any vascular compromise. On the resection specimen, the lesion size was measured as 5 × 3 × 3 mm, and the lesion was diagnosed as atypical adenomatous hyperplasia.

[Analysis] Atypical adenomatous hyperplasia (AAH), first described in the 1999 WHO classification, is pathologically defined as a small (usually less than 5 mm in diameter), limited, mild-to-moderate atypical proliferation of type II alveolar epithelial cells and/or Clara cells in the alveolar wall or the respiratory bronchiolar wall. AAH is mostly discovered incidentally in the surgically resected lung tissue due to other problems, especially primary lung cancer. The incidence of AAH ranges from 9.3% to 21.4% of cases resected from primary lung cancer, whereas the incidence of AAH in patients with benign or metastatic disease has been reported to be approximately 4.4% to 9.6%. Chapman et al. [11] reported that AAH was found more frequently in the lungs of adenocarcinoma (23.2%) compared with large cell undifferentiated carcinoma (12.5%) or squamous cell carcinoma (3.3%). Women with adenocarcinoma were more likely to have AAH (30.2%) than men with adenocarcinoma (18.8%). Due to the widespread use of CT in clinical practice and the large-scale screening of early lung cancer, the number of AAH lesions detected by radiology have been increasing.

AAH has been described as a focal nodular ground-glass opacity (GGO) lesion on CT. Ground-glass nodule (GGN) lesion is defined as hazy increased attenuation of the lung, but with preservation of bronchial and vascular margins. Almost all AAH appear to be pure GGN(pGGN) without any solid content. The pathological basis of pGGN is alveolar epithelial hyperplasia, the increase in the number of cells in the alveoli, thickening of the alveolar septum, and fluid accumulation in the bronchiole terminals. The interface between AAH and normal lung parenchyma is clear, and the edges are smooth. No blood vessel convergence or pleural retraction was detected. AAH has predominance for the upper lobes and can be either solitary or multifocal and does not change on the follow-up CT.

AAH is recognized as a preinvasive lesion of lung adenocarcinoma, which can be safely just

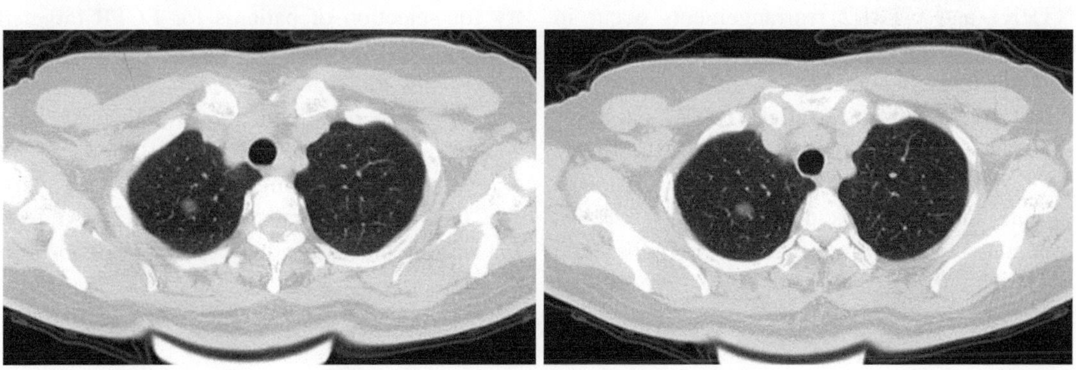

Fig. 1 Chest CT

followed by CT rather than surgical biopsy or resection. According to the tumor doubling time, a two- or three-year follow-up will be safe enough to confirm whether the lesion is AAH.

3.2 Case 2

A 43-year-old woman found a lung lesion on physical examination.

Chest CT: A pure GGO nodule of 15 mm in diameter in the right lower lung lobe (Fig. 2).

[Diagnosis] Adenocarcinoma in situ.

[Diagnosis Basis] The transverse CT scan shows a pure GGO nodule in the right lower lung lobe with clear boundary, regular shape. On the wedge resection specimen, the lesion was diagnosed as adenocarcinoma in situ (Fig. 3).

[Analysis] According to the 2015 WHO classification of lung adenocarcinoma, atypical adenomatous hyperplasia (AAH) and adenocarcinoma in situ (AIS) were defined as preinvasive lung adenocarcinoma lesions. In the 2021 WHO classification of lung tumors, they were categorized as precursor glandular lesions.

AIS was defined as a small (≤3 cm), localized adenocarcinoma with a pure lepidic growth that lacked stromal, vascular, alveolar space, or pleural invasion. Patterns of invasive adenocarcinoma (such as acinar, papillary, micropapillary, solid, colloid, enteric, fetal or invasive mucinous adenocarcinoma) and spread through air spaces are absent. If a tumor larger than 3 cm has been completely sampled histologically and shows no invasion, the tumor should be classified as "lepidic adenocarcinoma, suspect AIS."

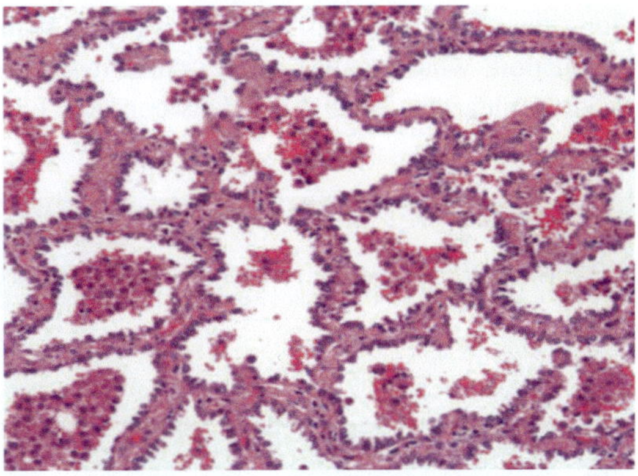

Fig. 3 Photomicrograph shows the lepidic growth pattern along alveolar septa with no identified focus of invasion

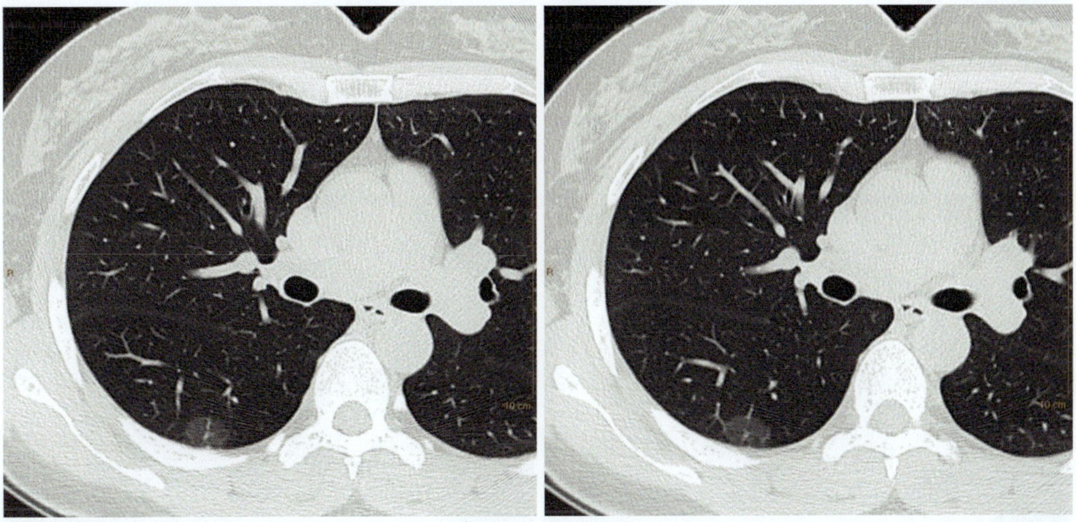

Fig. 2 Chest CT

AIS is subdivided into non-mucinous and mucinous variants. Most AIS are non-mucinous, which consists of type II pneumocytes and/or Clara cells. The rare cases of mucinous AIS consist of tall columnar cells and abundant cytoplasmic mucin. Nuclear atypia is absent or inconspicuous in both non-mucinous and mucinous AIS. Septal widening with sclerosis is common in AIS, particularly the non-mucinous variant. Most AIS patients are non-smokers and women. Mucinous AIS was significantly correlated with younger age, a TTF-1-negative cell lineage, and a wild-type EGFR. Both AAH and AIS demonstrate a replacing growth pattern along the alveolar lining, with no alveolar wall destruction, which makes it very challenging to make a clear-cut distinction between the two entities. Generally, AAH exhibits no attendant stromal thickening. In AIS, cell atypia may be more pronounced than in AAH.

On CT, the typical appearance of non-mucinous AIS is pure ground-glass nodule (pGGN) but sometimes as a part solid or occasionally a solid nodule. Mucinous AIS can appear as a solid nodule or consolidation (Fig. 4). The solid component represents fibrosis rather than invasion. AIS can be either single or multiple (Fig. 5).

It is often difficult to differentiate AAH from AIS. AAH usually has more air spaces and fewer cellular components than AIS, so that the density of AIS is slightly higher than that of AAH. AIS can also be distinguished from AAH on the basis of the mean CT attenuation. The

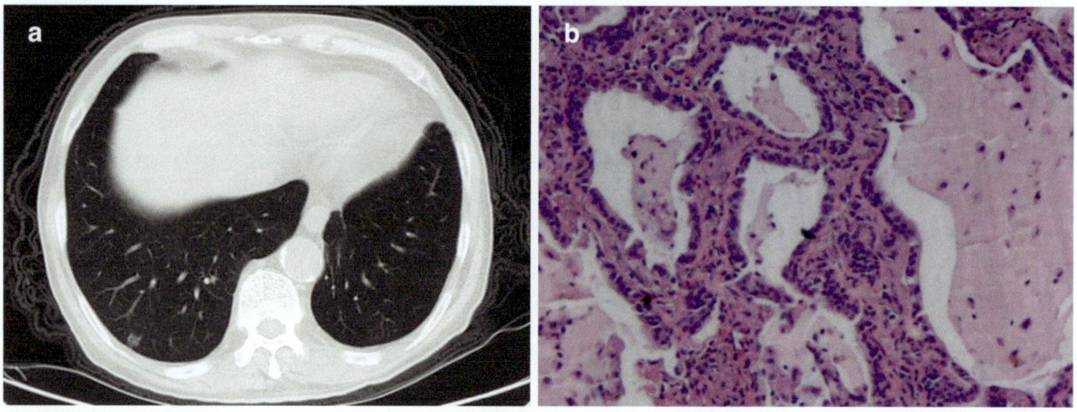

Fig. 4 A 73-year-old man with mucinous AIS. (**a**) CT scan shows a partly solid nodule in the right lower lobe. (**b**) Mucinous AIS consists of purely lepidic growth of tumor cells and intra-alveolar mucin. Neither stromal nor vascular invasion is seen

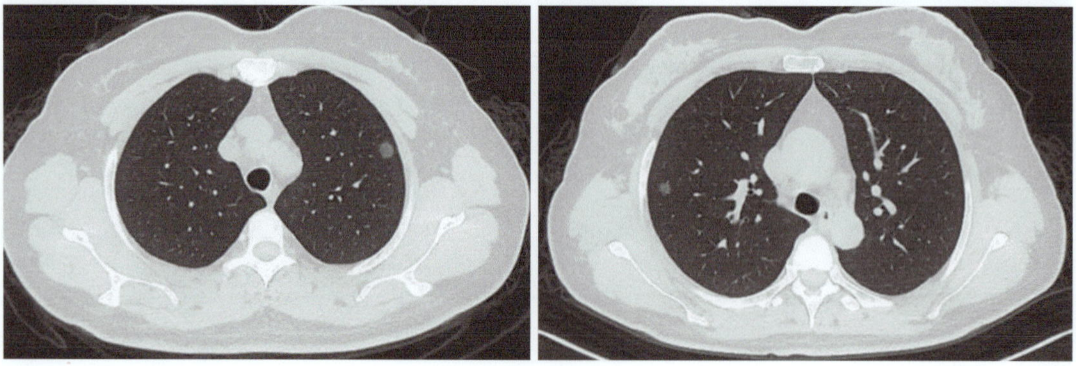

Fig. 5 A 47-year-old woman with AIS in the bilateral lungs

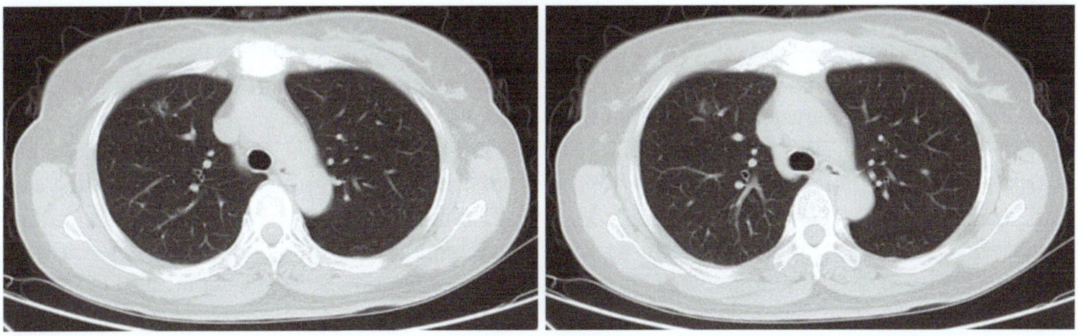

Fig. 6 Chest CT

mean CT attenuation of AAH is approximately −700 HU, which was significantly smaller than approximately −600HU for AIS. Kitami et al. [12] found that GGNs with a maximum diameter of ≤10 mm and CT value of ≤−600 HU are nearly always preinvasive lesions. The vacuole sign, a gassy, lucent shadow with a diameter of<5 mm, can also aid in the differentiation between AAH and AIS.

3.3 Case 3

A 51-year-old woman found a lung lesion on physical examination.

Chest CT: A GGO nodule in the right upper lung lobe (Fig. 6).

[Diagnosis] Minimally invasive adenocarcinoma.

[Diagnosis Basis] The transverse CT scan shows a GGO nodule in the upper lobe of right lung with bubble lucency and intact vessel distorted, supporting the diagnosis of lung adenocarcinoma. Patient underwent right upper lobectomy, the diameter of the lesion was approximately 7 mm, and the lesion was diagnosed as minimally invasive adenocarcinoma (Fig. 7).

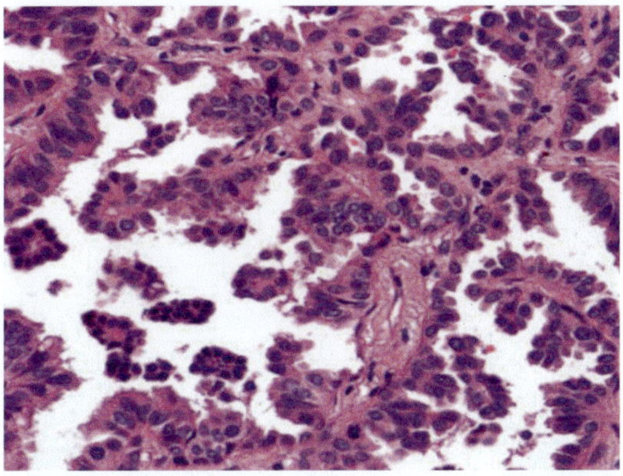

Fig. 7 The tumor shows a predominately lepidic growth pattern

[Analysis] MIA is a small (≤3 cm), solitary adenocarcinoma with a predominantly lepidic growth, showing ≤5 mm invasion along its greatest dimension, and lacking lymphatic, vascular, alveolar space, or pleural invasion. The invasive component to be measured includes any histologic subtype other than a lepidic pattern (such as acinar, papillary, micropapillary, solid, colloid, fetal, or invasive mucinous adenocarcinoma) or is defined as tumor cells infiltrating a myofibroblastic stroma. The cell type mostly non-mucinous (type II pneumocytes or Clara cells), but rarely may be mucinous (tall columnar cells with basal nuclei and abundant cytoplasmic mucin, sometimes resembling goblet cells) [7]. When there are multiple independent tumors, AIS and MIA should only be diagnosed if the lesions are considered to be synchronous primaries rather than intrapulmonary metastases. If a tumor larger than 3 cm has been completely sampled histologically and shows less than or equal to 0.5 cm of invasion, the tumor should be classified as "lepidic adenocarcinoma, suspect MIA."

The terms AIS and MIA are not suitable for diagnosis of small biopsies or cytology specimens. If there is a non-invasive pattern in a small biopsy, it should be referred to as a lepidic growth pattern. Similarly, if a cytology specimen exhibits AIS characteristics, the tumor should be diagnosed as an adenocarcinoma, possibly with a comment that this may represent, at least in part, AIS.

The imaging presentations of MIA can be pure GGO (Fig. 8) or part-solid nodule (Fig. 9) or even a solid nodule. Lee et al. [13] retrospectively investigated 55 pulmonary nodules in 52 patients pathologically confirmed as MIA, 53.8% were pure GGNs, 42.3% were part-solid GGNs, and 3.8% were solid nodules. Xiang et al. [14] suggested that the threshold of mean CT value for distinguishing between MIA and preinvasive lesions was −520 HU.

Pulmonary GGNs may histopathologically represent a variety of disorders such as lung adenocarcinoma, eosinophilic lung disease, pulmonary lymphoproliferative disorder, or organizing pneumonia/fibrosis. Henschke et al. [15] classified GGNs as solid, part-solid, or non-solid (pure GGO). They also reported that 63% of part-solid and 18% of non-solid nodules were malignant. Based on the presence of solid components in the

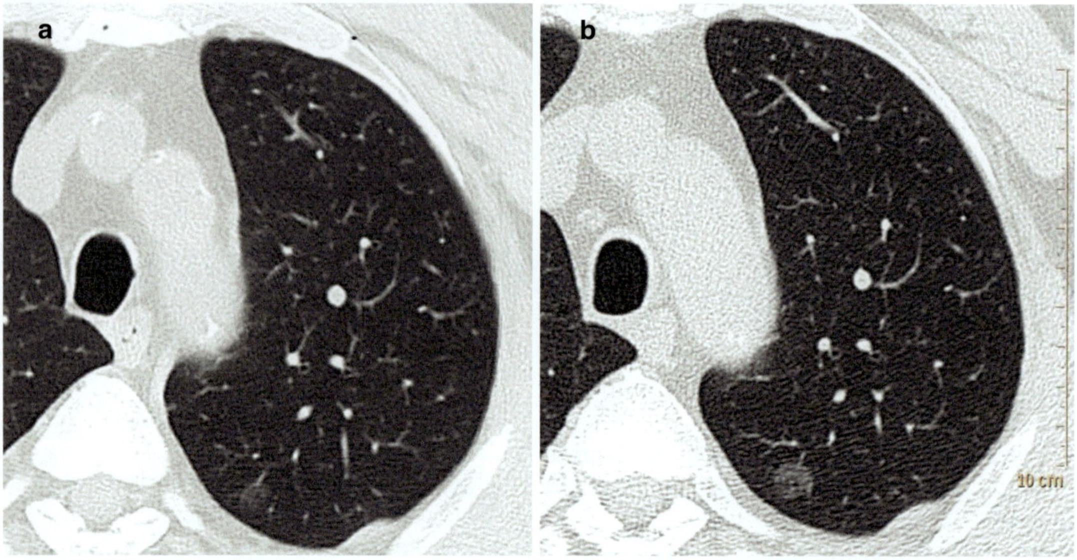

Fig. 8 A 50-year-old man with MIA showing GGO increase in size. (**a**) GGO in the left upper lobe, measuring 6 mm in diameter at detection. (**b**) Growth by 3 mm was confirmed after 9 months

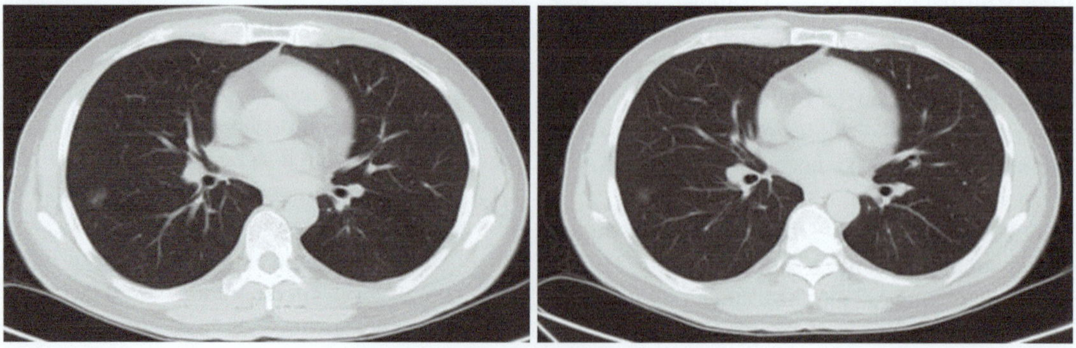

Fig. 9 A 57-year-old man with predominantly ground-glass with small central solid elements in the right lower lung lobe

nodules, GGNs are divided into two types: mixed GGO and pure GGO. AAH, AIS, MIA, and invasive adenocarcinoma (IAC) can be manifested as pure GGO or mixed GGO in CT imaging. AAH, AIS, and MIA grow along the walls of respiratory bronchioles and alveoli, most of them are pure GGO. If there is significant local fibroblast proliferation, local accumulation of tumor cells or collapse of alveolar walls, AAH, AIS, and MIA are usually manifested as mixed GGO. Kakinuma et al. [16] investigated that 7294 participants underwent screening for lung cancer with CT imaging, and identified 439 solitary pure GGNs 5 mm or smaller. Of the 439 pure GGNs, 394 were stable and 45 (10.3%) grew. Of the 45 pure GGNs that grew, 0.9% (four of 439) developed into adenocarcinomas (two minimally invasive and two invasive). In the four adenocarcinomas, the mean period between baseline CT screening and the appearance of solid components was 3.6 years. Their conclusion was that solitary pure GGNs of 5 mm or smaller detected by using CT screening should be rescanned 3.5 years later to search for development of a solid component. Yankelevitz et al. [17] investigated 57,496 participants underwent baseline and subsequent annual repeat CT screenings, and identified 2392 (4.2%) non-solid nodules, and pathologic pursuit led to the diagnosis of 73 cases of adenocarcinoma. A new non-solid nodule was identified in 485 (0.7%) of 64,677 annual repeat screenings, and 11 had a diagnosis of stage I adenocarcinoma; none were in nodules 15 mm or larger in diameter. Median time to treatment was 19 months. A solid component had developed in 22 cases prior to treatment (median transition time from non-solid to part-solid, 25 months). The lung cancer-survival rate was 100% with median follow-up since diagnosis of 78 month. They concluded that non-solid nodules of any size can be safely followed with CT at 12-month intervals to assess transition to part-solid. Surgery was 100% curative in all cases, regardless of the time to treatment. Ichinose et al. [18] examined 191 GGO lesions, including 114 pure GGO and 77 mixed lesions.160 patients underwent surgical resection. Among 114 pure GGO lesions, 14 (12%) were diagnosed as invasive lung cancer and 16 (14%) as MIA. Pure GGO lesions should be carefully monitored by periodic chest CT, and resection is recommended when they exhibit pleural indentation on HRCT or positivity on PET.

Approximately 10%–25% of pure GGNs increases in size or grow the solid component, while others remain unchanged for years. The Fleischner Society 2017 guidelines

suggest that pure GGNs smaller than 6 mm in diameter do not require routine follow-up. For pure GGNs 6 mm or larger, follow-up scanning is recommended at 6–12 months and then every 2 years thereafter until 5 years. To date, numerous reports have shown that pure GGNs that are 6 mm or larger may be followed safely for 5 years, with an average of 3–4 years typically required to establish growth or, less commonly, to diagnose a developing invasive carcinoma. For solitary part-solid nodules smaller than 6 mm, no routine follow-up is recommended. In practice, discrete solid components cannot be reliably defined in such small nodules, and they should be treated similar to the way in which pure ground-glass lesions of equivalent size are treated. For solitary part-solid nodules 6 mm or larger with a solid component less than 6 mm in diameter, follow-up is recommended at 3–6 months and then annually for a minimum of 5 years. Although part-solid nodules have a high likelihood of malignancy, nodules with a solid component smaller than 6 mm typically represent either AIS or MIA rather than invasive adenocarcinoma. For solitary part-solid nodules with a solid component 6 mm or larger, a short-term follow-up CT scan at 3–6 months should be considered to evaluate for persistence of the nodule. Abundant evidence has confirmed that the larger the solid component, the greater the risk of invasiveness and metastases. A solid component larger than 5 mm correlates with a substantial likelihood of local invasion [19].

Guidelines for the management of GGNs that have been stable for 5 years have not been determined. Lee et al. [20] conducted an observational study to investigate the natural course of GGNs that has had been stabilized for 5 years by low-dose CT. A total of 208 GGNs were detected in 160 participants. During a follow-up of 136 months, GGN growth was found in 27 (13.0%) GGNs. In approximately 95% of GGNs, the initial size was less than 6 mm, with 3.2 mm of growth over 8.5 years. Three out of 27 GGNs underwent biopsy and showed adenocarcinoma. In 8 of 27 cases, GGN growth preceded the development of a new solid component. In a multivariate analysis, bubble lucency, a history of cancer other than lung cancer, and development of a new solid component were important risk factors for GGN growth. They concluded that GGNs should not be ignored, even if it is smaller than 6 mm and stable for 5 years, especially when a new solid component appears during follow-up.

Wedge resection or segmentectomy is usually surgical method performed for AIS and MIA to maximize the preservation of functional lung parenchyma. After complete resection, the 5-year disease-free survival reaches 100% or nearly 100%. Since there is no regional lymph node metastasis or distant metastasis in AIS and MIA, it is no need for lymph node dissection during surgery.

Hu et al. [21] performed the analyses of multiregion whole-exome sequencing of 116 resected lung nodules including AAH (n = 22), AIS (n = 27), MIA (n = 54), and synchronous adenocarcinoma (ADC) (n = 13). They observed progressive genomic evolution at the single nucleotide level and demarcated evolution at the chromosomal level and supported the early lung carcinogenesis model from AAH to AIS, MIA, and ADC.

3.4 Case 4

A 65-year-old woman found a lung lesion for 2 months on physical examination.

Chest CT: A nodule in the right lower lung lobe (Fig. 10).

[Diagnosis] Invasive adenocarcinoma.

[Diagnosis Basis] The transverse CT scan shows a mixed GGO nodule in the lower lobe of right lung with lobulation, spiculation, air bronchogram, well-defined but coarse interface and pleural indentation, favoring the diagnosis of lung adenocarcinoma. Patient underwent right lower lobectomy, the lesion was approximately 3 × 2 × 1 cm, diagnosed as invasive adenocarcinoma (80% acinar type, and 20% lepidic type).

[Analysis] In the 2021 WHO classification, in addition to the rare variants, invasive adenocarcinoma is divided as non-mucinous and mucinous types. Invasive non-mucinous adenocarcinomas are the commonest subtype of lung cancer, consisting of malignant epithelial tumors with morphological or immunohistochemical evidence of glandular differentiation and not fulfilling criteria for any other type of adenocarcinoma, including lepidic, acinar, papillary, micropapillary, and solid growth patterns. Under the 2011 IASLC/ATS/ERS and 2015 WHO guidelines, invasive adenocarcinomas are classified according to the predominant subtype after evaluation of the tumor using comprehensive histologic subtyping to make a semiquantitative estimate of all of the different histologic patterns present in 5% increments. It is very useful to determine the predominant subtype when a tumor has two patterns with relatively similar percentages and allows reporting small amounts of components that may be prognostically important such as micropapillary or solid patterns. It also helps to distinguish multiple synchronous primary lung adenocarcinomas from a dominant tumor with pulmonary metastases.

Invasive adenocarcinoma is usually visualized as solid nodule, corresponding with the >5 mm of overt invasion seen on histopathology, but may also be part-solid nodule or occasionally GGN. Accepted predictors of malignancy include upper lobe location, size, and the presence of spiculation. For part-solid nodules, suspicious morphologic features include lobulated margins, air bronchograms, pleural tags, vascular convergence sign, and bubble-like lucencies (pseudocavitation), but none has been reliably shown to discriminate between benign and malignant nodules for these features. Spiculation (also called sunburst or corona radiata sign) is caused by

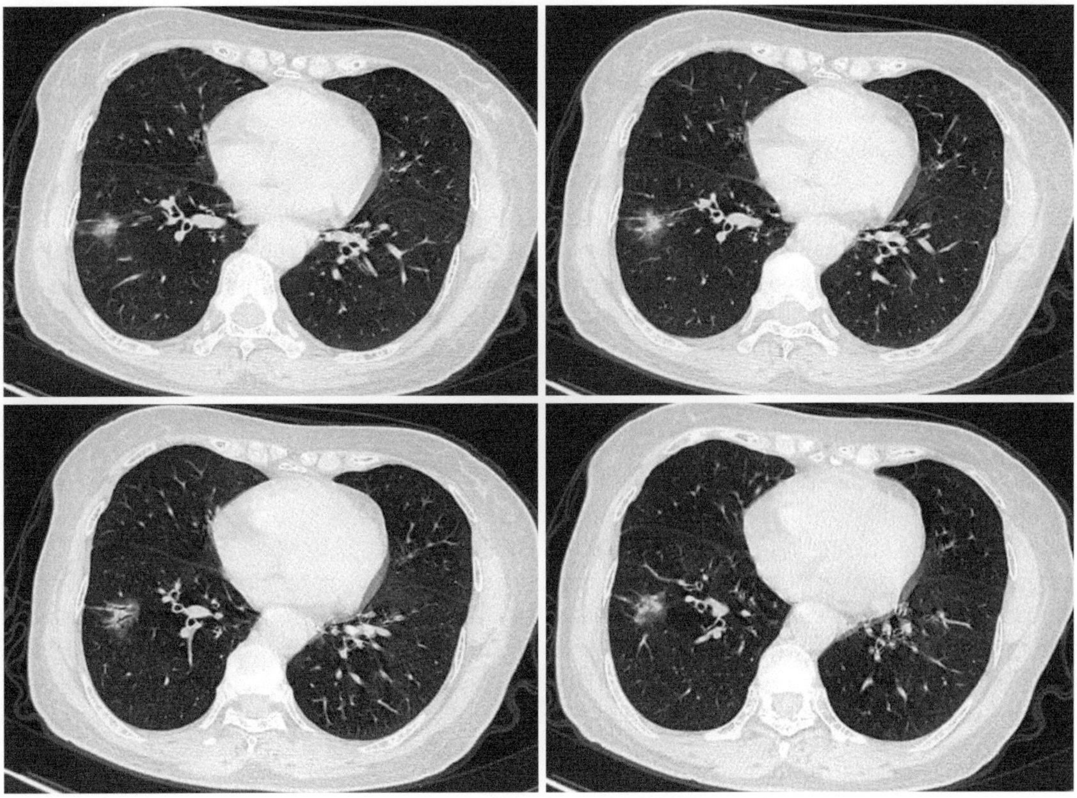

Fig. 10 Chest CT

interlobular septal thickening, fibrosis caused by obstruction of pulmonary vessels or lymphatic channels filled with tumor cells. A nodule with a spiculation is much more likely to be malignant than one with a smooth, well-defined margin. Lobulation is defined when portion of lesion's surface shows wavy or scalloped configuration. Lobulation in a nodule is attributed to different or uneven growth rates and is highly correlated with malignant tumors. Air bronchogram is defined when air-filled bronchus is present inside nodule, which strongly suggests invasive adenocarcinoma over MIA. Pleural tag is defined as one or more linear strands heading toward pleura. They correlate with thickening of the interlobular septa of the lung and can be caused by edema, tumor extension, inflammation, or fibrosis. Vascular convergence sign is described as vessels converging to a nodule without adjoining or contacting the edge of the nodule and is mainly seen in peripheral subsolid lesions. Bubble-like lucencies are areas of low attenuation due to small patent air-containing bronchi in the nodule. In subsolid nodules, bubble-like lucencies are slightly more common in invasive adenocarcinomas than in preinvasive lesions and are uncommon in non-neoplastic nodules.

Most studies have shown that lepidic adenocarcinomas are low grade; acinar and papillary tumors are intermediate grade; solid and micropapillary tumors are high grade. Patients with stage I lepidic predominant adenocarcinoma have an excellent prognosis; most of those tumors that recur have some high-risk factors, such as close margin in limited resection and the presence of micropapillary components or vascular and/or pleural infiltration. The solid and micropapillary subtypes are associated with poor prognosis, but their responsiveness to adjuvant chemotherapy has improved compared with acinar or papillary predominant tumors in surgically resected lung adenocarcinoma patients, based on disease-free survival and specific disease-free survival.

The grading system for lung adenocarcinoma has not been established. The IASLC pathology panel analyzed a multi-institutional study involving multiple cohorts of invasive pulmonary adenocarcinomas. A cohort of 284 stage I pulmonary adenocarcinomas was used as a training set to identify histologic features related to patient outcomes [22]. The best model was composed of a combination of predominant plus high-grade histologic pattern with a cutoff of 20% for the latter. The model consists of the following: grade 1, lepidic predominant tumor; grade 2, acinar or papillary predominant tumor, both with no or less than 20% of high-grade patterns; and grade 3, any tumor with 20% or more of high-grade patterns (solid, micropapillary, cribriform, and complex gland) [22]. The grading system is practical and prognostic for invasive pulmonary adenocarcinoma (IPA). Based on the grading system, Hou et al. [23] retrospectively analyzed 926 Chinese patients with completely resected stage I IPAs and classified them into three groups (grade 1, $n = 119$; grade 2, $n = 431$; grade 3, $n = 376$). In the multivariable analysis, the proposed grading system was independently associated with recurrence and death. Among patients with stage IB IPA ($N = 490$), the proposed grading system identified patients who could benefit from adjuvant chemotherapy but who were undergraded by the adenocarcinoma classification. The novel grading system not only demonstrated prognostic significance in stage I IPA but also provided clinical value for guiding therapeutic decisions regarding adjuvant chemotherapy.

3.5 Case 5

A 35-year-old woman found a lung lesion for 10 days on physical examination.

Chest CT: A nodule in the left upper lung lobe (Fig. 11).

[Diagnosis] Lepidic adenocarcinoma.

[Diagnosis Basis] The transverse CT scan shows a mixed GGO nodule in the upper lobe of left lung with well-defined interface. Patient underwent left upper lobectomy, the lesion was approximately 1.4 × 1.2 × 1.0 cm, and the final diagnosis was lepidic predominant adenocarcinoma.

[Analysis] According to the IASLC/ATS/ERS classification, the lepidic predominant pattern consists of three subtypes: AIS, MIA, and non-mucinous lepidic predominant invasive adenocarcinoma. Lepidic predominant adenocarcinoma (LPA), a non-mucinous entity, is defined as a predominant lepidic growth but with at least one focus of invasion measuring >5 mm. Any lepidic predominant tumors with lymphatic, vascular, pleural invasion, or tumor necrosis were diagnosed as lepidic predominant invasive tumors rather than AIS or MIA, regardless of the degree of invasion.

On CT, LPA can be shown as a part-solid nodule with variable proportions of ground-glass and solid components. Ko et al. [24] investigation showed that the mean solid to ground-glass component volume ratio for LPA was 14.5%, significantly higher than 8.2% in AIS/MIA. Lee et al. [25] retrospectively investigated the differentiating CT features between LPA and preinvasive lesions appearing as GGNs in 253 patients. They found that LPA is more likely to demonstrate a lobulated border and pleural retraction than the preinvasive lesions. In pure GGNs, preinvasive lesions were significantly smaller and more frequently non-lobulated than IPAs. The optimal cutoff size for preinvasive lesions was <10 mm. In part-solid GGNs, preinvasive lesions can be accurately differentiated from IPAs by the smaller lesion size, smaller solid proportion, nonspiculated margin, and non-lobulated border.

Several studies have demonstrated that the prognosis of LPA was more favorable. Yoshizawa et al. [26] reported a five-year survival rate of 90%. In 2014, Kadota et al. [27] retrospectively studied 1038 patients with stage I lung adenocarcinoma. Tumors were classified according to the IASLC/ATS/ERS classification: 2 were AIS, 34 MIA, and 103 LPA. Patients with LPA had an overall five-year recurrence rate of 8% compared with 19% in those with non-lepidic predominant tumors. The risk of recurrence varied based on the proportion of lepidic subtype present. Patients with >50% lepidic pattern tumors experienced no

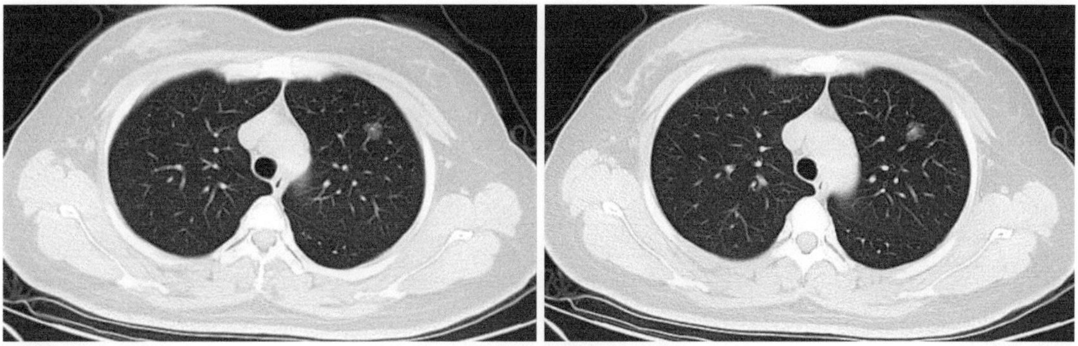

Fig. 11 Chest CT

recurrences (n = 84), those with >10% to 50% lepidic pattern tumors had an intermediate risk for recurrence (n = 344; 12%), and those with ≤10% lepidic pattern tumors had the highest risk (n = 610; 22%). Most patients with LPA who experienced a recurrence had potential risk factors, including sublobar resection with close margins (≤0.5 cm; n = 2), 20% to 30% micropapillary component (n = 2), and lymphatic or vascular invasion (n = 2).

Cox et al. [28] studied the association of extent of lung resection, pathologic nodal evaluation, and survival for patients with clinical stage I lepidic adenocarcinoma. Of the 1991 patients, 447 underwent sublobar resection and 1544 underwent lobectomy. Among patients who underwent lobectomy, 6% (n = 92) were upstaged because of positive nodal disease, with a median of seven lymph nodes sampled. In a multivariable analysis of a subset of patients, lobectomy was no longer independently associated with improved survival when compared with sublobar resection including lymph node sampling. They concluded that surgeons treating stage I lung adenocarcinoma patients with lepidic features should cautiously utilize sublobar resection rather than lobectomy, and they must always perform adequate pathologic lymph node evaluation including lymph node sampling.

Maurizi et al. [29] evaluated the role of a systematic lymphadenectomy in patients undergoing surgery for clinical stage I lung LPA. Only patients (n = 98) undergoing lobectomy or sublobar resection associated with systematic hilar-mediastinal nodal dissection were retrospectively enrolled in the study. Resection was lobectomy in 77.6% (76/98) and sublobar in 22.4% (n = 22). All the resections were complete (R0). Histology was LPA in 85 cases and MIA in 13 cases. At pathologic examination, N0 was confirmed in 78 patients (79.6%), while N1 in 12 (12.2%) and N2 in 8 (8.2%). At a median follow-up of 45.5 months, 26.5% of patients relapsed. The 5-year disease-free survival was 98.6% for stage I, 75% for stage II, and 45% for stage III. A complete nodal dissection can reveal occult nodal metastases in LPA patients and can improve the accuracy of pathologic staging. N1/N2 disease is a negative prognostic factor for this histology. A systematic lymph node dissection should be considered even in this setting.

3.6 Case 6

A 38-year-old man found a lung lesion for 2 months on physical examination.

Chest CT: A nodule in the right lower lung lobe (Fig. 12).

[Diagnosis] Acinar adenocarcinoma.

[Diagnosis Basis] The transverse CT scan shows an irregular nodule in the lower lobe of right lung with a prominent retraction of the adjacent fissure, favoring the diagnosis of lung adenocarcinoma. Lobectomy proved the malignant nature, showing an acinar adenocarcinoma.

[Analysis] Histopathologically, acinar-predominant adenocarcinoma consists mainly of glands, which are round to oval shaped with a central luminal space surrounded by tumor cells.

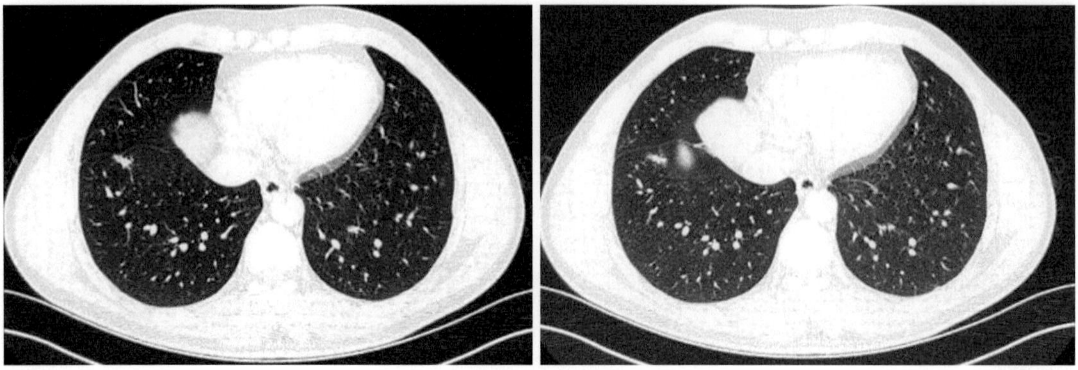

Fig. 12 Chest CT

The neoplastic cells and glandular spaces may contain mucin. It may be difficult to distinguish AIS with collapse from the acinar pattern. Invasive acinar adenocarcinoma is considered when the alveolar architecture is lost and/or myofibroblastic stroma is present. Acinar-predominant adenocarcinoma is probably the most prevalent subtype of pulmonary adenocarcinoma, accounting for 30%–40% of all invasive adenocarcinoma cases in some series. Duhig et al. [30] investigated 145 stage I adenocarcinoma cases. They found that the acinar pattern was the most common predominant architecture (44.4%), followed by papillary (22.8%) and solid (25.5%). There is no pure acinar pattern, but pure lepidic, papillary, and solid patterns were recorded. Warth et al. [31] evaluated 674 resected pulmonary adenocarcinoma cases. 248 cases (36.8%) were solid, followed by 207 (30.6%) acinar, 101 (15%) papillary, 55(8.2%) micropapillary, 35 (5.2%) lepidic, and 28 (4.2%) cribriform predominant.

Cribriform growth pattern is regarded as a variant of acinar adenocarcinoma and was first reported in lung cancer in 1978. The term cribriform is derived from the Latin cribrum (for "sieve"), which is defined by invasive back-to-back fused tumor glands with poorly formed glandular spaces lacking intervening stroma or invasive tumor nests of tumors cells that produce glandular lumina without solid components [30, 31]. Compared with common acinar pattern (tubular glands), cribriform growth pattern is associated with more aggressive histopathological structures, higher risk of recurrence, and shorter postoperative survival. These features are similar to solid or micropapillary adenocarcinoma. Cribriform growth pattern has been considered as a new pathologic subtype of lung adenocarcinoma.

3.7 Case 7

A 52-year-old man found a lung lesion on physical examination.

Chest CT: A lesion in the right middle lung lobe (Fig. 13).

[Diagnosis] Papillary adenocarcinoma.

[Diagnosis Basis] The transverse CT scan shows a 3.5 × 2 cm solid mass in the middle lobe of right lung with lobulated margins (red arrow) and internal vascular thickening (white arrow). Lobectomy revealed papillary predominant adenocarcinoma.

[Analysis] The Fleischner Society glossary of terms defines a lesion <3 cm in size as a nodule, whereas a lesion larger than 3 cm is referred to as a mass. Papillary predominant adenocarcinoma consists of a growth of glandular cells along central fibrovascular cores. The peak incidence of papillary adenocarcinoma patients ranges from 50 to 60 years old with a proneness to the female. The histological subtype in adenocarcinoma significantly correlated with the prognosis. Dong et al. [32] showed the 5-year survival rate of pap-

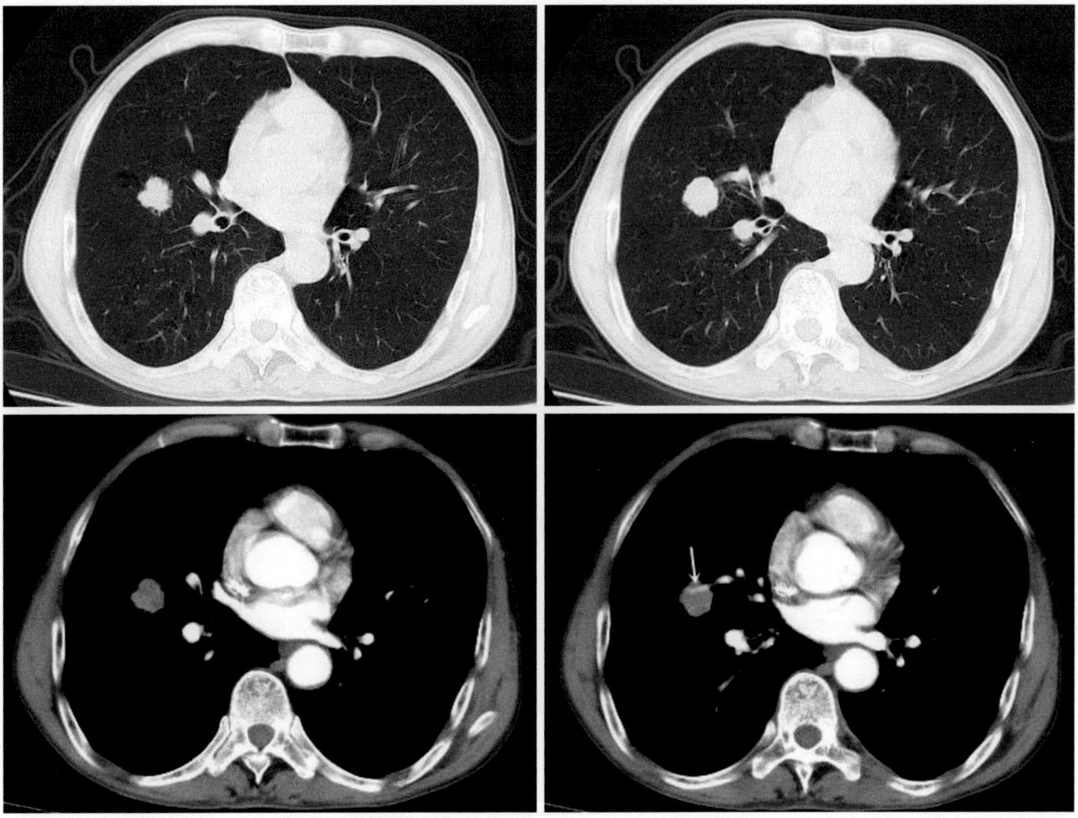

Fig. 13 Chest CT

illary predominant adenocarcinoma was 61.50% based on analyzing 226 Chinese papillary predominant adenocarcinoma patients. Sakurai et al. [33] retrospectively analyzed 2004 papillary adenocarcinoma patients, and the 5-year overall survival rate was 72.9%. Zhang et al. [34] retrospectively analyzed 3391 patients with primary pulmonary papillary predominant adenocarcinoma. Older age, larger lesions, lymph node invasion, distant metastases, and poor pathological differentiation are correlative with poor prognosis. Surgical intervention is beneficial for obtaining favorable prognosis. Chemotherapy or radiotherapy has no significant effects on patient survival.

The mean doubling time of tumors theoretically reflects the exponential growth of tumor cells and aids in predicting the likelihood of malignancy in pulmonary lesions. Henschke et al. [35] demonstrated that the volume doubling time (VDT) of lung cancer varies according to the lung cancer subtypes and CT features. Adenocarcinoma was the most frequent cell type (50%), followed by squamous cell carcinoma (19%), small cell carcinoma (19%), and cancers of other cell types (12%). The distribution of VDT by cell type was as follows: small cell carcinomas (median, 43 days), large cell/neuroendocrine carcinomas (median, 82 days), squamous cell carcinomas (median, 88 days), adenocarcinomas presenting with solid nodules (median, 140 days), and adenocarcinomas manifesting as subsolid nodules (median, 251 days). Park et al. [36] investigated differences in VDT between the predominant histologic subtypes of primary lung adenocarcinomas and to assess the correlation between VDT and prognosis. Among 268 patients, there were 30 lepidic, 87 acinar, 109 papillary, and 42 solid or micropapillary-predominant subtypes. The median VDT was

529 days for lung adenocarcinomas and 229 days for solid or micropapillary subtypes. Solid lesions (VDT, 248 days) had shorter VDTs than subsolid lesions (part-solid lesions, 665 days; non-solid lesions, 648 days). VDT (<400 days) was an independent risk factor for poor disease-free survival (DFS) and higher TNM stage.

3.8 Case 8

A 60-year-old woman found a lung lesion on physical examination.

Chest CT: An irregular lesion in the right upper lung lobe (Fig. 14).

[Diagnosis] Micropapillary adenocarcinoma.

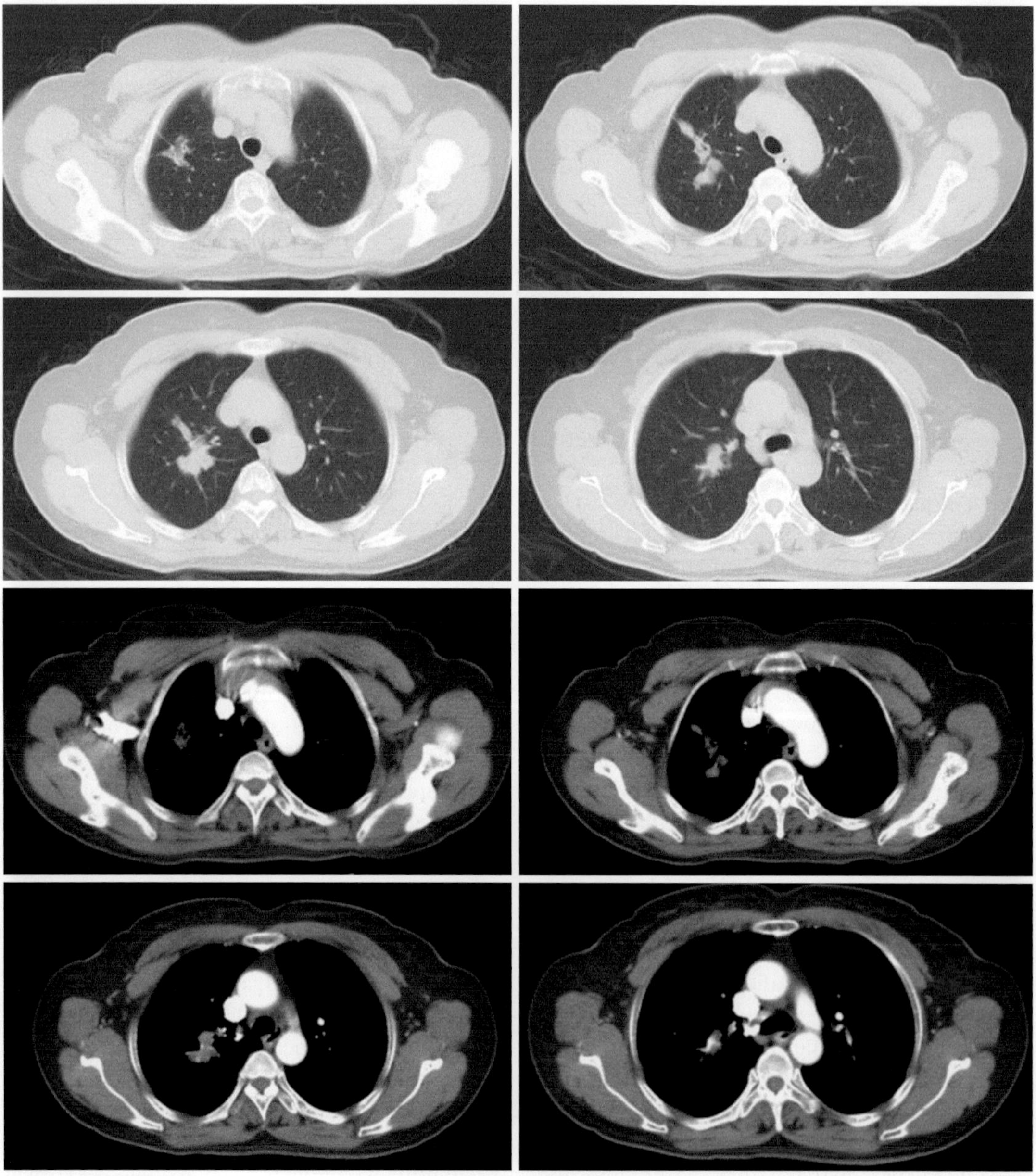

Fig. 14 Chest CT

[Diagnosis Basis] The transverse CT scan shows a lesion of 2.5 cm in diameter in the upper lobe of right lung with irregular shape, lobulated margins, bubble-like lucencies, pleural tags, and internal vascular distortion. She underwent right upper lobectomy. Specimens of cancer tissues showed adenocarcinoma with acinar (70%), invasive mucinous adenocarcinoma (20%), and micropapillary (10%) components, with visceral pleural invasion and peribronchial lymph node metastases (2/2).

[Analysis] Micropapillary-predominant adenocarcinoma has a unique growth pattern consisting of tumor cells growing in papillary tufts that lack fibrovascular cores, and is associated with a higher degree of aggressiveness. Micropapillary pattern (MPP) was first reported by McDivitt et al. [37] in breast carcinoma in 1982, and since then MPP has been reported in several other organs, including the urinary bladder and ovary. MPP was first reported in lung adenocarcinoma by Silver and Askin in 1997 [38]. They stated that 74% of papillary adenocarcinomas showed the MPP. Amin et al. [39] later studied 35 cases of primary lung adenocarcinoma with a micropapillary component. They found that MPP was not associated with any particular histologic subtype of lung adenocarcinoma. 33 of 35 patients (94%) developed metastases, primarily in the lymph nodes (26) and lung (17). Most metastases had a prominent micropapillary component, irrespective of the extent of the micropapillary carcinoma component in the primary lung tumor. They emphasized the importance of recognition of this histologic pattern, as those patients may have a higher risk of recurrence and thus require a close follow-up. Some studies further confirmed that smokers, lymphovascular invasion, visceral pleural invasion, and the presence of lymph node and intrapulmonary metastases are more frequently observed in MPP histologic subtype.

Micropapillary-predominant adenocarcinoma has been reported to have a poor prognosis with a tendency toward recurrence and metastasis. Tsubokawa et al. [40] retrospectively examined 347 consecutive patients with clinical stage IA lung adenocarcinoma who underwent complete resection. Patients with a higher ratio of MPP or papillary predominant subtypes have worse survival. Nitadori et al. [41] reported that the micropapillary histological subtype is a risk factor for recurrence after sublobar resection. Most recurrences (63.4%) were locoregional; micropapillary component of 5% or greater was statistically significantly associated with increased risk of local recurrence when the surgical margin was less than 1 cm. Sublobar resection may be insufficient for early-stage lung adenocarcinoma with micropapillary components because of the associated higher incidence of locoregional recurrence. Yoshida et al. [42] found that adenocarcinoma with a micropapillary component was more frequent in solid nodules (17.8%) than in either ground-glass nodules (1.5%) or part-solid nodules (5.3%) on high-resolution computed tomography (HRCT). In multivariate analysis, the HRCT finding was the only preoperative factor associated with a micropapillary component. Dai et al. [43] investigated the relationship between lymph node micrometastasis and histologic patterns of adenocarcinoma. Micropapillary component had been proven to be an independent predictor of increased frequency of micrometastasis. In micropapillary-positive patients, the presence of micrometastasis was correlated with a higher risk of locoregional recurrence rather than distant recurrence. Watanabe et al. [44] investigated the impact of MPP on the timing of postoperative recurrence using hazard curves. They found that patients with MPP retained a high risk of early postoperative recurrence, and risk of recurrence persisted over the long term. Even after complete resection in stage I lung adenocarcinoma patients, micropapillary component is still correlated with a poor prognosis.

As partial lung resection is associated with a poor prognosis in adenocarcinoma with micropapillary component, lobectomy followed by adjuvant chemotherapy is recommended.

3.9 Case 9

A 51-year-old man found a lung lesion on physical examination.

Chest CT: An oral nodule in the right lower lung lobe (Fig. 15).

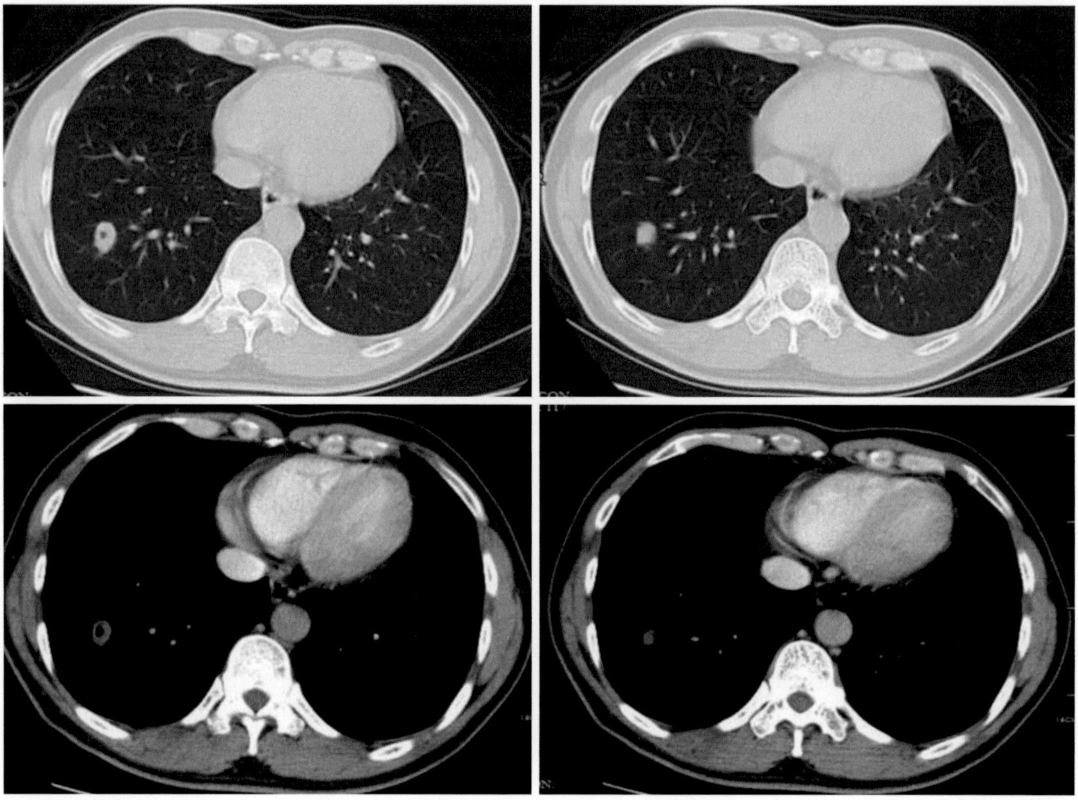

Fig. 15 Chest CT

[Diagnosis] Lung adenocarcinoma.

[Diagnosis Basis] The transverse CT scan shows a regular nodule in the lower lobe of right lung with smooth cavity. He underwent right lower lobectomy. The lesion was approximately 2.5 × 1.8 × 1.5 cm, diagnosed as invasive adenocarcinoma with micropapillary (50%), solid (40%), and acinar (10%) components, with necrosis, spread through air spaces, and lymph node metastases.

[Analysis] Tumor invasion in lung adenocarcinoma is defined as infiltration of stroma, blood vessels, or pleura. According to the 2015 WHO classification, tumor spread through air spaces (STAS) is defined as micropapillary clusters, solid nests, and/or single cancer cells spreading within air spaces beyond the edge of the main tumor. STAS was established as a new invasive pattern of adenocarcinoma. This concept is based on the fact that normal lung anatomy contains air spaces surrounded by the capillary network in the alveolar interstitium. The existence of mechanical forces, ranging from the inherent high flow velocities to the physics of breathing, to mechanical palpation of the surgeon during surgery, can certainly lend themselves to detach tumor clusters. These are usually identified within tumors, but are not identified as STAS until the tumor clusters appear outside the tumor periphery.

Prior to the definition of STAS, Shiono et al. [45, 46] in 2005 indicated aerogenous spreads with floating cancer cell clusters (ASFC) in cases with pulmonary metastases from colorectal cancer, and ASFC is unfavorable prognostic features. In 2013, Onzato et al. [47] proposed the concept of tumor islands, which was defined as a detached collection of tumor cells within alveolar spaces separated from the main tumor mass by a distance of at least a few alveoli. Tumor islands may be another pattern of tumor infiltration into the lung parenchyma. Lung adenocarcinomas with tumor islands were more likely to occur in smokers, exhibiting higher nuclear grade and a solid or micropapillary growth pattern, and harboring KRAS mutations. Tumor islands were significantly associated with a worse recurrence-free survival. Tumor islands seem to be a visual description of tumor cell clusters around the main tumor through STAS. If STAS is a dynamic process of tumor cell proliferation, then tumor islands can be regarded as an intuitive manifestation of tumor cells through STAS.

Some studies applied divergent definitions of STAS and/or related morphological features. In 2015, Kadota et al. [48] first suggested the possibility of STAS being a new pattern of invasion and defined it as the spread of tumor cells (as micropapillary structures, solid nests, or single cells) within air spaces beyond the edge of the primary tumor. They reviewed 411 resected small (less than or equal to 2 cm) stage I lung adenocarcinomas. STAS was observed in 155 cases (38%), and tumor cells were observed over 1 cm away from the edge of the tumor. STAS is usually found in the first alveolar layers close to the tumor but occasionally can be found more than 50 alveolar spaces away from the main tumor. They reported that lymphovascular invasion and high-grade morphologic pattern in main tumors were more frequently identified in STAS-positive tumors than in STAS-negative tumors and the presence of STAS is a significant risk factor of recurrence in small lung adenocarcinomas treated with limited resection. Warth et al. in 2015 [49] defined STAS as a detachment of small solid cell nests (at least 5 tumor cells) <3 alveolae away from the main tumor mass as limited STAS and tumor cell nests>3 alveolae away from the main tumor mass as extensive STAS. In the series of 569 resected pulmonary adenocarcinomas, limited (21.6%) or extensive (29%) STAS was present in roughly half of all adenocarcinomas. Tumors with STAS were much more prevalent in male sex, lymph node and distant metastasis, tumor stage, and high-grade histological patterns, and showed lower rates of EGFR but higher rates of BRAF mutations. The presence of STAS was associated with significantly reduced recurrence-free survival (RFS) and overall survival (OS) at any stage. In 2016, Morimoto et al. [50] proposed the concept of free tumor clusters (FTCs). They defined it to be a group of more than 3 small clusters containing <20 nonintegrated micropapillary tumor cells that were spreading within air spaces, >3 mm apart from the main tumor. The FTC does not contain solid nests or single cells. Coexistence of FTCs resulted in a further negative impact on postoperative prognosis among micropapillary component positive adenocarcinomas. In 2017, Uruga et al. [51] assessed semi-quantitatively small (≤2 cm) stage I lung adenocarcinomas surgically resected in the most prominent area as no STAS, low STAS (1–4 single cells or clusters of STAS), or high STAS (≥5 single cells or clusters of STAS). They found that one-third of resected small adenocarcinomas had high STAS, which was predictive of worse recurrence-free survival. Dai et al. [52] defined STAS as tumor cells observed within air spaces in the surrounding lung parenchyma beyond the edge of the main tumor. STAS was classified into three morphologic subtypes: single cells, micropapillary clusters, and solid nests. STAS could be considered as a factor in a staging system to predict prognosis more precisely, especially in lung adenocarcinomas larger than 2–3 cm. In 2018, Shiono et al. [53] assessed the prognostic impact of STAS in 329 patients with a sublobar resection for stage IA lung cancer versus 185 patients with a lobectomy. STAS is a prognostic factor of poor outcomes for sublobar resection in patients with lung cancer. Terada et al. [54] in 2019 showed that STAS invasion pattern was a significant risk factor for recurrence even in stage III (N2) adenocarcinoma.

STAS as an independent pathologic entity rather than an artifact caused by spreading through a knife surface is still controversial. Artifacts originate from loose tissue fragments in the lung. The concept of spread through a knife surface (STAKS) was first introduced by Thunnissen et al. [55], who pointed out that tumor cells could spread into alveolar spaces iatrogenically by the knife during pathological resection. Blaauwgeers et al. [56] prospectively investigated tumor clusters in tissue blocks. The first cut was made with a clean knife; the second cut was made in a parallel plane to the first. They discovered that the presence of loose tissue fragments in air spaces was more frequent in the latter blocks. Overall 93% of the loose tissue fragments could be explained by mechanical forces associated with tissue handling. However, Kadota et al. [48] and Warth et al. [49] demonstrated that STAS is not an artifact and provided the criteria for distinguishing artifacts from true STAS. Tumor floaters often presented at the edges of the tissue section or randomly scattered over tissue. The presence of jagged edges or linear strips represented tumor fragmentation or STAKS rather than STAS.

Lee et al. [57] retrospectively analyzed 316 surgically resected lung adenocarcinoma cases. STAS was found in 160 cases (50.6%). STAS was significantly associated with lymphovascular invasion, lymph node metastasis, higher stage, and high-grade histologic subtype. STAS was frequently observed in tumors with wild-type EGFR or ALK-rearrangement. Logistic regression analysis showed that STAS was significantly associated with absence of lepidic component, presence of micropapillary component, cribriform predominant type, lymphovascular invasion, and wild-type EGFR. Multivariate survival analysis confirmed that STAS was independently associated with shorter recurrence-free survival. STAS was also associated with recurrences to extrathoracic sites as well as intrathoracic sites. In 2019, Eguchi et al. [58] found that lobectomy was associated with better outcomes than sublobar resection in patients with T1 lung adenocarcinoma with STAS. Pathologists can recognize STAS on frozen sections. Their research suggested that the choice between limited resection and lobectomy could potentially be made intraoperatively on the basis of frozen section results. Yagi et al. [59] used high-resolution and high-quality three-dimensional (3D) reconstruction of images from immunohistochemical (IHC) and multiplex immunofluorescence (IF) experiments to analyze the spatial architecture of tumor cell clusters by STAS in the lung parenchyma. The 3D reconstructions confirmed that STAS tumor cells can attach to the alveolar walls rather than appearing free floating, as seen on the two-dimensional sections. This indicates that the tumor cells detach from the main tumor, migrate through air spaces, and reattach to the alveolar walls through vessel co-option, allowing them to survive and grow. This may explain that patients with STAS-positive tumors who undergo limited resection have a higher recurrence rate and poorer survival than those who undergo lobectomy.

Some studies reported detailed preoperative radiological features indicating the presence of STAS. Toyokawa et al. [60] analyzed the association of STAS with CT characteristics, such as vascular convergence, ground-glass opacity (GGO), air bronchogram, notch, pleural indentation, spiculation, and cavitation. The presence of notch and the absence of GGO were independently associated with the STAS phenomenon. Kim et al. [61] identified the features at CT that are predictive of STAS in surgically resected lung adenocarcinomas. They found that percentage of solid component was independently associated with STAS in lung adenocarcinomas. Both average and maximum diameter of solid component on CT were found to be predictors of STAS in pulmonary nodules by Kim et al. [61] and de Margerie-Mellon et al. [62] studies.

STAS has also been described in other primary lung cancers, most commonly in squamous cell carcinoma (SCC). Lu et al. [63] demonstrated for the first time that STAS is not limited to adenocarcinoma but is also a significant prognostic parameter for SCC by analyzing 445 resected stage I to III lung SCCs. STAS was present in 30% of the cases and the frequency increased with stage. The cumulative incidences of any recurrence, locoregional recurrence, distant recurrence, and lung cancer-specific death were significantly higher in patients with STAS compared with in those without STAS, whereas there was no statistically significant difference in overall survival. In multivariable models for any recurrence and lung cancer-specific death, STAS was an independent predictor for both outcomes. Kadota et al. [64] found that tumor STAS was an independent predictor of recurrence-free survival in patients with resected lung SCC and was associated with aggressive tumor behavior. Yanagawa et al. [65] in 2018 retrospectively reviewed 220 patients with lung SCC. They found that STAS was detected in 19.1% of surgical resected SCC, and it was associated with recurrence and worse survival in stage I SCC, but not in stage II and III SCC. Therefore, they suggested that STAS is a useful predictor of recurrence and prognosis in stage I lung SCC. Yokoyama et al. [66] found that tumor STAS in patients with pleomorphic carcinoma was shown to be associated with high recurrence rates and poor survival after surgical resection. Aly et al. [67] further investigated the prognostic importance of STAS in lung neuroendocrine tumors (NETs). They found that STAS is associated with early distant metastasis and worse lung cancer-specific cumulative incidence of death in patients with lung NETs. In patients with large cell neuroendocrine carcinoma (LCNEC) or small cell carcinoma (SCLC), STAS is an independent poor prognostic factor. Altinay et al. [68] investigated a retrospective series of 91 surgically resected atypical carcinoids (ACs). STAS was identified in 48% of ACs compared to 20.5% of typical carcinoids (TCs) and 71–88% of high-grade large and small cell carcinomas. In the carcinoid group, presence of STAS was significantly correlated with unfavorable parameters, such as positive nodal status, high tumor stage, high Ki-67 index, presence of angioinvasion, and with adverse disease outcome, shorter overall survival, and time to progression.

Chen et al. [69] performed the first systematic review and meta-analysis of STAS. The pooled results suggested that presence of STAS was associated with worse recurrence-free survival and overall survival in NSCLCs. Subgroup analysis by histology type indicated the presence of STAS was significantly associated with inferior recurrence-free survival in resected lung adenocarcinoma, lung SCC, and lung pleomorphic carcinoma. The presence of STAS was identified as a significant negative prognostic factor for overall survival in Japan and China, an almost significant factor in Germany, but a non-significant factor in the United States. One possible reason is that the presence of STAS is associated with lower EGFR mutations, and EGFR mutations in lung adenocarcinoma are more frequent in Asian patients than in Caucasian patients. In addition, the hazard ratio for recurrence-free survival seemed to be higher in adenocarcinoma than in SCC. STAS was also found to be a significant negative prognostic factor for overall survival in adenocarcinoma, but not in SCC. The reason for this is not known but differences in tumor progression might be a possible explanation. The alveolar filling type of lung SCCs, where tumor nests preserve the alveolar structure, had better recurrence-free survival than the expanding type, where tumor nests destroy the alveolar structure. Some cases of alveolar space-filling type SCC with STAS-like structure might have a better prognosis compared with adenocarcinoma. Liu et al. [70] further illuminated that the presence of STAS might be an unfavorable prognostic factor for patients with NSCLC through meta-analysis, including 3564 lung cancer patients from 12 individual studies.

In conclusion, there is a large amount of convincing evidence associating the existence of STAS with lower survival and suggesting that STAS is an independent prognostic factor, and has nothing to do with the stage of tumor. The standard of treatment for lung adenocarcinoma with STAS regardless of tumor size and lymph node metastasis may be lobectomy rather than sublobectomy because of the risk of local recurrence. More work should be done to improve the consensus on and identification of STAS.

3.10 Case 10

A 57-year-old man found a lung lesion on physical examination.

Chest CT: A regular lesion in the right upper lung lobe (Fig. 16).

[Diagnosis] Invasive adenocarcinoma.

[Diagnosis Basis] The transverse CT scan shows a lesion in the upper lobe of right lung with lobulated margins and pleural retraction. He underwent right upper lobectomy. The lesion was approximately 1.5 × 1.5 × 1.5 cm, diagnosed as invasive adenocarcinoma with acinar (85%), papillary (5%), and micropapillary (5%) components, with visceral pleural invasion.

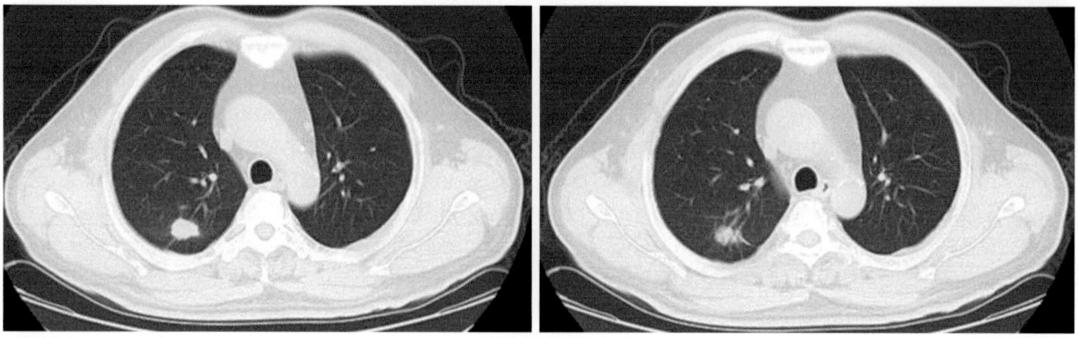

Fig. 16 Chest CT

[Analysis] The visceral pleura is composed of a single layer of mesothelial cells located on a basement membrane, a submesothelial connective tissue layer, an elastic fiber layer, and a connective tissue layer that separates the elastic layer from the lung parenchyma which is demarcated by a layer of pneumocytes resting on a thin basement membrane.

Pleural invasion is classified into four groups on the basis of pathologic findings. PL0 defined tumor within the subpleural lung parenchyma or superficial invasion into the connective tissue beneath the elastic layers. Tumor invades beyond the thick elastic layer of the visceral pleura is categorized as PL1. Tumor invasion to the visceral pleural surface is PL2 and invasion to the parietal pleura is PL3. Among these, both PL1 and PL2 are considered visceral pleural invasion (VPI). The use of elastic stains is recommended when the invasion beyond the elastic layer is not clear on hematoxylin eosin stains alone.

VPI is a poor prognostic factor of non-small cell lung cancer (NSCLC) patients and is defined as a factor to be upstaged from T1 to T2 in the seventh and eighth edition of the TNM classification for lung cancer. Patients with pleural invasion should be indicated for lobectomy rather than sublobar resection. Jiang et al. [71] investigated the impact of visceral pleural invasion in node-negative NSCLC in 13 relevant studies involving 27,171 patients. The number of patients with VPI was 5821 (21%). VPI was a significant adverse prognostic factor with reduced overall survival, including patients with tumor size ≤3 cm. VPI together with tumor size has a synergistic effect on the survival of node-negative NSCLC. The impact of VPI on survival increases with the size of the tumor. Stage IB NSCLC patients with larger tumor size with VPI might be considered for adjuvant chemotherapy after surgical resection and need careful preoperative evaluation and postoperative follow-up.

Dziedzic et al. [72] investigated the risk factors for local and distant recurrence after surgical treatment for NSCLC in a group of 14,578 patients. Of these patients, 2816 (19.3%) experienced recurrence of primary cancer. Local or distant recurrence was found in 20.5% and 79.5% of patients, respectively. In the series, 6.3% (917/14,578) of patients showed VPI. 16% (450/2816) showed VPI in the group of patients with recurrence, whereas in the group of patients without recurrence, VPI was present in only 4.4% (521/11,762). Multivariate analysis indicated that the presence of VPI is an independent prognostic factor (HR, 1.17).

Although at clinical staging VPI can be assumed by some imaging features, including direct pleural contact of the tumor, pleural retraction, and pleural tags, VPI is still a pathological descriptor. Hsu et al. [73] retrospectively investigated the association of pleural tags with VPI of NSCLC that does not abut the pleural surface. In 141 patients, 44 patients (31.2%) have VPI proved by pathologic analysis. They classified pleural tags into three types: type 1, one or more linear pleural tag; type 2, one or more linear pleural tag with soft tissue component at the pleural end; and type 3, one or more soft tissue cord-like pleural tag. In the absence of pleural tags, no pleural invasion was observed. Type 2 pleural tags were moderately associated with VPI. PL1 and PL2 cannot be distinguished by type 2 pleural tags. Ahn et al. [74] studied 188 T1-sized peripheral pulmonary nodular adenocarcinomas. In part-solid nodules, the CT features of pleural contact, pleural thickening, solid proportion greater than 50%, and nodule size greater than 20 mm were shown to be significant indicators of VPI. The specificity was 99.2% when all variables were used in combination. Kim et al. [75] retrospectively studied 695 patients with clinical T1 stage lung adenocarcinoma. They found that the accuracy of CT features of pathological visceral pleural invasion (pVPI) was 62.7%–72.3%. CT features of pVPI were not independent prognostic factors for disease-free survival in clinical T1 lung adenocarcinomas. This research does not support the use of CT features of VPI as T2 descriptors in the clinical staging of lung cancer. Yip et al. [76] determined long-term survival of VPI and parenchymal invasion (PAI) (angiolymphatic and/or vascular) on survival of NSCLCs less than 30 mm in maximum diameter. They found that the frequency of PAI versus VPI was significantly higher in patients with solid nodules than in those with subsolid nodules, and correspondingly, Kaplan-Meier lung cancer survival was significantly higher among patients with subsolid nodules. Multivariable Cox regression indicated that only tumor diameter and PAI remained significant, whereas VPI was not significant. Nodule consistency on CT was a more significant prognostic indicator than either PAI or VPI. They suggest that NSCLC patients with VPI and a maximum tumor diameter of 30 mm or less not be upstaged to T2.

In future, novel techniques and more reasonable experimental design may provide more accurate information for predicting pleural invasion and may improve the diagnostic accuracy and clinical outcomes in patients with lung cancer.

3.11 Case 11

A 60-year-old man found a lung lesion on physical examination.

Chest CT: A regular lesion in the right lower lung lobe (Fig. 17).

[Diagnosis] Invasive mucinous adenocarcinoma.

[Diagnosis Basis] The transverse CT scan shows a mixed GGN in the lower lobe of right lung with lobulated margins, spiculation and bubble-like lucencies, suggesting the diagnosis of lung adenocarcinoma. There is a low-density area (red arrow) at the lower edge of the nodule, indicating the diagnosis of invasive mucinous adenocarcinoma. He underwent a right lower lobectomy. The lesion was approximately 2.5 × 2.0 × 1.8 cm, diagnosed as invasive mucinous adenocarcinoma with visceral pleural invasion.

[Analysis] Mucinous lung adenocarcinoma is relatively rare, accounting for 3% to 10% of invasive adenocarcinomas.

Invasive mucinous adenocarcinoma (IMA) is diagnosed based on components of columnar or goblet cells with abundant intracellular or extracellular mucus and with invasive adenocarcinoma patterns, such as lepidic, acinar, papillary, micropapillary, and solid predominant patterns. IMA can be divided into two groups based on the percentage of mucinous pattern: pure mucinous (>90% invasive mucinous pattern, lepidic predominant pattern) and mixed mucinous/non-mucinous (≥10% of non-mucinous invasive component). The lepidic growth pattern is a characteristic feature of IMAs, which is why they were formerly termed mucinous bronchioloalveolar carcinomas (BACs).

Compared with other lung adenocarcinoma subtypes, IMA shows different clinical, immunohistochemical, and molecular features. IMA occurs at a greater frequency in female and non-smoking patients. Ichinokawa et al. [77] selected 46 cases of adenocarcinoma with a goblet cell-type component of ≥90% from 2228 cases of surgically resected primary lung adenocarcinoma, showing a significantly higher rate of tumor location on the left side, in the lower lobe and pathological stage I. Furthermore, IMA displayed a lower frequency of central fibrosis, plural invasion, pulmonary metastasis, lymphatic permeation, and vascular invasion. IMA showed local recurrence in two of 46 cases (4.3%) and no incidents of distant metastasis. IMA is associated with immunohistochemical profiles that differ from non-mucinous adenocarcinomas, including

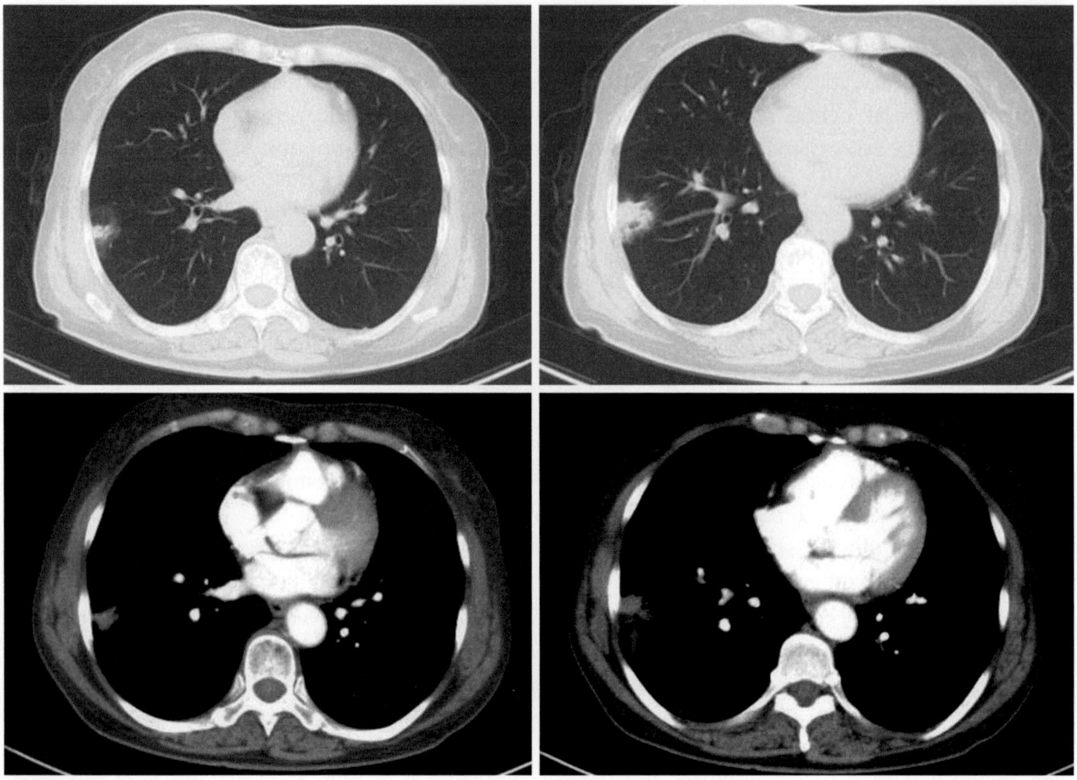

Fig. 17 Chest CT

lack of expression of TTF-1 and Napsin A, and expression of cytokeratin 7(~88%), cytokeratin 20(~54%), and CDX2 focal. Loss of TTF-1 expression has been associated with adverse prognosis. IMA selectively expresses hepatocyte nuclear factor 4α (HNF4α), a transcription factor presents in normal and malignant gastrointestinal mucosa, which could distinguish IMA from other mucin-producing adenocarcinomas. Multiple reports indicate that IMA is associated with KRAS mutation but not EGFR mutation. Kadota et al. [78] found that IMA was associated with KRAS transition mutations (G → A) but not transversion mutations (G → T or G → C) compared with nonmucinous tumors. Among IMA with KRAS mutation, a pure mucinous pattern was more common than a mixed mucinous/nonmucinous pattern. IMA is associated with decreased or absent expression of the transcription factor NK2 homeobox 1 (NKX2-1). NKX2-1(also known as TTF-1) encodes a homeobox-containing transcription factor with physiologic roles in lung development and function. The expression of NKX2-1 protein product TTF-1 (homeobox protein Nkx-2.1) is organ specific and restricted to thyroid, lung, and regions of the brain, and TTF-1 immunohistochemical analysis is frequently used to distinguish carcinomas of pulmonary and thyroid origin. Maeda et al. [79] demonstrated that NKX2-1 inhibits Kras(G12D)-driven mucinous pulmonary adenocarcinoma. Hwang et al. [80] found that frameshift or nonsense mutations in NKX2-1 occurred in about 19% (4/21) of IMAs by next-generation sequencing and Sanger sequencing. The TTF-1 protein was not expressed because of these mutations, which is a common finding in IMAs. Their finding supported NKX2-1 as a lineage-specific tumor suppressor gene in lung carcinogenesis. In IMAs, loss of TTF-1 expression owing to NKX2-1 mutation would derepress the transcription of these downstream genes, accounting for the presence of HNF4α and MUC5AC in these tumors. NKX2-1 mutations appear to be specific for pulmonary IMAs, and if present, it may be helpful to distinguish primary mucinous lung neoplasm from metastatic mucinous neoplasm to the lung.

In Shim et al. study [81], KRAS mutations were the most common variant, accounting for 63% of all cases. NRG1 fusions were second most common, accounting for 7%. When all fusion cases were combined, they accounted for 13% of all cases. G12D (42%) and G12V (31%) were the most common variants observed in mucinous tumors, while G12C was the most common in lung adenocarcinoma. KRAS mutations G12D and G12V are frequently observed in mucinous colorectal or pancreatobiliary tumors, suggesting that IMA of lung may be biologically more similar to pancreatobiliary and intestinal tract cancers. Within the KRAS-negative cases, they found numerous potentially targetable gene fusions and mutations, including CD74-NRG1, VAMP2-NRG1, TRIM4-BRAF, TPM3-NTRK1, and EML4-ALK gene fusions and ERBB2, BRAF, and PIK3CA mutations. Chang et al. [82] analyzed 200 IMAs by 410-gene DNA NGS (n = 136) or hotspot 8-oncogene genotyping (n = 64). Mutually exclusive driver alterations were identified in 96% of IMAs, including KRAS mutations (76%), NRG1 fusions (7%), ERBB2 alterations (6%), and other less common events. In addition, whole-transcriptome sequencing identified a novel NRG2 fusion (F11R-NRG2). Compared with KRAS-mutant IMAs, NRG1-rearranged tumors exhibited several more aggressive characteristics, including worse recurrence-free survival.

IMAs rarely express TP53 mutations, which may reflect the lower mutation burden of IMAs compared with that of invasive non-mucinous adenocarcinomas (INMAs). Kawai et al. [83] considered that pure goblet cell-type IMA can progress to scant-mucinous adenocarcinoma and that TP53 mutation might be a factor involved in such progression. IMAs rarely exhibit PD-L1 and predominantly occur in people who are not heavy smokers.

The prognosis of IMA is controversial. Several studies indicated that patients with mucinous BAC show poorer prognosis than those with non-mucinous BAC. Russell et al. [84] classified lung adenocarcinoma according to the 2011 IASLC/ATS/ERS classification scheme. They confirmed that the new subtypes of AIS, MIA, and LPA had a 5-year survival approaching 100%, whereas micropapillary predominant and solid with mucin-predominant adenocarcinomas were associated with particularly poor survival, with 38% and 39%, respectively. Papillary predominant and acinar-predominant adenocarcinomas had an intermediate prognosis, with 71% and 68%, respectively. This effect persisted after controlling for stage. IMA and colloid adenocarcinoma had 51% 5-year survival. Yoshizawa et al. [85] validated the new adenocarcinoma classification with a North American data set comprising 514 stage I lung adenocarcinomas. They found that AIS and MIA had 100% 5-year disease-free survival; non-mucinous lepidic-predominant, papillary-predominant, and acinar-predominant with 90, 83, and 84% 5-year disease-free survival, respectively; and IMA, colloid predominant, solid predominant, and micropapillary predominant, with 75, 71, 70, and 67% 5-year disease-free survival, respectively. On the contrary, Warth et al. [86] reported that IMAs show better prognosis than conventional non-mucinous adenocarcinomas. Watanabe et al. [87] classified IMA as "solitary-type" or "pneumonic-type" tumors based on the thin-section computed tomography findings. The 5-year overall survival and relapse-free survival rates in patients with solitary-type tumors were 83.3% and 88.8%, respectively, while those with pneumonic-type tumors were 20.0% and 0%, respectively. The median follow-up time for surviving patients was 81 months.

Lee et al. [88] studied 81 patients with a solitary IMA of the lung and compared the prognosis of IMAs with that of non-mucinous adenocarcinomas. They found that patients with IMA showed longer disease-free survival (DFS) than did those with non-mucinous adenocarcinomas, whereas overall survival (OS) did not differ significantly. In their study, only 5% of patients with IMA had lymph node metastasis. In solitary IMA, tumor size and maximum standardized uptake value are the factors related to mitigating

DFS and tumor size is the only predictor for reduced OS. Watanabe et al. [87] and Lee et al. [88] studies also revealed that solitary-type IMA is far more common than pneumonic-type IMA. Cha et al. [89] investigated the clinical course of stage IV IMAs and compared the findings with those of stage IV invasive non-mucinous adenocarcinomas (INMAs). KRAS mutations were noted in 60.0% of the examined IMAs. The OS of untreated IMA patients was significantly better than that of untreated INMA patients. Compared with untreated IMA patients, IMA patients treated with non-TKI chemotherapy did not improve their OS. In Shimizu et al. [90] study, the prognosis of resected IMA of the lung was relatively good, because lung IMA was not associated with lymph node metastasis. However, pneumonic-type IMA had a higher rate of intrathoracic metastasis and was associated with a poor prognosis.

In summary, patients with IMA showed comparable survival outcome to those with INMAs, and IMA is classified as an intermediate-grade tumor group among all invasive adenocarcinomas. IMA patients have a low chance of receiving targeted therapy because of the rare occurrence or absence of targetable mutations. Surgery may be the treatment of choice for solitary-type IMAs.

3.12 Case 12

A 68-year-old woman complained of cough and expectoration for more than half a year.

Chest CT: A consolidation in the right middle lung lobe (Fig. 18).

[Diagnosis] Invasive mucinous adenocarcinoma.

[Diagnosis Basis] The transverse CT scan shows a dense consolidation in the middle lobe of right lung with areas of ground-glass attenuation, bulging of the interlobar fissure, air broncho-

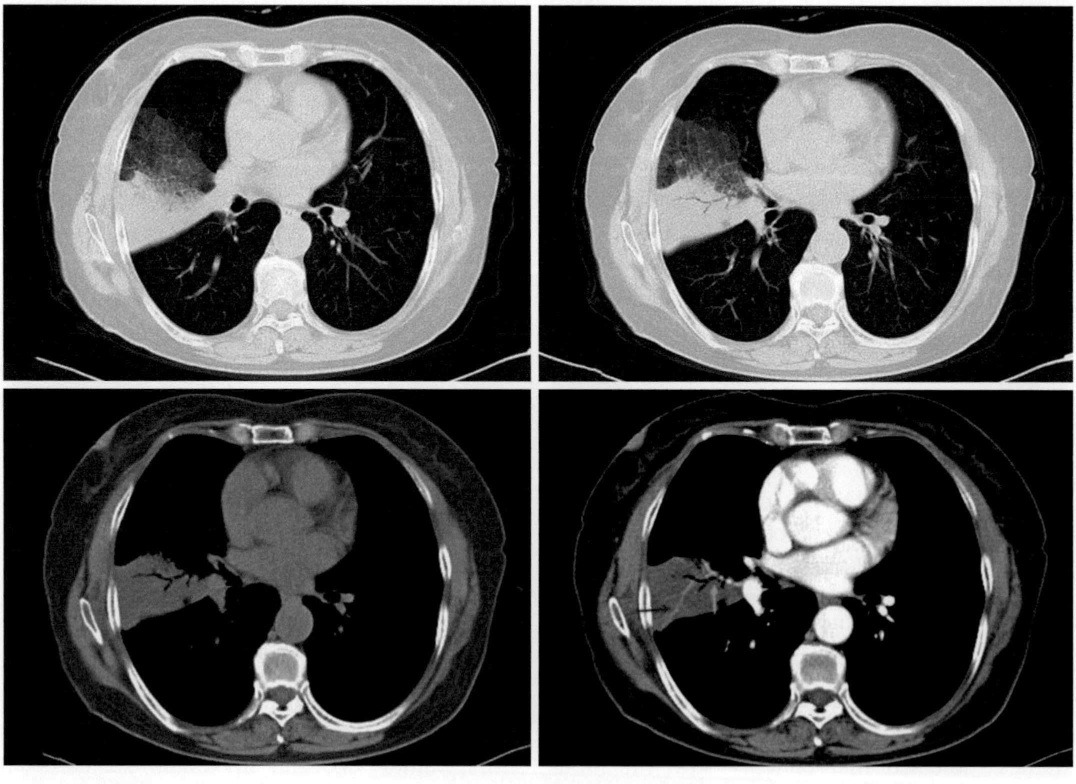

Fig. 18 Chest CT

grams (green arrow) and angiogram sign (red arrow), suggesting the diagnosis of invasive mucinous adenocarcinoma. She underwent a right middle lobectomy, diagnosed as invasive mucinous adenocarcinoma.

[Analysis] CT appearance of IMA could be solitary nodules or masses ("solitary type") or a segmental or lobar consolidation ("pneumonic type"). There tendency for multicentric, multilobar, and bilateral lung involvement may reflect aerogenous dissemination. The CT features of IMA include relatively well-defined GGO margins, multiple cysts, cavities, or bubble-like lucencies, "leafless tree" air bronchogram, bulging of the interlobar fissure, slight enhancement and low-density area, and angiogram sign.

IMA could present GGO by endogenous aspiration of mucin from the tumor cells. The appearance of remote GGO from consolidation, and absence of pleural and bronchial thickening adjacent to the area of consolidation, differentiates pneumonic-type IMA from infectious pneumonia.

Airspace lesions in IMA were formed by dilation of the bronchioles, dilated alveolar spaces resulting from accumulated mucin, and tumor-free regions consisting of normal alveolar spaces. There were less lesions with tumor necrosis. The bubble-like lucencies (or pseudocavitations) in the consolidation or nodule were observed in 40–78% of IMA cases, which is caused by patent small airways and areas of focal emphysema within the nodule or distended alveolar spaces within papillary regions of tumor growth. The bronchus in the area of consolidation is often patent and has the appearance of a leafless tree.

Due to the unique lepidic growth, IMA seldom obliterates the original architecture of the lung, including the bronchus within the tumor. As the tumor fills the alveolar spaces and infiltrates the alveolar septa and bronchial walls, IMA had air bronchograms with a stretched, sweeping, narrowed appearance, widening of the branch angle at bifurcations, and bulging of the fissure. Bulging fissure is one of the characteristic findings of IMA and can be caused by mucin production in the tumor, resulting in swelling of the lobe.

Usually, normal soft tissue shows an attenuation value of approximately 40 HU. As mucin shows a lower CT attenuation than the tumor cells and soft tissue, MIA is expected to show a relatively low mean attenuation value.

CT angiogram sign is the ability to see normal pulmonary vasculature within parenchymal consolidations. It was initially described as a specific sign of lobar bronchoalveolar cell carcinoma and has reported recently to be seen in both benign and malignant entities, including IMA, pneumonia, pulmonary edema, obstructive pneumonitis due to central lung tumors, lymphoma, and metastasis from gastrointestinal carcinomas. Angiogram sign within a hypoattenuated consolidation with an air bronchogram probably indicates a mucinous carcinoma with lepidic growth.

3.13 Case 13

A 60-year-old man complained of cough and expectoration for more than half a year.

Chest CT: Multiple consolidations, nodules, and ground-glass opacity shadows in bilateral lungs (Fig. 19).

[Diagnosis] Invasive mucinous adenocarcinoma.

[Diagnosis Basis] The transverse CT scan shows consolidations and nodules in bilateral lungs with areas of ground-glass attenuation, bubble-like lucencies, air bronchograms, angiogram sign, suggesting the diagnosis of invasive mucinous adenocarcinoma. Lung biopsy revealed mucinous adenocarcinoma of lung origin.

[Analysis] Pulmonary IMAs often present with spatially separate lung lesions. Yang et al. [91] evaluated clonal relationship between such lesions by comparative genomic profiling. In 24 IMAs patients, 19 had contralateral lesions. Except for one patient, all other patients shared matching driver alterations, including KRAS (n = 19), NRG1 (n = 2), ERBB2 (n = 1), or BRAF (n = 1). In addition, Shared driver alterations were accompanied by up to 4 (average 2.6) other identical mutations in patients with paired tumors profiled

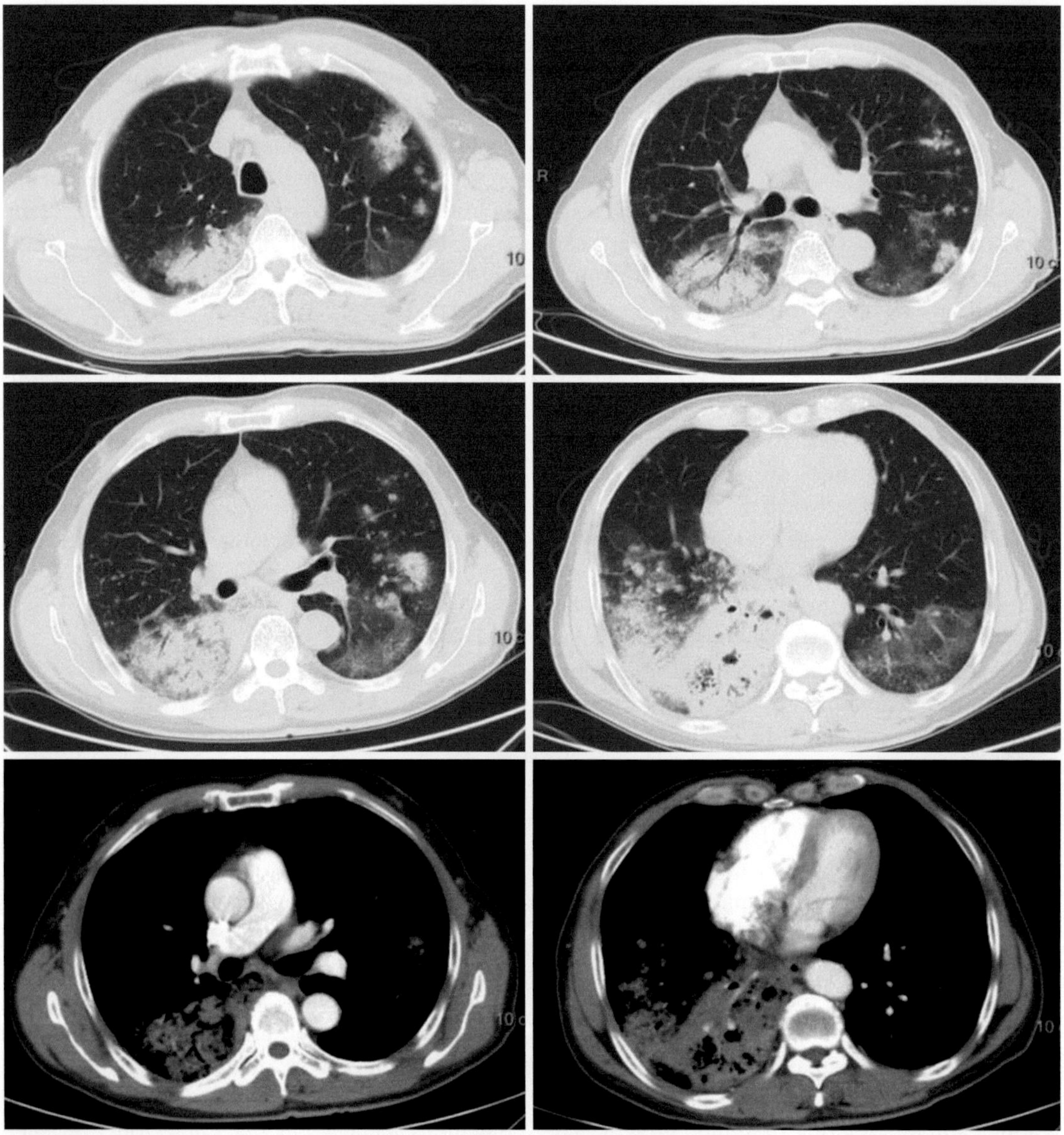

Fig. 19 Chest CT

by NGS (n = 12), further supporting the clonal relationship between the tumors. Comparative molecular profiling indicates that nearly all separate pulmonary IMA lesions represent intrapulmonary spread caused by a single tumor and documents a subset with a remarkably protracted course of intrapulmonary progression.

Pneumonic-type adenocarcinoma (P-ADC) is defined as pulmonary adenocarcinoma with a pneumonia-like area of infiltrate/consolidation, with no prior diagnosis of thoracic or extrathoracic adenocarcinoma. Histologically, this is usually predominant lepidic growth, with partial filling of alveolar air spaces by mucin or tumor cells. So most P-ADC s are IMAs, particularly with the 2015 WHO classification. On the contrary, some historical studies reported that pneumonic-type lung cancer consisted of approximately 45% (26%–57%) mucinous, 40% (29%–53%) non-mucinous, and 15% (12%–21%) mixed adenocarcinoma.

Owing to the bronchogenic dissemination and air space spread of the IMA, it is difficult to differentiate pneumonia radiologically.

Recurrent and long-lasting infectious symptoms, such as cough, sputum, and dyspnea, etc., suggest the possibility of P-ADC. The excessive cough and white sputum were more common in patients with pneumonic-type compared with solitary-type. This may be because the pneumonic-type is related to higher stage and uncontrolled growth of tumor cells, which may cause excessive production of mucus and discharge through the upper airways. Fine-needle aspiration cytology or lung biopsy is necessary for tumor diagnosis.

Wislez et al. [92] reported that the median survival time of P-ADC after diagnosis was 10.5 months (range 1–150 months). The most effective treatment option for P-ADC is surgical resection. The 5-year survival rate of surgically treated P-ADC patients and nonsurgical treatment patients is approximately 30% to 68% and 14% to 60%, respectively.

3.14 Case 14

A 26-year-old woman complained of cough for 1 week.

Chest CT: An oral mass in the left lower lung lobe, with heterogeneous enhancement (Fig. 20).

[Diagnosis] Fetal lung adenocarcinoma.

[Diagnosis Basis] She underwent a left lower lobectomy. Pathology analysis showed a tumor consisting of tubular to cribriform glands with endometrioid morphology. The glands consisted of columnar cells with basally located nuclei with occasional nuclear clearing and numerous mitotic figures (Fig. 21). Immunohistochemistry analysis showed tumor cells positive for TTF-1, β-catenin, and synaptophysin, and negative for chromogranin A, ER, and PR. The final diagnosis was low-grade fetal lung adenocarcinoma.

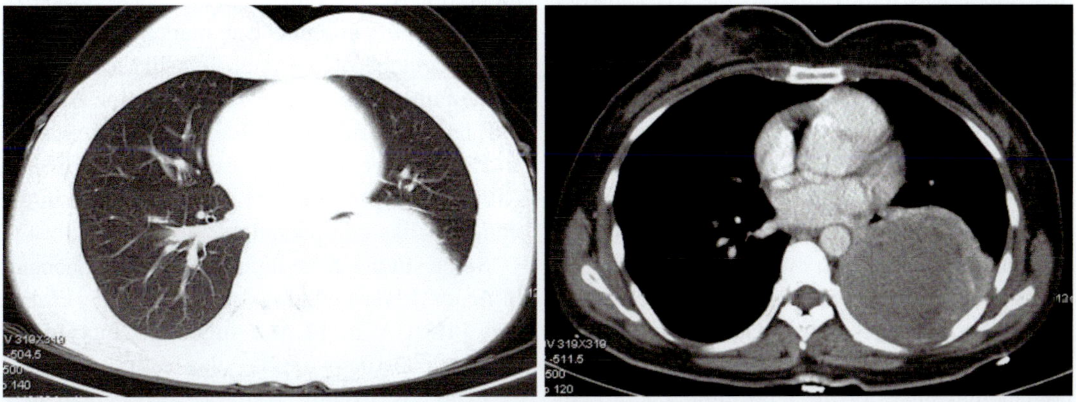

Fig. 20 Chest CT

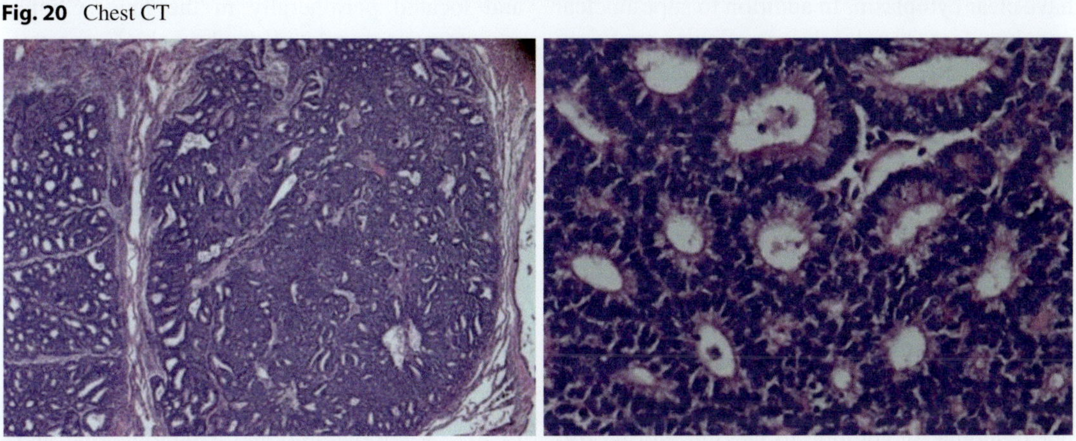

Fig. 21 L-FLAC shows complex glandular structures, with prominent morule formation (3, 10×; 4, 40×)

[Analysis] Fetal lung adenocarcinoma (FLAC) is extremely rare and accounts for approximately 0.1%–0.5% of all primary lung neoplasms. In 1945 and 1952, Barnard [93] first applied the term "embryoma" to this tumor. In 1961, Spencer [94] introduced the term pulmonary blastoma (PB), because it is a biphasic lung tumor comprising an epithelial component surrounded by mesenchymal stroma that resembled Wilms' tumor of the kidney. In 1982, Kradin et al. [95] found the tumor lacking the sarcomatous areas integral to the concept of blastoma. So they suggested that the designation pulmonary endodermal tumor resembling fetal lung may better describe this neoplasm. In 1984, Kodama et al. [96] introduced the phrase "well-differentiated fetal adenocarcinoma of the lung" (WDFA) to categorize this tumor because it is a rare glycogen-rich tumor that closely resembles fetal lung tissue at 10–15 week gestation with neuroendocrine differentiation. In the 1999 WHO classification, this tumor was removed from the PB category and classified as a variant of lung adenocarcinoma. According to clinicopathological features and biological behaviors, the tumor was further classified into two subtypes: low-grade FLAC(L-FLAC) and high-grade FLAC (H-FLAC) in the 2004 WHO classification.

FLAC resembles fetal lung in its pseudoglandular stage (8–16 weeks of gestation). FLAC consists of complex glandular structures that comprises glycogen rich, non-ciliated cells resembling a developing epithelium in the pseudoglandular phase of the fetal lung. These cells have clear cytoplasm. In addition to supranuclear or subnuclear vacuoles, large vesicular nuclei are seen. L-FLAC (WDFA) has low nuclear atypia and morule formation and has a pure pattern. The neoplastic glands are typically enveloped by a loose fibromyxoid stroma with spindle cells. H-FLAC generally displays at least 50% fetal morphology and often together with other conventional types of lung adenocarcinoma (lepidic, papillary, acinar, micropapillary, and solid patterns). Occasionally, H-FLAC is combined with other carcinoma components, such as large cell neuroendocrine carcinoma and enteric adenocarcinoma. In addition to lacking morule formation, H-FLAC has prominent nuclear atypia and nucleoli, accompanied by necrosis and frequent mitosis.

Two subtypes of FLAC also show differences in their immunohistochemical staining. L-FLAC constantly exhibits aberrant cytoplasm/nuclear distribution of β-catenin and frequent β-catenin gene mutations. On the contrary, H-FLAC shows a membranous staining for β-catenin while lacking β-catenin gene mutations. The Wnt signaling pathway is important during embryogenesis, but when altered can lead to tumor formation. The Wnt signaling component upregulation such as β-catenin has been known for L-FLAC. L-FLAC exhibits lower expression of p53, which in contrast, is commonly overexpressed in H-FLAC. High p53 expression is correlated with poor differentiation, smoking history, advanced stage, and low survival rate in patients with lung adenocarcinoma. Both L-FLAC and H-FLAC show positive neuroendocrine markers (chromogranin A and synaptophysin). The grade of positivity of neuroendocrine markers depends on the percentage of the fetal lung-like component in the tumor. Morita et al. [97] and Suzuki et al. [98] have reported that α-fetoprotein, glypican 3, and SALL4 are frequently expressed in H-FLAC, with a more prominent expression profile in the non-fetal-like components.

Some studies have reported lower frequencies of major driver mutations such as KRAS, EGFR, and PIK3CA in FLAC, suggested that FLAC may have distinctive molecular features.

FLAC is usually solitary, well-demarcated, and located peripherally in the lung. Clinical symptoms are related to bronchial irritation, including chest pain, dyspnea, cough, and hemoptysis. Approximately 25%–40% of patients are asymptomatic. L-FLAC is generally found in young patients in the third-fourth decade with a slight female predominance. The initial diagnosis of L-FLAC occurs during the early stages (I-II). H-FLAC mostly occurs in elderly male smokers around the sixth to seventh decade of life, presenting advanced-stage disease (stage III-IV) and a poorer prognosis.

Surgical resection is the standard treatment for FLAC. Radiotherapy and chemotherapy have been used as adjuvant therapy, although they have shown limited effect in some reports. Thoracic lymphadenopathy, metastasis at diagnosis, and tumor recurrence are poor prognostic factors for FLAC. L-FLAC probably has a better prognosis than the stage-matched conventional pulmonary adenocarcinoma.

3.15 Case 15

A 67-year-old man complained of right-side chest pain for 2 days.

Chest CT: A regular lesion in the right lower lung lobe (Fig. 22).

[Diagnosis] Pulmonary enteric adenocarcinoma.

[Diagnosis Basis] The transverse CT scan shows a nodule in the lower lobe of right lung with lobulated margins and spiculation, suggesting the diagnosis of lung adenocarcinoma. He underwent a right lower lobectomy and systemic lymph node dissection, using video-assisted thoracic surgery (VATS). The lesion was approximately 2.0 cm with a white-gray surface, pathology analysis showed colorectal carcinoma-like components. Immunohistochemistry analysis showed tumor cells positive for TTF-1, Napsin A, Villin, CEA, and CK7 and negative for CK-20 and CDX2. The final diagnosis was pulmonary enteric adenocarcinoma, and metastasis has not been found in mediastinal lymph nodes.

[Analysis] Colloid and enteric-type adenocarcinomas are thought to have similar origins to pulmonary IMA due to identical molecular profiles with approximately half of the cases harboring KRAS mutations.

In 1991, pulmonary enteric adenocarcinoma (PEAC) was first described by Tsao and Frasein [99] who reported a "primary well-differentiated pulmonary adenocarcinoma with enteric differ-

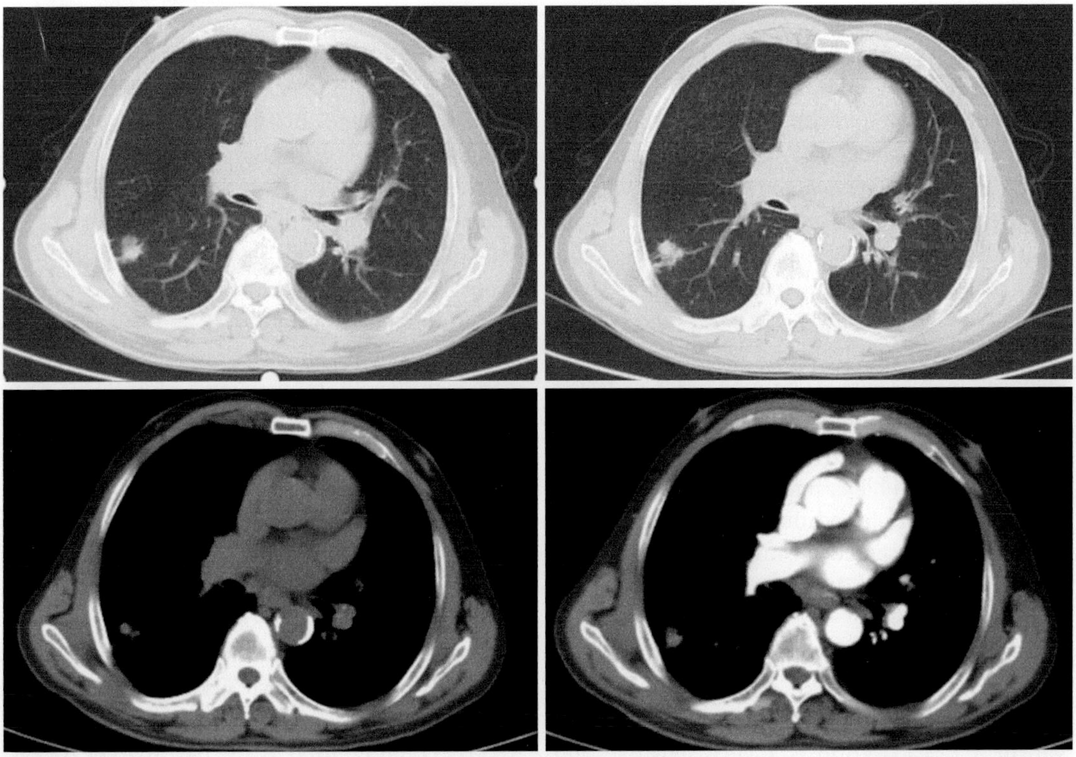

Fig. 22 Chest CT

entiation" after the histological examination of a lung nodule excised from the right upper lobe in a 40-year-old man and formulated the diagnosis of "primary pulmonary adenocarcinoma with enteric differentiation," and was officially declared for the first time as a separate variant of invasive lung adenocarcinoma in the international multidisciplinary classification of lung adenocarcinoma in 2011 and subsequently proposed in the 2015 WHO classification.

PEAC is defined as the intestinal differentiation component in lung adenocarcinoma exceeds 50%, together with the positive immunohistochemistry staining for at least one marker of enteric differentiation, namely cytokeratin 20 (CK20), Caudal Type Homeobox (CDX2), and/or Mucin 2 (MUC2). PEAC is histologically heterogeneous with some component that resembles primary lung adenocarcinoma such as lepidic growth. The enteric pattern is composed of glandular and/or papillary structures sometimes with a cribriform pattern, lined by neoplastic cuboidal to columnar cells with nuclear pseudostratification, luminal necrosis, and prominent nuclear debris, goblet and Paneth cells. Poorly differentiated tumors may also have a solid pattern.

Although PEAC has its own pathological features, it is difficult to distinguish from lung metastatic colorectal cancers (MCC) by histopathology alone. Immunohistochemical markers play an important role in distinguishing PEAC from other histological subtype of lung adenocarcinoma and MCC. PEAC expresses immunoreactivity for CK20, CDX-2, MUC2, and Villin, which are not usually expressed in pulmonary adenocarcinomas but are common to MCC. Wang et al. [100] found that PEAC showed positive staining for CK20, CDX-2, MUC2, and Villin in 22.2%, 66.7%, 44.4%, and 66.7%, respectively. Zhao et al. [101] found that 89.28% (25/28) of PEAC cases presented positivity for Villin, and 80% of cases with both CK20- and CDX-2-negative expressions were Villin-positive. Lin et al. [102] confirmed the frequent expression of CDX2(90.0%), followed by Villin (80.0%), CK20(70.0%), CK7(30.0%), TTF-1(30.0%), and Napsin A (25%). Villin is a very sensitive and relatively specific marker of gastrointestinal adenocarcinomas and proved to be a very sensitive and helpful enteric marker in the differential diagnosis between PEAC and other lung adenocarcinomas. The positive staining for CK7 and TTF-1 in approximately half cases also helps in the distinction from MCC. CK7-negative PEAC cases may occur and CK7 expression has been described in up to 17% of colorectal cancers. Chen et al. [103] found that the combination of CK7+/CDX2+ acquired high sensitivity (71.3%) and specificity (82%) in differential diagnosis of PEAC from colorectal adenocarcinoma.

Palmirotta et al. [104] summarized 295 patients from 58 published articles and found that the most represented immunohistochemical markers were CEA (93.5%), CK7 (81.8%), CDX2 (80.7%), and Villin (76.6%), whereas a minor expression was observed for MUC5A5 (47.8%), CK20 (47.0%), SP-A(42.1%), MUC2 (37.4%), TTF1 (35.4%), and Napsin A (28.7%). They also recorded the majority of mutations in KRAS (38.5%), MMR (32.4%), ERBB2 (22.5%), and EGFR (13.3%) genes, whereas the translocation of EML4-ALK was detected in 9.4% of cases (N = 117). Less common were BRAF (2.0%, N = 102) and NRAS (2.0%, N = 49) mutations. They further analyzed the potential differences between PAEC diagnosed in Asia and in European/North American countries. Most PAEC cases (185/295) were described in Asia. They observed a high similarity between the two groups, in terms of TTF1, MUC2, MUC5A5, Villin, Napsin A, and SP-A expression. On the other hand, they found a significantly higher rate of CK20-positive tumors in the Asian population, whereas CK7 and CDX2 were significantly more expressed in PAEC samples from Europe and North America, as compared with those reported in Asia.

Recently, alternative methods for the differential diagnosis of PEAC and MCC have been explored. Cadherin-17 (CDH17) and SATB homeobox 2 (SATB2) immunoexpression have been demonstrated in colorectal adenocarcinoma. Bian et al. [105] found that CDH17 and SATB2 are highly expressed in MCC but rarely expressed in PEAC, and the combination of CDH17 and SATB2 could be used as the best marker for distinguishing PEAC from MCC. Matsushima et al.

[106] found that β-catenin and SATB2 are useful immunohistochemical markers for differentiating between PEAC and MCC by eight samples of PEAC. Immunohistochemically, the positive rates of PEAC for each antibody were as follows: CK7, 88%; CK20, 88%; TTF-1, 13%; β-catenin, 0% (0/8, strong nuclear expression); and SATB2, 13%. The positive rates of MCC for these antibodies were 10%, 95%, 5%, 55%, and 100%, respectively. The result indicated that β-catenin and SATB2 are useful immunohistochemical markers for differentiating PEAC from MCC. Jurmeister et al. [107] reported that DNA methylation profiling could reliably distinguish PEAC from MCC.

The main treatment for PEAC is surgery and systemic chemotherapy. The colorectal cancer chemotherapy regimens were not effective in PEAC patients, and carboplatin combined with paclitaxel is the most commonly used regimen, which is typical adjuvant treatment for primary lung adenocarcinoma. Although different genetic mutations were detected in PEAC patients, targeted therapy is currently not feasible.

3.16 Case 16

A 51-year-old man found a lung lesion on physical examination.

Chest CT: A cystic airspace in right lower lobe (Fig. 23).

[Diagnosis] Lung cancer associated with cystic airspaces.

[Diagnosis Basis] CT scan shows cystic airspace with thin wall in right lower lung lobe, surrounded by solid, irregularly marginated nodule. The histopathologic diagnosis of the lesion was adenocarcinoma.

[Analysis] Lung cancer associated with cystic airspaces (LC-CAS), also known as cystic or pericystic lung cancer, is a rare radiological entity that comprises primary lung cancer associated with a "cystic airspace" on CT, accompanied by consolidation and/or ground glass. The term cystic airspace indicates discrete air-filled areas in the lung including congenital cysts, emphysematous bullae, fibrotic cysts, bronchiectatic airways, subpleural blebs, and cystic dilation of the distal airway from a small cancer caused by obstruction. Cyst was defined as air-containing spaces surrounded by a thin wall, less than 2 mm.

The exact carcinogenic mechanism remains unclear. LC-CAS was first described by Womack et al. in 1941 [108]. They assigned the cause of LC-CAS to a previously existing congenital malformation. Anderson and Pierce in 1954 [109] described 6 cases of carcinoma of the bronchus in which the radiological appearance was that of a thin-walled cavity or cyst. They suggested that this variety of bronchial carcinoma may arise when a thin layer of malignant cells grows into and lines a pre-existing cavity. The cavity is formed either by pressure changes consequent on a valvular obstruction to a bronchus by a small nodule of growth, or by inflammatory changes in the proximity of but not involving the neoplasm.

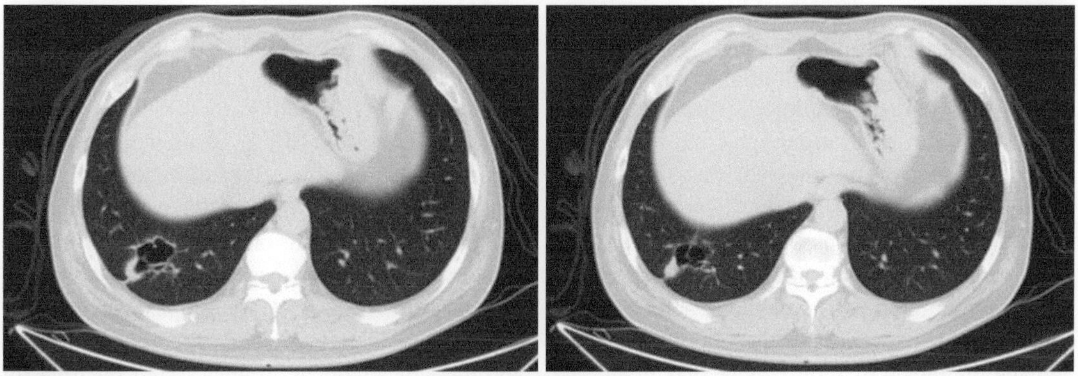

Fig. 23 Chest CT

Bass and Singer in 1951 [110] first reported lung cancer associated with bullous lung disease. Goldstein et al. [111] in 1968 described the clinical and roentgenographic features of 18 patients with bronchogenic carcinoma associated with giant bullous disease. The incidence of bulla associated carcinoma was 3.8% (18 cases out of 411). They speculated that constitutional factors may cause bullous disease and simultaneously may also predispose the patient to lung cancer. Maki et al. [112] in 2006 reviewed retrospectively 20 patients with CT appearances of bronchogenic carcinoma associated with bullous lung disease. They could be classified into 3 types; nodule or mass extruding from the bullous wall, nodule or mass confined within the bullous lumen, and soft tissue density extending along the bullous wall. Lantuejoul et al. [113] in 2007 reviewed 7 cases of type 1 congenital cystic adenomatoid malformation (CCAM) with adenocarcinoma. Type 1 CCAM mucinous cells share the same differentiation profile with corresponding mucinous BAC, consistent with a common bronchial origin. Kaneda et al. [114] in 2010 studied retrospectively 545 cases with primary lung cancer and found 19 cases of cancer adjoined a bulla. Bulla/cancer incidence was 3.5%. They reviewed 95 cases in Japan from 1974, most of the cases were heavy smokers. Smoking is a common causative factor for both bulla and lung cancer. They speculated that limited air flow in areas of compressed parenchyma and connective tissues surrounding a pulmonary bulla may lead to deposits of microorganisms on the wall of the bulla with repeated infection. Repeated inflammatory process may lead to a fibrous scar to form around the bulla. This may cause accumulation of carcinogen in the bulla. Farooqi et al. [115] in 2012 found that the pathologic findings correlated well with the radiographic findings of a large dominant cystic airspace associated with carcinoma (3.7%), but that the histological features of the cystic lesions were variable. CT scans showed the initial cystic airspace had a thin wall (median diameter, 1.0 mm) that subsequently became thicker; eventually the nodule appeared and the diagnosis of lung cancer was made. 19 out of 26 patients (73%) developed emphysema, suggesting that emphysema is an independent risk factor for lung cancer because it increases the likelihood of lung cancer four-fold to five-fold and may be a contributing factor to the development of malignancy. Mascalchi et al. [116] in 2015 used a 4-type classification to describe the morphologic CT features of LC-CAS based on the initial scheme of Maki. Type I corresponds to the presence of a nodule extruding from the cystic airspace wall; type II corresponds to a nodule confined within the lumen of the cystic airspace; type III corresponds to a soft tissue density extending along the wall of the cystic airspace; and type IV corresponds to solid or non-solid tissue intermixed within cluster of multiple cystic airspaces. Type III and IV are most common, and type II occurs less frequently. In the series, 6 out of 24 lesions showed an increase in size of the cystic airspace, which was presumably caused by a valve mechanism on the distal airway connected with the cystic airspace. Fintelmann et al. [117] in 2017 found that cystic airspaces were associated with 1% of NSCLC cases. 97% patients had a smoking history. Twenty of 30 cases demonstrated increased soft tissue due to wall thickening, increased loculations, enlargement and/or increased attenuation of a mural nodule, or replacement by a mass. Cystic airspaces on CT can be caused by a check-valve mechanism obstructing the small airways, lepidic growth of adenocarcinoma in an area of emphysema, cystification of tumor due to degeneration, or adenocarcinoma growing along the wall of a pre-existing bulla.

Most studies showed that adenocarcinoma is the predominant histological type in LC-CAS with up to 80% and 88% in the largest studies (by Fintelmann [117] and Farooqi [115]). In the study by Farooqi [115], 23 cases were of adenocarcinoma, squamous cell carcinoma in one case, non-small cell carcinoma in one case, and atypical carcinoid tumor in one case. In the study by Fintelmann [117], 24 cases were of adenocarcinomas, 4 squamous cell carcinomas, and 2 poorly differentiated carcinomas. Fourteen of 26 tumors and 64% of adenocarcinomas tested positive for an alteration of KRAS with or without other alterations. In a small series by Guo et al. [118] of 15 patients (Asian origin), histological analysis showed that 11 cases were of adenocarcinoma, two of squamous cell carcinoma, one of adenosquamous cell carcinoma, and one of large cell carcinoma. EGFR and KRAS mutations were detected in eight cases. Three patients showed an EGFR mutation affecting exons 19 (n = 2 deletion) and 21 (n = 1 L858R) mutation. There was no KRAS mutation in all eight patients. In the study by Snoeckx [119], histopathological analysis showed 11 adenocarcinoma and 2 squamous cell carcinoma cases. In the 11 patients with adenocarcinoma, mutational analysis information was available for 10 patients (91%) 0.5 out of 10 patients showed different molecular alterations: an EGFR exon 18 mutation, ROS1 rearrangement, and BRAF mutation in one patient each. Two patients showed KRAS mutations. Toyokawa et al. investigated the occurrence of programmed death-ligand 1 (PD-L1) expression in "emphysematous bullae-associated lung adenocarcinomas." They found that emphysematous bullae-associated lung adenocarcinomas express PD-L1 protein more frequently than those without emphysematous bullae. In the study by Haider et al. [120], all patients (n = 11) had a history of smoking. Adenocarcinomas with lepidic, papillary, and acinar-predominant patterns were found in nine patients (81.8% cases), while two patients demonstrated squamous cell carcinomas on histology. In the meta-analysis by Mendoza et al. [121], most patients were current or previous smokers (127/192, 66.1%). The common histology was adenocarcinoma (289/328, 88.1%) and squamous cell carcinoma (30/328, 9.1%). The most common driver mutations were EGFR (46/122, 37.7%) and KRAS (21/122, 17.2%).

The morphological classification of LC-CAS was proposed in 2006 by Maki and updated in 2015 by Mascalchi. Mendoza et al. [121] found that the cysts in LC-CAS commonly had non-uniform (104/114; 91.2%) and thick (83/222; 37.4%) walls, irregular margins (53/142; 37.3%), and were unilocular (173/272; 63.6%). Most LC-CAS had a nodular component (210/328; 64.0%). Over time, the nodule component of most LC-CAS developed or enlarged (61/89, 68.5%), approximately half (43/89, 48.3%) had interval wall thickening, and a minority evolved into completely solid lesions (11/89, 12.4%). The cystic component may increase (36/89, 40.4%), decrease (28/89, 31.5), or remain stable (24/89, 27.0%) in size (Figs. 24, 25, 26). It is difficult to differentiate between benign and malignant cystic airspace by 18F-FDG-PET, because infectious (including fungal) diseases, inflammatory abnormalities, and granulomatous diseases can also show high uptake. LC-CAS can be indolent, and long-term surveillance with imaging should be considered if not resected.

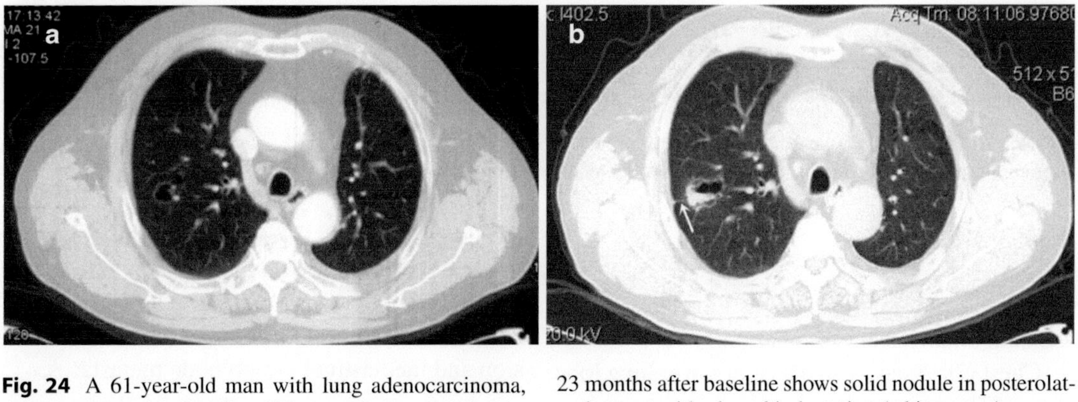

Fig. 24 A 61-year-old man with lung adenocarcinoma, type I pattern. (**a**) Baseline CT scan shows a cystic airspace with thin wall in right upper lobe. (**b**) CT scan 23 months after baseline shows solid nodule in posterolateral aspect with pleural indentation (white arrow)

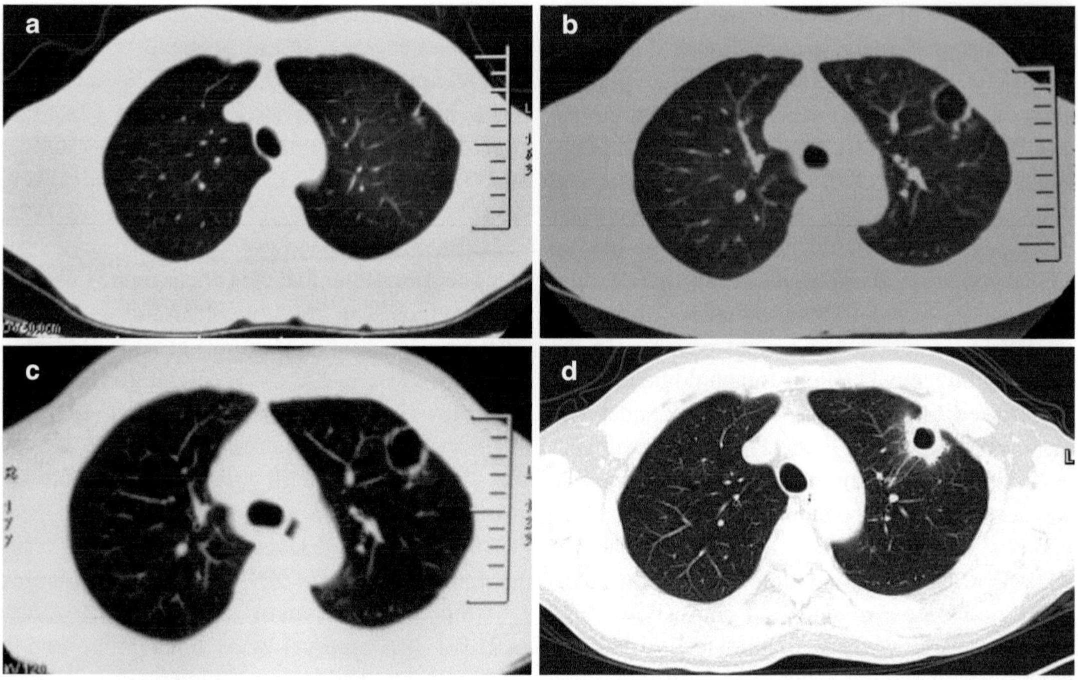

Fig. 25 A 61-year-old man with lung adenocarcinoma, type III pattern. (**a**) CT scan shows cystic airspace with thin wall in left upper lobe on November 21, 2011. (**b**) CT scan shows that the size of the airspace had increased and a solid component has appeared adjacent to the chest wall on April 25, 2016. (**c**) CT scan shows that the airspace and the solid component have further increased on February 17, 2017. (**d**) CT scan shows that the solid component surrounded the airspace and became thicker, and the cystic airspaces shrunk on March 5, 2017

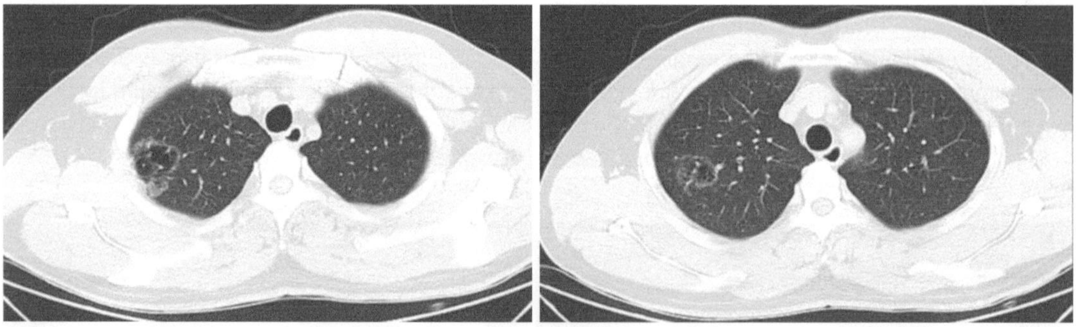

Fig. 26 A 42-year-old man with lung adenocarcinoma, type IV pattern. CT scan shows a lesion in the right upper lobe containing several cystic airspaces, which is demarcated by a thin wall

3.17 Case 17

A 53-year-old man found a lung lesion for 1 month on physical examination.

Chest CT: A cavity in the right lower lung lobe (Fig. 27).

[Diagnosis] Lung adenocarcinoma with cavity.

[Diagnosis Basis] CT scan shows a right lower lobe cavitary lesion with pleural indentation. The histopathologic diagnosis of the lesion was acinar adenocarcinoma with visceral pleural invasion and mediastinal lymph node metastases.

[Analysis] Radiographically, cavity is defined as a gas-filled space within an area of pulmonary

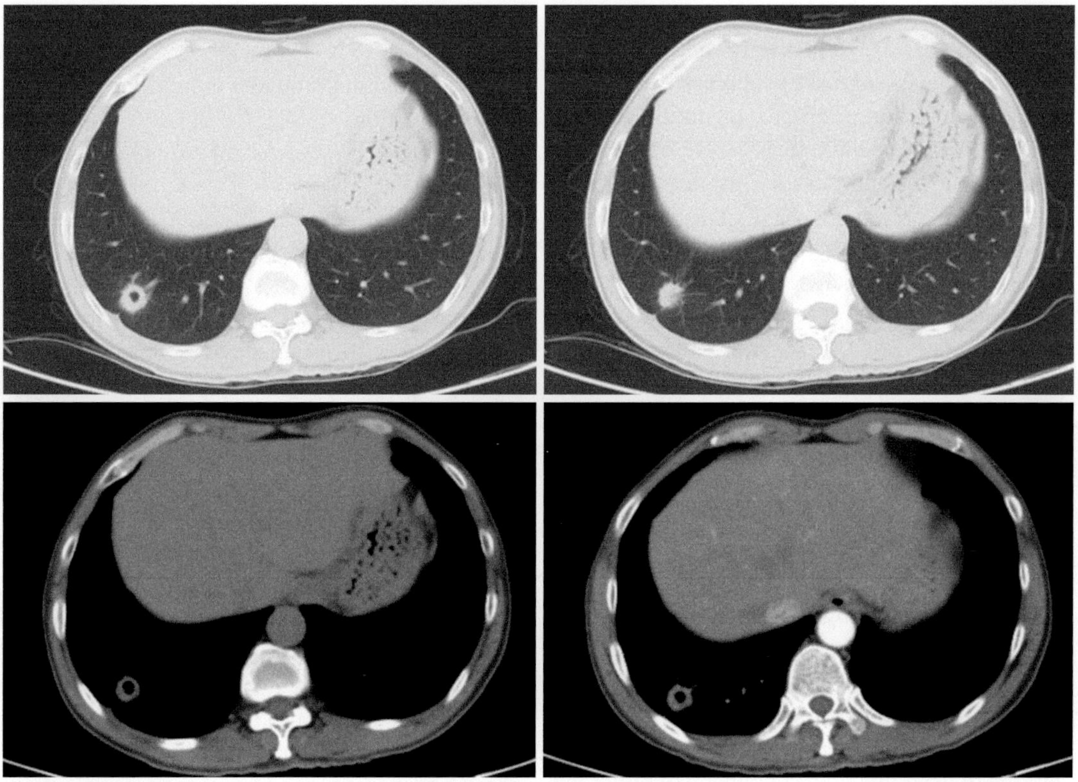

Fig. 27 Chest CT

consolidation, a mass or a nodule. It is often reported in cavities with wall thickness of >4 mm and is often difficult to accurately differentiate cavity from cyst because of overlap in their etiology and pathophysiology.

Lung cancer with cavity is fairly common and is most prevalent in squamous cell carcinoma, followed by adenocarcinoma; no cavity is detected in small cell carcinoma. As the prevalence of lung adenocarcinoma increases, lung adenocarcinoma with cavity has also increased, with an incidence of 5.7% to 14.9%.

Woodring et al. [122] reported that maximum cavity wall thickness provided a more reliable indication to distinguish between benign lesions and malignant lesions in a study of 65 cases of solitary lung cavities. All lesions in which the thickest part of the cavity wall was 1 mm were benign. Of the lesions whose thickest measurement was 4 mm or less, 92% were benign. Of the lesions 5–15 mm, 51% were benign and 49% malignant. Of those greater than 15 mm, 95% were malignant. Watanabe et al. [123] in 2015 studied 2316 primary lung adenocarcinoma patients with surgical resection. Among these cases, 143 (6.2%) were diagnosed as cavitary adenocarcinoma based on high-resolution computed tomography scans. The most prevalent histologic subtype of cavitary adenocarcinoma was the papillary type (41.3%,59/143), followed by the solid type(21.0%,30/143), the lepidic type(10.5%,15/143), the acinar type (10.5%,15/143), and the micropapillary type (7.0%,10/143). Compared with non-cavitary adenocarcinoma, cavitary adenocarcinoma tended to be larger and were significantly associated with a worse prognosis, male sex, smoking history, tumor in the lower lobe, lymph node metastasis, advanced tumor stage, and postoperative recurrence. Watanabe et al. in 2016 [124] categorized surgically resected cavitary adenocarcinoma patients into two groups stratified by the cutoff value of 4 mm of cavity wall thickness. The thick-walled group (>4 mm) had a higher frequency of solid predominant tumors, vascular invasion, necrosis, lymphatic invasion, obstructive pneumonia, intracavity abscess, and bronchiolar obstruction. Lepidic predominant and papillary predominant patterns were more common in the thin-walled group(≤4 mm). Multivariate analysis revealed cavity wall thickness to be an independent prognostic factor, particularly for early-stage cancer. The 5-year overall survival of stage I patients with thin-wall and thick-wall was 91.5% and 70.1%, respectively. Shigefuku et al. [125] reported that neither whole tumor size nor lymph node metastasis was a prognostic factor for overall survival in NSCLCs with cavity formation in univariate analysis. Only maximum cavity wall thickness was a significant prognostic factor by multivariate analysis.

Although the pathogenesis of cavitary adenocarcinoma is often difficult to ascertain, several mechanisms of cavity development in primary lung cancer have been explained. The cavity might be caused by necrosis of the primary cancer growth itself due to the occlusion of either the feeding vessels within the tumor or a check-valve mechanism of the conducting bronchus, or it originated in the wall of a pre-existing cystic lesion, or it might develop by neoplastic cell autophagy due to a particular enzymatic system secreted by tumor cells. In addition, Zhang et al. [126] reported that the number of tumor blood vessels decreased with increasing tumor size in NSCLC, so inadequate vascularization might partly account for cavity formation in lung carcinoma.

In summary, cavitary adenocarcinoma has worse prognostic characteristics than non-cavitary adenocarcinoma. Cavitary lung cancer can be indicated by the following clinical signs: uneven thickening of cavity wall; the formation of wall nodules; the presence of compartments in the cavity; cavity accompanied by mediastinal lymph nodes or distant organ metastasis; cavity enlargement under long-term observation.

3.18 Case 18

A 77-year-old man found a lung lesion on physical examination.

Chest CT: A lesion in right upper lobe (Fig. 28).

[Diagnosis] Lung adenocarcinoma.

[Diagnosis Basis] CT scan shows a right upper lobe lesion with pseudocavitation, air bronchograms, angiogram sign, and pleural indentation. The histopathologic diagnosis of the lesion was lung adenocarcinoma.

[Analysis] The Fleischner Society glossary of terms defines pseudocavity as an oval or round area of low attenuation in lung nodules, masses, or areas of consolidation, representing spared parenchyma, normal or ectatic bronchi, or focal emphysema rather than cavitation. The diameter of pseudocavities is usually less than 1 cm. They have been described in patients with adenocarcinoma and benign conditions such as infectious pneumonia.

Tailor et al. [127] found that pseudocavitation at CT is more common in primary lung adenocarcinoma than in other types of NSCLC. Among adenocarcinomas, the pseudocavitation sign was more frequent in tumors with lepidic growth versus those without lepidic growth [10/24 (41.7%) vs. 9/62 (14.5%)], indicating a correlation between the imaging finding of pseudocavitation and the pathologic finding of lepidic growth. Utrera Pérez et al. [128] analyzed whether the presence of pseudocavitation was associated with size, the histologic type, or EGFR positivity of the tumor as well as with the sex or age of the patient. They found that pseudocavitation was present in 15% of the tumors and was significantly more common in adenocarcinomas (24.1%), although it was present in 9.8% of the epidermoid carcinomas and in 3% of the microcytic carcinomas. In the resected adenocarcino-

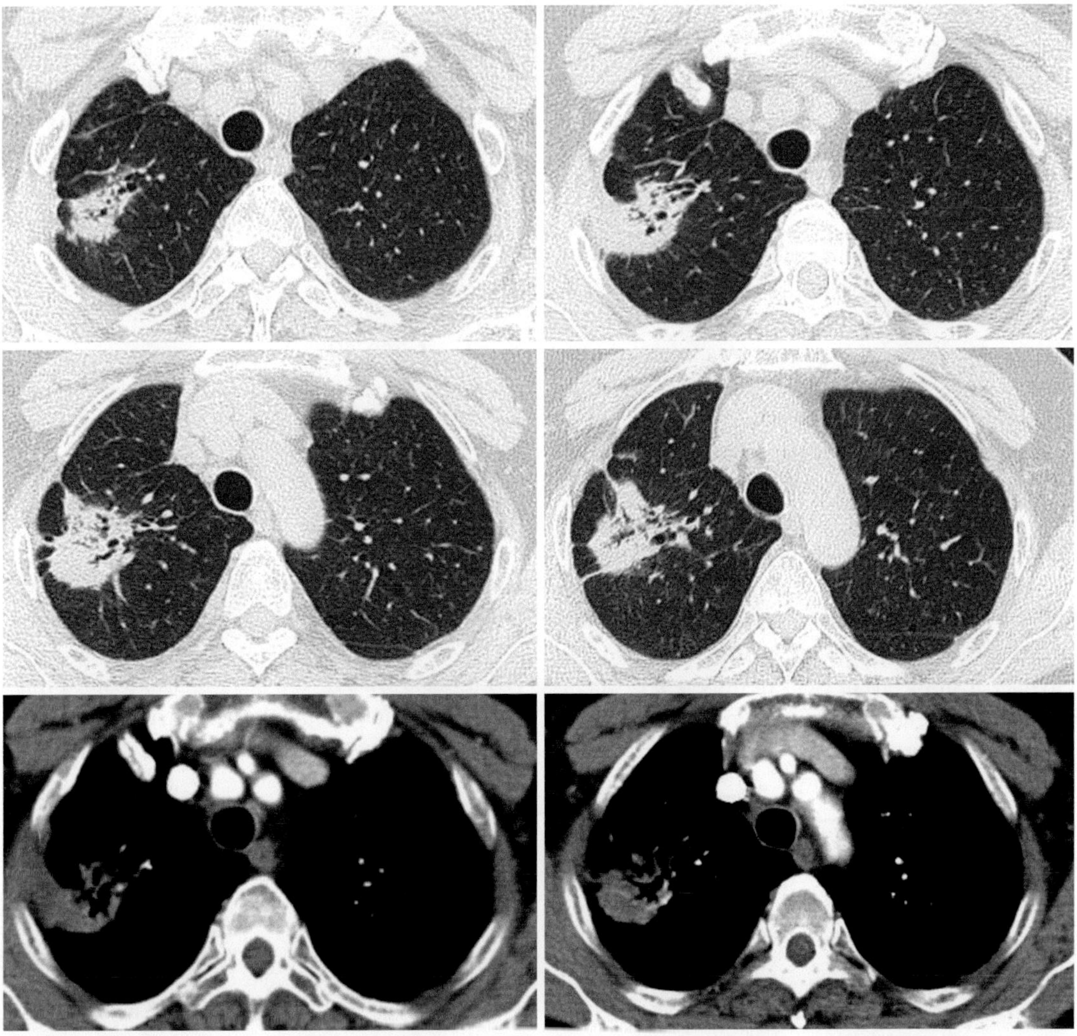

Fig. 28 Chest CT

mas, 65% (13/20) of the tumors with pseudocavitation had lepidic growth; the prevalence of pseudocavitation was 40.6% (13/32) in tumors with lepidic growth, 31.5% (6/19) in those with acinar growth, 33% (1/3) in those with papillary growth. Pseudocavitation was not observed in solid adenocarcinoma or mucinous adenocarcinoma. Pseudocavitation was significantly more common in women (29%); no differences were found with respect to age, size, or EGFR positivity.

In summary, pseudocavitation is more common in adenocarcinomas with lepidic growth and in women.

3.19 Case 19

A 56-year-old man complained of dry cough for 1 month.

Chest CT: Bilateral multiple cavities, nodules, and mass (Fig. 29).

[Diagnosis] Lung adenocarcinoma with multiple cavitary metastases.

[Diagnosis Basis] CT scan shows bilateral multiple cavities, nodules, and mass with pseudocavitations in the right upper lobe. Computed tomography-guided percutaneous lung biopsy revealed invasive lung adenocarcinoma.

[Analysis] The most frequent etiologies of cavitary lesions are abscess, cavitary tumors, bacterial and fungal infections. Spontaneous cavitation in the primary lung cancer is very common, but cavitary lesions are present in only 4% of metastatic nodules and multiple cavitary lesions are rarely seen in primary lung adenocarcinoma.

The possible mechanisms of cavitation include ischemic necrosis, check-valve obstruction, and disruption of the alveolar wall by a tumor. Based on the finding that multiple cavitary metastases were fused, necrosis was probably the main cause of cavitation in this case. These cavitations usually have irregular or spiculated inner or outer margins.

3.20 Case 20

A 58-year-old man found a lung lesion on physical examination.

Chest CT: A solid mass with pleural tags in right upper lobe (Fig. 30).

[Diagnosis] Lung adenocarcinoma with dry pleural dissemination.

[Diagnosis Basis] CT scan shows a solid mass with pleural tags, spiculation, cavity, and necrosis (white arrow) in right upper lobe and multiple

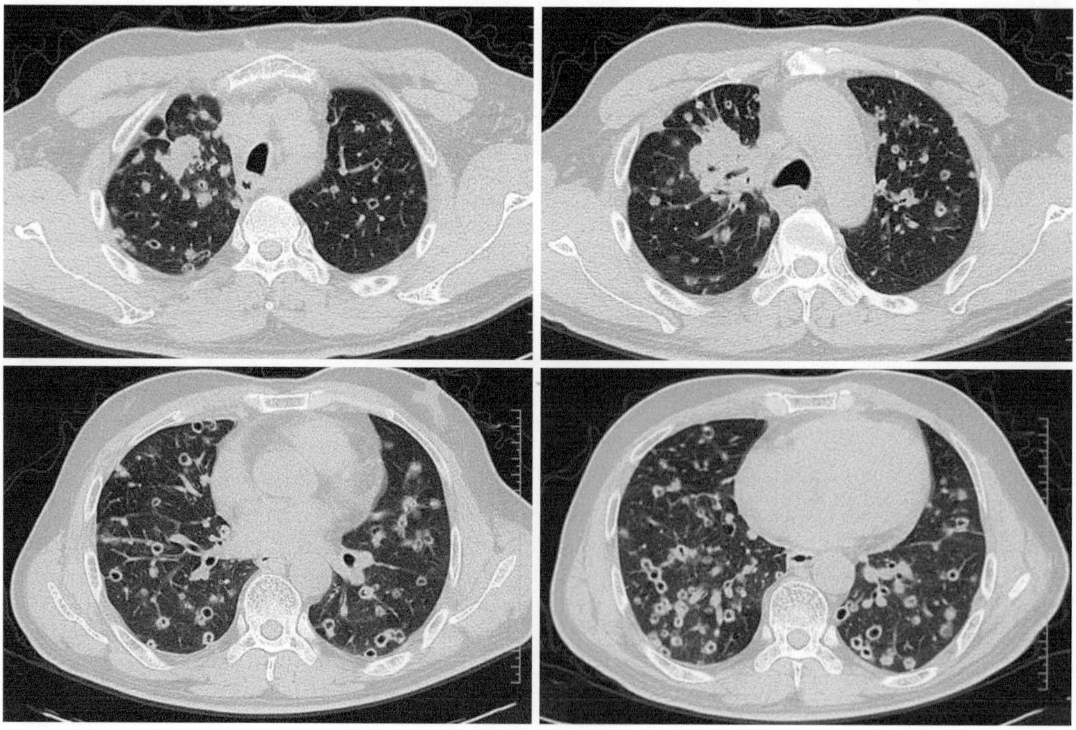

Fig. 29 Chest CT

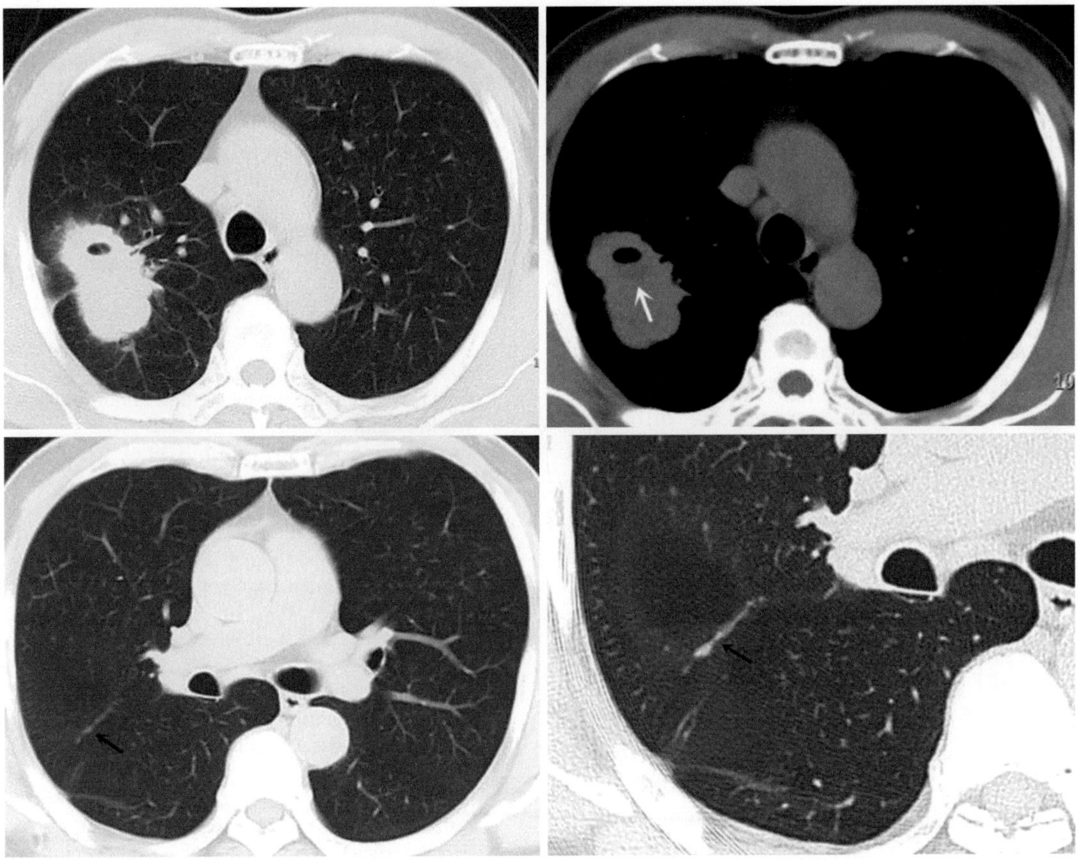

Fig. 30 Chest CT

small nodules within major fissures on the right side (black arrow), considering the possibility of metastasis. Almost all fissural nodular metastases are lung adenocarcinoma, and a few are adenosquamous carcinoma. The pathology of the patient outside the hospital was poorly differentiated squamous cell carcinoma, but the imaging shows lung adenocarcinoma with dry pleural dissemination. After pathology consultation and immunohistochemistry, the final diagnosis was poorly differentiated adenocarcinoma.

[Analysis] Pleural dissemination is one of the important modes of metastasis and also a poor prognostic factor for NSCLC. Adenocarcinoma is the most common primary lung cancer that metastasized to the pleura, with or without effusion. Pleural metastasis of lung cancer is divided into wet pleural dissemination (WPD) and dry pleural dissemination (DPD). DPD in NSCLC is defined as solid pleural metastases without pleural malignant effusion and is a condition occurring in M1a stage.

The CT findings of dry pleural dissemination include small nodules along the mediastinal, costal, or diaphragmatic pleural surfaces and small nodules or irregular nodular thickening in fissures. Mori et al. [129] found that thin-section CT provided more useful information than thick-section CT for the evaluation of pleural dissemination in lung cancer. Shim et al. [130] retrospectively analyzed the CT findings of pathologically proved DPD in 8 of 172 patients with peripheral adenocarcinoma of the lung. The CT findings of DPD were pleural small nodules (n = 8) and uneven (n = 4) or band-like (n = 3) fissural thickening. CT can image DPD of morphologic multiple small pleural or fissural nodules with a diameter of less than 5 mm or uneven or band-like pleural or fissural thickening, because the lungs provide a natural high contrast. When six or more pleural or fissural nodules and uneven pleural or fissural thickening are observed at CT in the ipsilateral pleura in patients with peripheral pulmonary adenocarcinoma, pleural dissemination should be considered despite the absence of pleural effusion. Nonmalignant pleural or fissural nodules include intrapulmonary lymph nodes, nodular fissural thickenings, anthracofibrotic nodules, or granulomas. Kim et al. [131] compared prognostic differences between DPD and WPD in patients with NSCLC and reviewed the applicability of CT findings of DPD for rendering the diagnosis of this disease. Median survival after initial presentation was significantly longer in patients with DPD than in patients with WPD; it was 38 months in patients with DPD and 13 months in patients with WPD. CT was helpful in identifying DPD in 90% (18/20) of patients with pathologically proved DPD. Multiple pleural or fissural nodules were noted on CT images in 80% (16/20) of patients. Uneven or band-like pleural thickening was recognized in 15 (75%) patients. They believed that patients with DPD show better survival than patients with WPD. CT can effectively indicate the presence of DPD preoperatively.

Malignant pleural dissemination is generally considered as a contraindication to surgery. A few studies have reported relatively better prognosis of patients with intraoperatively diagnosed DPD. Li et al. [132] retrospectively evaluated 43 lung adenocarcinoma patients with pleural seeding diagnosed unexpectedly during surgery. Their study showed that the progression-free and overall survival after main tumor and visible pleural nodule resection in patients with lung adenocarcinoma with intraoperatively diagnosed pleural seeding were improved. Kim et al. [133] in 2020 retrospectively reviewed 104 patients with NSCLC and DPD confirmed by surgery. The most common histologic type was adenocarcinoma in 95 (91.3%) patients. Almost half of all patients with NSCLC and DPD experienced malignant pleural effusion (MPE), and 14.4% patients developed symptomatic MPE requiring invasive procedures. MPE in DPD did not affect the survival in NSCLC patients.

In summary, primary tumor resection might be a treatment option in patients with unexpected intraoperatively proven malignant pleural nodules.

References

1. WHO. Histological typing of lung tumors. Geneva: World Health Organization (WHO); 1967.
2. WHO. Histological typing of lung tumors. Geneva: World Health Organization (WHO); 1981.
3. Travis WD, Colby TV, Corrin B, et al. Histological typing of lung and pleural tumors. Berlin: Springer; 1999.
4. Travis WD, Brambilla E, Muller-Hermelink HK, et al. Pathology and genetics. Tumors of the lung, pleura, thymus and heart. Lyon, France: IARC Press; 2004.
5. Liebow AA. Bronchiolo-alveolar carcinoma. Adv Intern Med. 1960;10:329–58.
6. Noguchi M, Morikawa A, Kawasaki M, et al. Small adenocarcinoma of the lung. Histologic characteristics and prognosis. Cancer. 1995;75:2844–52.
7. Travis WD, Brambilla E, Noguchi M, et al. International association for the study of lung cancer/American thoracic society/European respiratory society international multidisciplinary classification of lung adenocarcinoma. J Thorac Oncol. 2011;6:244–85.
8. Travis WD, Brambilla E, Burke AP, et al. WHO classification of tumors of the lung, pleura, thymus and heart. 4th ed. Lyon: International Agency for Research on Cancer; 2015. p. 9–96.
9. Hong DS, Fakih MG, Strickler JH, et al. $KRAS^{G12C}$ inhibition with Sotorasib in advanced solid tumors. N Engl J Med. 2020;383:1207–17.
10. Kalemkerian GP, Narula N, Kennedy EB, et al. Molecular testing guideline for the selection of patients with lung cancer for treatment with targeted tyrosine kinase inhibitors: American Society of Clinical Oncology endorsement of the College of American Pathologists/International Association for the Study of Lung Cancer/Association for Molecular Pathology Clinical Practice Guideline Update. J Clin Oncol. 2018;36:911–9.
11. Chapman AD, Kerr KM. The association between atypical adenomatous hyperplasia and primary lung cancer. Br J Cancer. 2000;83:632–6.
12. Kitami A, Sano F, Hayashi S, et al. Correlation between histological invasiveness and the computed tomography value in pure ground-glass nodules. Surg Today. 2016;46:593–8.
13. Lee SM, Goo JM, Lee KH, et al. CT findings of minimally invasive adenocarcinoma (MIA) of the

lung and comparison of solid portion measurement methods at CT in 52 patients. Eur Radiol. 2015;25:2318–25.
14. Xiang W, Xing Y, Jiang S, et al. Morphological factors differentiating between early lung adenocarcinomas appearing as pure ground-glass nodules measuring ≤10 mm on thin-section computed tomography. Cancer Imaging. 2014;14:33.
15. Henschke CI, Yankelevitz DF, Mirtcheva R, et al. CT screening for lung cancer: frequency and significance of part-solid and nonsolid nodules. AJR. 2002;178:1053–7.
16. Kakinuma R, Muramatsu Y, Kusumoto M, et al. Solitary pure ground-glass nodules 5 mm or smaller: frequency of growth. Radiology. 2015;276:873–82.
17. Yankelevitz DF, Yip R, Smith JP, et al. CT screening for lung cancer: nonsolid nodules in baseline and annual repeat rounds. Radiology. 2015;277:555–64.
18. Ichinose J, Kohno T, Fujimori S, et al. Invasiveness and malignant potential of pulmonary lesions presenting as pure ground-glass opacities. Ann Thorac Cardiovasc Surg. 2014;20:347–52.
19. MacMahon H, et al. Guidelines for management of incidental pulmonary nodules detected on CT images: from the Fleischner Society 2017. 2017. doi: https://doi.org/10.1148/radiol.2017161659.
20. Lee HW, Jin KN, Lee JK, et al. Long-term follow-up of ground-glass nodules after 5 years of stability. J Thorac Oncol. 2019;14:1370–7.
21. Hu X, Fujimoto J, Ying L, et al. Multi-region exome sequencing reveals genomic evolution from preneoplasia to lung adenocarcinoma. Nat Commun. 2019;10:2978.
22. Moreira AL, Ocampo PSS, Xia Y, et al. A grading system for invasive pulmonary adenocarcinoma: a proposal from the International Association for the Study of Lung Cancer Pathology Committee. J Thorac Oncol. 2020;15:1599–610.
23. Hou L, Wang T, Chen D, et al. Prognostic and predictive value of the newly proposed grading system of invasive pulmonary adenocarcinoma in Chinese patients: a retrospective multicohort study. Mod Pathol. 2022;10
24. Ko JP, Suh J, Ibidapo O, et al. Lung adenocarcinoma: correlation of quantitative CT findings with pathologic findings. Radiology. 2016;280:931–9.
25. Lee SM, Park CM, Goo JM, et al. Invasive pulmonary adenocarcinomas versus preinvasive lesions appearing as ground-glass nodules: differentiation by using CT features. Radiology. 2013;268:265–73.
26. Yoshizawa A, Motoi N, Riely GJ, et al. Impact of proposed IASLC/ATS/ERS classification of lung adenocarcinoma: prognostic subgroup and implications for further revision of staging based on analysis of 514 stage I cases. Mod Pathol. 2011;24:653–64.
27. Kadota K, Villena-Vargas J, Yoshizawa A, et al. Prognostic significance of adenocarcinoma in situ, minimally invasive adenocarcinoma, and nonmucinous lepidic predominant invasive adenocarcinoma of the lung in patients with stage I disease. Am J Surg Pathol. 2014;38:448–60.
28. Cox ML, Yang CJ, Speicher PJ, et al. The role of extent of surgical resection and lymph node assessment for clinical stage I pulmonary Lepidic adenocarcinoma: an analysis of 1991 patients. J Thorac Oncol. 2017;12:689–96.
29. Maurizi G, D'Andrilli A, Argento G, et al. Complete lymphadenectomy for clinical stage I lepidic adenocarcinoma of the lung: is it justified? Semin. Thorac Cardiovasc Surg. 2022;8:S1043-0679(22)00050-8.
30. Duhig EE, Dettrick A, Godbolt DB, et al. Mitosis trumps T stage and proposed international association for the study of lung cancer/American thoracic society/European respiratory society classification for prognostic value in resected stage 1 lung adenocarcinoma. J Thorac Oncol. 2015;10:673–81.
31. Warth A, Muley T, Kossakowski C, et al. Prognostic impact and clinicopathological correlations of the cribriform pattern in pulmonary adenocarcinoma. J Thorac Oncol. 2015;10:638–44.
32. Dong Y, Li Y, Jin B, et al. Pathologic subtype-defined prognosis is dependent on both tumor stage and status of oncogenic driver mutations in lung adenocarcinoma. Oncotarget. 2017;8:82,244–55.
33. Sakurai H, Asamura H, Miyaoka E, et al. Differences in the prognosis of resected lung adenocarcinoma according to the histological subtype: a retrospective analysis of Japanese lung cancer registry data. Eur J Cardiothorac Surg. 2014;45:100–7.
34. Zhang Y, Xie H, Zhang Z, et al. The characteristics and nomogram for primary lung papillary adenocarcinoma. Open Med (Wars). 2020;15:92–102.
35. Henschke CI, Yankelevitz DF, Yip R, et al. Lung cancers diagnosed at annual CT screening: volume doubling times. Radiology. 2012;263:578–83.
36. Park S, Lee SM, Kim S, et al. Volume doubling times of lung adenocarcinomas: correlation with predominant histologic subtypes and prognosis. Radiology. 2020;295:1–10.
37. McDivitt RW, Boyce W, Gersell D. Tubular carcinoma of the breast. Clinical and pathological observations concerning 135 cases. Am J Surg Pathol. 1982;6:401–11.
38. Silver SA, Askin FB. True papillary carcinoma of the lung: a distinct clinicopathologic entity. Am J Surg Pathol. 1997;21:43–51.
39. Amin MB, Tamboli P, Merchant SH, et al. Micropapillary component in lung adenocarcinoma: a distinctive histologic feature with possible prognostic significance. Am J Surg Pathol. 2002;26:358–64.
40. Tsubokawa N, Mimae T, Sasada S, et al. Negative prognostic influence of micropapillary pattern in stage IA lung adenocarcinoma. Eur J Cardiothorac Surg. 2016;49:293–9.
41. Nitadori J, Bograd AJ, Kadota K, et al. Impact of micropapillary histologic subtype in selecting

limited resection vs lobectomy for lung adenocarcinoma of 2 cm or smaller. J Natl Cancer Inst. 2013;105:1212–20.
42. Yoshida Y, Nitadori JI, Shinozaki-Ushiku A, et al. Micropapillary histological subtype in lung adenocarcinoma of 2 cm or less: impact on recurrence and clinical predictors. Gen Thorac Cardiovasc Surg. 2017;65:273–9.
43. Dai C, Xie H, Kadeer X, et al. Relationship of lymph node micrometastasis and micropapillary component and their joint influence on prognosis of patients with stage I lung adenocarcinoma. Am J Surg Pathol. 2017;41:1212–20.
44. Watanabe K, Sakamaki K, Ito H, et al. Impact of the micropapillary component on the timing of recurrence in patients with resected lung adenocarcinoma. Eur J Cardiothorac Surg. 2020;58:1010–8.
45. Shiono S, Ishii G, Nagai K, et al. Predictive factors for local recurrence of resected colorectal lung metastases. Ann Thorac Surg. 2005;80:1040–5.
46. Shiono S, Ishii G, Nagai K, et al. Histopathologic prognostic factors in resected colorectal lung metastases. Ann Thorac Surg. 2005;79:278–82.
47. Onozato ML, Kovach AE, Yeap BY, et al. Tumor islands in resected early-stage lung adenocarcinomas are associated with unique clinicopathologic and molecular characteristics and worse prognosis. Am J Surg Pathol. 2013;37:287–94.
48. Kadota K, Nitadori J, Sima CS, et al. Tumor spread through air spaces is an important pattern of invasion and impacts the frequency and location of recurrences after limited resection for small stage I lung adenocarcinomas. J Thorac Oncol. 2015;10:806–14.
49. Warth A, Muley T, Kossakowski CA, et al. Prognostic impact of intra-alveolar tumor spread in pulmonary adenocarcinoma. Am J Surg Pathol. 2015;39:793–801.
50. Morimoto J, Nakajima T, Suzuki H, et al. Impact of free tumor clusters on prognosis after resection of pulmonary adenocarcinoma. J Thorac Cardiovasc Surg. 2016;152:64–72.
51. Uruga H, Fujii T, Fujimori S, et al. Semiquantitative assessment of tumor spread through air spaces (STAS) in early-stage lung adenocarcinomas. J Thorac Oncol. 2017;12:1046–51.
52. Dai C, Xie H, Su H, et al. Tumor spread through air spaces affects the recurrence and overall survival in patients with lung adenocarcinoma >2 to 3 cm. J Thorac Oncol. 2017;12:1052–60.
53. Shiono S, Endo M, Suzuki K, et al. Spread through air spaces is a prognostic factor in sublobar resection of non-small cell lung cancer. Ann Thorac Surg. 2018;106:354–60.
54. Terada Y, Takahashi T, Morita S, et al. Spread through air spaces is an independent predictor of recurrence in stage III (N2) lung adenocarcinoma. Interact Cardiovasc Ther. 2019;29:442–8.
55. Thunnissen E, Blaauwgeers HJ, de Cuba EM, et al. Ex vivo artifacts and histopathologic pitfalls in the lung. Arch Pathol Lab Med. 2016;140:212–20.
56. Blaauwgeers H, Flieder D, Warth A, et al. A prospective study of loose tissue fragments in non-small cell lung cancer resection specimens: an alternative view to "spread through air spaces". Am J Surg Pathol. 2017;41:1226–30.
57. Lee JS, Kim EK, Kim M, et al. Genetic and clinicopathologic characteristics of lung adenocarcinoma with tumor spread through air spaces. Lung Cancer. 2018;123:121–6.
58. Eguchi T, Kameda K, Lu S, et al. Lobectomy is associated with better outcomes than sublobar resection in spread through air spaces (STAS)-positive T1 lung adenocarcinoma: a propensity score-matched analysis. J Thorac Oncol. 2019;14:87–98.
59. Yagi Y, Aly RG, Tabata K, et al. Three-dimensional histologic, Immunohistochemical, and multiplex immunofluorescence analyses of dynamic vessel co-option of spread through air spaces in lung adenocarcinoma. J Thorac Oncol. 2020;15:589–600.
60. Toyokawa G, Yamada Y, Tagawa T, et al. Computed tomography features of resected lung adenocarcinomas with spread through air spaces. J Thorac Cardiovasc Surg. 2018;156:1670–6.
61. Kim SK, Kim TJ, Chung MJ, et al. Lung adenocarcinoma: CT features associated with spread through air spaces. Radiology. 2018;12(289):831–40.
62. de Margerie-Mellon C, Onken A, Heidinger BH, et al. CT manifestations of tumorspread through airspaces in pulmonary adenocarcinomas presenting as subsolid nodules. J Thorac Imaging. 2018;33:402–8.
63. Lu S, Tan KS, Kadota K, et al. Spread through air spaces (STAS) is an independent predictor of recurrence and lung cancer specific death in squamous cell carcinoma. J Thorac Oncol. 2017;12:223–34.
64. Kadota K, Kushida Y, Katsuki N, et al. Tumor spread through air spaces is an independent predictor of recurrence-free survival in patients with resected lung squamous cell carcinoma. Am J Surg Pathol. 2017;41:1077–86.
65. Yanagawa N, Shiono S, Endo M, et al. Tumor spread through air spaces is a useful predictor of recurrence and prognosis in stage I lung squamous cell carcinoma, but not in stage II and III. Lung Cancer. 2018;120:14–21.
66. Yokoyama S, Murakami T, Tao H, et al. Tumor spread through air spaces identifies a distinct subgroup with poor prognosis in surgically resected lung pleomorphic carcinoma. Chest. 2018;154:838–47.
67. Aly RG, Rekhtman N, Li X, et al. Spread through air spaces (STAS) is prognostic in atypical carcinoid, large cell neuroendocrine carcinoma, and small cell carcinoma of the lung. J Thorac Oncol. 2019;14:1583–93.
68. Altinay S, Metovic J, Massa F, et al. Spread through air spaces (STAS) is a predictor of poor outcome in atypical carcinoids of the lung. Virchows Arch. 2019;475:325–34.
69. Chen D, Mao Y, Wen J, et al. Tumor spread through air spaces in non-small cell lung cancer: a system-

atic review and meta-analysis. Ann Thorac Surg. 2019;108:945–54.
70. Liu H, Yin Q, Yang G, et al. Prognostic impact of tumor spread through air spaces in non-small cell lung cancers: a meta-analysis including 3564 patients. Pathol Oncol Res. 2019;25:1303–10.
71. Jiang L, Liang W, Shen J, et al. The impact of visceral pleural invasion in node-negative non-small cell lung cancer: a systematic review and meta-analysis. Chest. 2015;148:903–11.
72. Dziedzic DA, Rudzinski P, Langfort R, et al. Risk factors for local and distant recurrence after surgical treatment in patients with non-small-cell lung cancer. Clin Lung Cancer. 2016;175:e157–67.
73. Hsu JS, Han IT, Tsai TH, et al. Pleural tags on CT scans to predict visceral pleural invasion of non-small cell lung cancer that does not abut the pleura. Radiology. 2016;279:590–6.
74. Ahn SY, Park CM, Jeon YK, et al. Predictive CT features of visceral pleural invasion by T1-sized peripheral pulmonary adenocarcinomas manifesting as subsolid nodules. AJR Am J Roentgenol. 2017;209:561–6.
75. Kim H, Goo JM, Kim YT, et al. CT-defined visceral pleural invasion in T1 lung adenocarcinoma: lack of relationship to disease-free survival. Radiology. 2019;2923:1–9.
76. Yip R, Ma T, Flores RM, et al. Survival with parenchymal and pleural invasion of non-small cell lung cancers less than 30 mm. J Thorac Oncol. 2019;145:890–902.
77. Ichinokawa H, Ishii G, Nagai K, et al. Clinicopalhological charaeteristics of primary lung adenocarcinoma predominantly composed of goblet cells in surgically resected cases. Pathol Int. 2011;6:423–9.
78. Kadota K, Yeh YC, D'Angelo SP, et al. Associations between mutations and histologic patterns of mucin in lung adenocarcinoma: invasive mucinous pattern and extracellular mucin are associated with KRAS mutation. Am J Surg Pathol. 2014;388:1118–27.
79. Maeda Y, Tsuchiya T, Hao H, et al. Kras(G12D) and Nkx2-1 haploinsufficiency induce mucinous adenocarcinoma of the lung. J Clin Invest. 2012;12212:4388–400.
80. Hwang DH, Sholl LM, Rojas-Rudilla V, et al. KRAS and NKX2-1 mutations in invasive mucinous adenocarcinoma of the lung. J Thorac Oncol. 2016;114:496–503.
81. Shim HS, Kenudson M, Zheng Z, et al. Unique genetic and survival characteristics of invasive mucinous adenocarcinoma of the lung. J Thorac Oncol. 2015;10:1156–62.
82. Chang JC, Offin M, Falcon C, et al. Comprehensive molecular and clinicopathologic analysis of 200 pulmonary invasive mucinous adenocarcinomas identifies distinct characteristics of molecular subtypes. Clin Cancer Res. 2021;27:4066–76.
83. Kawai H, Sugano M, Nakano N, et al. A case of invasive mucinous adenocarcinoma of the lung showing stepwise progression at the primary site. Lung Cancer. 2019;136:94–7.
84. Russell PA, Wainer Z, Wright GM, et al. Does lung adenocarcinoma subtype predict patient survival?: a clinicopathologic study based on the new International Association for the Study of Lung Cancer/American Thoracic Society/European Respiratory Society international multidisciplinary lung adenocarcinoma classification. J Thorac Oncol. 2011;6:1496–504.
85. Yoshizawa A, Motoi N, Riely GJ, et al. Impact of proposed IASLC/ATS/ERS classification of lung adenocarcinoma: prognostic subgroups and implications for further revision of staging based on analysis of 514 stage I cases. Mod Pathol. 2011;24:653–64.
86. Warth A, Muley T, Meister M, et al. The novel histologic International Association for the Study of Lung Cancer/American Thoracic Society/European Respiratory Society classification system of lung adenocarcinoma is a stage-independent predictor of survival. J Clin Oncol. 2012;30:1438–46.
87. Watanabe H, Saito H, Yokose T, et al. Relation between thin-section computed tomography and clinical findings of mucinous adenocarcinoma. Ann Thorac Surg. 2015;993:975–81.
88. Lee HY, Cha MJ, Lee KS, et al. Prognosis in resected invasive mucinous adenocarcinomas of the lung: related factors and comparison with resected nonmucinous adenocarcinomas. J Thorac Oncol. 2016;11:1064–73.
89. Cha YJ, Kim HR, Lee HJ, et al. Clinical course of stage IV invasive mucinous adenocarcinoma of the lung. Lung Cancer. 2016;102:82–8.
90. Shimizu K, Okita R, Saisho S, et al. Clinicopathological and immunohistochemical features of lung invasive mucinous adenocarcinoma based on computed tomography findings. Onco Targets Ther. 2017;10:153–63.
91. Yang SR, Chang JC, Leduc C, et al. Invasive mucinous adenocarcinomas with spatially separate lung lesions: analysis of clonal relationship by comparative molecular profiling. J Thorac Oncol. 2021;16:1188–99.
92. Wislez M, Massiani MA, Milleron B, et al. Clinical characteristics of pneumonic-type adenocarcinoma of the lung. Chest. 2003;123:1868–77.
93. Barnard WG. Embryoma of lung. Thorax. 1952;7:299–301.
94. Spencer H. Pulmonary blastomas. J Pathol Bacteriol. 1961;82:161–6.
95. Kradin RL, Young RH, Dickersin GR, et al. Pulmonary blastoma with argyrophil cells and lacking sarcomatous features (pulmonary endodermal tumor resembling fetal lung). Am J Surg Pathol. 1982;6:165–72.
96. Kodama T, Shimosato Y, Watanabe S, et al. Six cases of well-differentiated adenocarcinoma simulating fetal lung tubules in pseudoglandular stage.

Comparison with pulmonary blastoma. Am J Surg Pathol. 1984;8:735–44.
97. Morita S, Yoshida A, Goto A, et al. High-grade lung adenocarcinoma with fetal lung-like morphology: clinicopathologic, immunohistochemical, and molecular analyses of 17 cases. Am J Surg Pathol. 2013;37:924–32.
98. Suzuki M, Nakatani Y, Ito H, et al. Pulmonary adenocarcinoma with high-grade fetal adenocarcinoma component has a poor prognosis, comparable to that of micropapillary adenocarcinoma. Mod Pathol. 2018;31:1404–17.
99. Tsao MS, Fraser RS. Primary pulmonary adenocarcinoma with enteric differentiation. Cancer. 1991;68:1754–7.
100. Wang CX, Liu B, Wang YF, et al. Pulmonary enteric adenocarcinoma: a study of the clinicopathologic and molecular status of nine cases. Int J Clin Exp Pathol. 2014;7:1266–74.
101. Zhao L, Huang S, Liu J, et al. Clinicopathological, radiographic, and oncogenic features of primary pulmonary enteric adenocarcinoma in comparison with invasive adenocarcinoma in resection specimens. Medicine (Baltimore). 2017;96:e8153.
102. Lin L, Zhuang W, Wang W, et al. Genetic mutations in lung enteric adenocarcinoma identified using next-generation sequencing. Int J Clin Exp Pathol. 2017;109:9583–90.
103. Chen M, Liu P, Yan F, et al. Distinctive features of immunostaining and mutational load in primary pulmonary enteric adenocarcinoma: implications for differential diagnosis and immunotherapy. J Transl Med. 2018;16:81.
104. Palmirotta R, Lovero D, D'Oronzo S, et al. Pulmonary enteric adenocarcinoma: an overview. Expert Rev Mol Med. 2020;22:e1.
105. Bian T, Zhao J, Feng J, et al. Combination of cadherin-17 and SATB homeobox 2 serves as potential optimal makers for the differential diagnosis of pulmonary enteric adenocarcinoma and metastatic colorectal adenocarcinoma. Oncotarget. 2017;8:63442.
106. Matsushima J, Yazawa T, Suzuki M, et al. Clinicopathological, immunohistochemical, and mutational analyses of pulmonary enteric adenocarcinoma: usefulness of SATB2 and beta-catenin immunostaining for differentiation from metastatic colorectal carcinoma. Hum Pathol. 2017;64: 179–85.
107. Jurmeister P, Schöler A, Arnold A, et al. DNA methylation profiling reliably distinguishes pulmonary enteric adenocarcinoma from metastatic colorectal cancer. Mod Pathol. 2019;32:855–65.
108. Womack NA, Graham EA. Epithelial metaplasia in congenital cystic disease of the lung: its possible relation to carcinoma of the bronchus. Am J Pathol. 1941;17:645–654.5.
109. Anderson HJ, Pierce JW. Carcinoma of the bronchus presenting as thin-walled cysts. Thorax. 1954;9:100–5.
110. Bass HE, Singer E. Co-existing lobar adenocarcinoma and cystic disease of the lung. Ann Intern Med. 1951;34:498–507.
111. Goldstein MJ, Snider GL, Liberson M, et al. Bronchogenic carcinoma and giant bullous disease. Am Rev Respir Dis. 1968;97:1062–70.
112. Maki D, Takahashi M, Murata K, et al. Computed tomography appearances of bronchogenic carcinoma associated with bullous lung disease. J Comput Assist Tomogr. 2006;30:447–52.
113. Lantuejoul S, Nicholson AG, Sartori G, et al. Mucinous cells in type 1 pulmonary congenital cystic adenomatoid malformation as mucinous bronchioloalveolar carcinoma precursors. Am J Surg Pathol. 2007;31:961–9.
114. Kaneda M, Tarukawa T, Watanabe F, et al. Clinical features of primary lung cancer adjoining pulmonary bulla. Interact Cardiovasc Thorac Surg. 2010;10:940–4.
115. Farooqi AO, Cham M, Zhang L, et al. Lung cancer associated with cystic airspaces. AJR Am J Roentgenol. 2012;199:781–6.
116. Mascalchi M, Attinà D, Bertelli E, et al. Lung cancer associated with cystic airspaces. J Comput Assist Tomogr. 2015;39:102–8.
117. Fintelmann FJ, Brinkmann JK, Jeck WR, et al. Lung cancers associated with cystic airspaces: natural history, pathologic correlation, and mutational analysis. J Thorac Imaging. 2017;32:176–88.
118. Guo J, Liang C, Sun Y, et al. Lung cancer presenting as thin-walled cysts: an analysis of 15 cases and review of literature. Asia Pac J Clin Oncol. 2016;12:e105–12.
119. Snoeckx A, Reyntiens P, Pauwels P, et al. Molecular profiling in lung cancer associated with cystic airspaces. Acta Clin Belg. 2019;113:1–4.
120. Haider E, Burute N, Harish S, et al. Lung cancer associated with cystic airspaces: characteristic morphological features on CT in a series of 11 cases. Clin Imaging. 2019;56:102–17.
121. Mendoza DP, Heeger A, Mino-Kenudson M, et al. Clinicopathologic and longitudinal imaging features of lung cancer associated with cystic airspaces: a systematic review and meta-analysis. AJR Am J Roentgenol. 2021;216:318–29.
122. Woodring JH, Fried AM, Chuang VP. Solitary cavities of the lung: diagnostic implications of cavity wall thickness. AJR Am J Roentgenol. 1980;135:1269–71.
123. Watanabe Y, Kusumoto M, Yoshida A, et al. Surgically resected solitary cavitary lung adenocarcinoma: association between clinical, pathologic, and radiologic findings and prognosis. Ann Thorac Surg. 2015;99:968–74.
124. Watanabe Y, Kusumoto M, Yoshida A, et al. Cavity Wall thickness in solitary cavitary lung adenocarcinomas is a prognostic indicator. Ann Thorac Surg. 2016;102:1863–71.
125. Shigefuku S, Kudo Y, Yunaiyama D, et al. Prognostic factors for surgically resected non-small cell

lung cancer with cavity formation. J Thorac Dis. 2018;10:973–83.
126. Zhang L, Yankelevitz DF, Henschke CI, et al. Variation in vascular distribution in small lung cancers. Lung Cancer. 2010;68:389–93.
127. Tailor TD, Schmidt RA, Eaton KD, et al. The pseudocavitation sign of lung adenocarcinoma: a distinguishing feature and imaging biomarker of lepidic growth. J Thorac Imaging. 2015;305:308–13.
128. Utrera Pérez E, Trinidad López C, González Carril F, et al. Can pseudocavitation in lung tumors predict the diagnosis of adenocarcinoma with lepidic growth? Radiologia. 2019;615:396–404.
129. Mori K, Hirose T, Machida S, et al. Helical computed tomography diagnosis of pleural dissemination in lung cancer: comparison of thick section and thin-section helical computed tomography. J Thorac Imaging. 1998;13:211–8.
130. Shim SS, Lee KS, Kim BT, et al. Integrated PET/CT and the dry pleural dissemination of peripheral adenocarcinoma of the lung: diagnostic implications. J Comput Assist Tomogr. 2006;30:70–6.
131. Kim YK, Lee HY, Lee KS, et al. Dry pleural dissemination in non-small cell lung cancer: prognostic and diagnostic implications. Radiology. 2011;260:568–74.
132. Li C, Kuo SW, Hsu HH, et al. Lung adenocarcinoma with intraoperatively diagnosed pleural seeding: is main tumor resection beneficial for prognosis? J Thorac Cardiovasc Surg. 2018;155:1238–49.
133. Kim W, Park IK, Park S, et al. Clinical course of non-small cell lung cancer patients with dry pleural dissemination: retrospective observational study. Medicine (Baltimore). 2020;99:1–6.

Squamous Cell Carcinoma

Song Zhang

Squamous cell carcinoma (SCC) is the second most common histological type of lung cancer and accounts for approximately 20%–30% of NSCLC cases. SCC is more common in men than women and is strongly associated with a history of cigarette smoking which increases burden of somatic mutations.

1 Pathophysiology

SCC of the lung originates from the transformation of the squamous cells lining the airways. Squamous cells are thin, flat cells distributed in many organs of the human body. The main causative agent of cellular transformation is tobacco smoke, which contains more than 300 harmful agents and 40 potential carcinogens. The characteristics of transformed squamous cells are keratinization and/or intercellular bridges and typically exhibit a high degree of mutation frequency. When a minimum of 10% of the tumor bulk of resected samples exhibits transformation features such as keratinization or intracellular bridges, the diagnosis of SCC can be confirmed.

S. Zhang (✉)
Department of Respiratory and Critical Care Medicine, Shandong Provincial Hospital Affiliated to Shandong First Medical University, Jinan, Shandong, China

2 Classification

In the 2004 WHO classification, SCC was classified into papillary, clear cell, small cell, and basaloid subtypes; nevertheless, this was not very meaningful as the papillary, clear cell, and small cell subtypes are very uncommon. SCC was graded by the degree of keratinization into well, moderately, and poorly differentiated. In the well-differentiated SCC, there were tumor nests composed of differentiated keratinocyte-like tumor cells with prominent keratinization (layered and cytoplasmic keratin) and intercellular bridges. In the poorly differentiated SCC, squamous structure was only noticeable in a small area of the tumor. The moderately differentiated SCC showed an intermediate degree of squamous differentiation that was between well and poorly differentiated tumors [1].

In the 2005 Head and Neck WHO classification of nasopharyngeal carcinomas, tumors were classified as nonkeratinizing, keratinizing, and basaloid SCCs. Tumors were classified as having a keratinizing subtype when there was greater than or equal to 5% keratinizing pattern of the entire tumor, whereas nonkeratinizing subtypes were defined as having less than 5% keratinizing pattern. The basaloid pattern was defined as tumor nests showing prominent peripheral palisading of tumor cells with scanty cytoplasm (high nuclear/cytoplasmic ratio) and a greater amount of hyperchromatic nuclei [2].

S. Zhang (ed.), *Diagnostic Imaging of Lung Cancers*, https://doi.org/10.1007/978-981-99-6815-2_2

In the 2015 WHO classification, SCC was reclassified as keratinizing, nonkeratinizing, and basaloid subtypes, with the nonkeratinizing tumors requiring immunohistochemistry proof of squamous differentiation, similar to the Head and Neck WHO classification of nasopharyngeal carcinomas. Tumors are classified as keratinizing SCC if any amount of keratinization is present and basaloid SCC if basaloid component is greater than 50% of the tumor with minimal areas of squamous differentiation. In tumors with 50% or less of a basaloid component, this can be acknowledged in the diagnosis "with basaloid features." In the absence of unequivocal keratinization, immunohistochemistry with positive squamous markers such as p40, p63, or CK5/6 is required to diagnose nonkeratinizing SCC.

In the 2021 WHO classification, lymphoepithelial-like carcinoma is renamed as lymphoepithelial carcinoma and classified as a type of SCC with diffuse positive staining for CK5/6, p40, p63, distinct syncytial growth pattern, variable lymphoplasmacytic infiltrate, and frequent association with Epstein–Barr virus [3].

3 Molecular Pathology

EGFR and MET mutations, and ALK or ROS1 rearrangements, can occur in pulmonary SCC, especially among young nonsmoking patients. Meng et al. [4] identified 31 cases of ALK rearrangement in SCC patients through a literature search. These fusion genes typically appear in a younger age-group with a mean age of 55.6 years and non-smokers (18/31, 58.1%). A total of 20 cases received an ALK inhibitor as first- or second-line treatment, of which 11 were partial response (PR), 4 were stable disease (SD), and 5 were progressive disease (PD). SCC patients with ALK rearrangement obtained clinical benefit from ALK inhibitor therapy, especially those who were non-smokers and whose tumors had been identified by IHC+/FISH+.

LUX-Lung 8 was a randomized, controlled, phase 3 study comparing afatinib and erlotinib as second-line treatment of patients with advanced squamous cell carcinoma (SCC) of the lung. Patients with stage IIIB or IV lung SCC who had progressed after at least four cycles of platinum-based chemotherapy were enrolled. 795 eligible patients were randomly assigned (1:1) to receive afatinib (40 mg per day) or erlotinib (150 mg per day) until disease progression. Goss et al. [5] reported the final overall survival (OS) and safety analyses of LUX-Lung 8. Afatinib significantly prolonged OS compared with erlotinib (median 7–8 months vs 6–8 months). 5.3% (21/398) of afatinib-treated patients and 3.3% (13/397) of erlotinib-treated patients achieved long-term benefit; median OS was 34.6 months and 20.1 months, respectively. Among 132 patients who received afatinib treatment and underwent tumor genetic analysis, ERBB family mutations were more common in patients with long-term benefit than in the overall population (50% vs 21%). They concluded that afatinib is a treatment option for pulmonary SCC patients progressing on chemotherapy who are ineligible for immunotherapy, particularly those with ERBB family genetic aberrations.

4 Immune Checkpoint Inhibitors

In recent years, immune checkpoint inhibitor (ICI) has made remarkable progress in NSCLC including SCC. ICIs therapy is associated with good effects in NSCLC patients with a smoking history. Nivolumab and pembrolizumab, anti-programmed cell death 1 (PD-1) antibodies, and atezolizumab and durvalumab, anti-programmed cell death ligand 1 (PD-L1) antibodies, have been approved in some countries.

CheckMate 017 is a phase 3 study evaluated the efficacy and safety of nivolumab, as compared with docetaxel in patients with previously treated, advanced squamous cell NSCLC. Nivolumab was significantly better in overall survival, response rate, and progression-free survival than docetaxel, regardless of PD-L1 expression level [6].

KEYNOTE 407 is a phase 3 clinical trial of chemotherapy plus either pembrolizumab (n = 278) or placebo (n = 281) for SCC. Pembrolizumab plus carboplatin and paclitaxel/nab-paclitaxel(chemotherapy) significantly improved overall survival (OS) and progression-free survival (PFS) compared with placebo plus chemotherapy in patients with previously untreated metastatic squamous NSCLC [7].

In recent years, there has been significant development in the treatment of SCC of the lung. Many other clinical trials are underway to find the best treatment.

5 Case Analysis

5.1 Case 1

A 60-year-old man complained of cough for 1 year.

Chest CT: Mucus-filled dilated bronchi (black arrow) of the right upper lobe and a mass within the right main bronchus (white arrow) (Fig. 1).

[Diagnosis] Central squamous cell cancer of the lung.

[Diagnosis Basis] The transverse CT scan shows finger-in-glove sign and tree-in-bud pattern, suggesting the diagnosis of central lung cancer. Bronchoscopic examination revealed total occlusion of the right superior lobar bronchus by a polypoid mass, and endobronchial forceps biopsy specimen of the tumor showed squamous cell lung cancer.

[Analysis] Lung tumors are divided into central and peripheral types according to the location of primary site. Generally, when the tumor is located in the inner one-third of the lung field on a CT scan, it is considered to be the central, and when the tumor is located in the outer two-thirds, it is considered to be peripheral. Central lung cancer was also defined as a tumor confirmed by bronchoscopy between the orifice of the lobar bronchus and sub-segmental bronchus.

The progression of SCC in the central airway is considered to be a gradual and stepwise epithelial change from normal mucosa to preneoplastic lesions, then to carcinoma in situ

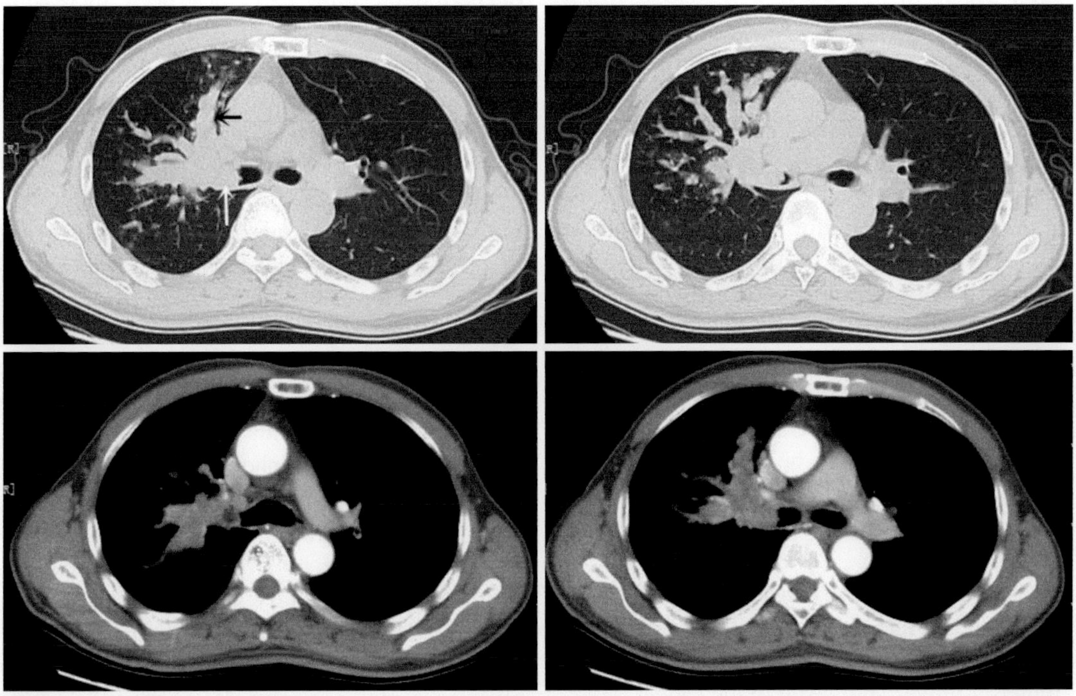

Fig. 1 Chest CT

and invasive lesion. Several sequential molecular abnormalities, such as 3p loss of heterozygosity, 9p loss of heterozygosity, methylation of tumor suppressor gene, telomerase activation, and 5q loss of heterozygosity, contribute to the development of invasive carcinoma.

SCC in the central airway is described as masses involving lobar or segmental bronchi, accompanied by obstructive pneumonia or atelectasis, and commonly presenting necrosis or cavitation. This case showed evidence of mucoid impaction in a patient with lung SCC. Mucoid impaction is a clinical radiographic syndrome and is defined as airway filling by mucoid secretions, usually accompanied by bronchial dilatation. Glazer et al. [8] suggested that this process may be caused by abnormal mucociliary transport and excessive production of mucus. It may occur in a number of obstructive or non-obstructive diseases of the bronchi and most commonly occurs in patients with inflammatory conditions such as allergic bronchopulmonary aspergillosis (ABPA)/mycosis (ABPM). However, as in this case, it is also found in patients with benign and malignant conditions causing airway obstruction. The term "finger-in-glove" was first used by Mintzer et al. [9] in 1978 to describe a case of ABPA. The "finger-in-glove" sign is defined as branching tubular opacities that extend peripherally from the direction of the hilum. It mostly implies benign endobronchial lesions, such as mucoid impaction, and may occasionally imply neoplastic disorders [10]. The incidence of finger-in-glove sign in central lung cancer was found to be obviously relative to pathological type and was frequently detected in patients with SCC. The reason may be related to the fact that SCC usually originates from the bronchial epithelium and tends toward an intraluminal growth.

Central SCC of the lung easily causes bronchial stenosis and occlusion at an early stage, leading to obstructive mucoid impaction and "finger-in-glove" sign distal to the cancer.

5.2 Case 2

A 58-year-old man complained of fever for 1 month.

Chest CT: A mass in the right lower lobe (Fig. 2).

[Diagnosis] Squamous cell lung cancer.

[Diagnosis Basis] The transverse CT scan shows the tumor in the right lower lobe with smooth margin, vascular bundle thickening (red arrow), bronchial cut-off sign (white arrow), and heterogeneous enhancement (central hypoattenuation areas), suggesting the diagnosis of lung cancer. He underwent a right lower lobectomy. The lesion was approximately 4 × 4 × 3.5 cm, diagnosed as moderately and poorly differentiated SCC with necrosis.

[Analysis] SCC can be divided into central and peripheral types based on the tumor location. Traditionally, about 70% of SCC arises from central portion of the lung, whereas the remaining 30% from periphery in literature. The incidence of peripheral lung SCC has been increasing recently, accounting for around 50% of all SCCs of the lung in some reports. Central- and peripheral-type SCC have different clinicopathological and biological features.

In 2003, Funai et al. [11] first evaluated the clinicopathologic factors in the peripheral type of lung SCC. Although the patient population of the peripheral type was older, with a lower pathologic stage, lower lymphatic vessel involvement, and lymph node metastasis than that of the central type, the Kaplan–Meier survival proportions did not differ significantly between these two groups. Based on the histologic growth pattern, they classified the peripheral type into three subgroups as follows: (1) the alveolar space-filling type, (2) the expanding type, and (3) the combined type. These tumors with alveolar space-filling type are solitary and show growth by filling the alveolar space separated by thin preexisting septa without the destruction of the alveolar septa. The alveolar space-filling type

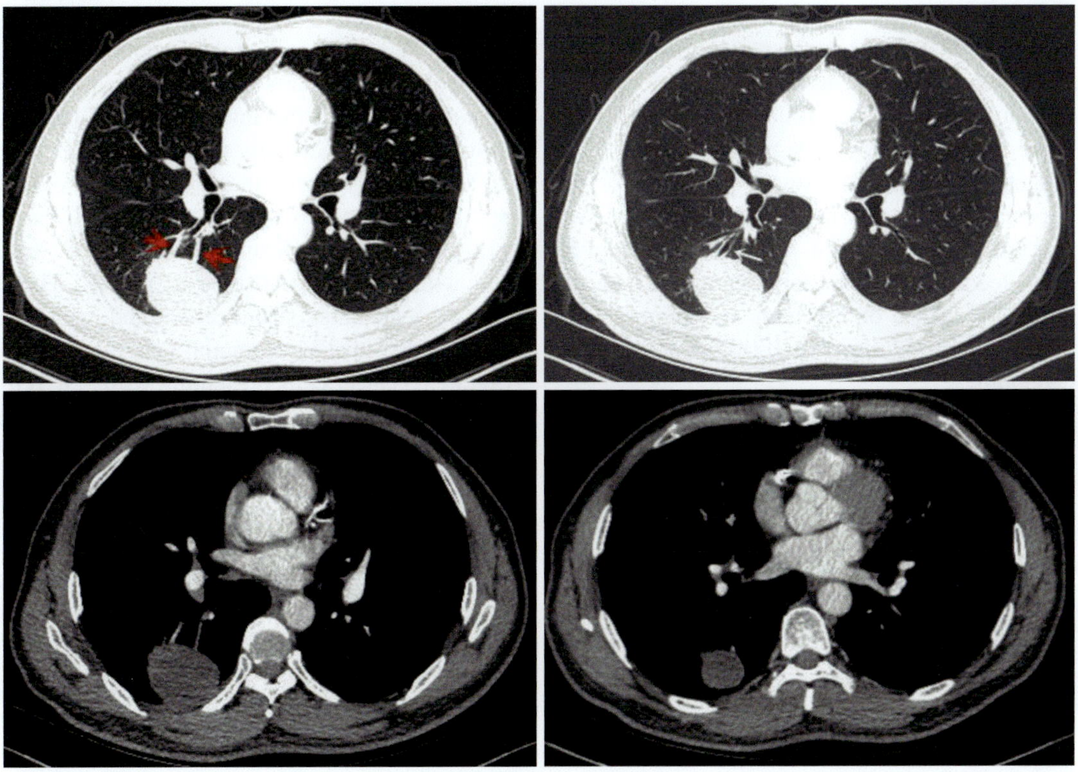

Fig. 2 Chest CT

showed neither lymphatic vessel invasion nor lymph node metastasis, had the most favorable prognosis, showed 100% 5-year survival and thought to be classified as a peripheral incipient SCC. They considered that central and peripheral types of lung SCC have different clinicopathologic characteristics and should be classified in different categories.

In 2006, Maeshima et al. [12] evaluated various clinicopathologic parameters in 101 peripheral lung SCC patients, defined as tumors located in or more peripheral to the fourth branching bronchus, with diameter 30 mm or less. Multivariate analysis showed that the size of the minimal tumor nest (MTN), a background of usual interstitial pneumonia (UIP) and lymph node metastasis were significant prognostic factors. MTN sizes were defined as large (>6 tumor cells), small (2–5 tumor cells), or single cell. Tumors with a single cell invasive component appear to be highly malignant and should be distinguished from invasive cancers with a low malignant potential (tumors with large or small tumor nest components). Saijo et al. [13] investigated differences between the properties and phenotypes of peripheral-type and central-type SCC by performing an immunohistochemical analysis. The results of the clinicopathological study showed that the patients with peripheral-type SCC were significantly older than the patients with central-type SCC and that squamous metaplasia was predominant in central-type SCC than in peripheral-type SCC. CK7 expression was more predominant in peripheral-type SCC than in central-type SCC, and CK19 expression was more predominant in central-type SCC than in peripheral-type SCC.

In 2009, Yousem [14] claimed that predominance of alveolar filling pattern was found in peripheral-type SCC and approximately one fourth of SCCs had 20% of their gross diameters composed of carcinoma cells filling airspaces with preserved alveolar architecture; on the other hand, infiltrating pattern predominated in central-type SCC.

In 2011, Watanabe et al. [15] evaluated various clinicopathological parameters in 81 patients with peripheral-type SCCs, which are defined as tumors located in or more peripheral from the third branching bronchus, measuring 30 mm or less in diameter. They found that the alveolar space-filling ratio is a significantly favorable prognostic factor for small peripheral type. Especially the focally invasive tumors with alveolar space-filling ratio of 70% or more might be classified as a microinvasive carcinoma of the peripheral SCCs of the lung and tumors with alveolar space-filling ratio 100% as noninvasive carcinoma.

In 2013, Hayashi et al. [16] first compared the immunophenotypes of central and peripheral pulmonary SCCs. There may not be biological or prognostic differences between the two except in ways of proliferation. Only the presence of emphysema, interstitial fibrosis, and entrapped pneumocytes inside the tumor showed statistic predominance in peripheral SCC. Emphysema and fibrosis may increase the risk of peripheral SCC occurrence.

In 2017, Zhang et al. [17] investigated clinicopathologic features, status of common driver mutations, and immunophenotypes of peripheral-type SCC compared to central-type SCC. They found that peripheral-type SCC shared some features with adenocarcinoma when compared to central-type SCC, including peripheral tumor location, female gender, never-smoking status, and a higher proportion of EGFR mutations.

Based on the above studies, the growth pattern of peripheral lung SCC is divided into two types: alveolar space-filling (ASF) growth and alveolar space-destructive (ASD) growth. The growth pattern of ASD type has no morphologic findings of alveolar space-filling characteristics; instead, it is characterized by stromal reactions such as inflammatory cell infiltration and fibroblast recruitment. The ASF type seemingly displays "less aggressive phenotype." In 2019, Omori et al. [18] further investigated the clinicopathological differences between cancer cells displaying ASF and ASD growth. They analyzed 155 peripheral SCC patients measuring 30 mm or less in diameter. The proportion of ASF in the total tumor area (%ASF) was determined using digital image analysis. The ASF ≤30% group showed a significantly higher ratio of lymphovascular invasion. Immunohistochemical staining revealed that the expression level of the invasive-related marker, laminin-5, in cancer cells within the ASD area was significantly higher than that within the ASF area. In addition, cases with a larger ASD area (>1.0 cm^2) had a significantly worse survival than those with a smaller ASD area (≤1.0 cm^2). These results revealed that cancer cells in the ASD area have a higher invasive potential than those in the ASF area. Cancer cells presenting with ASF represent a "less invasive phenotype" in peripheral SCC.

In 2020, Sung et al. [19] found that stages of peripheral SCCs were significantly lower than central SCCs. Cystic change of the mass, presence of interstitial fibrosis, and anthracosis in the background lung were significantly associated with the peripheral SCCs. Lower stage is a favorable factor for survival but more frequent interstitial fibrosis and older age are unfavorable factors in peripheral SCCs. Cytokeratin-7 positivity was also higher in peripheral SCCs with cutoffs of both 10% and 50%. Among the 72 evaluated cases, only one observed pathogenic mutation in EGFR and KRAS. Multivariate Cox analysis revealed that peripheral type is associated with better disease-free survival.

In summary, lung SCC may have different histological patterns and show different growth behaviors (polypoid and/or infiltrative growth in central lesions, expanding and/or alveolar space-filling in peripheral lesions), the different clinicopathological and biological features of central- and peripheral-type SCC need further investigation.

5.3 Case 3

A 60-year-old man complained of cough and expectoration for 3 months.

Chest CT: A mass in the dorsal segment of the left lower lobe (Fig. 3).

[Diagnosis] Squamous cell lung cancer.

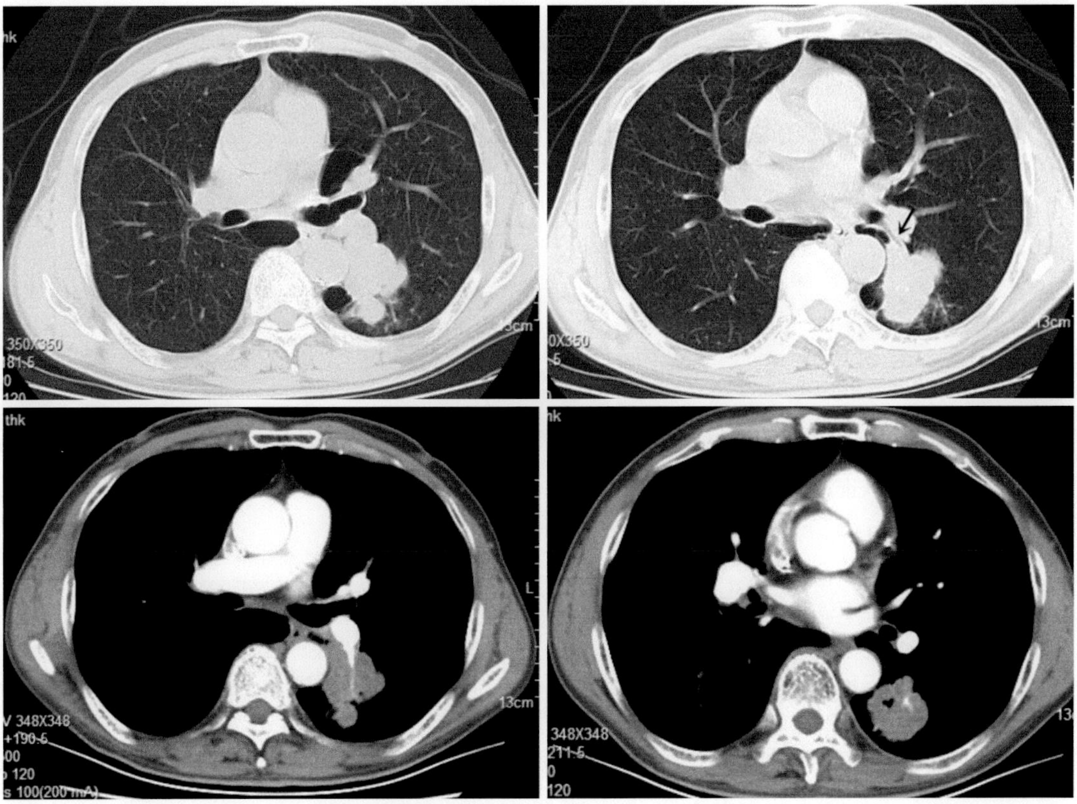

Fig. 3 Chest CT

[Diagnosis Basis] The transverse CT scan shows the tumor in the dorsal segment of the left lower lobe with deep lobulated margin, pleural retraction, eccentric cavity, and bronchial cut-off sign (black arrow), suggesting the diagnosis of lung tumor. Percutaneous pulmonary biopsy of the tumor showed squamous cell lung cancer.

[Analysis] Tsuboi et al. [20] first classified the tumor–bronchus relationship into four types: type I-bronchial lumen is patent up to the tumor mass; at the tumor-bronchus junction, the tumor tissue replaces the bronchial lining; type II-a bronchus is contained in the tumor mass; type III-a bronchus is compressed and narrowed by the tumor but the bronchial mucosa is intact; type IV-the proximal bronchial tree is so narrowed by peribronchial or submucosal spread of the tumor or by the enlarged nodes that endoscopic biopsy instruments cannot reach the lesion.

Qiang et al. [21] investigated the relationship between solitary pulmonary nodules (SPN) and bronchi and its value in predicting the nature of the SPN. They identified five types of tumor-bronchus relationships. Type I: the bronchus was obstructed abruptly by the SPN; type II: the bronchus penetrated into the SPN with tapered narrowing and interruption; type III: the bronchial lumen shown within the SPN was patent and intact; type IV: the bronchus ran around the periphery of the SPN with intact lumen; type V: the bronchus was displaced, compressed, and narrowed by the SPN. Malignant nodules were most commonly of type I (58.5%), secondly of type IV (26.4%), and rarely of type V (1.9%). Benign nodules were most often of type V (36.0%), followed by type III (20.0%), type I (16.0%), and there were no type II. Types I, II, and IV were more common in malignant nodules, whereas type V was seen more frequently in

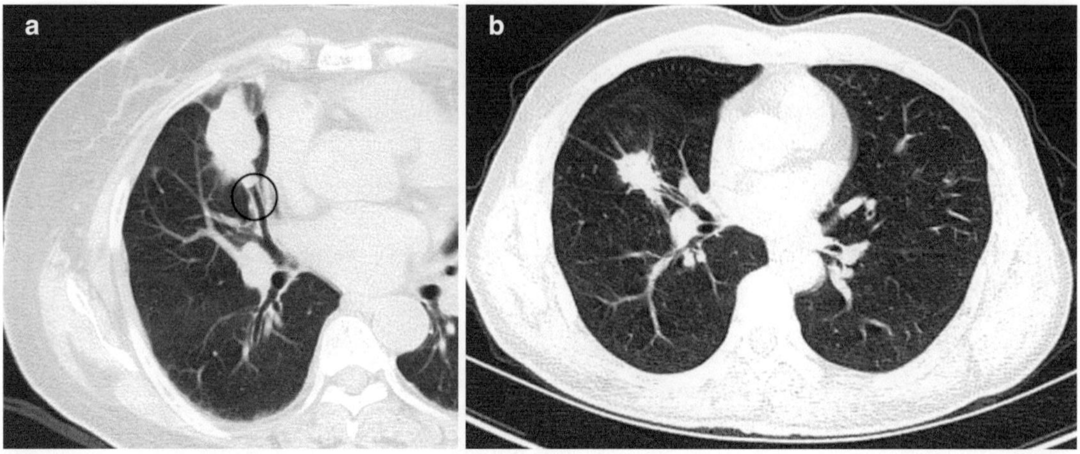

Fig. 4 (**a**) Bronchial cut-off sign is shown in a case of SCC. (**b**) Bronchial cut-off sign is shown in a case of adenocarcinoma

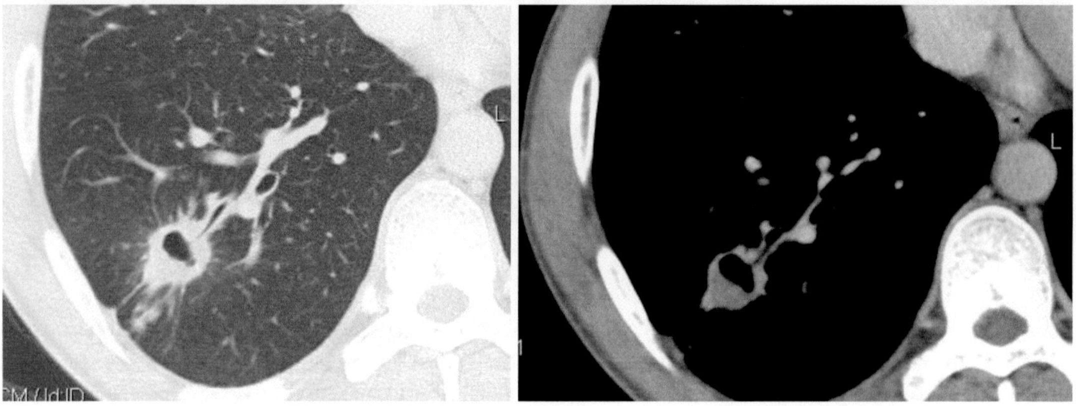

Fig. 5 Draining bronchus is shown in a a case of pulmonary tuberculosis

benign nodules. There was no statistically significant difference between the two groups regarding type III.

The bronchus cut-off sign revealed that the tumor cells invaded along the alveolar structure and peripheral bronchiole. The tumor tissue was exposed to the bronchial lumen resulting in the bronchus cut-off at the edge of the tumor. Bronchial cut-off sign on CT scans is more common in SCC cases than in adenocarcinoma cases (Fig. 4a, b). Pulmonary tuberculosis shows the draining bronchus on CT scans (Fig. 5), and most of them are no obvious bronchus cut-off sign, which can be distinguished from the tumor.

5.4 Case 4

A 60-year-old man with a history of smoking.

Chest CT: A mass in the right lower lobe (Fig. 6).

[Diagnosis] Squamous cell lung cancer.

[Diagnosis Basis] The transverse CT scan shows the tumor in the right lower lobe with lobulated margin, pleural indentation, cavity, and short burrs, suggesting the diagnosis of lung tumor. Percutaneous pulmonary biopsy of the tumor showed squamous cell lung cancer.

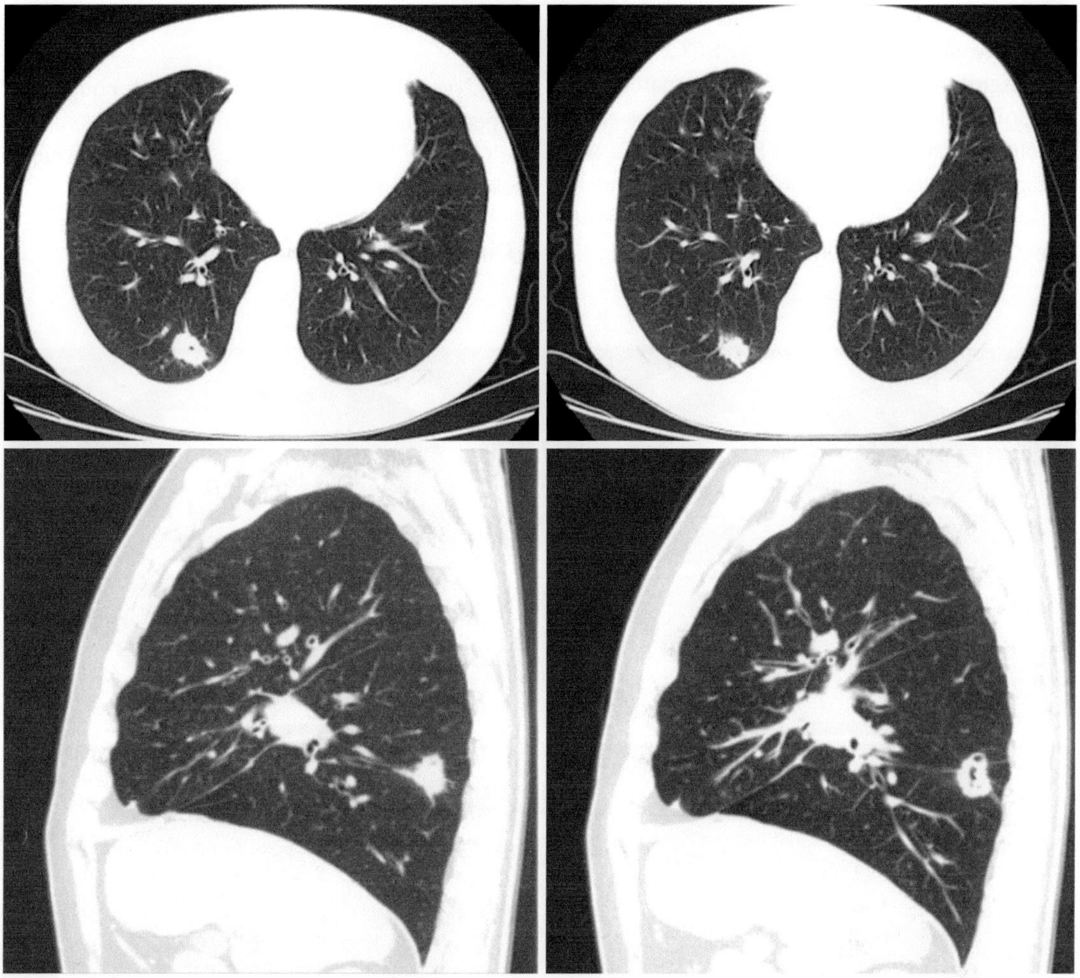

Fig. 6 Chest CT

[Analysis] The early invasiveness of peripheral lung tumor mainly includes the invasion of the peripheral structures, such as intra-alveolar invasion, interlobular septal invasion, pleural invasion, and local bronchial lumen invasion. CT signs include short burrs, lobulation sign, vacuole sign, vessel sign, pleural indentation, bronchial stiffness, traction, narrowing, and truncation.

It is clinically important to distinguish lung adenocarcinoma from SCC. CT scan is the most economical, effective, noninvasive, and quick diagnostic way for lung cancer. Yue et al. [22] retrospectively compared 275 cases (259 adenocarcinoma and 16 SCC). They found that adenocarcinomas were more likely to have deep lobulated margin, vascular bundle thickening, and pleural indentation compared with SCC. The characteristics, including tumor size, location of the tumor, bronchial cut-off sign, dilated bronchial arteries, short burrs, or spinous processes, were no significant difference. Kosaka et al. [23] identified the clinicopathological differences between patients with small-sized peripheral SCC and adenocarcinoma. The results revealed that patients with SCC exhibited higher rates of pleural invasion, vascular invasion, lymphatic invasion, and postoperative recurrence compared with adenocarcinoma patients. The incidence of pleural invasion, vascular invasion, and lymphatic invasion, and the rate of postoperative recurrence in patients with solid adenocarcinomas were similar to those with SCC, but were also significantly higher when compared with non-solid adenocarcinomas patients. The study concluded that patients with SCC and solid adenocarcinoma may not be suitable candidates for sublobar resection, despite exhibiting small tumors that are located in the peripheral lung.

5.5 Case 5

A 53-year-old man complained of cough and expectoration for half a year.

Chest CT: A mass with an irregular-shaped cavity in the right lower lobe (Fig. 7).

[Diagnosis] Squamous cell lung cancer.

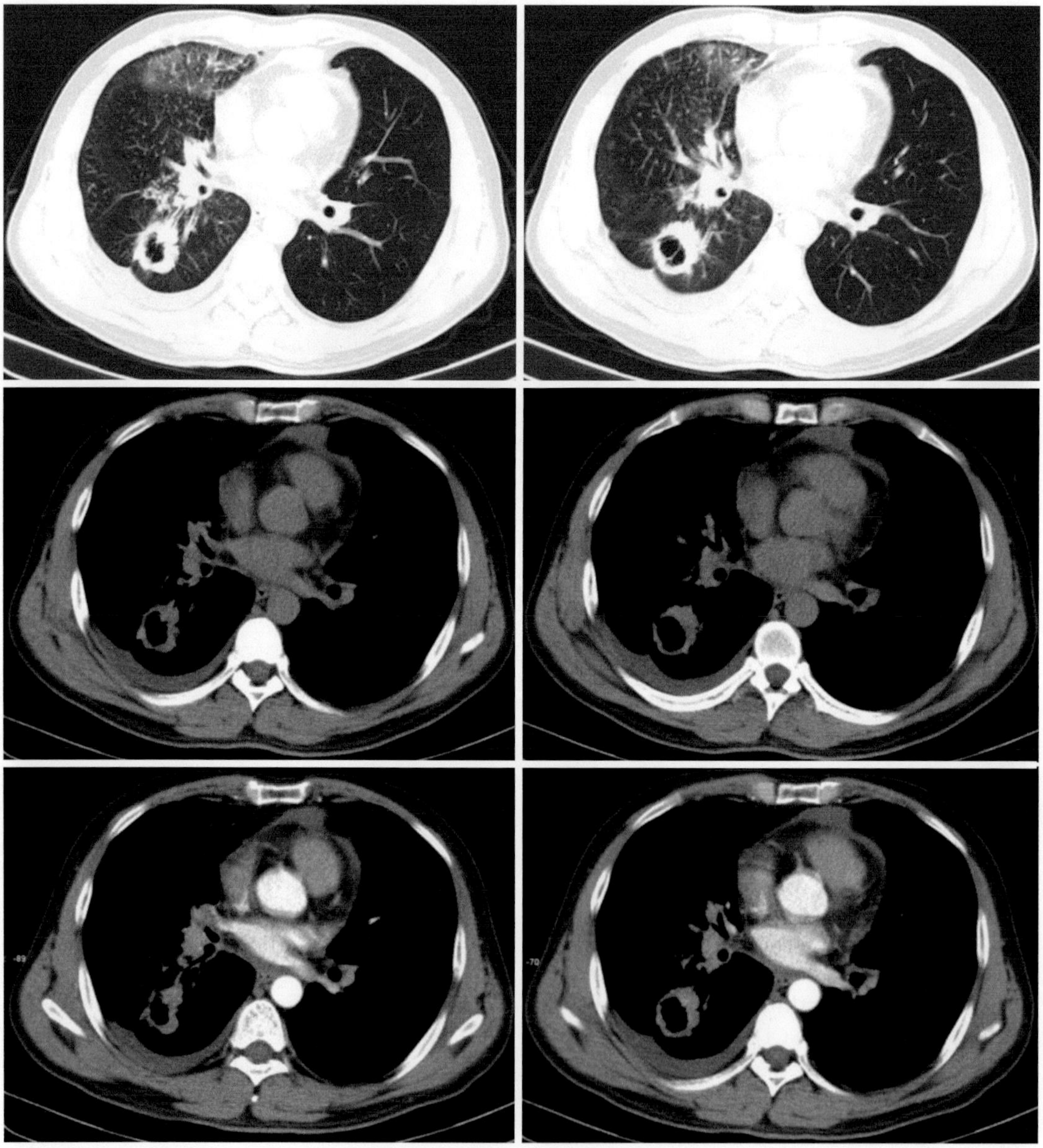

Fig. 7 Chest CT

[Diagnosis Basis] The transverse CT scan shows the tumor in the right lower lobe with lobulated margin, bronchial cut-off sign, pleural indentation, cavity with central septation, and hydrothorax, suggesting the diagnosis of lung tumor. Percutaneous pulmonary biopsy of the tumor showed squamous cell lung cancer.

[Analysis] Cavitation occurs in approximately 10%–22% of diagnosed cases of lung cancer. Cavitation is more common in SCC than in adenocarcinoma and other types of cancer. Lung cancer patients with cavitary lesions are usually attributed to worse prognosis. Cavitation in SCCs mainly consists of necrosis, which is caused by a bronchial obstruction and the vascular involvement of tumor cells leading to ischemia. Usui et al. [24] investigated the difference in the clinicopathological implications of vascular involvement between SCC. They found that the difference in cancer-free survival between vascular involvement-positive and -negative patients was statistically significant for adenocarcinoma, but it was not significant for SCC. SCC was then divided into two groups: large-vessel invasion (LVI; 1000 μm or more) and small-vessel invasion (SVI; less than 1000 μm). The LVI group showed a significantly higher incidence of cavity formation and distant metastasis. A check-valve mechanism can be another reason of cavity development in lung cancer and is observed in both adenocarcinoma and SCC.

Koenigkam et al. [25] characterized the morphological CT features of pulmonary SCC submitted to therapeutic resection. Cavitation correlated negatively with overall, disease-specific and disease-free survival, independent from age, gender, tumor pathological stage, size, and location. Compared with adenocarcinoma, peripheral SCC presented less round but more ovoid shape, more lobulated but less concave margins, more mixed predominant margins but less spiculated, less semi-solid, less homogeneous, less undetermined enhancement, more cavitation, rare internal air bronchograms, and less pleural tags. Kunihiro et al. [26] retrospectively evaluated the high-resolution CT findings of tumors with cavitation in 60 patients. They found that the cavity wall tends to be thicker in SCCs than in adenocarcinomas, and the presence of ground-glass opacity and intratumoral bronchiectasis is strongly suggestive of adenocarcinoma.

Lung cancer with solitary cavitation is a big challenge for clinicians and radiologists. Cavitation accompanied by uneven thickening of the cavity wall or wall nodules, an enhance in the wall and central solid tissue or septation indicated potential lung cancer.

5.6 Case 6

A 78-year-old man complained of cough and expectoration for a month.

Chest CT: A mass with cavitation in the right lower lobe (Fig. 8).

[Diagnosis] Squamous cell lung cancer.

[Diagnosis Basis] The transverse CT scan shows the tumor in the right lower lobe with cavitation and hydrothorax. Emphysema is observed around the tumor. Percutaneous pulmonary biopsy of the tumor showed squamous cell lung cancer.

[Analysis] Cigarette smoking is the highest risk factor for chronic obstructive pulmonary disease (COPD) and lung cancer. COPD is an independent risk factor for lung cancer. Young et al. [27] found that the prevalence of COPD in newly diagnosed lung cancer cases was six-fold greater than in matched smokers after controlling for important variables.

de Torres et al. [28] studied a cohort of 2507 COPD patients without initial clinical or radiologic evidence of lung cancer, and 215 patients with COPD developed lung cancer. The incidence is 16.7 cases per 1000 person-years. The most frequent type was SCC (44%). Lung cancer incidence was lower in patients with worse severity of airflow obstruction. Smith et al. [29] determined the relationship between emphysema on chest CT and lung cancer histology. They found that emphysema was associated

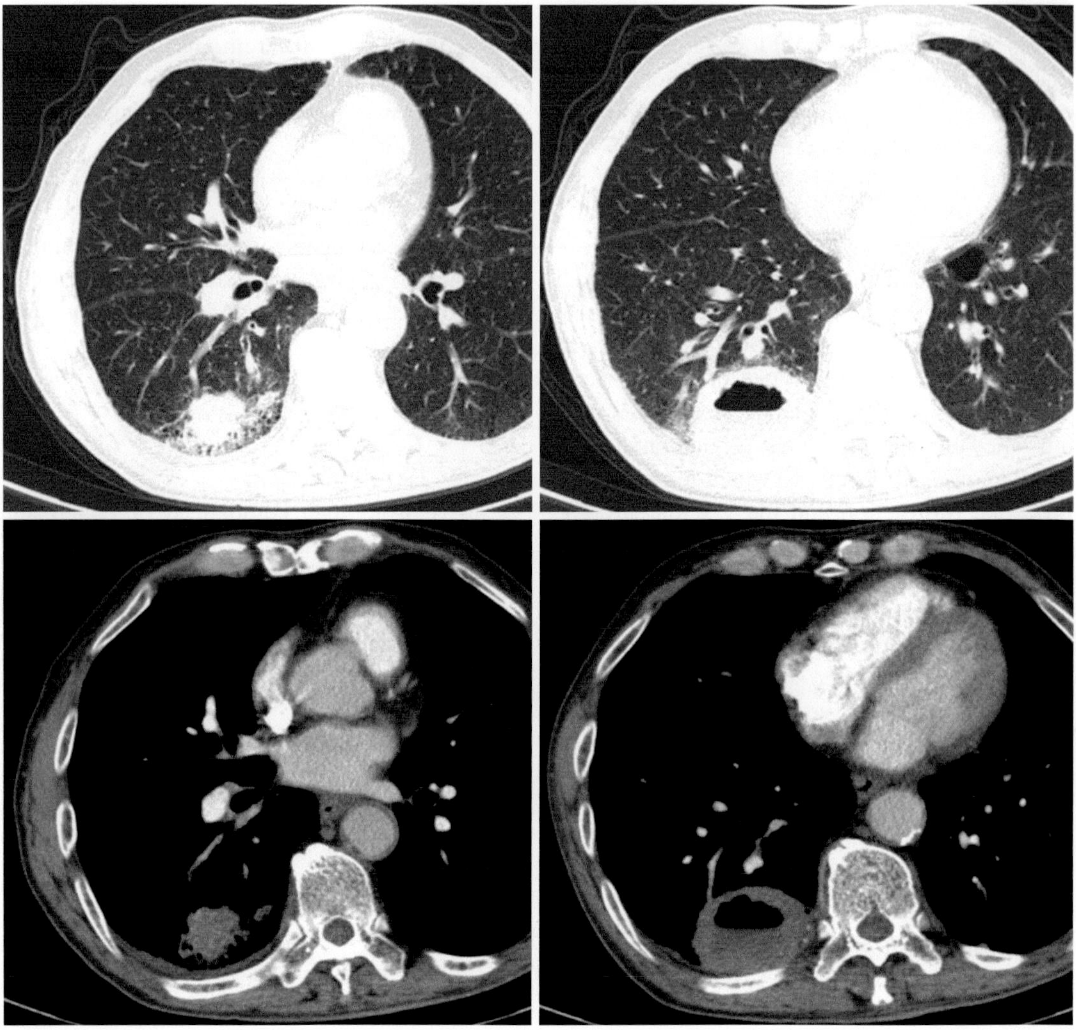

Fig. 8 Chest CT

with SCC after adjustment for age, sex, COPD and smoking history, but not other common subtypes. Shin et al. [30] further demonstrated that peripheral lung cancer from emphysema areas was associated with SCC, and adenocarcinoma was the most likely histologic subtype of peripheral lung cancers originating from areas without emphysema. Kim et al. [31] suggested that CT-emphysema score is significantly associated with poor prognosis in patients with advanced SCC.

One possible mechanism for the poor prognosis associated with emphysema in SCC involves the relationship between the tumor microenvironment and the clinicopathologic aggressiveness of the cancer. Matrix metalloproteinases (MMPs) play an important role in tumor growth and the multistep processes of invasion and metastasis. MMP can proteolytically process substrates in the extracellular milieu, and thereby promote tumor progression. The production and activation of MMPs also play an important role in the pathogenesis of emphysema. Murakami et al. [32] found that the expression of MMP-9 in intratumoral stromal cells is associated with the clinicopathologic aggressiveness of lung cancer and is predominantly found in tumors arising in emphysematous lungs.

References

1. Travis WD, Muller-Hermelink HK, Harris CC, et al. WHO classification of tumours of the lung, thymus and heart. 4th ed. Lyon, France: International Agency for Research on Cancer; 2004.
2. Barnes L, Eveson JW, Reichart P, Sidransky D. Pathology and genetics of head and neck tumours. Lyon, France: International Agency for Research on Cancer; 2005.
3. Nicholson AG, Tsao MS, Beasley MB, et al. The 2021 WHO classification of lung tumors: impact of advances since 2005. J Thorac Oncol. 2022;17:362–87.
4. Meng Q, Dong Y, Tao H, et al. ALK-rearranged squamous cell carcinoma of the lung. Thorac Cancer. 2021;12:1106–14.
5. Goss GD, Cobo M, Lu S, et al. Afatinib versus erlotinib as second-line treatment of patients with advanced squamous cell carcinoma of the lung: final analysis of the randomised phase 3 LUX-Lung 8 trial. EClinicalMedicine. 2021;37:100940.
6. Brahmer J, Reckamp KL, Baas P, et al. Nivolumab versus docetaxel in advanced squamous-cell non-small-cell lung cancer. N Engl J Med. 2015;373:123–35.
7. Paz-Ares L, Luft A, Vicente D, et al. Pembrolizumab plus chemotherapy for squamous non-small cell lung cancer. N Engl J Med. 2018;379:2040–51.
8. Glazer HS, Anderson DJ, Sagel SS. Bronchial impaction in lobar collapse: CT demonstration and pathologic correlation. AJR Am J Roentgenol. 1989;153:485–8.
9. Mintzer RA, Neiman HL, Reeder MM. Mucoid impaction of a bronchus. JAMA 1978;240:1397–8.
10. Martinez S, Heyneman LE, McAdams HP, et al. Mucoid impactions: finger-in-glove sign and other CT and radiographic features. Radiographics. 2008;28:1369–83.
11. Funai K, Yokose T, Ishii G, et al. Clinicopathologic characteristics of peripheral squamous cell carcinoma of the lung. Am J Surg Pathol. 2003;27:978–84.
12. Maeshima AM, Maeshima A, Asamura H, et al. Histologic prognostic factors for small-sized squamous cell carcinomas of the peripheral lung. Lung Cancer. 2006;52:53–8.
13. Saijo T, Ishii G, Nagai K, et al. Differences in clinicopathological and biological features between central-type and peripheral-type squamous cell carcinoma of the lung. Lung Cancer. 2006;52:37–45.
14. Yousem SA. Peripheral squamous cell carcinoma of lung: patterns of growth with particular focus on airspace filling. Hum Pathol. 2009;40:861–7.
15. Watanabe Y, Yokose T, Sakuma Y, et al. Alveolar space filling ratio as a favorable prognostic factor in small peripheral squamous cell carcinoma of the lung. Lung Cancer. 2011;732:217–21.
16. Hayashi T, Sano H, Egashira R, et al. Difference of morphology and immunophenotype between central and peripheral squamous cell carcinomas of the lung. Biomed Res Int. 2013;2013:157838.
17. Zhang Y, Zheng D, Li Y, et al. Comprehensive investigation of clinicopathologic features, oncogenic driver mutations, and immunohistochemical markers in peripheral lung squamous cell carcinoma. J Thorac Dis. 2017;9:4434–40.
18. Omori T, Aokage K, Nakamura H, et al. Growth patterns of small peripheral squamous cell carcinoma of the lung and their impacts on pathological and biological characteristics of tumor cells. J Cancer Res Clin Oncol. 2019;145:1773–83.
19. Sung YE, Cho U, Lee KY. Peripheral type squamous cell carcinoma of the lung: clinicopathologic characteristics in comparison to the central type. J Pathol Transl Med. 2020;54:290–9.
20. Tsuboi E, Ikeda S, Tajima M, et al. Transbronchial biopsy smear for diagnosis of peripheral pulmonary carcinoma. Cancer. 1967;20:687–98.
21. Qiang JW, Zhou KR, Lu G, et al. The relationship between solitary pulmonary nodules and bronchi: multislice CT-pathological correlation. Clin Radiol. 2004;59:1121–7.
22. Yue JY, Chen J, Zhou FM, et al. CT-pathologic correlation in lung adenocarcinoma and squamous cell carcinoma. Medicine (Baltimore). 2018;97:50.
23. Kosaka T, Shimizu K, Nakazawa S, et al. Clinicopathological features of small-sized peripheral squamous cell lung cancer. Mol Clin Oncol. 2020,12:69–74.
24. Usui S, Minami Y, Shiozawa T, et al. Differences in the prognostic implications of vascular invasion between lung adenocarcinoma and squamous cell carcinoma. Lung Cancer. 2013;82:407–12.
25. Koenigkam Santos M, Muley T, Warth A, et al. Morphological computed tomography features of surgically resectable pulmonary squamous cell carcinomas: impact on prognosis and comparison with adenocarcinomas. Eur J Radiol. 2014;837:1275–81.
26. Kunihiro Y, Kobayashi T, Tanaka N, et al. High-resolution CT findings of primary lung cancer with cavitation: a comparison between adenocarcinoma and squamous cell carcinoma. Clin Radiol. 2016;7111:1126–31.
27. Young RP, Hopkins RJ, Christmas T, et al. COPD prevalence is increased in lung cancer, independent of age, sex and smoking history. Eur Respir J. 2009;34:380–6.
28. de Torres JP, Marín JM, Casanova C, et al. Lung cancer in patients with chronic obstructive pulmonary

disease- incidence and predicting factors. Am J Respir Crit Care Med. 2011;184:913–9.
29. Smith BM, Schwartzman K, Kovacina B, et al. Lung cancer histologies associated with emphysema on computed tomography. Lung Cancer. 2012;761:61–6.
30. Shin B, Shin S, Chung MJ, et al. Different histological subtypes of peripheral lung cancer based on emphysema distribution in patients with both airflow limitation and CT-determined emphysema. Lung Cancer. 2017;104:106–10.
31. Kim YS, Kim EY, Ahn HK, et al. Prognostic significance of CT-emphysema score in patients with advanced squamous cell lung cancer. J Thorac Dis. 2016;88:1966–73.
32. Murakami J, Ueda K, Sano F, et al. Pulmonary emphysema and tumor microenvironment in primary lung cancer. J Surg Res. 2016;200:690–7.

Small Cell Lung Carcinoma

Song Zhang

Small cell lung carcinoma (SCLC) represents approximately 13% of newly diagnosed lung cancers and is the most common primary pulmonary neuroendocrine tumor derived from bronchial epithelial cells. SCLC is characterized by a rapid doubling time, high growth fraction (the ratio of proliferating cells to total cells), and a propensity for early development of widespread metastases (most commonly to the brain, liver, or bone), resulting in a 95% mortality rate. Approximately 60%–70% of patients have metastatic disease at initial diagnosis.

1 Etiology

Cigarette smoking (heavy smoking) is responsible for approximately 95% cases of SCLC. Women who begin smoking at an early age are more susceptible to SCLC. Over the past few decades, the incidence in women is increasing, and the male-to-female incidence ratio is now 1:1, even though the overall incidence and mortality of SCLC have declined. The decline in smoking rates (especially white men), the replacement of low-tar filtered and "light" cigarettes, and changes in the pathological criteria of SCLC are reasonable explanation for this trend. SCLC patients should strongly advocate smoking cessation.

Other risk factors for the incidence of SCLC include exposures to radon, arsenic, halogenated ethers, chromium, asbestos, polyaromatic hydrocarbons, and vinyl chloride.

2 Classification

SCLC was first described in 1879 and classified as a lymphosarcoma. In the 1981 WHO classification [1], SCLC was subdivided into 3 categories, including oat cell, intermediate cell, and combined cell types. In 1988, the International Association for the Study of Lung Cancer (IASLC) groups classified SCLC into pure small cell, non-pure small cell /large cell, and combined small cell types [2]. In the 1999 WHO classification, WHO/IASLC retained the combined small cell type and deleted non-pure small cell / large cell type, SCLC included pure and combined subsets.

Combined small cell lung carcinoma (C-SCLC) is defined as SCLC combined with any elements of NSCLC and represents approximately 30% of cases of SCLC. The NSCLC component is typically composed of adenocarcinoma, squamous cell carcinoma (SCC), large cell carcinoma (LCC), large cell neuroendocrine carcinoma (LCNEC), or less commonly sarco-

S. Zhang (✉)
Department of Respiratory and Critical Care Medicine, Shandong Provincial Hospital Affiliated to Shandong First Medical University,
Jinan, Shandong, China

S. Zhang (ed.), *Diagnostic Imaging of Lung Cancers*, https://doi.org/10.1007/978-981-99-6815-2_3

matoid or giant cell carcinoma. C-SCLC is diagnosed irrespective of cell amounts when SCLC combined with adenocarcinoma, SCC or sarcomatoid carcinoma, but at least 10% LCC (or LCNEC) is required for the diagnosis of C-SCLC. Furthermore, more than two components can also be observed.

3 Pathology

The pathological changes of SCLC are characterized by small blue cells with scant cytoplasm, ill-defined cell borders, finely granular nuclear chromatin, and absent or inconspicuous nucleoli. Cell size is usually set at <3 small resting lymphocytes. SCLC cells are round, oval, or spindle-shaped with high mitotic counts and extensive necrosis. The high nuclear-to cytoplasmic ratio and paucity of nucleoli in SCLC are the most useful characteristics for distinguishing SCLC from LCNEC.

Immunohistochemistry (IHC) is helpful to establish the diagnosis of SCLC. Nearly all SCLCs are positive for cytokeratin, epithelial membrane antigen, and thyroid transcription factor-1 (TTF-1) and negative for Napsin A. Cytokeratin staining is necessary for small cell neoplasm to distinguish SCLC from lymphoid tumor (namely small lymphocytic lymphoma), especially when the sample derives from a mediastinal mass. Markers of neuroendocrine differentiation, including chromogranin A, neuron-specific enolase (NSE), neural cell adhesion molecule (NCAM; CD56), and synaptophysin, are also positive in most SCLCs cases. Synaptophysin and chromogranin A are the first-choice markers, rather than CD56 (which is highly sensitive but poorly specific) and NSE (which is of limited specificity in cytological and histological samples). However, neuroendocrine markers alone cannot be used to distinguish SCLC from NSCLC, because approximately 10% of NSCLCs will be positive for at least 1 of these markers and fewer than 10% of SCLCs are negative for all neuroendocrine markers. The Ki-67 proliferation index ranges from 50% to 100% for SCLC and can be used to differentiate SCLC from carcinoid tumors, especially in small biopsy samples with crushed or necrotic tumor cells in which counting mitotic figures is difficult.

Common genetic lesions in SCLC include simultaneous pathognomonic inactivation of the tumor suppressor genes TP53 and RB1, MYC family copy number gain, and inactivating mutations in epigenetic readers and writers as well as NOTCH family members. The retinoblastoma protein (pRB), together with p16, and cyclin D1 are major components of the RB pathway, which controls the G1 checkpoint of the cell cycle. Biallelic inactivation of RB1 gene results in uncontrolled proliferation in aggressive solid tumors. Yuan et al. [3] applied immunohistochemical techniques to study the expression of pRB, p16, and cyclin D1 in 161 samples of primary SCLC and 20 samples of NSCLC. pRB and cyclin D1 staining was negative in 161 specimens of SCLC, and p16 expression was observed in 153 samples. Compared with SCLC, 16 out of 20 NSCLC cases exhibited pRB expression and 15 showed cyclin D1 expression, but only very weak p16 staining was found in 5 samples. These observations could provide additional criteria for distinguishing between SCLC and NSCLC. Biallelic TP53 and RB1 gene inactivation is consistently associated with SCLC, resulting in pRB loss and p53 overexpression in almost all SCLC.IHC staining with specific monoclonal antibodies can easily assess pRB and p53.

4 Clinical Features

The most common symptoms due to local primary tumor growth include cough, chest pain, hemoptysis, and dyspnea. Symptoms such as weight loss, fatigue, and anorexia are often present due to systemic disease.

Patients with primary tumor invasion or regional lymphatic metastases may present with specific symptoms. For instance, 10% of patients related to superior vena cava syndrome due to local invasion into mediastinum or lymphadenopathy in right paratracheal region. Invasion of the esophagus, left vocal cord paralysis, and phrenic nerve can result in dysphagia, hoarseness, and hemidiaphragm elevation, respectively. Extrathoracic (hematogenous) metastases can manifest as bone pain, jaundice, pruritus, seizures, changes in mental status, and/or ataxia. Bone, liver, the central nervous system, lymph node, adrenal glands, subcutaneous tissue, and pleura are common sites of metastasis.

5 Paraneoplastic Syndromes

Many paraneoplastic neurologic and endocrine syndromes are very commonly associated with SCLC.

Neurologic paraneoplastic syndromes, including Lambert-Eaton myasthenic syndrome, encephalomyelitis, and sensory neuropathy, are thought to occur through autoimmune mechanisms when antibodies bind to both the SCLC and the central nervous system. Patients with Lambert-Eaton syndrome present with weakness of proximal muscles of the lower and upper extremities with relative sparing of respiratory and bulbar muscles caused by antibodies directed against the voltage-gated calcium channels. Electromyography is used for definitive diagnosis. Paraneoplastic encephalomyelitis and sensory neuropathy are caused by the production of anti-Hu antibodies (anti-Hu) and anti-Purkinje cell antibodies (cerebellar degeneration) that cross-reacts with both SCLC antigens and human neuronal RNA-binding proteins, resulting in multiple neurologic deficits. Neurologic paraneoplastic syndromes are usually progressive and are independent of the cancer and outcomes of cancer therapy. Rare neurologic disorders seen in SCLC include cerebellar degeneration, retinal blindness, opsoclonus, and stiff person syndrome.

SCLC cells sometimes produce polypeptide hormones, including vasopressin and adrenocorticotropic hormone, which cause hyponatremia of malignancy and Cushing syndrome, respectively. The paraneoplastic endocrine syndromes related to peptide production by the tumor usually abate with effective treatment of cancer.

6 Staging

SCLC is usually categorized as either limited-stage SCLC (LS-SCLC) or extensive-stage SCLC (ES-SCLC) by the Veterans Administration Lung Cancer Study Group (VALSG) staging system in 1957.The system classified patients based on whether all known tumors can be treated within a single radiation port or not. LS-SCLC was defined as tumor that is confined to one hemithorax (with or without local extension) with no distant extrathoracic metastatic diseases. Regional and ipsilateral supraclavicular lymph nodes were classified as LS-SCLC if they could be included in a single safe and adequate radiation port. ES-SCLC was defined as tumor that cannot be classified as limited, including malignant pleural or pericardial effusions, contralateral hilar or supraclavicular lymph nodes, and hematogenous metastases [4]. In 1989, the International Association of Lung Cancer (IASLC) modified the VALSG staging system, contralateral mediastinal or supraclavicular lymph nodes and ipsilateral pleural effusions independent of cytological findings were classified under LS-SCLC. Only patients with distant metastasis were considered as ES-SCLC. Micke et al. [5] retrospectively analyzed 109 SCLC patients and found that the IASLC staging criteria for SCLC patients have a higher prognostic impact than the VALSG system.

The IASLC has recommended that the current seventh edition of the American Joint Committee on Cancer (AJCC) tumor-node-metastasis (TNM) staging system for lung cancer replaces the VALSG system for the staging of SCLC. In this system, stage I-III is equivalent to LS-SCLC and stage IV is equivalent to ES-SCLC.

In SCLC patients, except for rare limited-stage diseases that can be treated surgically, the purpose of staging is to determine whether treatment is with chemotherapy and radiation for limited-stage diseases or with chemotherapy alone for extensive-stage diseases.

7 Radiographic Features

Most of SCLCs arise from main stem or lobar bronchus, the tumor tends to grow in the bronchial submucosa and subsequently metastasizes to the hilar and mediastinal lymph nodes. The most common CT feature of SCLC is a large mass located within the central region of the chest (Fig. 1) or a mass with hilar or mediastinal lymphadenopathy (Fig. 2). Contrast-enhanced CT scan may reveal the extent of mediastinal invasion, including the trachea, esophagus (Fig. 3), heart, and vessels (Fig. 4). Centrally tumor can also result in atelectasis of either a lobe or the entire lung (Fig. 5).

Peripheral SCLCs typically manifest as a well-defined nodule or mass with little spiculated sign, pleural indentation, and internal necrosis. Most peripheral SCLC is round or ovoid, some are irregular or vermiform shape (Fig. 6).

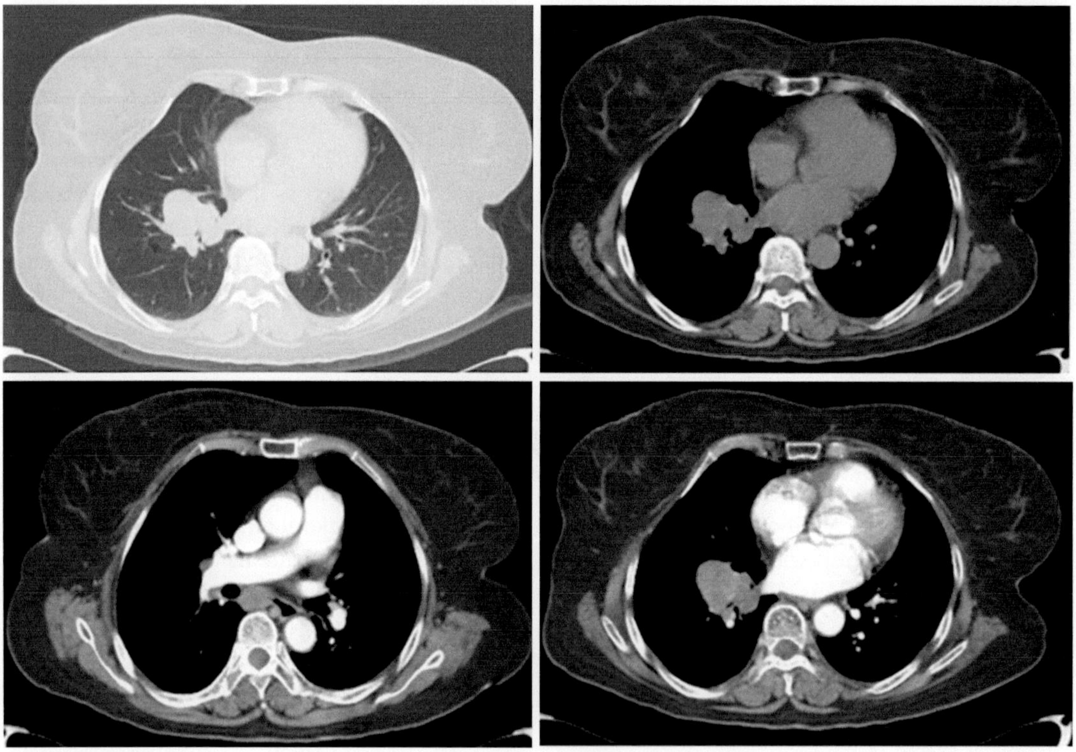

Fig. 1 SCLC in a 67-year-old woman. Contrast-enhanced CT scan shows a large soft-tissue mass in the right perihilar lung

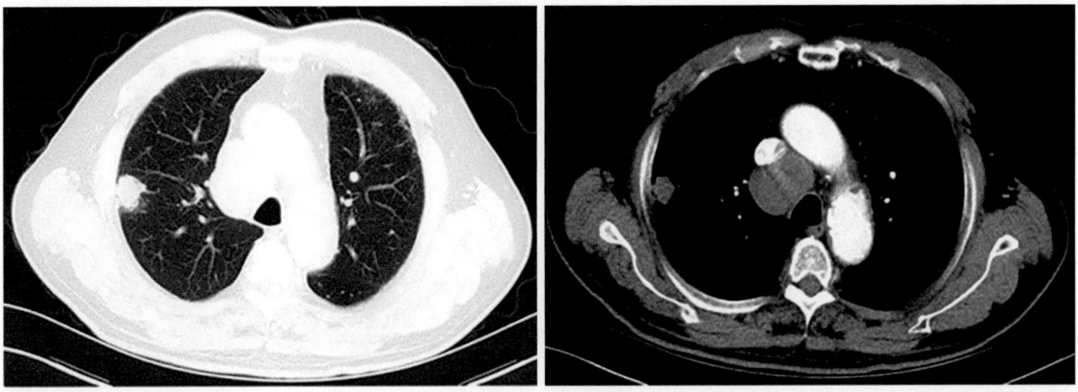

Fig. 2 SCLC in a 65-year-old man. Contrast-enhanced CT scan shows a lesion in the right upper lobe with mediastinal lymphadenopathy

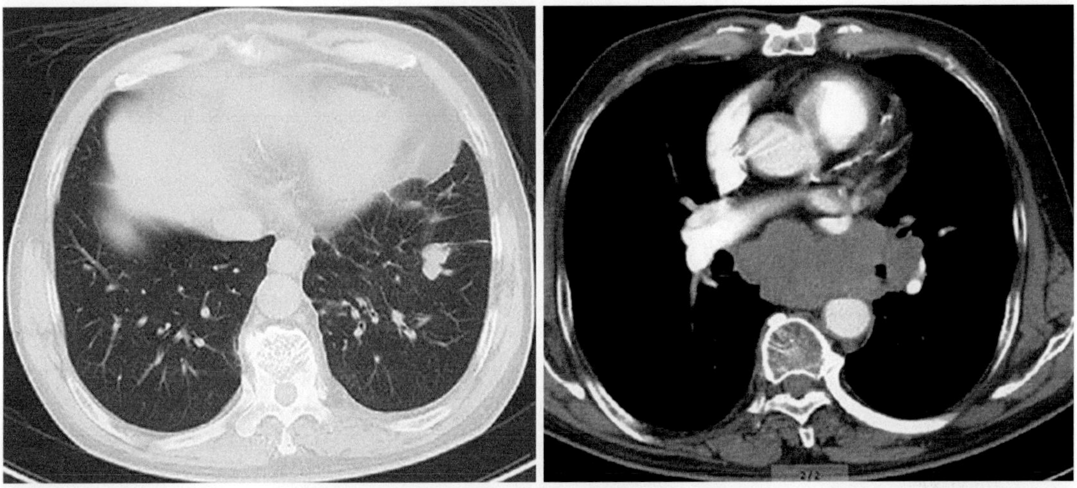

Fig. 3 A 73-year-old man complained of dysphagia for 1 week. Contrast-enhanced CT scan shows a mass in the left lower lobe with middle to posterior mediastinal lymphadenopathy, invading the heart and esophagus

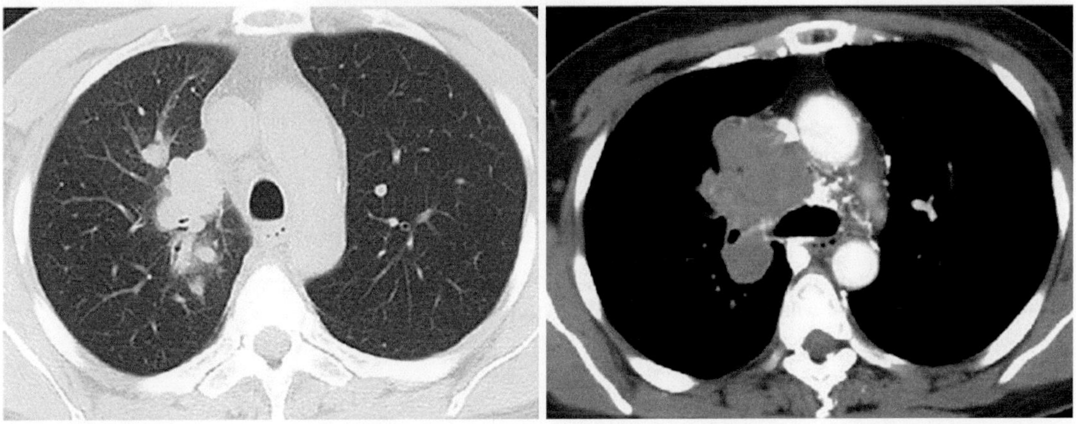

Fig. 4 A 43-year-old woman complained of facial edema for 3 months. Contrast-enhanced CT scan shows a large soft-tissue mass in the mediastinum, invading and obliterating the superior vena cava

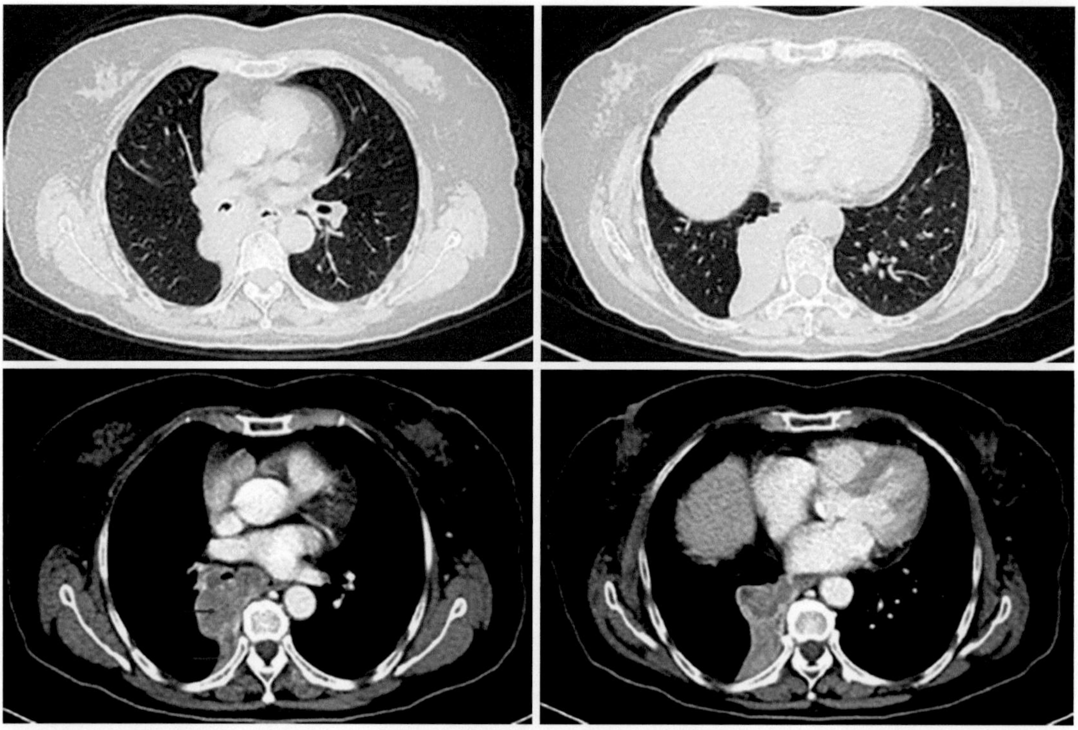

Fig. 5 SCLC in a 64-year-old woman. Contrast-enhanced CT scan shows a primary tumor in the posterior mediastinum (red arrow), resulting in atelectasis of the right lower lobe (blue arrow)

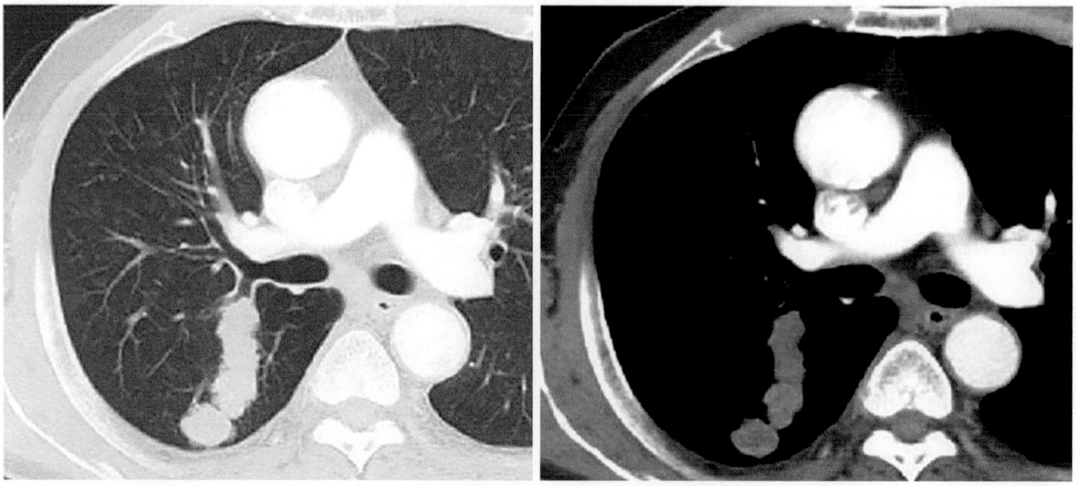

Fig. 6 SCLC in a 64-year-old man. Contrast-enhanced CT scan shows a well-defined, vermiform soft-tissue density mass in the right lower lobe with mediastinal lymphadenopathy

8 Treatment

At present, surgery is not a major treatment for most patients with SCLC. Primary surgical resection with adjuvant chemotherapy is considered only in patients with stage I (T1-2 N0) SCLC. Chemotherapy is an essential component of treatment for all SCLC patients. Radiotherapy has a potential role in all patients with SCLC, as part of either definitive or palliative therapy. More than 50% of patients with SCLC occur intracranial metastases. Prophylactic craniocerebral irradiation (PCI) is effective in decreasing the incidence of brain metastasis.

The standard treatment for LS-SCLC is 4–6 cycles of chemotherapy with cisplatin (or carboplatin) and etoposide, thoracic radiotherapy initiated early with the first cycle of chemotherapy. Prophylactic craniocerebral irradiation (PCI) is recommended in the subset of patients with good response to initial treatment. Approximately 25% of LS-SCLC can be cured by chemoradiotherapy.

Current first-line treatment for ES-SCLC is platinum-based doublet chemotherapy with either cisplatin or carboplatin in combination with etoposide. Patients who achieve a good response to initial treatment and a good performance status are considered for PCI and/or thoracic radiotherapy. Even though first-line standard therapy has good initial response rate of 60%–80%, the prognosis is poor because of relapse shortly after treatment, with overall survival of 10–12 months.

The only approved second-line therapy for patients with recurrent SCLC is topotecan, with response rates of 6%–12% in chemorefractory disease and 15%–37% in chemosensitive disease. Chemorefractory disease and chemosensitive disease defined as relapse within 3 months or beyond 3 months, respectively. Other chemotherapeutic agents for the second-line and beyond including paclitaxel, docetaxel, irinotecan, gemcitabine, temozolomide, vinorelbine, and bendamustine.

Over the past two decades, there were no advancements in the treatment of SCLC. Unlike NSCLC, the targeted therapy for SCLC has not yet been determined. Immune checkpoint pathways, involving the cytotoxic T-lymphocyte-associated protein 4 (CTLA-4) and programmed cell death protein-1 (PD-1) receptors and their ligands, inhibit the T-cell immune response and represent important biomarkers in different tumor types, used for prognostic and therapeutic purposes. Immune checkpoint inhibitors have shown promise in the treatment of ES-SCLC.

The IMpower133 trial [6] found that combining atezolizumab to chemotherapy in the first-line treatment of ES-SCLC led to significantly longer overall survival and progression-free survival than chemotherapy alone (mOS 12.3 months vs.10.3 months, mPFS 5.2 months vs. 4.3 months).This trial is a landmark achievement because it is the first significant improvement in the systemic treatment of untreated SCLC since the advent of platinum-containing combinations in the 1980s.The CASPIAN trial assessed durvalumab, with or without tremelimumab, in combination with etoposide plus either cisplatin or carboplatin (platinum-etoposide) in treatment-naive patients with ES-SCLC [6]. The median overall survival was 13.0 months in the durvalumab plus platinum-etoposide group versus 10.3 months in the platinum-etoposide group, with 34% versus 25% of patients alive at 18 months. The result suggested that first-line durvalumab plus platinum-etoposide significantly improved overall survival in patients with ES-SCLC compared with a clinically relevant control group [7]. The CheckMate 032 trial is a phase 1/2, multicenter, open-label study of nivolumab(anti-PD1) ± ipilimumab(anti-CTLA-4) in SCLC or other advanced/metastatic solid tumors previously treated with one or more platinum-based chemotherapies. Ready et al. [8] reported results of third- or later-line nivolumab monotherapy treatment in SCLC. The objective response rate was 11.9% with a median duration of response of 17.9 months. At 6 months, 17.2% of patients were progression-free. The 12-month and 18-month overall survival rates were 28.3% and 20.0%, respectively. These results confirmed that nivolumab monotherapy is an effective third- or later-line treatment for this patient population. Cope et al. [9] found that nivolumab ± ipilimumab had a more durable tumor response and more favorable long-term survival compared with chemotherapies (topotecan via intravenous and amrubicin) for recurrent SCLC. Goodman et al. [10] defined tumor mutational burden (TMB) as the total number of somatic missense mutations, and patients were divided into tertiles: low, 0 to <143 mutations; medium, 143 to 247 mutations; and high, ≥248 mutations. Hellmann et al. [11] used whole exome sequencing to evaluate the impact of TMB on efficacy of nivolumab ± ipilimumab in patients with SCLC from the nonrandomized or randomized cohorts of CheckMate 032. The study showed that TMB could serve as a predictive biomarker in SCLC. Nivolumab plus ipilimumab appeared to provide a greater clinical benefit than nivolumab monotherapy in the high tumor mutational burden tertile. These differences were most striking in the combination group. The 1-year survival of the highest TMB tertile was 62.4%, while the middle and lowest tertile were 19.6% and 23.4%, respectively. The KEYNOTE-028 study [12] and phase II KEYNOTE-158 study [13] showed that pembrolizumab showed durable antitumor activity in a subset of patients with recurrent or metastatic SCLC who had undergone two or more previous lines of therapy, regardless of PD-L1 expression. In summary, PD-1 inhibitors (durvalumab, pembrolizumab, nivolumab) and PD-L1 inhibitor (atezolizumab) are approved for use in recurrent or metastatic SCLC.

Approximately 3%–10% of EGFR-mutant NSCLCs undergo transformation to SCLC. Marcoux et al. [14] retrospectively studied patients with EGFR-mutant SCLC. EGFR mutations included exon 19 deletion (69%), L858R (25%), and other (6%). All patients received one or more EGFR tyrosine kinase inhibitor before SCLC transformation. Median time to transformation was 17.8 months. Median overall survival since diagnosis was 31.5 months, whereas median survival since the time of SCLC transformation was 10.9 months. Fifty-nine patients had tissue genotyping at first evidence of SCLC. All maintained their founder EGFR mutation, and 15 of 19 with previous EGFR T790M positivity were T790 wild-type at transformation. Other recurrent mutations included Rb1, TP53, and PIK3CA. Responses to platinum-etoposide and taxanes are frequent, but checkpoint inhibitors yielded no responses. CNS metastases were frequent after transformation. The optimal strategies for this group need to better elucidate.

Recent transcriptional data revealed intertumoral heterogeneity of SCLC. Rudin et al. [15] proposed a working nomenclature for SCLC subtypes defined by relative expression of four factors: ASCL1 (achaete-scute homologue 1; also known as ASH1), NEUROD1 (neurogenic differentiation factor 1), POU2F3 (POU class 2 homeobox 3), and YAP1 (yes-associated protein 1). Baine et al. [16] analyzed the expression of ASCL1, NEUROD1, POU2F3, and YAP1 by immunohistochemistry in 174 patient samples with SCLC. They found that ASCL1 was expressed in 69% of cases, followed by 17% NEUROD1. POU2F3 was detected in 7% of SCLC and was mutually exclusive of ASCL1 and NEUROD1. YAP1 was expressed at low levels, mainly in combined SCLC, and was not exclusive of other subtypes. Both ASCL1-dominant and NEUROD1-dominant subtypes were associated with neuroendocrine marker high/TTF-1 high/DLL3 high profile, whereas POU2F3 and other ASCL1/NEUROD1 double-negative tumors were neuroendocrine marker low/TTF-1 low/DLL3 low. They confirmed that ASCL1/NEUROD1 double-negative tumors represent a distinct neuroendocrine-low subtype of SCLC, which is either uniquely associated with POU2F3 or lacks a known dominant regulator. Owonikoko et al. [17] found that the SCLC-YAP1 subtype was associated with high expression of interferon-γ response genes, and HLA and T-cell receptor genes and enrichment in long-term survivors. Some studies found that the YAP1 subtype is not a separate group but overlaps with the other three. Gay et al. [18] identified four subtypes of SCLC defined largely by differential expression of transcription factors ASCL1 (SCLC-A), NEUROD1 (SCLC-N), and POU2F3 (SCLC-P) or low expression of ASCL1, NEUROD1, and POU2F3 ("triple negative"

SCLC) with a marked "inflamed" gene signature (SCLC-I). SCLC-I exhibits the greatest benefit from the addition of immunotherapy to chemotherapy, while the other subtypes each have distinct vulnerabilities. Due to SCLC-I representing a highly platinum-resistant subtype, cisplatin treatment of SCLC-A patient-derived xenografts induces intratumoral shifts toward SCLC-I, supporting subtype switching as a mechanism of acquired platinum resistance.

9 Case Analysis

9.1 Case 1

A 54-year-old man complained of cough and expectoration for 2 months.

Chest CT: A mass in the left lower lobe with hilar and mediastinal lymphadenopathy (Fig. 7).

[Diagnosis] Small cell lung carcinoma.

[Diagnosis Basis] The transverse CT scan shows a left lower lobe mass with ipsilateral mediastinal conglomerate mass, encasing the left main bronchus (blue arrow) and invading the left main pulmonary arteries (red arrow), suggesting the diagnosis of SCLC. Bronchoscope biopsy specimen showed small cell lung carcinoma.

[Analysis] CT features of SCLC have been reported in a few studies. In 1999, Hashimoto et al. [19] retrospectively reviewed CT findings of 38 patients with pathologically proven SCLC.23 cases (61%) were central type and 15 cases (39%) were peripheral type. The most typical sign of SCLC is a bulky central mass that represents metastasis to the hilar and/or mediastinal lymph nodes (22 central tumors, 5 peripheral tumors). In 2006, Kazawa et al. [20] classified the spread patterns of SCLC into 8 different type by the CT imaging: central perihilar type, central + mediastinal extension type, peripheral type,

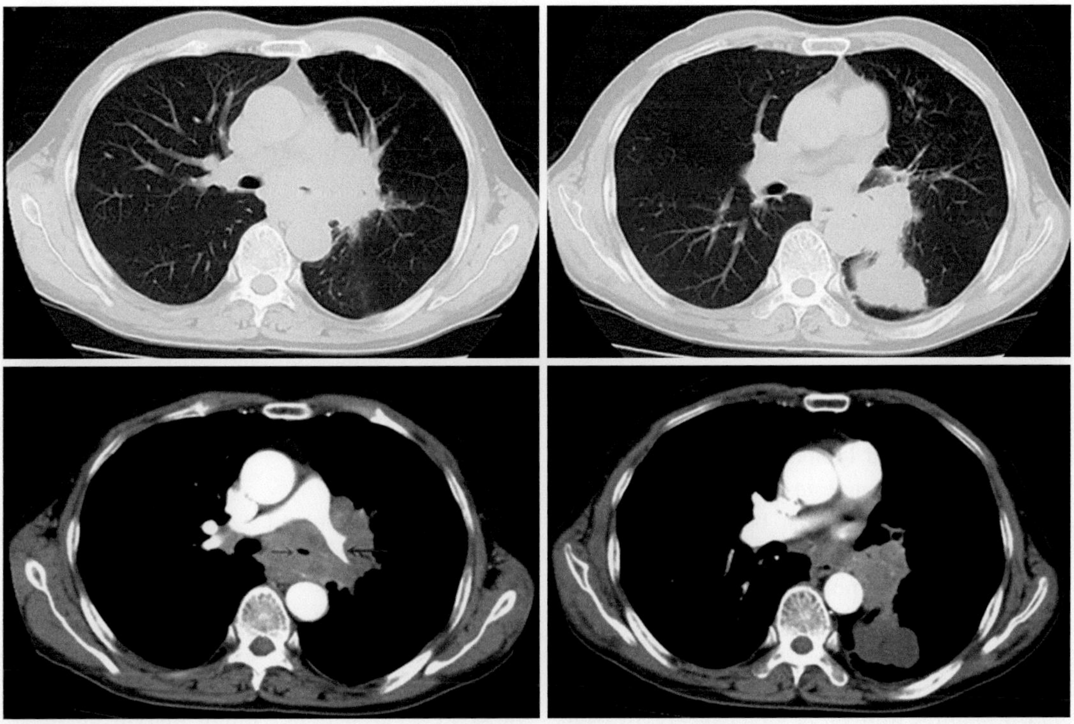

Fig. 7 Chest CT

peripheral + mediastinal extension type, lymphangitic spread type, pleural dissemination type, lobar replacement type, and air-space consolidation type. The most common manifestation was central mass + mediastinal extension type (29.4%), followed by central perihilar mass (17.6%), peripheral mass + mediastinal extension (20.6%), and peripheral mass (10.3%). Peribronchial extension and great vessel wall involvement, such as main pulmonary artery, superior vena cava, and peri−/intra-cardial extension, were commonly observed in advanced stage. In 2016, Lee et al. [21] retrospectively reviewed in 142 patients with pathologically proven SCLC. The recognizable CT features of SCLC were a hilar mass with mediastinal conglomerate mass. Most of the hilar masses showed 2 or more bronchial stenoses/obstructions. Vascular invasion and concomitant parenchymal findings were observed commonly. Most cases of peripheral SCLC manifested as a lobulated mass rather than a spiculated mass.

CT features of SCLC are useful for early diagnosis in order to predict SCLC and manage patients.

9.2 Case 2

A 73-year-old man complained of cough, expectoration, and haemoptysis for 1 month.

Chest CT: A mass in the left lower lobe (Fig. 8).

[Diagnosis] Small cell lung carcinoma.

[Diagnosis Basis] The transverse CT scan shows a well-defined, vermiform soft-tissue density mass with hilar lymphadenopathy in the left lower lung, elongated in the direction of the course of broncho-vascular bundles, suggesting the diagnosis of SCLC. Percutaneous lung biopsy specimen of the tumor showed small cell lung carcinoma.

[Analysis] Peripheral SCLC often shows different CT features from other lung cancers. In 1999, Yabuuchi et al. [22] investigated 12 patients with surgically resected and histologically proven peripheral SCLC. They concluded that a homogenous mass without necrosis is the most characteristic feature of peripheral SCLC on CT and mostly tumors have well-defined margins and lobulation. In 2007, Sone et al. [23] noted that irregularly shaped nodular lesions (vermiform, pine-cone-like, or tandem-like nodular lesions) with a branching pattern and a lobular margin are more frequently than a rounded mass with notched margin in peripheral SCLC on CT. Such appearance may be caused by tumor growth along the long axis of the bronchial wall in the lung periphery. In 2015, Kobayashi et al. [24] retrospectively reviewed the HRCT findings of 33 patients with peripheral SCLC measuring 30 mm or less. Vermiform/branching and polygonal shape were observed in 33.3% and 21.2% of cases, respectively. The vermiform/branching shape is more frequently observed in non-stage I than in stage I tumors. The vermiform/branching shape may correspond to tumor extension along the bronchial wall, suggesting the presence of relatively advanced disease, including hilar and mediastinal lymph node metastasis.

In summary, when peripheral SCLC grows along the bronchial/blood vessel wall, it is oppressed by the surrounding tissues and grows unbalanced, which may be the reason why peripheral SCLC may be multinodular or vermiform shape.

9.3 Case 3

A 60-year-old man complained of bloody sputum for 5 months.

Chest CT: A mass in the left upper lobe (Fig. 9).

[Diagnosis] Combined small cell lung carcinoma.

[Diagnosis Basis] The transverse CT scan shows a well-defined, spindle left upper lobe soft-tissue density mass, suggesting the diagnosis of SCLC. The patient's tumor marker levels are normal. Percutaneous lung biopsy specimen of

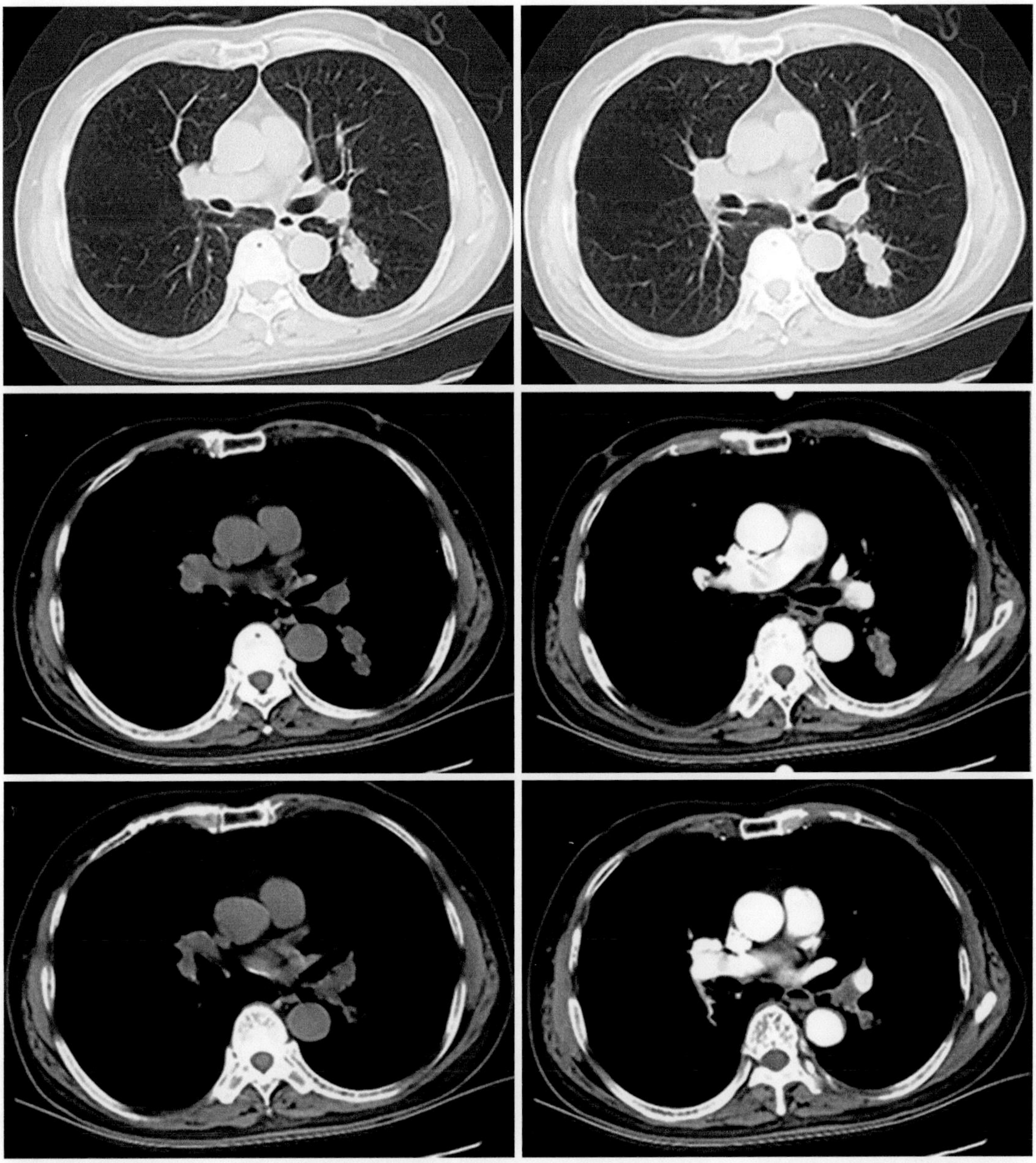

Fig. 8 Chest CT

the tumor showed combined small cell lung carcinoma (SCLC combined with adenocarcinoma, C-SCLC). The patient received 2 cycles of chemotherapy, and the lesion was significantly reduced (Fig. 10).

[Analysis] Some studies have shown that the subcomponents of C-SCLC originate from a common precursor tumor cell or a collision of multiple primaries growing at a same site. C-SCLC has similar clinical features compared with pure SCLC. Most C-SCLC patients are male and approximately 70% C-SCLC patients have a history of smoking. Men et al. [25] investigated the clinical features and prognostic factors of C-SCLC. They found that smoking, advanced

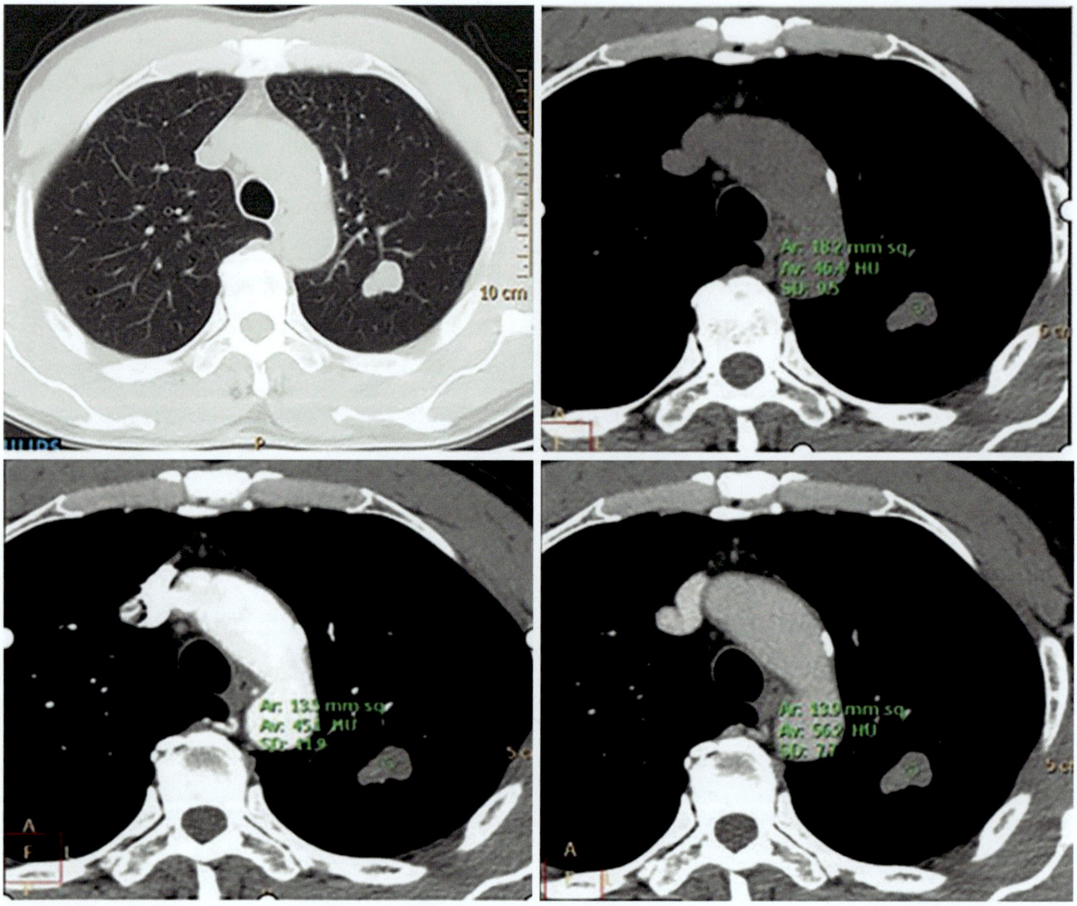

Fig. 9 Chest CT

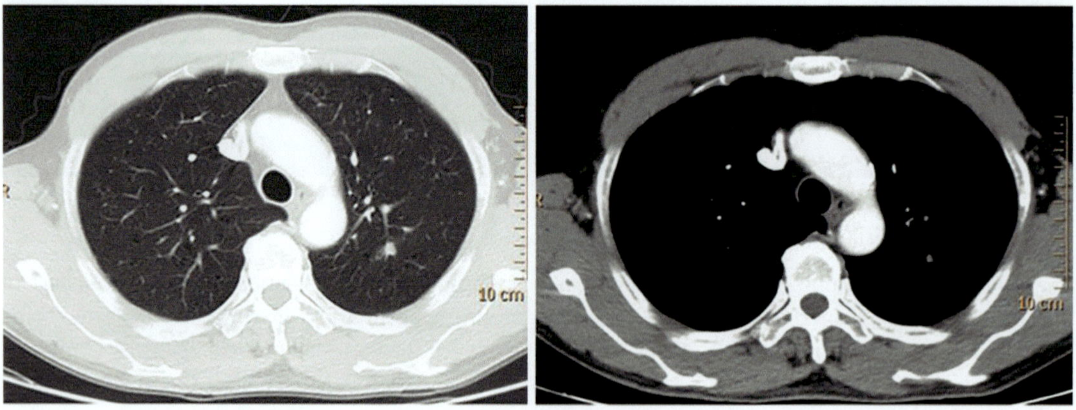

Fig. 10 The lesion was significantly reduced after 2 cycles of chemotherapy

TNM stage, positive resection margin, and positive lymph nodes ratio >10% are poor prognostic factors.

C-SCLC shows decreased responsiveness to chemotherapy because of the NSCLC component. Babakoohi et al. [26] analyzed 1628 consecutive cases of lung cancer (1200 NSCLC, 428 SCLC) and identified 22 patients with C-SCLC. They found that C-SCLC patients carry a better prognosis than those with pure SCLC and are more likely to undergo surgery. Men et al. [25] also suggested that C-SCLC has a relatively early stage and good prognosis, which may be due to the underestimated diagnosis in non-surgical patients. While a study by Zhao et al. [27] showed that the median survival times of patients with pure SCLC and C-SCLC were 58 months and 26 months, respectively. They suggested that C-SCLC was associated with decreased overall survival compared with pure SCLC. These studies showed that C-SCLC is in a relatively early stage at diagnosis and may benefit from surgery.

References

1. The World Health Organization histological typing of lung tumours. 2nd ed. Am J Clin Pathol 1982, 77:123–36
2. Hirsch FR, Matthews MJ, Aisner S, et al. Histopathologic classification of small cell lung cancer. Changing concepts and terminology. Cancer. 1988;62:973–7.
3. Yuan J, Knorr J, Altmannsberger M, et al. Expression of p16 and lack of pRB in primary small cell lung cancer. J Pathol. 1999;189:358–62.
4. Stahel RA, Ginsberg R, Havemann K, et al. Staging and prognostic factors in small cell lung cancer: a consensus report. Lung Cancer. 1989;5:119–26.
5. Micke P, Faldum A, Metz T, et al. Staging small cell lung cancer: veterans administration lung study group versus International Association for the Study of Lung Cancer–what limits limited disease? Lung Cancer. 2002;37:271–6.
6. Horn L, Mansfield AS, Szczęsna A, et al. First-line atezolizumab plus chemotherapy in extensive-stage small-cell lung cancer. N Engl J Med. 2018;379:2220–9.
7. Paz-Ares L, Dvorkin M, Chen Y, Reinmuth N, et al. Durvalumab plus platinum-etoposide versus platinum-etoposide in first-line treatment of extensive-stage small-cell lung cancer (CASPIAN): a randomised, controlled, open-label, phase 3 trial. Lancet. 2019;394:1929–39.
8. Ready N, Farago AF, de Braud F, et al. Third-line Nivolumab monotherapy in recurrent SCLC: CheckMate 032. J Thorac Oncol. 2019;14:237–44.
9. Cope S, Keeping ST, Goldgrub R, et al. Indirect comparison of nivolumab ± ipilimumab (CheckMate 032) versus other treatments for recurrent small-cell lung cancer. J Comp Eff Res. 2019;8:733–51.
10. Goodman AM, Kato S, Bazhenova L, et al. Tumor mutational burden as an independent predictor of response to immunotherapy in diverse cancers. Mol Cancer Ther. 2017;16:2598–608.
11. Hellmann MD, Callahan MK, Awad MM, et al. Tumor mutational burden and efficacy of nivolumab monotherapy and in combination with ipilimumab in small-cell lung cancer. Cancer Cell. 2018;33:853–61. e4.
12. Ott PA, Elez E, Hiret S, et al. Pembrolizumab in patients with extensive-stage small-cell lung cancer: results from the phase Ib KEYNOTE-028 study. J Clin Oncol. 2017;35:3823–9.
13. Chung HC, Piha-Paul SA, Lopez-Martin J, et al. Pembrolizumab after two or more lines of prior therapy in patients with advanced small-cell lung cancer (SCLC): results from the KEYNOTE-028 and KEYNOTE-158 studies. J Thorac Oncol. 2019;15:618–27.
14. Marcoux N, Gettinger SN, O'Kane G, et al. EGFR-mutant adenocarcinomas that transform to small-cell lung cancer and other neuroendocrine carcinomas: clinical outcomes. J Clin Oncol. 2019;37:278–85.
15. Rudin CM, Poirier JT, Byers LA, et al. Molecular subtypes of small cell lung cancer: a synthesis of human and mouse model data. Nat Rev Cancer. 2019;19:289–97.
16. Baine MK, Hsieh MS, Lai WV, et al. SCLC subtypes defined by ASCL1, NEUROD1, POU2F3, and YAP1: a comprehensive Immunohistochemical and histopathologic characterization. J Thorac Oncol. 2020;15:1823–35.
17. Owonikoko TK, Dwivedi B, Chen Z, et al. YAP1 expression in SCLC defines a distinct subtype with T-cell-inflamed phenotype. J Thorac Oncol. 2021;16:464–76.
18. Gay CM, Stewart CA, Park EM, et al. Patterns of transcription factor programs and immune pathway activation define four major subtypes of SCLC with distinct therapeutic vulnerabilities. Cancer Cell. 2021;39:346–60.e7.
19. Hashimoto M, Heianna J, Okane K, et al. Small cell carcinoma of the lung: CT findings of parenchymal lesions. Radiat Med. 1999;17:417–21.
20. Kazawa N, Kitaichi M, Hiraoka M, et al. Small cell lung carcinoma: eight types of extension and spread on computed tomography. J Comput Assist Tomogr. 2006;30:653–61.
21. Lee D, Rho JY, Kang S, et al. CT findings of small cell lung carcinoma: can recognizable features be found? Medicine(Baltimore). 2016;95:e5426.

22. Yabuuchi H, Murayama S, Sakai S, et al. Resected peripheral small cell carcinoma of the lung: computed tomographic-histologic correlation. J Thorac Imag. 1999;14:105–8.
23. Sone S, Nakayama T, Honda T, et al. CT findings of early-stage small cell lung cancer in a low-dose CT screening programme. Lung Cancer. 2007;56:207–15.
24. Kobayashi T, Tanaka N, Matsumoto T, et al. HRCT findings of small cell lung cancer measuring 30 mm or less located in the peripheral lung. Jpn J Radiol. 2015;33:67–75.
25. Men Y, Hui Z, Liang J, et al. Further understanding of an uncommon disease of combined small cell lung cancer: clinical features and prognostic factors of 114 cases. Chin J Cancer Res. 2016;28:486–94.
26. Babakoohi S, Fu P, Yang M, et al. Combined SCLC clinical and pathologic characteristics. Clin Lung Cancer. 2013;14:113–9.
27. Zhao X, McCutcheon JN, Kallakury B, et al. Combined small cell carcinoma of the lung: is it a single entity? J Thorac Oncol. 2018;13:237–45.

Large Cell Neuroendocrine Carcinoma

Song Zhang

Large cell neuroendocrine carcinoma (LCNEC) is a relatively rare subset of lung cancers, accounting for 15% of neuroendocrine tumors and approximately 3% of primary lung cancers. The current WHO classification defines LCNEC as NSCLC with neuroendocrine morphology and the expression of neuroendocrine markers. LCNEC is often associated with male sex, older age (median age is 65 years), and exposure to tobacco smoke.

1 Classification

In 1991, LCNEC was first described by Travis et al. [1] as poorly differentiated high-grade neoplasms, which are morphologically distinct from SCLC, and retain demonstrable neuroendocrine differentiation by immunohistochemistry or electron microscopy. In 1999 and 2004 WHO classification, LCNEC was classified as a variant of large cell carcinoma (LCC), a subtype of NSCLC. In the 2015 WHO classification of tumors of the lung, for the first time, neuroendocrine tumors were categorized in one category, including typical carcinoid tumor, atypical carcinoid tumor, LCNEC, and SCLC. In the 2021 WHO classification, lung neuroendocrine neoplasms were categorized as neuroendocrine tumors including low-grade typical carcinoid and intermediate-grade atypical carcinoid, and high-grade neuroendocrine carcinomas including LCNEC and SCLC.

LCNEC can contain components of adenocarcinoma, squamous cell carcinoma, giant cell carcinoma, or spindle cell carcinoma, which is called combined LCNEC. Adenocarcinoma is the most common histological type found in combination with LCNEC.LCNEC may also be combined with SCLC and is classified under the term "combined SCLC and LCNEC." Pulmonary combined tumors generally occur in the setting of high-grade carcinomas and not in carcinoids, which differs from digestive and pancreatic neuroendocrine neoplasms, where all of tumors can contain an exocrine glandular component, termed "mixed neuroendocrine/non-neuroendocrine neoplasm" (MiNEN).

2 Pathology

According to the 2015 WHO classification [2], the diagnostic criteria of LCNEC were large cell size, typically necrosis, low nuclear/cytoplasm ratio, presence of neuroendocrine morphology (palisading, organoid nesting, trabeculae, and/or rosettes), high mitotic rate, defined as >10 mitoses/2 mm^2 and immunohistochemical expression

S. Zhang (✉)
Department of Respiratory and Critical Care Medicine, Shandong Provincial Hospital Affiliated to Shandong First Medical University, Jinan, Shandong, China

S. Zhang (ed.), *Diagnostic Imaging of Lung Cancers*, https://doi.org/10.1007/978-981-99-6815-2_4

of at least one neuroendocrine marker such as chromogranin A, synaptophysin, CD56/NCAM (neural cell adhesion molecule). TTF-1 is present in approximately half of LCNEC cases, and Napsin A is infrequently present. The Ki-67 labeling index was used as an indicator of high-grade malignancy.

The difference between LCNEC and SCLC is based on distinctive non-small cell cytomorphological features, including the presence of prominent nucleoli and/or vesicular chromatin and/or abundant cytoplasm.

3 Molecular Subtypes

LCNEC has unique gene profile and transcription profile. The common molecular alterations in LCNEC included TP53 (64–92%), RB1 (19–42%), STK11 (17–33%), KEAP1 (19–31%), PIK3CA (3–7%), and KRAS (4–24%).

Rekhtman et al. [3] segregated LCNEC into 2 major and 1 minor subsets: SCLC-like, characterized by TP53 + RB1 co-mutation/loss and other SCLC-type alterations, including MYCL amplification; NSCLC-like, characterized by the lack of co-altered TP53 + RB1 and nearly universal occurrence of NSCLC-type mutations (KRAS, STK11, and KEAP1); and carcinoid-like, characterized by MEN1 mutations and low mutation burden. SCLC-like and NSCLC-like subsets revealed several clinicopathologic differences, including higher proliferative activity in SCLC-like tumors and exclusive adenocarcinoma-type differentiation marker expression in NSCLC-like tumors. Although exhibiting predominant similarity with lung adenocarcinoma, NSCLC-like LCNEC harbored several distinctive genomic alterations, including more frequent mutations in NOTCH family genes (28%), which may be key regulators of neuroendocrine differentiation. They suggested that LCNEC is a biologically heterogeneous group of tumors, comprising distinct subsets with genomic signatures of SCLC, NSCLC (predominantly adenocarcinoma), and rarely, highly proliferative carcinoids.

George et al. [4] categorized LCNEC genomic subtypes as type I (NSCLC type) with TP53 and STK11/KEAP1 alterations and type II (SCLC type) with TP53 and RB1 alterations. Despite the same genomic changes as adenocarcinomas and squamous cell carcinomas, no transcriptional relationship was found, whereas LCNECs formed distinct transcriptional subgroups with closest similarity to SCLC. Although type I LCNECs and SCLCs exhibit a neuroendocrine profile with ASCL1 high/DLL3 high/NOTCH low, type II LCNECs have TP53 and RB1 alterations and differ from most SCLC tumors with reduced neuroendocrine markers, a pattern of ASCL1 low/DLL3 low/NOTCH high, and an upregulation of immune-related pathways. They concluded that LCNECs comprise two molecularly defined subgroups, and distinguishing them from SCLC may allow stratified targeted treatment of high-grade neuroendocrine lung tumors.

4 Treatment

Currently, there are no standard treatment guidelines for LCNEC. An operable tumor surgery is advocated for early stage tumors. Some reports indicated that adjuvant chemotherapy may have a beneficial effect on survival. Filosso et al. [5] collected retrospectively 400 patients with LCNEC operated on in 14 thoracic surgery institutions worldwide between 1992 and 2014. They observed weak evidence of a higher overall survival in patients receiving adjuvant chemotherapy. Kujtan et al. [6] evaluated the impact of systemic chemotherapy on patients with stage I LCNEC who have undergone surgical resection. They found that survival was improved in patients who received chemotherapy in both stage IA and stage IB LCNEC. Ramanet al [7]. reported that LCNEC patients who underwent an operation generally experienced worse survival by stage than that of adenocarcinoma patients but experienced improved survival compared with SCLC patients. Medically fit patients with both early and locally advanced LCNEC should be offered surgery, with guideline-concordant induction or adjuvant therapy.

For advanced disease, as LCNEC exhibits clinicopathologic features of both NSCLC and SCLC, the optimal chemotherapy treatment for LCNEC remains unclear. Because of the clinical similarity of LCNEC to SCC, American Society of Clinical Oncology Clinical Practice Guideline Update Committee believes a platinum plus etoposide or the same treatment as other patients with nonsquamous carcinoma may be administered (type: informal consensus; evidence quality: low; strength of recommendation: weak). However, the National Comprehensive Cancer Network (NCCN) groups LCNEC into the same treatment guidelines as those used for NSCLC.

Molecular LCNEC subtypes potentially have a different response to chemotherapy regimens, with SCLC-like subtype more favorable toward etoposide and NSCLC-like toward gemcitabine/taxanes. Derks et al. [8] found that patients with LCNEC tumors that carry a wild-type RB1 gene or express the RB1 protein do better with NSCLC-GEM/TAX (platinum + gemcitabine or taxanes) treatment than with SCLC-PE (platinum-etoposide) chemotherapy. However, no difference was observed for RB1 mutated or with lost protein expression. Zhuo et al. [9] reported that the overall survival of patients with SCLC-like LCNEC is shorter than that of patients with NSCLC like LCNEC despite higher response rate (RR) to chemotherapy. Furthermore, compared with pemetrexed-platinum and gemcitabine/taxane-platinum doublets, treatment with etoposide-platinum was associated with superior response and survival in SCLC-like LCNEC, while treatment with gemcitabine/taxane-platinum led to a shorter survival compared with etoposide-platinum or pemetrexed-platinum in NSCLC-like LCNEC patients.

The role of radiotherapy in the treatment of local or advanced pulmonary LCNEC is still unclear, but the administration of radiotherapy according to NSCLC guidelines in LCNEC patients appears reasonable. Limonnik et al. [10] compared outcomes in patients receiving chemotherapy and chemoradiotherapy (CRT). They found that definitive CRT was an independent predictor of increased overall survival in patients with locally advanced LCNEC of the lung. May et al. [11] reported that radiotherapy was associated with improved survival for non-surgical patients in stage I and II disease, but not for those who underwent surgery. For patients with stage III disease, radiotherapy was associated with improved survival in surgical and non-surgical patients.

Immunotherapy in LCNEC has been assessed in clinical studies. Some studies report that NSCLC-like LCNEC can be expected to respond to a DLL3 inhibitor, and SCLC-like LCNEC can be expected to respond to immunotherapy.

5 Prognosis

LCNEC is one of the most aggressive lung cancers, characterized by widely disseminated metastases and a poor prognosis. Previous studies reported the overall survival (OS) rate of 5 years was 15%–57%. Kinslow et al. [12] revealed that median survival time from diagnosis is 9.7 months and 54.6% of patients have stage IV LCNEC at the time of diagnosis. Stage I-III LCNEC behaves similarly to NSCLC, whereas stage IV is more akin to SCLC. Lowczak et al. [13] reported that patients treated with negative resection margin, with lower clinical stage, without lymph node metastasis, and with size of primary tumor $\leq$4 cm showed significantly better OS and progression-free survival (PFS). The main risk factors with an adverse effect on survival were advanced clinical stage and positive resection margin.

6 Case Analysis

A 61-year-old man with a 100-pack year smoking history who presented cough and expectoration for 2 months.

Chest CT: A mass in the left lung (Fig. 1).

[Diagnosis] Large cell neuroendocrine carcinoma.

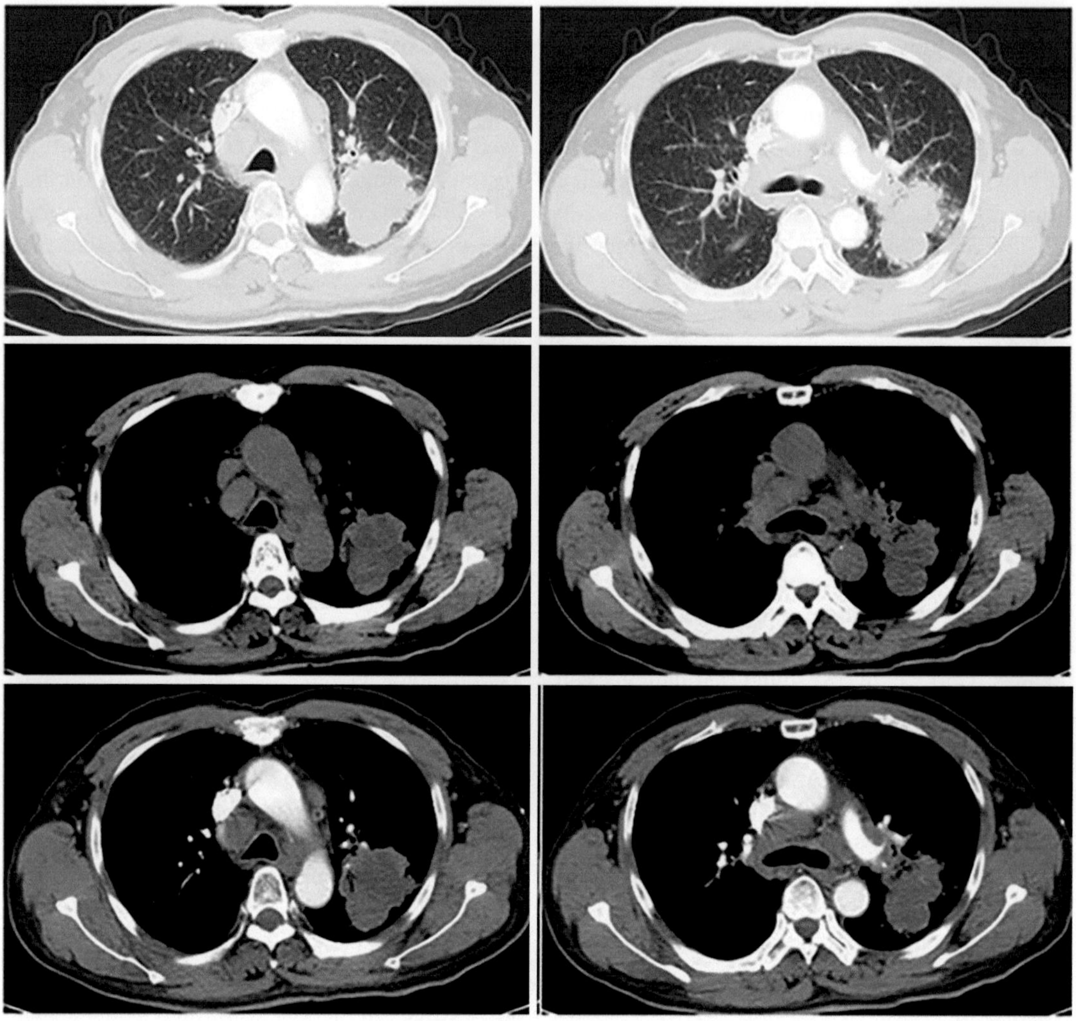

Fig. 1 Chest CT

[Diagnosis Basis] The tumor is located peripherally, exhibits a lobulated and well-defined margin, no burr, cavitation, pleural indentation sign, and vascular cluster sign, which does not support the diagnosis of lung adenocarcinoma. Pulmonary sarcoma is rarely associated with lymph node metastasis, and more likely to be associated with pleural metastasis. In this case, the mediastinal lymph nodes are significantly enlarged, which does not support the diagnosis of pulmonary sarcoma. The lesions are large, and the mediastinal lymph nodes have no obvious fusion trend, which does not meet the characteristics of small cell lung cancer. Elderly man with long-term smoking history, obvious necrosis in the lesion, and visible calcification (red arrow), need to consider the possibility of squamous cell carcinoma and large cell neuroendocrine carcinoma. Necrosis can be observed in the lesion, but there is no obvious cavitation, which is more in line with the diagnosis of large cell neuroendocrine carcinoma. The pathology of percutaneous lung biopsy revealed that the cancer cells were loosely arranged, round, oval, and fusiform, with consistent size and obvious atypia (Fig. 2). Immunohistochemistry confirmed a neuroendo-

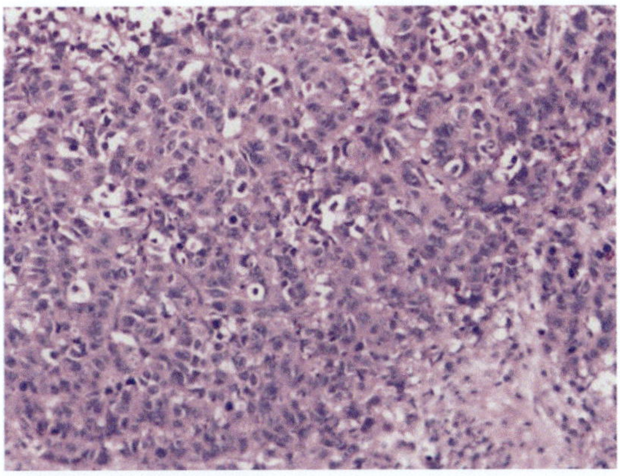

Fig. 2 The morphologic features of LCNEC

crine origin with positive CD56, synaptophysin, chromogranin A, and TTF-1 markers consistent with LCNEC.

[Analysis] This patient had a significant smoking history and presented with nonspecific symptoms of most lung tumors. Paraneoplastic syndromes are less common in patients with LCNEC.

Unlike SCLC, LCNEC is more commonly located peripherally (64%) and less likely to have hilar/mediastinal lymphadenopathy. Some studies revealed that peripheral lesion is lobulated nodule or mass with clear boundaries and short burrs, which are similar to those of peripheral SCLC and poorly differentiated adenocarcinoma. The mean SUVmax is consistent with malignant tumors. Cavitation (0%–3%), calcification (6.5%–21%), and air-bronchogram (7%–9.7%) are the rare CT findings of LCNEC. Cavitation and necrosis may be due to high mitotic rate and angioinvasion. Nevertheless, no special imaging feature could be used to distinguish LCNEC from other lung tumors. Lee et al. [14] evaluated whether CT and FDG PET findings can help predict the clinical outcome. They reported that female gender, a larger tumor diameter, no lobulated margin, and higher SUVmax were poor prognostic factors.

Immunohistochemistry of the patient's lung tissue is positive for CD56, synaptophysin, and chromogranin A, which indicates neuroendocrine origin. TTF-1 is also positive, which confirms primary lung origin. Minami et al. [15] found that small-sized (≤30 mm) LCNEC positive for three neuroendocrine markers (chromogranin A, synaptophysin, and CD56) had a poor prognosis and high rate of lymph node metastasis. There were some similarities in clinicopathological features between small-sized triple-positive LCNEC and small-sized SCLC. They believed that the findings may provide new insights into treatment strategies for LCNEC, such as surgical indication and adjuvant chemotherapy.

It is difficult to diagnosis LCNEC by puncture biopsy or frozen pathology, and a definite diagnosis relies on postoperative paraffin-embedded pathological sections with immunohistochemical staining. Currently, there is no entirely sensitive and specific immunohistochemistry marker to distinguish LCNEC from SCLC. Napsin A is one of the potential useful markers. Rekhtman et al. [16] found that Napsin A was expressed in 15% of LCNEC, whereas all carcinoids and SCLC were consistently negative. Thus, weak Napsin A labeling could serve as a helpful clue for the diagnosis of LCNEC.

References

1. Travis WD, Linnoila RI, Tsokos MG, et al. Neuroendocrine tumors of the lung with proposed criteria for large-cell neuroendocrine carcinoma. An ultrastructural, immunohistochemical, and flow cytometric study of 35 cases. Am J Surg Pathol. 1991;15:529–53.
2. WHO Classification of Tumours Editor Board. WHO classification of tumour of the lung, pleura, thymus and heart. International Agency for Research on Cancer: Lyon, France; 2015.
3. Rekhtman N, Pietanza MC, Hellmann MD, et al. Next-generation sequencing of pulmonary large cell neuroendocrine carcinoma reveals small cell carcinoma-like and non-small cell carcinoma-like subsets. Clin Cancer Res. 2016;22:3618–29.
4. George J, Walter V, Peifer M, et al. Integrative genomic profiling of large-cell neuroendocrine carcinomas reveals distinct subtypes of high-grade neuroendocrine lung tumors. Nat Commun. 2018;9:1048.
5. Filosso PL, Guerrera F, Evangelista A, et al. Adjuvant chemotherapy for large-cell neuroendocrine lung carcinoma: results from the European Society for Thoracic Surgeons Lung Neuroendocrine tumors retrospective database. Eur J Cardiothorac Surg. 2017;52:339–45.

6. Kujtan L, Muthukumar V, Kennedy KF, et al. The role of systemic therapy in the management of stage I large cell neuroendocrine carcinoma of the lung. J Thorac Oncol. 2018;13:707–14.
7. Raman V, Jawitz OK, Yang CJ, et al. Outcomes for surgery in large cell lung neuroendocrine cancer. J Thorac Oncol. 2019;14:2143–51.
8. Derks JL, Leblay N, Thunnissen E, et al. Molecular subtypes of pulmonary large-cell neuroendocrine carcinoma predict chemotherapy treatment outcome. Clin Cancer Res. 2018;24:33–42.
9. Zhuo M, Guan Y, Yang X, et al. The prognostic and therapeutic role of genomic subtyping by sequencing tumor or cell-free DNA in pulmonary large-cell neuroendocrine carcinoma. Clin Cancer Res. 2020;26:892–901.
10. Limonnik V, Abel S, Finley GG, Long GS, et al. Factors associated with treatment receipt and overall survival for patients with locally advanced large cell neuroendocrine carcinoma of the lung: a National Cancer Database analysis. Lung Cancer. 2020;150:107–13.
11. May MS, Kinslow CJ, Adams C, et al. Outcomes for localized treatment of large cell neuroendocrine carcinoma of the lung in the United States. Transl Lung Cancer Res. 2021;10:71–9.
12. Kinslow CJ, May MS, Saqi A, et al. Large-cell neuroendocrine carcinoma of the lung: a population-based study. Clin Lung Cancer. 2020;21:e99–e113.
13. Lowczak A, Kolasinska-Cwikla A, Osowiecka K, et al. Outcomes of patients with pulmonary large cell neuroendocrine carcinoma in I-IV stage. Medicina (Kaunas). 2021;57:118.
14. Lee KW, Lee Y, Oh SW, et al. Large cell neuroendocrine carcinoma of the lung: CT and FDG PET findings. Eur J Radiol. 2015;84:2332–8.
15. Minami K, Tanaka Y, Ogawa H, et al. Neuroendocrine marker staining pattern categorization of small-sized pulmonary large cell neuroendocrine carcinoma. Thorac Cancer. 2019;10:2152–60.
16. Rekhtman N, Pietanza CM, Sabari J, et al. Pulmonary large cell neuroendocrine carcinoma with adenocarcinoma-like features: napsin A expression and genomic alterations. Mod Pathol. 2018;31:111–21.

Carcinoid Tumor

Song Zhang

Carcinoid tumors are slow-growing neoplasms stemming from neuroendocrine cells, which can secrete a variety of peptides and neuroamines. The common primary sites are the gastrointestinal tract followed by the tracheobronchial tree, small bowel, colon, appendix, rectum, stomach, or thymus.

Pulmonary neuroendocrine neoplasms arise from bronchial mucosal cells known as enterochromaffin cells or Kulchitsky cells and are currently classified as low-grade typical carcinoid, intermediate-grade atypical carcinoid, and the high-grade LCNEC and SCLC. Typical and atypical carcinoid tumors are classified based on the presence of mitosis and necrosis. LCNEC and SCLC are distinguished based on cytological criteria (cell size, nuclear features).

1 Classification

Carcinoid tumors were first described in 1888 by Otto Lubarsch. The term carcinoid, or carcinoma-like, was coined by Siegfried Oberndorfer in 1907 when he described a distinct intestinal tumor that was biologically less aggressive than intestinal adenocarcinoma. Kramer classified this tumor among the so-called bronchial adenomas to signify its relatively indolent behavior in 1930. Hamperl initially distinguished bronchial carcinoids from other bronchial neoplasms in 1937. The term carcinoid has been maintained during all WHO classifications published since 1967 [1]. In 1970, pulmonary neuroendocrine neoplasms were classified into three categories: typical carcinoid, atypical carcinoid, and SCLC. In 1991, Travis et al. [2] proposed 4 categories of pulmonary neuroendocrine neoplasms: typical carcinoid, atypical carcinoid, LCNEC, and SCLC. In the 1999 WHO classification, the diagnostic criteria separating typical carcinoid from atypical carcinoid were introduced, allowing sharp morphological definition of typical versus atypical carcinoids, and atypical carcinoids versus LCNEC. Diffuse idiopathic neuroendocrine cell hyperplasia (DIPNECH), considered a preneoplastic processes, was also introduced. In the 2004 WHO classification, typical carcinoid and atypical carcinoid were categorized together under the heading of carcinoid tumors; LCNEC was retained as a subtype of LCC, and SCLC was retained as an independent category. All four tumors were characterized by varying degrees of neuroendocrine morphologic features histologically. In the 2015 WHO classification, neuroendocrine tumors were categorized together in one category. In the 2021 WHO classification, carcinoid tumors included typical carcinoid / neuroendocrine tumor, grade 1 and atypical carcinoid/

S. Zhang (✉)
Department of Respiratory and Critical Care Medicine, Shandong Provincial Hospital Affiliated to Shandong First Medical University, Jinan, Shandong, China

S. Zhang (ed.), *Diagnostic Imaging of Lung Cancers*, https://doi.org/10.1007/978-981-99-6815-2_5

neuroendocrine tumor, grade 2. LCNEC and SCLC corresponded to grade 3 neuroendocrine carcinoma.

2 Pathology

The histologic appearance of pulmonary carcinoid (PC) is characterized by tumor cells with eosinophilic cytoplasm, finely granular chromatin, and inconspicuous or absent nucleoli. These cells have characteristic neuroendocrine morphology and growth patterns, including organoid, trabecular, palisading, rosette-like, and other arrangements [3].

In the 2004 WHO classification, typical carcinoid was defined as a neuroendocrine tumor with less than two mitoses per 2 mm^2 (10 high-power fields), measuring 5 mm or more, and lacking any evidence of necrosis; atypical carcinoid was defined as a neuroendocrine tumor with either 2 to 10 mitoses 2 mm^2 or necrosis. Compared with LCNEC and SCLC, PCs do not occur in combination with other types of carcinoma. Accurate sub-classification of PCs into typical or atypical carcinoids may not be possible on small biopsy specimens as mitotic activity and necrosis may be present only focally within a given tumor.

In the 2015 WHO classification, it recommends that mitoses should be counted in the areas of highest activity and per 2 mm^2 rather than 10 high-power fields for the aim of avoiding discrepancies due to the different microscope models. In tumors that are near the cutoffs of 2 or 20 mitoses per 2 mm^2, at least three sets of 2 mm^2 should be counted and the mean used for determining the mitotic rate, rather than the single highest rate. For typical and atypical carcinoids, mitotic rate and necrosis status should be included in pathology reports [3].

In the 2021 WHO classification, DIPNECH was defined by pathological and clinical criteria: histologically, it is a multifocal hyperplasia of pulmonary neuroendocrine cells associated with tumorlets and constrictive bronchiolitis. It needs to be distinguished from localized reactive neuroendocrine cell hyperplasia secondary to various non -neoplastic conditions [4]. The term "carcinoid tumor not otherwise specified (NOS)" was recommended for small samples from primary or metastatic neuroendocrine tumors and the mitotic count and the presence of any foci of necrosis with a comment if the findings raise concern for AC should be recorded.

According to mitosis, Ki-67 labeling index, and/or the presence of necrosis, neuroendocrine neoplasms are graded as G1, G2, or G3 in many organ systems. Typical and atypical carcinoids are closest to the G1 and G2 gastroenteropancreatic neuroendocrine tumors, respectively. The category of G3 atypical carcinoid in the lung is not a validated entity and not recognized in the 2015 WHO classification. Ki-67 labeling index is usually less than 5% in typical carcinoid and is higher in atypical carcinoid, usually between 5% and 20%. The role of Ki-67 in lung neuroendocrine neoplasms is mainly to separate the PCs from the high-grade LCNEC and SCLC, especially in small biopsies with crushed and/or necrotic tumor cells. Ki-67 labeling index exceeding 30% is usually indicative of a high-grade LCNEC or SCLC.Ki-67 is not recommended to distinguish the typical carcinoids from atypical carcinoids in the 2015 WHO classification.

Some neuroendocrine neoplasms are characterized by the well differentiated, organoid morphology of carcinoids, with an elevated proliferative activity as documented by a mitotic count exceeding 10 mitosis/2 mm^2 and a high Ki-67 index (>20%–30%). The current recommendation is to label such tumors as LCNEC (based on the high mitotic count), if available, add a note specifying the carcinoid morphology and the Ki-67 index. These tumors with a 20% greater Ki-67 index and a smaller mitotic index, with 10 mitosis/2 mm^2 are described as highly proliferative carcinoids.

In summary, it is difficult to distinguish typical carcinoid from atypical carcinoid in small biopsy and cytology, the diagnostic criteria still rely on histology and require a surgical specimen.

3 Epidemiology

PCs account for approximately 20%–30% of all neuroendocrine neoplasms and represent only 1%–2% of all lung cancers. Typical carcinoids are more prevalent than atypical carcinoids, accounting for approximately 90% of PCs. The age-adjusted incidence rate of PCs is 0.2–2/100000 population/year in the western hemisphere.

PCs prevail slightly in women over men, in whites over other ethnicities including Hispanic and Asian people. On average, they are up to a decade younger at diagnosis than those with other lung cancer, with around 45 years of age for typical carcinoid and one decade later for atypical carcinoid. PCs are the most common primary pulmonary neoplasm diagnosed in children and adolescents, with typical carcinoid prevailing by far over atypical carcinoid.

Cigarette smoking is always a consideration in bronchopulmonary tumors. In contrast to LCNEC and SCLC, the majority of PC patients are more common in light smokers or non-smokers, although atypical carcinoid patients seem to be slightly more frequent in smokers.

4 Molecular Features

PCs appear to have their own unique molecular landscape compared to high-grade LCNEC and SCLC and NSCLCs. The introduction of high-throughput next generation sequencing (NGS) techniques has provided a means to investigate the genomic profiling of PCs.

Fernandez-Cuesta et al. [5] sequenced the whole exome of 69 PCs. They found that chromatin-remodeling is the most frequently mutated pathway in PCs; the genes MEN1, PSIP1, and ARID1A were recurrently affected by mutations. Specifically, covalent histone modifiers and subunits of the SWI/SNF complex are mutated in 40% and 22.2% of the cases, respectively. In contrast to LCNEC and SCLC, TP53 and RB1 mutations are rare events, suggesting that these genes are not main drivers in PCs. They detected 529 non-synonymous mutations in 494 genes, which translates to a mean somatic mutation rate of 0.4 mutations per megabase (Mb), which is much lower than the rate observed in other lung tumors. This high mutation rate of G:C > A:T transitions is characteristic of smoking exposure, which can explain that PCs are more common in non-smokers.

Swarts et al. [6] found that 13% of PCs harbor MEN1 mutation associated with reduced mRNA expression and poor prognosis. Similarly, in mutation-negative tumors, low MEN1 gene expression correlates with an adverse disease outcome.

Simbolo et al. [7] sequenced 148 lung neuroendocrine tumors comprising 53 typical carcinoids, 35 atypical carcinoids, 27 LCNLCs, and 33 SCLCs. Carcinoids and carcinomas shared the majority of altered genes but with different prevalence rates. When mutations and copy number changes were combined, MEN1 alterations were almost exclusive to carcinoids, whereas alterations of TP53 and RB1 cell cycle regulation genes and PI3K/AKT/mTOR pathway genes were significantly enriched in carcinomas. Conversely, mutations in chromatin-remodeling genes, including those encoding histone modifiers and members of SWI-SNF complexes, were found at similar rates in carcinoids (45.5%) and carcinomas (55.0%), suggesting a major role in lung neuroendocrine tumors pathogenesis. In addition, MEN1 mutation was associated with poor prognosis in atypical carcinoid.

Overall, MEN1 is the most frequently somatically mutated gene in carcinoids (11%–22%), usually accompanied by loss of heterozygosity. MEN1 is a molecular adaptor that acts as a scaffold protein assembling the MEN1-MLL-PSIP1 ternary complex, which promotes the expression of CDKN1B and CDKN2C, both of them cell cycle inhibitor genes. MEN1 gene mutations and reduced gene expression have been associated with poor prognosis and shorter survival in PCs.

5 Clinical Features

PCs are divided into central or peripheral depending on their site of origin within the bronchial tree. Approximately 80% of PCs are located centrally, and 20% are peripheral. Patients with central lesions often cause symptoms related to airway obstruction, including cough, hemoptysis, dyspnea, chest pain, wheezing, and recurrent pneumonia. Patients with peripheral lesions usually are asymptomatic. In a population-based study in Denmark [8], 24% of typical carcinoid and 7% of atypical carcinoid are incidentally identified at autopsy. All PCs are malignant and have the potential to metastasize.

Approximately 5% of cases of PCs are associated with multiple endocrine neoplasia type 1 (MEN1), usually typical carcinoid with a smaller number of atypical carcinoid. MEN1 is investigated by family history, clinical examination, and laboratory screening including intact parathyroid hormone, ionized calcium, and prolactin. If family history indicates a MEN1 syndrome or a second MEN1 feature is present, MEN1 gene mutation screening should be carried out.

Because of the relative paucity of serotonin secretion, carcinoid syndrome occurs in <5% of PCs, especially in atypical carcinoids with liver metastases and high tumor burden. 24 h urine 5-hydroxyindoleacetic acid measurement is measured. Cushing's syndrome occurs in 1%–6% of PCs, and measurements recommended include serum cortisol, 24 h urine free cortisol, and adrenocorticotropic hormone (ACTH). Other rare endocrine manifestations include acromegaly, hypercalcemia, and hypoglycemia.

6 Radiographic Features

The majority of typical carcinoids are centrally, and atypical carcinoids located peripherally in the lungs. Peripheral PCs usually present in CT as spherical masses with clear borders (Fig. 1). Lobulation (mainly slight lobulation) (Fig. 2) and burr can be seen in some cases. Individuals may have pleural depression (Fig. 3), which resembles lung adenocarcinoma. Carcinoids grow slowly, with few cystic degeneration, necrosis (Fig. 4), and cavity formation. Dystrophic calcification is found in 11% of patients and can be central or peripheral (Fig. 5). Most carcinoid tumors are supplied by bronchial artery with good blood circulation. Enhanced CT scan often shows round foci with clear contrast medium uptake (>50 HU) and usually detectable relationship to bronchi (Fig. 6). In carcinoids that originate from larger airways, the endobronchial portion of the tumor is often smaller than the extrabronchial/parenchymal portion, showing a typical "iceberg sign" (Fig. 7).

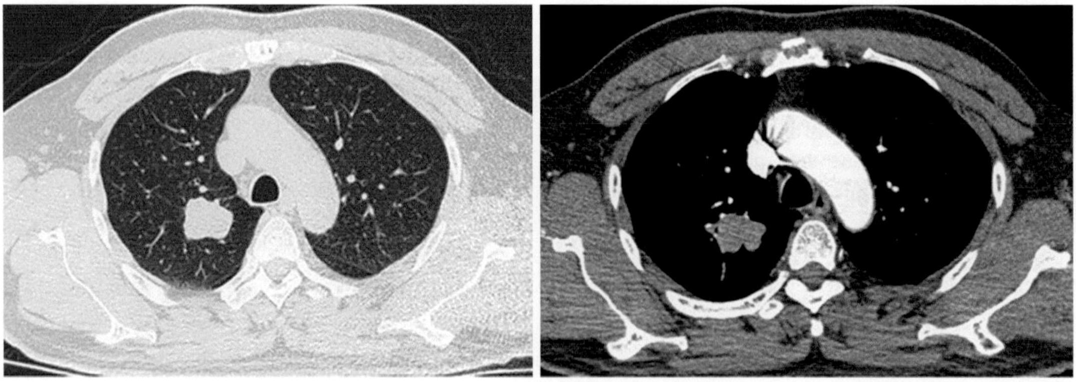

Fig. 1 Peripheral typical carcinoid in a 48-year-old man. Contrast-enhanced CT scan shows a soft-tissue mass in the right upper lung

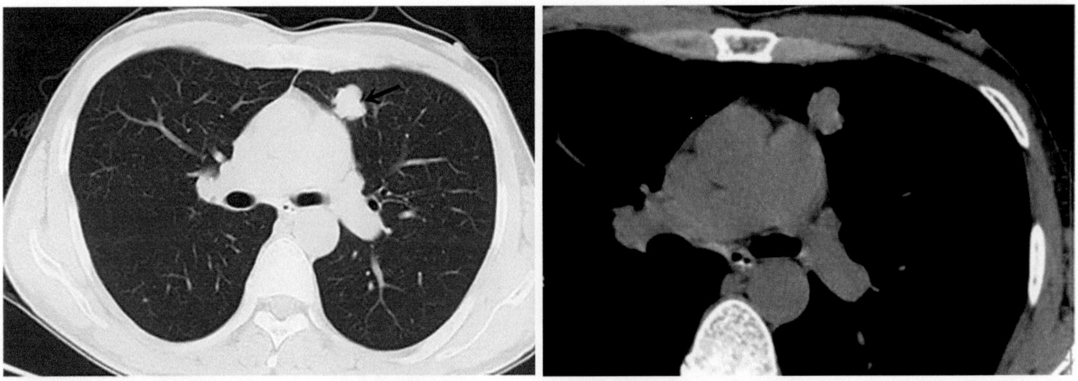

Fig. 2 Peripheral atypical carcinoid in a 40-year-old woman. Contrast-enhanced CT scan shows a soft-tissue mass with deep lobulation (black arrow)

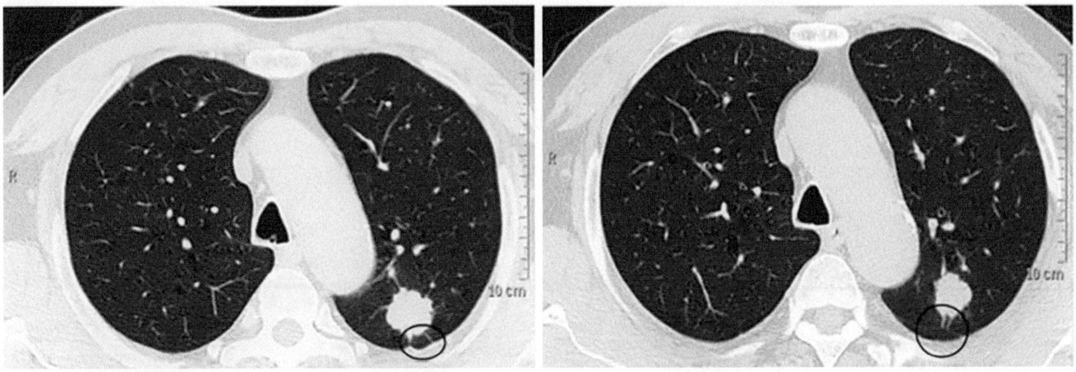

Fig. 3 Peripheral atypical carcinoid in a 60-year-old man. CT scan shows a soft-tissue mass with pleural depression in the left upper lung

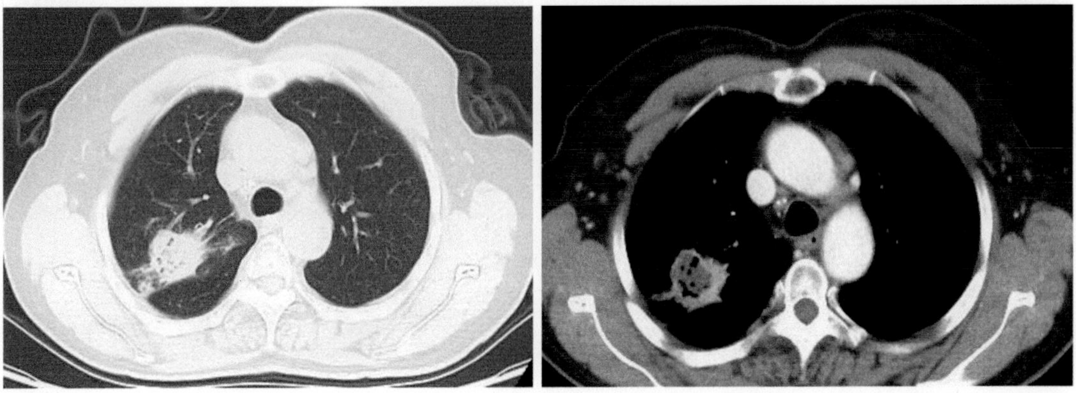

Fig. 4 Peripheral atypical carcinoid in a 75-year-old woman. Contrast-enhanced CT scan shows a soft-tissue mass with necrosis in the right upper lung

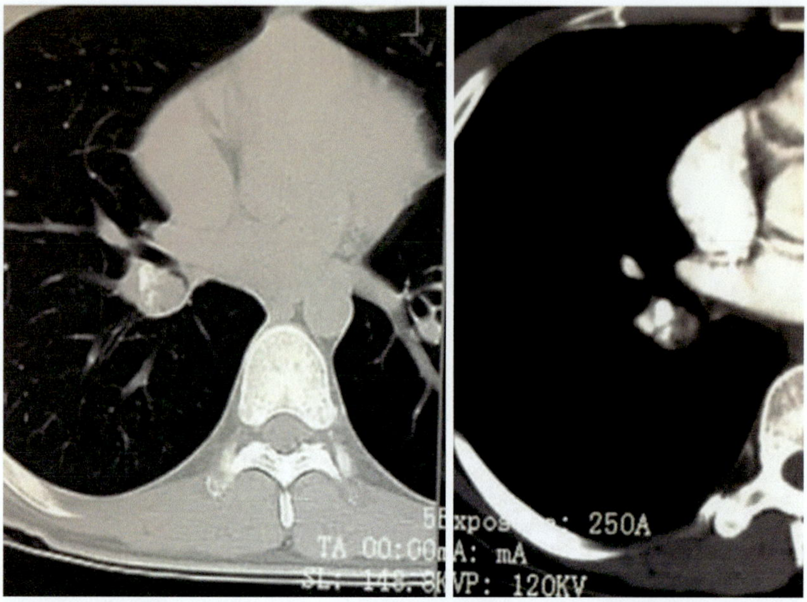

Fig. 5 Central typical carcinoid with eccentric calcifications

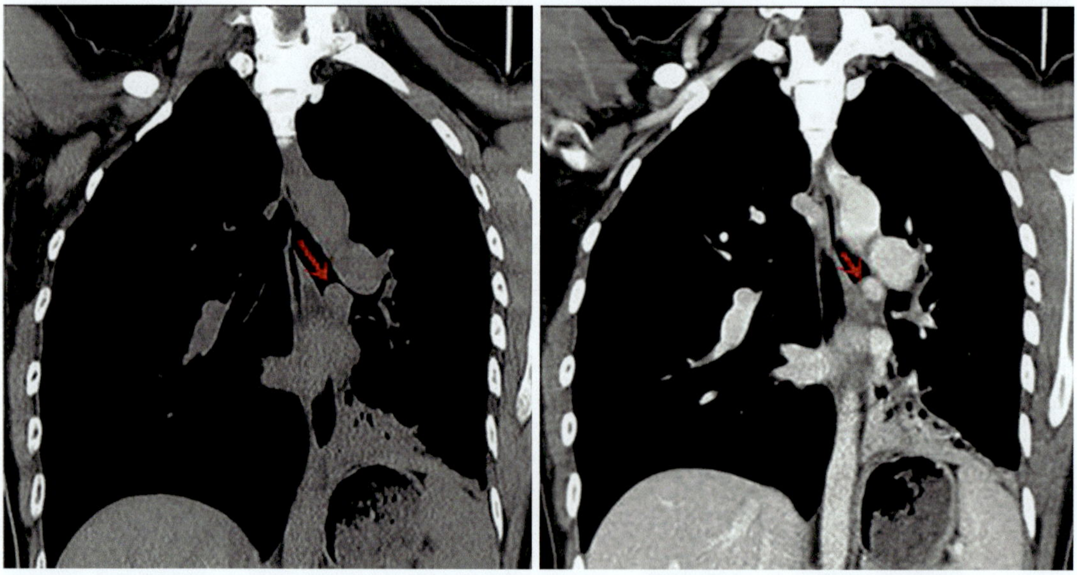

Fig. 6 Central typical carcinoid in a 20-year-old woman. The CT values of usual scan and enhanced scan are 29 and 122HU, respectively

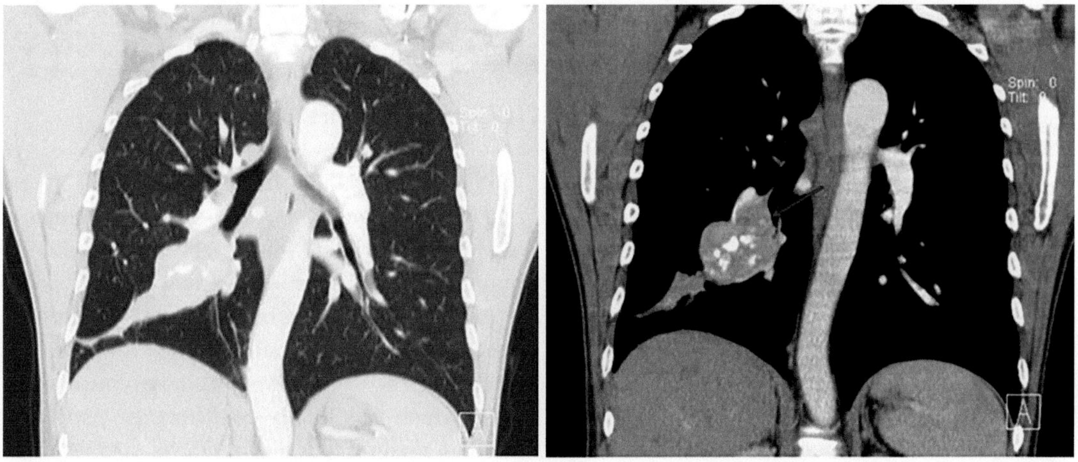

Fig. 7 Central typical carcinoid with calcifications, iceberg sign, and obstructive atelectasis

7 Treatment

Surgery is the mainstay for the treatment of PCs with the aim of removing the tumor and preserving as much lung tissue as possible. Lobectomy and pneumonectomy are the most common options for atypical carcinoid. Bronchial sleeve resection which involves removal of less tissue is suitable for typical carcinoid as they are not as aggressive as atypical carcinoid. Complete anatomic resection and systematic nodal dissection are recommended in patients with peripheral PCs. Resection of metastases should be considered with the aim of curative intent. Caplin et al. [9] recommend that somatostatin scintigraphy SPECT/CT is useful to determine the N and M stage in the preoperative phase, especially in well-differentiated carcinoids; FDG-PET/CT might be useful in intermediate or poorly differentiated tumors. Additionally, whenever available, ^{68}Gallium-DOTA-PET should be preferentially performed, because it is more sensitive than scintigraphy when investigating possible metastases.

In advanced and unresectable PCs, systemic therapies with the aim of controlling tumor growth include somatostatin analogs (SSAs), everolimus, peptide receptor radionuclide therapy (PRRT), chemotherapy, and molecular-targeted therapy. Somatostatin receptors (SSTRs) often show surface overexpression in low-grade lung neuroendocrine tumors. SSAs bind to SSTRs, blocking the release of peptides and amines, and helping to control symptoms. SSAs have been considered as first-line systemic antiproliferative treatment in unresectable PCs. Lung neuroendocrine tumors have shown increased activation of the mTOR (mechanistic target of rapamycin) signaling pathway. So the mTOR inhibitor everolimus is potential therapy for patients with a lung carcinoid tumor. PRRT delivers a radiolabeled agent to a specific target (such as SSTRs) and is an option in patients with strong expression of SSTRs. Systemic chemotherapy has been the standard for advanced unresectable progressive PCs. The most common cytotoxic regimen is cisplatin-etoposide or carboplatin-etoposide, which has been demonstrated limited effects. Temozolomide has shown most clinical benefit. In cases of atypical carcinoids showing aggressive characteristics, negative SSTRs expression, and Ki-67 less than 15%, temozolomide-based chemotherapy is recommended as a last line of therapy. Locoregional or radiotargeted therapies should be considered for metastatic PCs.

8 Prognosis

Typical carcinoid patients have a favorable prognosis, with a 5-year overall survival of 87%–100% after radical surgery. Atypical carcinoid patients are worse, averaging 60%–70% survival at 5 years. Several clinical factors can impact prognosis, including age, gender, previous malignancies, peripheral tumor, TNM stage, and performance status [10].

9 Case Analysis

9.1 Case 1

A 27-year-old woman complained of recurrent hemoptysis for 2 years.

Chest CT: A highly enhanced endoluminal nodule in the left middle bronchus (Fig. 8).

[Diagnosis] Central carcinoid.

[Diagnosis Basis] A young woman has a 2-year history of hemoptysis. The CT scan shows a well-circumscribed, round, completely endoluminal nodule, supporting the diagnosis of benign or low-grade tumors. Combined with the obvious enhancement of the lesion, it suggested that the tumor may be carcinoid, especially typical carcinoid, which was finally confirmed by pathology after surgical resection (Fig. 9).

[Analysis] Most central carcinoids are typical carcinoid tumors, leading to cough, fever, expectoration, wheezing, dyspnea, hemoptysis, chest

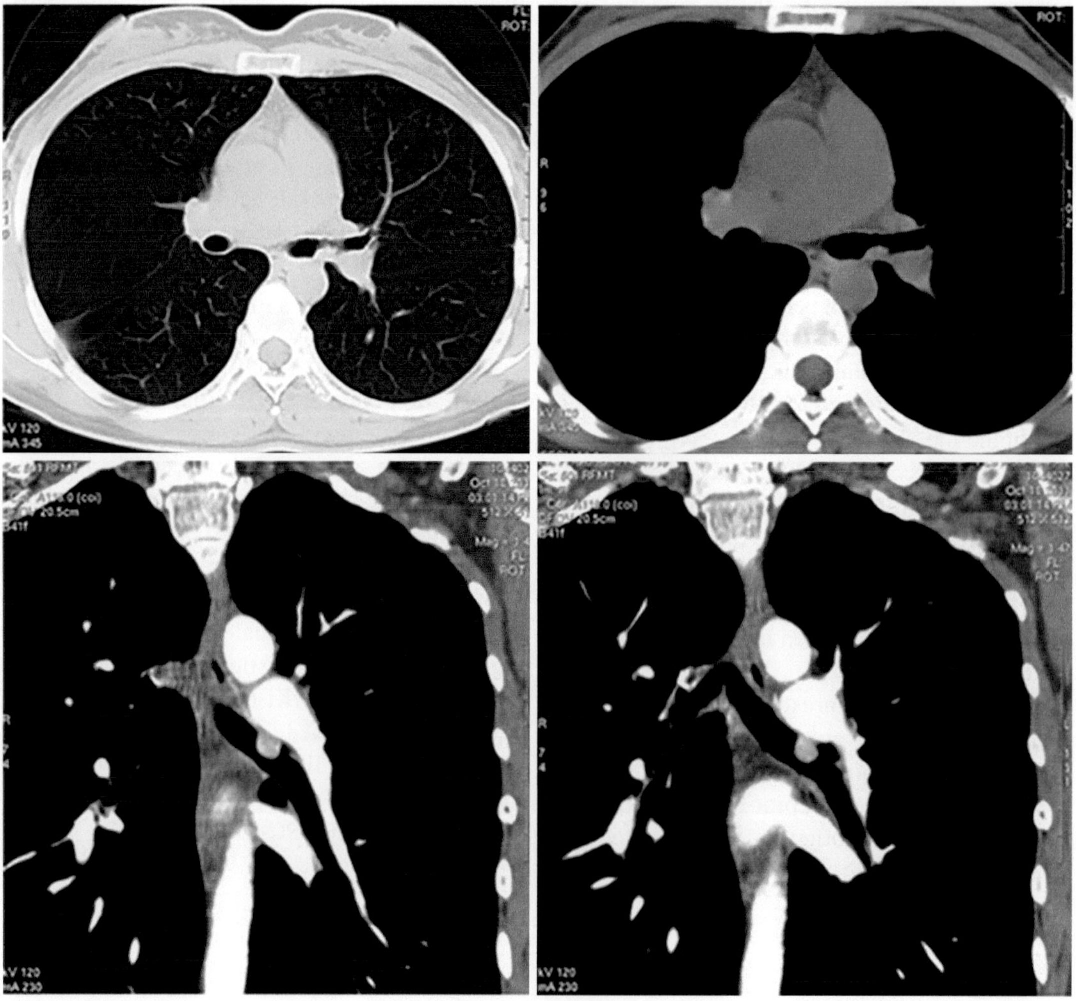

Fig. 8 Chest CT

pain, and recurrent pneumonia due to bronchospasm and obstruction. The triad of cough, hemoptysis, and pneumonia is common symptoms of central carcinoids. Hemoptysis occurs in at least 50% of patients because of the highly vascular nature of carcinoid tumors. About 25% of patients are asymptomatic, which are found incidentally. Because carcinoid tumors are rare, they are generally not considered as a differential diagnosis in young patients like our case. So most intrabronchial carcinoid tumors are misdiagnosed or diagnosed late. Patients with recurrent respiratory symptoms should be thoroughly investigated with radiological examination and bronchoscopy followed by tissue biopsy for accurate and early diagnosis.

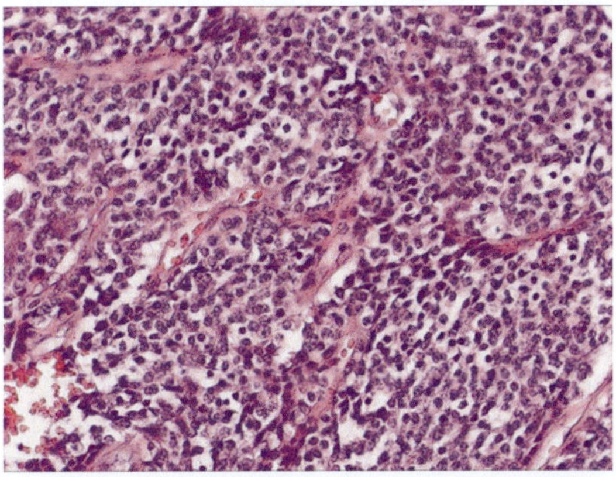

Fig. 9 Histologic section shows that tumor cells arrange in trabecular and glandular pattern. The tumor cells are uniform round and no evidence of mitosis and necrosis

Some small central carcinoids are located entirely within the bronchial lumen without extraluminal components. The tumor is usually a well-defined, round, or ovoid nodule. Ancillary CT features of endobronchial carcinoid tumors include obstructive pneumonitis, secretion-filled bronchi (mucoid impaction), atelectasis, and air trapping caused by ball-valve mechanism (Fig. 10). Central carcinoids also may be hilar or perihilar mass with a close anatomic relationship to the bronchus. Bronchoscopy is helpful in detecting bronchial carcinoids, and most bronchial carcinoids are located centrally within reach of a bronchoscope. Bronchial carcinoid usually appears as a smooth, cherry red, endobronchial nodule or mass, attached to the bronchus by a broad base, may have a polypoid appearance (Fig. 11).

Diagnosis can be confirmed by bronchoscopic biopsy. Due to the highly vascular nature of carcinoids, massive hemorrhage following endoscopic biopsy has occasionally been reported. Bronchoscopic resection might be a feasible option in patients with entirely intraluminal carcinoid tumors without evidence of bronchial wall involvement or suspicious lymphadenopathy. Hemorrhage during resection is a potential complication and may lead to airway compromise. Thus, rigid bronchoscopy is preferable against flexible bronchoscopy. Once the diagnosis is confirmed, surgical resection using bronchoplastic techniques (i.e., sleeve, wedge, or flap resection)

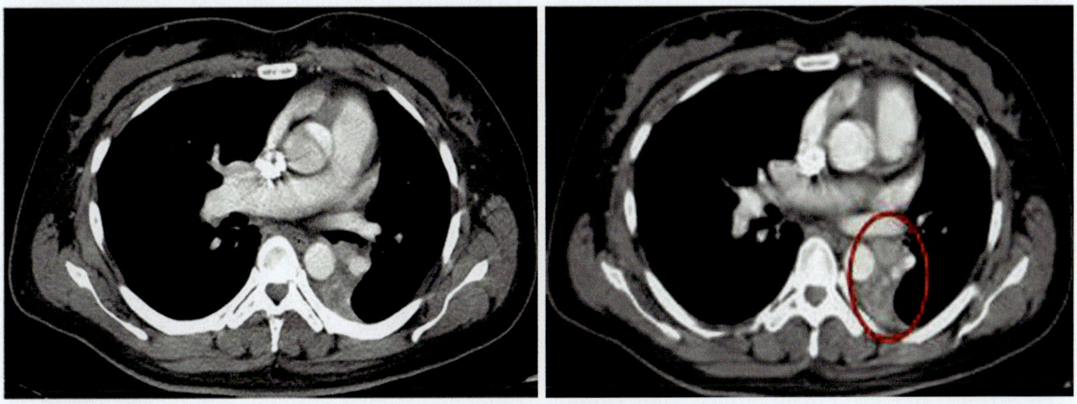

Fig. 10 Central typical carcinoid in a 42-year-old woman. Contrast-enhanced CT scan shows a soft-tissue mass in the left lower lung with atelectasis (red circle)

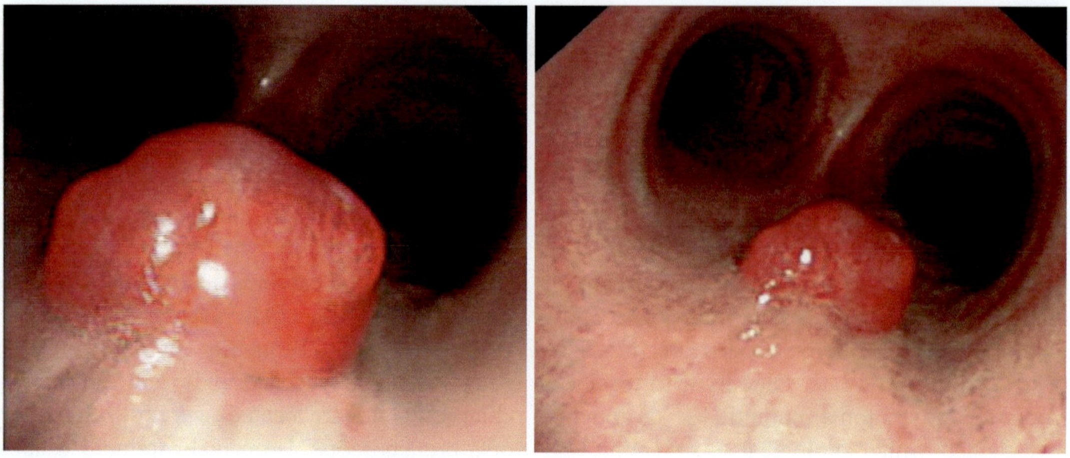

Fig. 11 Bronchoscopy appearance of bronchial carcinoid

to preserve lung parenchyma is the preferred treatment of choice.

9.2 Case 2

A 48-year-old man complained of cough, expectoration, and hemoptysis for half a month.

Chest CT: A mass in the left middle lobe, the CT attenuations of the four-phase dynamic scan were 33.0, 40.8, 59.35, and 59.5HU, respectively (Fig. 12).

[Diagnosis] Right middle lobe carcinoid tumor.

[Diagnosis Basis] This case is a lesion at the right hilum of lung, crossing the interlobar fissure (orange arrow), without lobulation, spiculation, or pleural depression. These features do not support the diagnosis of lung adenocarcinoma. The lesions have uniform density and smooth border, supporting the possibility of benign lesion or low-grade tumor. There is no fat density and calcification in the lesion, which do not support the diagnosis of hamartoma. The presence of calcification does not differentiate carcinomas from hamartomas. Carcinoids tended to have eccentric calcification more frequently than hamartomas. Overlying vessel sign (red arrow) and prominent artery sign (green arrow) conform to the imaging features of pulmonary sclerosing pneumocytoma (PSP). However, PSP mostly occurs in young women, the gender of this case does not match. The lesion causes compression and displacement of the lower trachea (black circle), but not obstructing the bronchus (pink arrow). MPR reconstruction shows that the lesion is mainly located outside the lumen (yellow arrow), resulting in stenosis of the bronchial lumen (blue arrow), suggesting that the lesion is more closely related to the trachea. Multiple continuous blood vessels (purple arrows) are more in line with the diagnosis of lung carcinoid rather than PSP. Ultimately, the postoperative pathology of the patient was right middle lobe carcinoid tumor.

[Analysis] Carcinoid and PSP are very similar in density, morphology, margin, calcification, location, and enhancement characteristics. The peripheral blood vessels of lung carcinoid tumor can also be compressed and displaced, and prominent artery sign can also appear due to highly vascular nature. Intraluminal growth is rare in PSP. On CT, PSP generally has no discernible well-developed blood vessels. In this case, the intratumoral blood vessels are clearly visible, which does not support the diagnosis of PSP. Carcinoids are rich in blood supply, and obvious vascular shadows can be seen on imag-

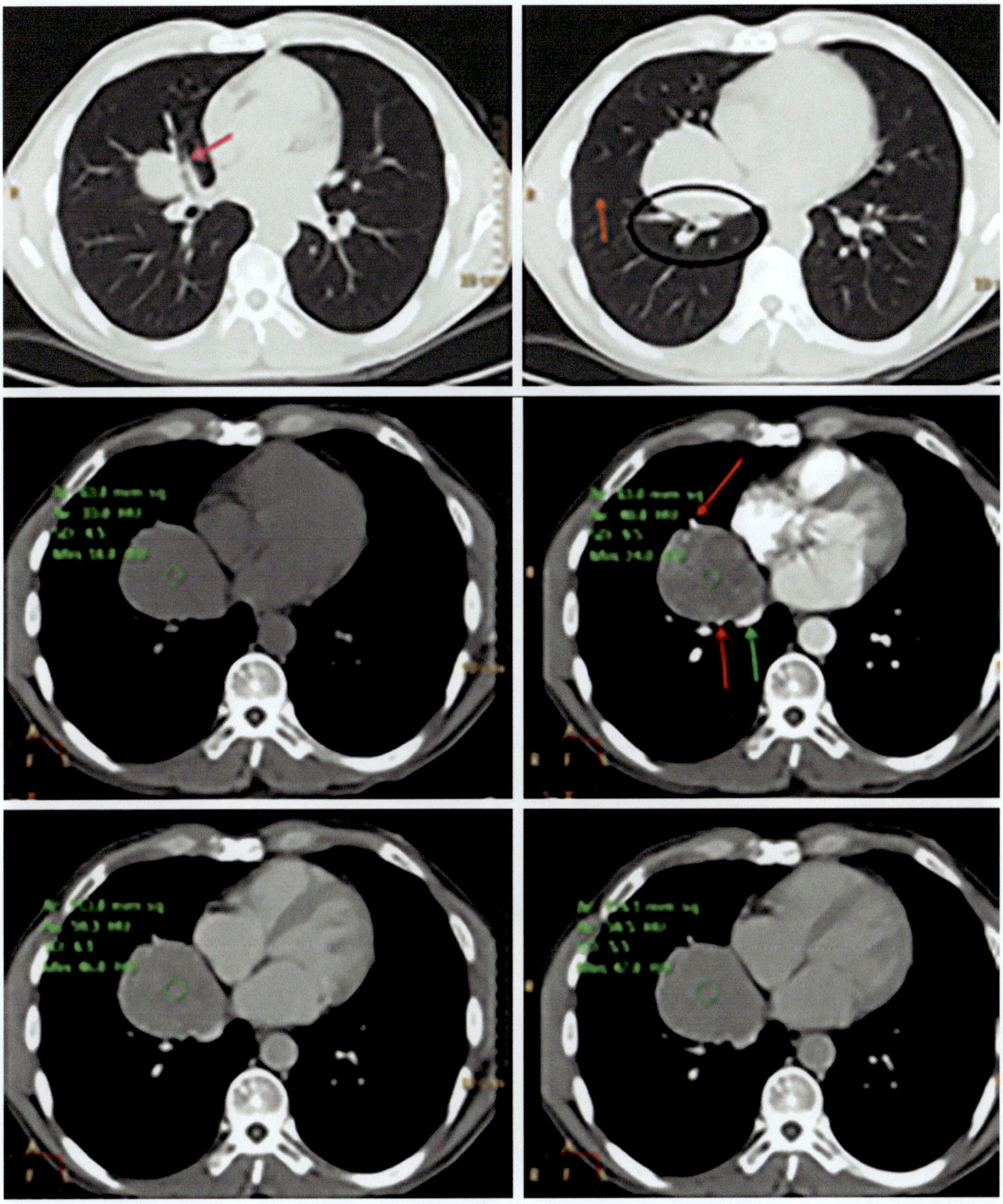

Fig. 12 Chest CT

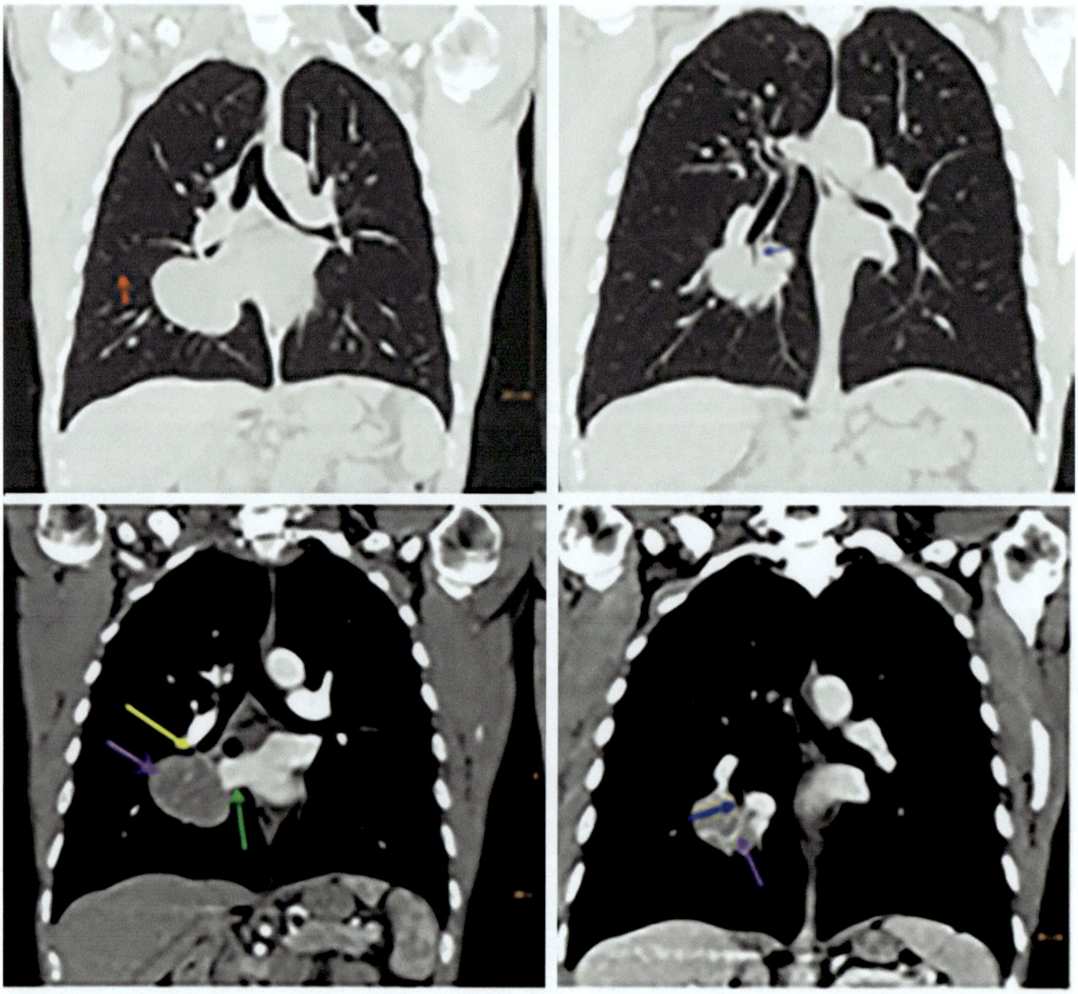

Fig. 5.12 (continued)

ing or pathology (Fig. 13), which is helpful for the distinction between them.

9.3 Case 3

A 33-year-old man complained of cough and expectoration for half a month. Ultrasound of the neck revealed multiple lymphadenopathies in the right supraclavicular region.

Chest CT: A lesion in the right lower lobe with enlarged mediastinal and right hilar lymph nodes, and obstructive pneumonia (Fig. 14).

[Diagnosis] Carcinoid tumor.

[Diagnosis Basis] The patient underwent transbronchial lung biopsy (TBLB) and transbronchial needle aspiration (TBNA). Bronchoscopy showed that the bronchial lumen of the right lower lobe was stenosis by external pressure, with a degree of 90%. Histopathological report of TBLB specimens in the right lower lobe and immunohistochemistry were consistent with typical carcinoid. TBNA (group 4R lymph node) specimen showed a small amount of bronchial mucosal tissue with fibrinoid exudate. The biopsy

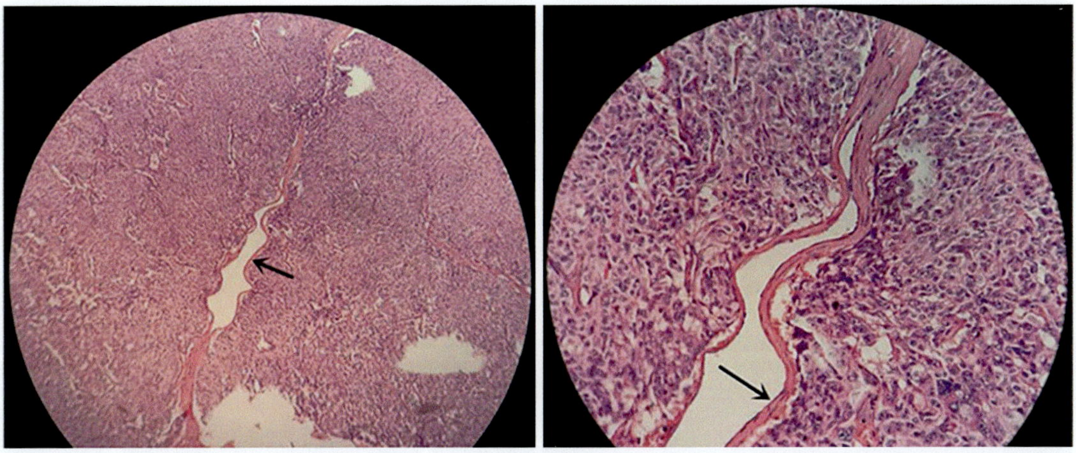

Fig. 13 Pathological manifestations of atypical carcinoid tumor with obvious vascular shadows (black arrows)

specimen of the right supraclavicular lymph node showed lymphoid hyperplasia, which was considered to be reactive lymphoid hyperplasia, with more plasma cell infiltration.

[Analysis] Typical and atypical carcinoids have similar radiologic features. Diagnosis relies on contrast-enhanced CT scan to show endobronchial nodule, hilar or perihilar mass, enlarged mediastinal lymph nodes, tumor relationship to bronchi and smaller nodules beyond subsegmental bronchus lesions. Bronchoscopy is the best choice for tissue diagnosis.

According to the degree of differentiation and lymph node metastasis, the prognosis of typical carcinoid is better than that of atypical carcinoid, with a 10-year survival rate of more than 80%. Although the overall survival rate is high, typical carcinoids metastasize in 10–15% of cases and atypical carcinoids in up to 50%, and recurrence may still occur many years after completion of primary treatment. Metastases usually occur in the mediastinal lymph nodes, followed by the liver and bone. Although hilar and mediastinal lymph nodes are the most common metastatic sites for typical carcinoids, most lymphadenopathies result from reactive inflammatory reaction. This may explain why histopathological studies of lymph nodes in the mediastinal and supraclavicular regions of our patient were negative for metastasis.

9.4 Case 4

A 70-year-old man complained of chest pain for 3 days.

Chest CT: A mass in the left lower lobe with obvious necrosis, the CT attenuations of the three-phase dynamic scan were 17, 20, and 21 HU in the central area and 65, 63, and 63 HU in the peripheral area, respectively (Fig. 15).

[Diagnosis] Peripheral carcinoid tumor.

[Diagnosis Basis] This case is an elderly man with a mass in the lower lobe of the left lung with distal pneumonitis (white arrow). The patient's short medical history and no obvious fever do not support the diagnosis of community-acquired pneumonia. Pulmonary tuberculosis may have a peripheral ring-enhancement, but often without the overlying vessel sign (green arrow). When a large area of necrosis occurs in a lung abscess, the patient often has symptoms such as fever, and most of the patients have comfortable thick-walled cavities, which is not suitable for this case. Most PSPs have obvious enhancement and delayed enhancement, but obvious necrosis is rare. The enhancement pattern and degree of necrosis in this case do not support the diagnosis. In this case, the bronchial compression of the posterior basal segment of the left lower lobe was visible (red arrow), suggesting that the lesion is

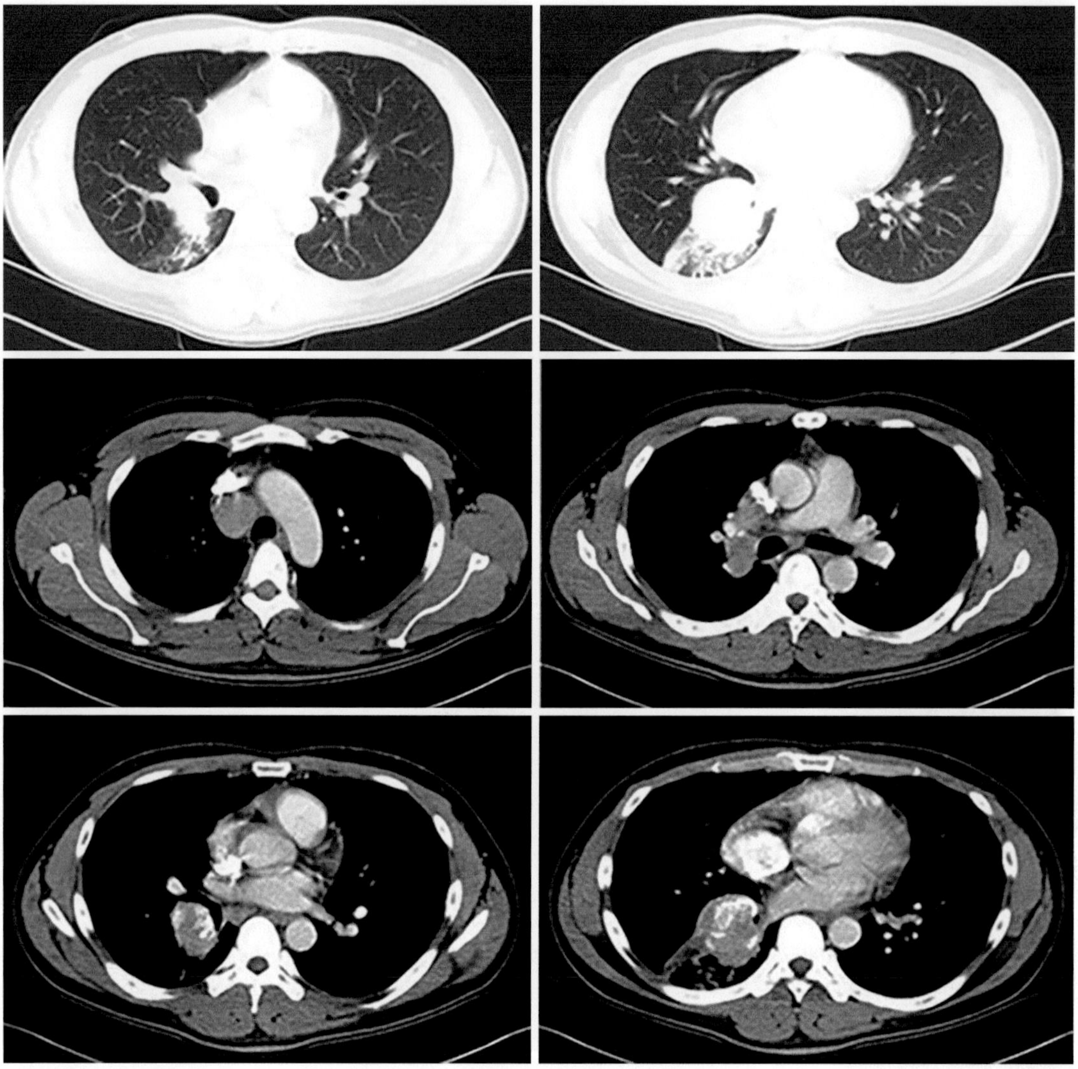

Fig. 14 Chest CT

closely related to the trachea, and combined with the abundant blood vessels around the lesion, carcinoid tumors should be considered. The patient underwent surgical resection. The lesion was located in the left lower lobe with an incomplete capsule. The cut surface was pale-yellow, soft, and mostly necrotic. The tumor involved the visceral pleura, and there was no implantation metastasis. Histopathologic study of the excised mass revealed atypical carcinoid tumor with infarction. Immunohistochemistry was positive for CD56, chromogranin A, NSE, and synaptophysin, and Ki-67 index was 2%. No mediastinal lymph nodes were involved (Figs. 16 and 17).

[Analysis] Atypical carcinoids are mostly located in the periphery and rarely present with any symptoms. Contrast-enhanced CT scan demonstrates atypical carcinoids present as solitary pulmonary nodule or mass lesion.

Many studies have confirmed that typical and atypical carcinoids are distinct disease entities, and as such treated accordingly. Thakur et al. [11] performed a retrospective analysis of all

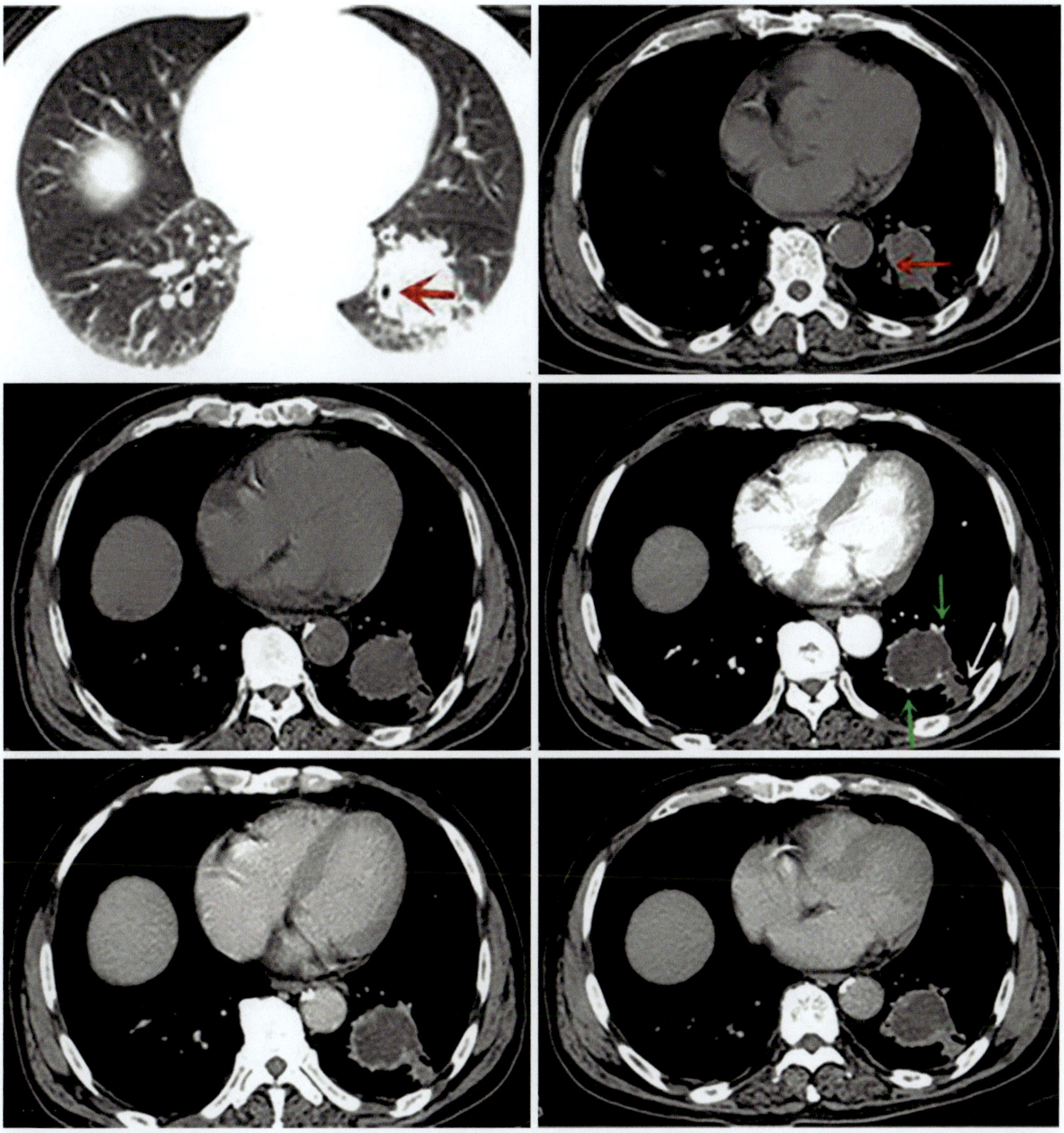

Fig. 15 Chest CT

patients who underwent surgical resection of lung carcinoid tumors across multiple institutions in Melbourne, Australia. They found that atypical histology and lymph node involvement were significant prognostic factors, and sublobar resection should not be considered in patients with either of the above features. Typical carcinoid tumor without nodal involvement may be appropriate for sublobar resection. Walters et al. [12] evaluated 816 atypical and 5688 typical carcinoid patients aged 18 years or more. They concluded that increasing age, comorbidities, and stage were identified as significant predictors of mortality in atypical patients in a multivariate analysis. The extent of surgical resection (lobectomy versus sublobar resection) was not identified as a predictor of survival in atypical carcinoid tumors.

Compared with typical carcinoid, atypical carcinoid was significantly more aggressive, with a higher frequency of nodal (50%) and distant (20%) metastases (Fig. 18). In atypical carci-

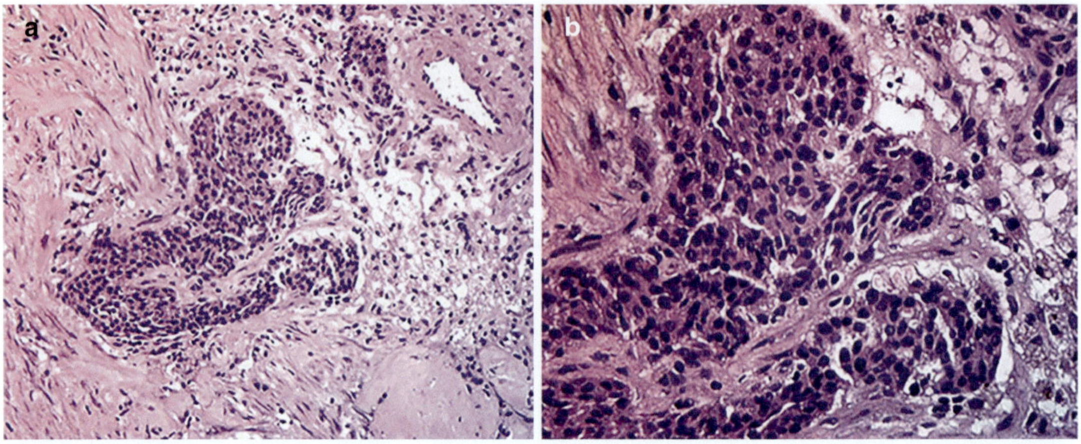

Fig. 16 (**a**) Histologic section shows uniform round cells disposed in nests and trabeculae(original magnification, ×20; hematoxylin-eosin stain). (**b**) Tumor cells with abundant cytoplasm and moderately pleomorphic nuclei(original magnification, ×40; hematoxylin-eosin stain)

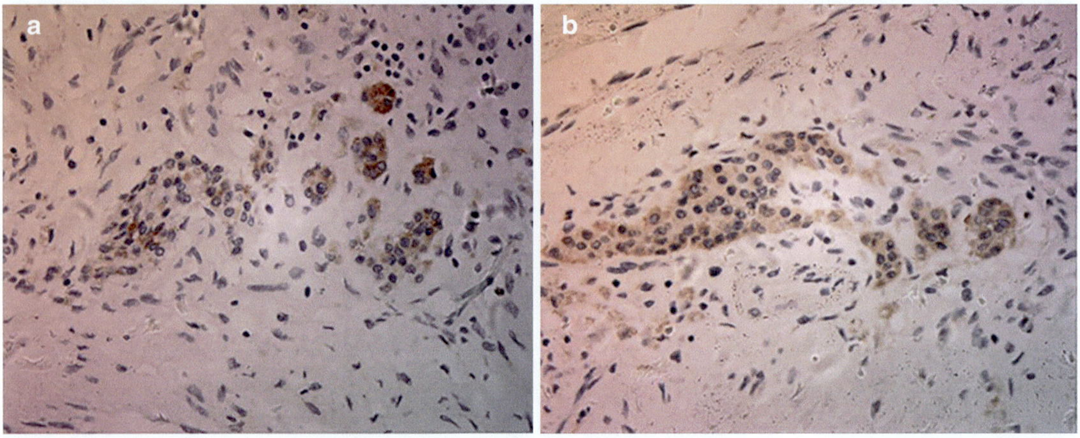

Fig. 17 (**a**) Immunohistochemistry shows cytoplasmic positivity for chromogranin A. (**b**) Immunohistochemistry shows cytoplasmic positivity for synaptophysin

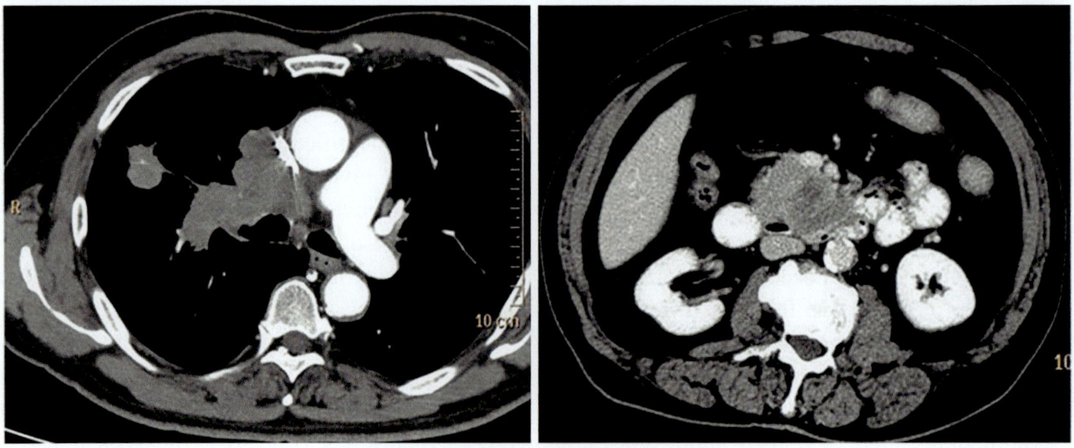

Fig. 18 A 74-year-old man with pulmonary atypical carcinoid. CT scan shows mediastinal and pancreatic metastases

noids, ipsilateral mediastinal lymph node metastases (N2) are found in up to 21% of patients. Contralateral mediastinal lymph nodes (N3) are extremely rare in lung carcinoids. Further research on the optimal surgical management is warranted.

Atypical carcinoid has a worse prognosis and higher recurrence rate than typical carcinoid. The 10-year survival was 82%–88.9% for typical carcinoid and 50%–56% for atypical carcinoid.

References

1. Williams ED, Sandler M. The classification of carcinoid tumors. Lancet. 1963;1:238–9.
2. Travis WD, Linnoila RI, Tsokos MG, et al. Neuroendocrine tumors of the lung with proposed criteria for large cell neuroendocrine carcinoma. An ultrastructural, immunohistochemical, and flow cytometric study of 35 cases. Am J Surg Pathol. 1991;15:529–53.
3. WHO Classification of Tumours Editorial Board. WHO classification of tumours of the lung, pleura, thymus and heart. Lyon, France: International Agency for Research on Cancer; 2015.
4. WHO Classification of Tumours Editorial Board. Thoracic tumours. 5th ed. Lyon, France: International Agency for Research on Cancer; 2021.
5. Fernandez-Cuesta L, Peifer M, Lu X, et al. Frequent mutations in chromatin-remodelling genes in pulmonary carcinoids. Nat Commun. 2014;27:3518.
6. Swarts DR, Scarpa A, Corbo V, et al. MEN1 gene mutation and reduced expression are associated with poor prognosis in pulmonary carcinoids. J Clin Endocrinol Metab. 2014;99:E374–8.
7. Simbolo M, Mafficini A, Sikora KO, et al. Lung neuroendocrine tumors: deep sequencing of the four World Health Organization histotypes reveals chromatin-remodelling genes as major players and a prognostic role for TERT, RB1, MEN1 and KMT2D. J Pathol. 2017;241:488–500.
8. Skuladottir H, Hirsch FR, Hansen HH, et al. Pulmonary neuroendocrine tumors: incidence and prognosis of histological subtypes. A population-based study in Denmark. Lung Cancer. 2002;37:127–35.
9. Caplin ME, Baudin E, Ferolla P, et al. Pulmonary neuroendocrine (carcinoid) tumors: European neuroendocrine tumor society expert consensus and recommendations for best practice for typical and atypical pulmonary carcinoids. Ann Oncol. 2015;26:1604–20.
10. Filosso PL, Guerrera F, Evangelista A, et al. Prognostic model of survival for typical bronchial carcinoid tumours: analysis of 1109 patients on behalf of the European Association of Thoracic Surgeons (ESTS) Neuroendocrine tumours working group. Eur J Cardiothorac Surg. 2015;48:441–7.
11. Thakur S, Florisson D, Telianidis S, et al. Pulmonary carcinoid tumors: a multi-Centre analysis of survival and predictors of outcome following sublobar, lobar, and extended pulmonary resections. Asian Cardiovasc Thorac Ann. 2021;29:532–40.
12. Walters SL, Canavan ME, Salazar MC, et al. A national study of surgically managed atypical pulmonary carcinoid tumors. Ann Thorac Surg. 2021;112:921–7.

Large Cell Carcinoma

Song Zhang

Pulmonary large cell carcinoma (LCC) is one of the three major histological subtypes of non-small cell lung cancer (NSCLC) along with adenocarcinoma and squamous cell carcinoma. With the development of pathological, genomic, and clinical progression, LCC has been reclassified into more specific pathological entities, resulting in LCC becoming one of the rarest subtypes of NSCLC.

1 Classification

In 1967, the first edition of the World Health Organization (WHO) classification of lung tumors was published and classified lung carcinoma into four categories: adenocarcinoma, squamous cell carcinoma, small cell carcinoma (SCLC), and LCC. LCC included those tumors that lacked characteristics of other lung cancer types, including the variant giant cell carcinoma, clear cell carcinoma, and LCC with mucin-like features.

In the 1981 WHO classification, the diagnosis of LCC with mucin-like content was reclassified under the adenocarcinoma category as solid carcinoma with mucus formation.

S. Zhang (✉)
Department of Respiratory and Critical Care Medicine, Shandong Provincial Hospital Affiliated to Shandong First Medical University, Jinan, Shandong, China

In the 1999 WHO classification, LCC included large-cell neuroendocrine carcinoma (LCNEC), lymphoepithelial-like carcinoma (LELC), and basaloid carcinoma. Giant cell carcinoma was removed as a variant.

In the 2004 WHO classification, LCC is considered a poorly differentiated or undifferentiated carcinoma of the lung lacking the cytologic and architectural features of small cell carcinoma and glandular or squamous differentiation. LCC included several variants such as LCNEC, basaloid carcinoma, lymphoepithelioma-like carcinoma, clear cell carcinoma, and LCC with rhabdoid phenotype. It acknowledged the close morphologic overlap between the undifferentiated form of LCC and solid subtype adenocarcinoma, and recommended the use of mucin stains to distinguish the two.

There was no role for immunohistochemistry (IHC) using adenocarcinoma or squamous markers in assessing these tumors in the 2004 WHO classification. However, some studies have shown that about 60%–70% of LCC should be considered as poorly differentiated adenocarcinoma, 10%–20% squamous cell carcinoma, and 5% LCNEC, only a small subset of LCC remain undifferentiated based on different immunohistochemical features.

The 2015 WHO classification emphasized the significance of immunohistochemical features in tumor classification. Solid-grown

S. Zhang (ed.), *Diagnostic Imaging of Lung Cancers*, https://doi.org/10.1007/978-981-99-6815-2_6

tumors were classified as solid adenocarcinoma, nonkeratinizing squamous cell carcinoma, and neuroendocrine carcinoma depending on the outcome of TTF-1 (with or without Napsin A), P40 (with or without cytokeratin 5/6), or neuroendocrine (chromogranin A, synaptophysin, CD56) marker staining, respectively. LCC subtypes from the 2004 WHO classification were reclassified as follows. LCNEC was moved to the neuroendocrine tumor group. Basaloid carcinoma was moved to a subtype of squamous cell carcinoma. Lymphoepithelioma-like carcinoma was moved to a group of other and unclassified carcinomas. Clear cell carcinoma and rhabdoid phenotype were regarded as a cytologic change rather than a specific histologic subtype. Only those NSCLC with negative or unclear immunophenotypes were classified as LCC with null immunohistochemical features.

2 Pathology

The entity LCC can only be diagnosed on surgical specimens, so this term should not be applied to small biopsies or cytological samples, where NSCLC lacking any specific morphologic criteria must be diagnosed as NSCLC, not otherwise specified (NSCLC-NOS).

Currently, the histopathological diagnosis of classic LCC is a tumor featuring round to polygonal cells, arranged in cohesive or even discohesive sheets or nests with prominent nucleoli and a moderate amount of cytoplasm, without the presence of differentiating features such as any gland or mucin formation seen in adenocarcinoma or small cells with scant cytoplasm, any keratinization or intercellular bridges seen in squamous cell carcinoma, and salt-and-pepper-type chromatin that would classify it as SCLC (Figs. 1a, b and 2a, b).

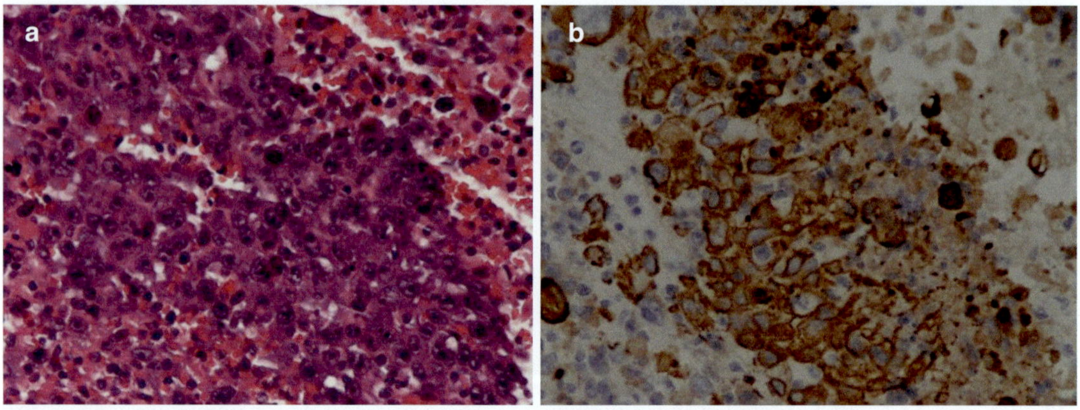

Fig. 1 (**a**) Hematoxylin-eosin staining of a large cell carcinoma. (**b**) CK immunostaining is positive

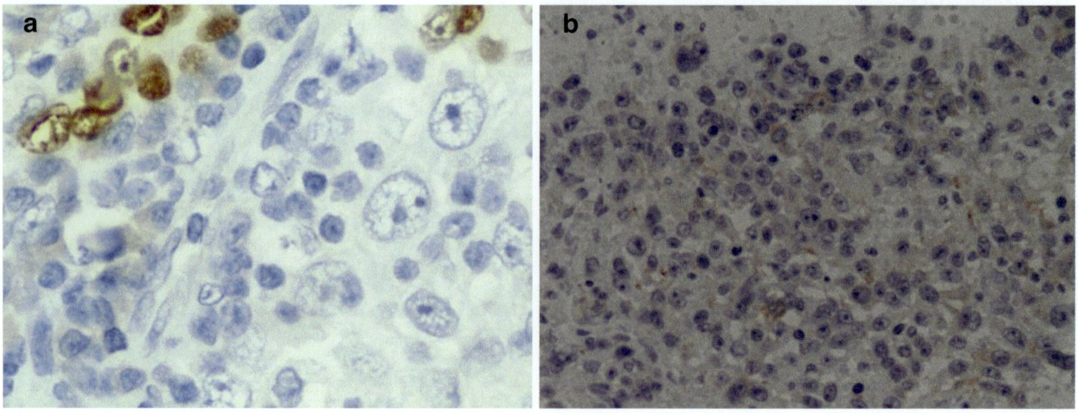

Fig. 2 (**a**) TTF-1 immunostaining is negative. (**b**) Synaptophysin immunostaining is negative

3 Radiographic Features

On CT, most of the LCC of the lung is similar to other common NSCLCs, often manifesting as a single, peripheral nodule or mass with irregular shape and margins. The tumor diameter often exceeded 4 cm, which is larger than that of lung adenocarcinoma, but no significant difference compared with lung squamous cell carcinoma. The lesion mostly has signs of lobulation without air bronchogram, bulky lymphadenopathy, cavitation, and calcification (Fig. 3). Inhomogeneous enhancement was seen in enhanced CT scan. LCC is prone to necrosis, which is closely related to its low degree of differentiation and rapid growth (Fig. 4). LCC has a high degree of malignancy and rapid proliferation (Fig. 5). In some cases, the pleura can be invaded, and regional lymph nodes and distant metastases can occur.

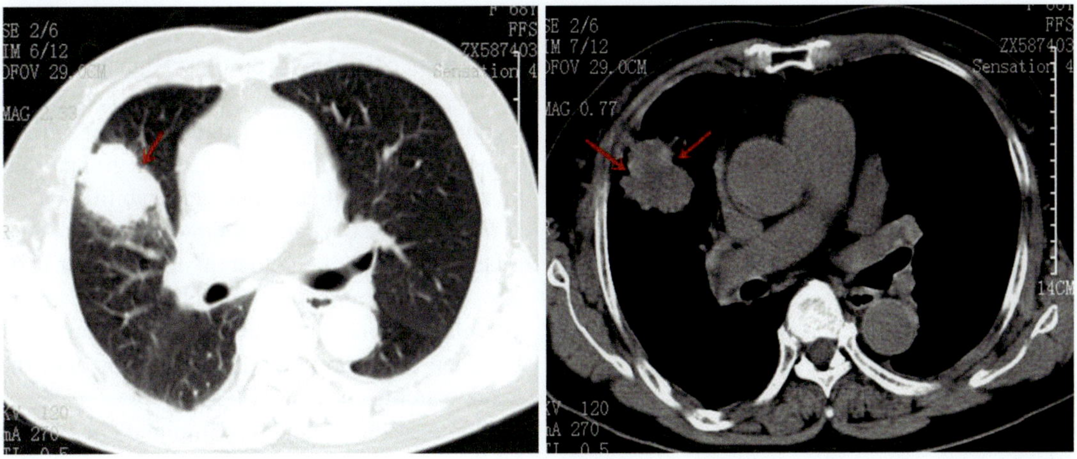

Fig. 3 Peripheral LCC in a 68-year-old man. CT scan shows a soft-tissue mass with deep lobulation (red arrow)

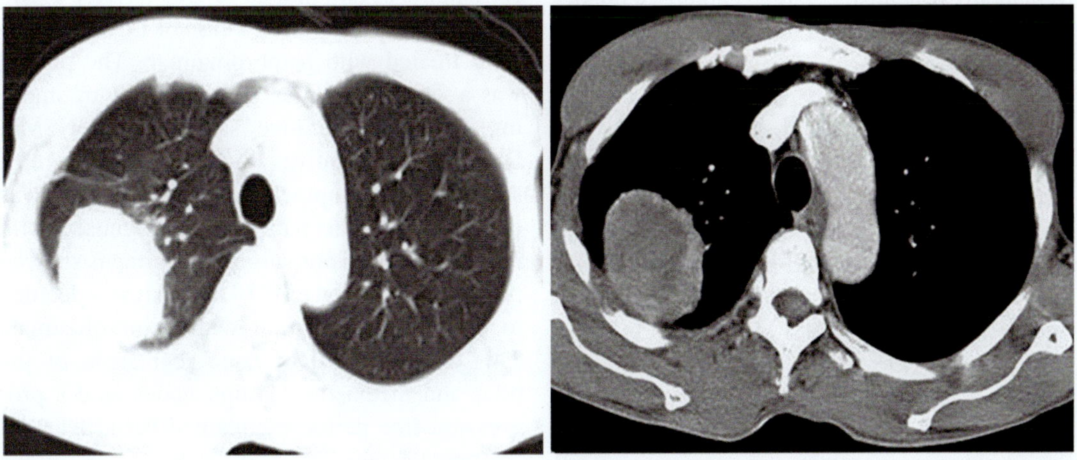

Fig. 4 Peripheral LCC in a 53-year-old man. Contrast-enhanced CT scan shows a soft-tissue mass with necrosis

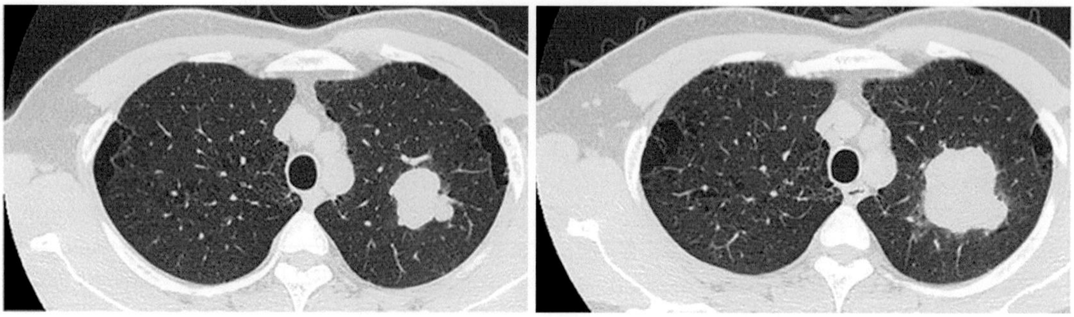

Fig. 5 Peripheral LCC in a 48-year-old man. CT scan shows a soft-tissue mass in the left upper lobe with significant increase after 1 month

4 Treatment

According to the diagnostic criteria of the 2015 WHO classification, the incidence of LCC has declined sharply. Currently, there are no standard treatment guidelines for LCC. Its options are generally based on the treatment experience of NSCLC. An operable tumor surgery is advocated for early stage LCCs. Chen et al. [1] reviewed a consecutive cohort of 789 resected NSCLC cases. They found that 59 cases (7.5%) lacked morphologic differentiation. According to the 2015 WHO lung tumor classification, these cases were identified and further characterized by immunohistochemistry. Molecular alterations were investigated by multiple technologies including immunohistochemistry, target capture sequencing, and fluorescence in situ hybridizations. With use of immunohistochemistry, 20 cases (33.9%) were reclassified as adenocarcinoma (LCC-AD), 14 (23.7%) were reclassified as squamous cell carcinoma (LCC-SqCC), and 25 (42.4%) remained LCC-Null. Characteristic alterations of adenocarcinoma (EGFR, KRAS, ALK, ROS1, and STK11) were detected in the LCC-AD subgroup but not in LCC-SqCC, whereas squamous-lineage alterations (PIK3CA, FGFR1, SOX2, and AKT1) were detected in the LCC-SqCC subgroup but not in the LCC-AD. Although some LCC-Null tumors exhibited a genetic profile similar to either adenocarcinoma or squamous cell carcinoma, more than half of the LCC-Null group were completely devoid of recognizable lineage-specific genetic profiles. High expression of programmed death-ligand 1 (PD-L1) and high frequency of cell cycle regulatory gene alterations were found in the LCC-Null group, suggesting potential therapeutic vulnerabilities. LCC is not sensitive to chemotherapy. To date, no specific or standard chemotherapy regimen for LCC has been recommended in NSCLC treatment guidelines. This comprehensive molecular study by Chen et al. provided further insight into the genetic architecture of LCC.

Some studies found that immune checkpoint inhibitors (ICIs) may be effective for LCC. Ooi et al. [2] reported an 80-year-old woman with pulmonary LCC who was successfully treated with pembrolizumab but developed sclerosing cholangitis as an immune-related adverse event. Okabe et al. [3] reported a case of LCC successfully treated with pembrolizumab. The patient was a 58-year-old man with a history of smoking. The postoperative stage was T3N2M0. During postoperative adjuvant chemotherapy, swelling of the supraclavicular lymph node was observed, and the patient was diagnosed with recurrence. Previous surgical specimens showed positive expression of PD-L1, and it was decided to commence treatment with pembrolizumab. This treatment led to rapid regression of the hilar and mediastinal lymph nodes, and a progression-free period maintained for at least 24 treatment cycles.

Treatment with ICIs may be an option for patients with PD-L1 positive LCC.

5 Prognosis

The prognosis of LCC depends on the tumor, node, and metastasis (TNM) staging at the time of diagnosis. LCC is prone to regional lymph node and distant metastasis and has always represented a histological type with poor prognosis. Patients with LCC was associated with significantly worse survival than patients with other histologic subtypes of NSCLC according to the new diagnostic criteria.

6 Case Analysis

6.1 Case

A 67-year-old man complained of hemoptysis for 1 month.

Chest CT (January 12, 2016): A nodule in the left upper lobe with a size of 1.68 × 1.87 cm, the CT attenuations of the three-phase dynamic scan were 38.8, 27.3, and 36.6 HU, respectively (Fig. 6).

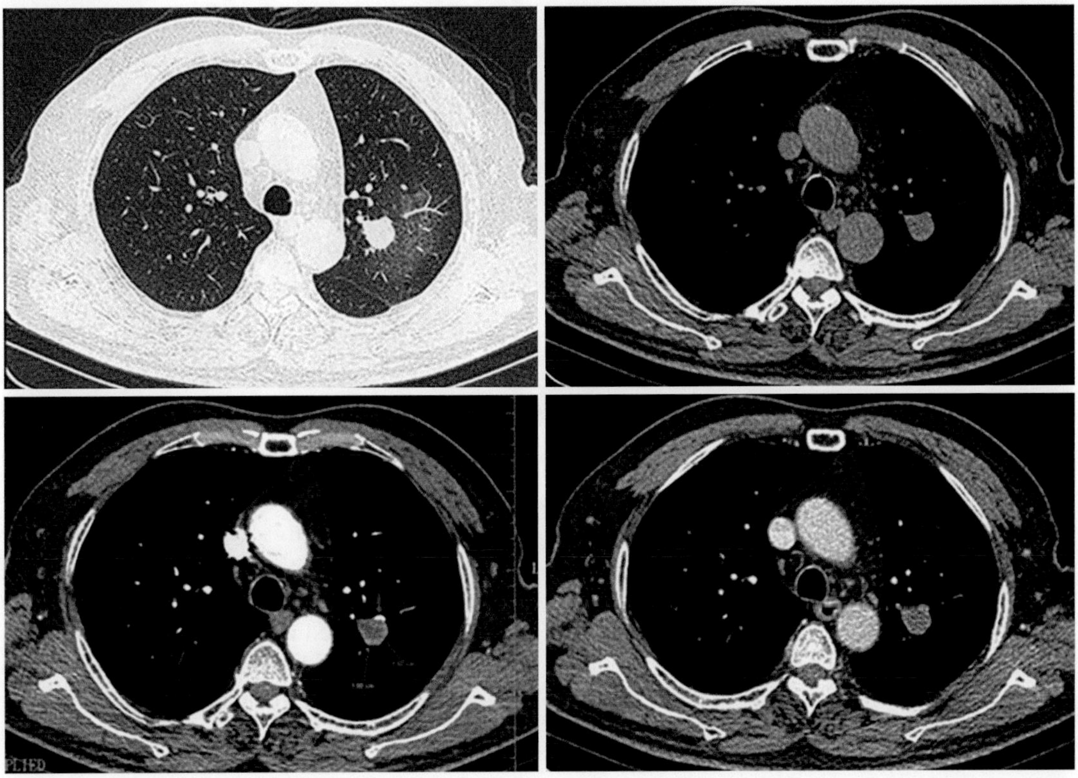

Fig. 6 Chest CT (January 12, 2016)

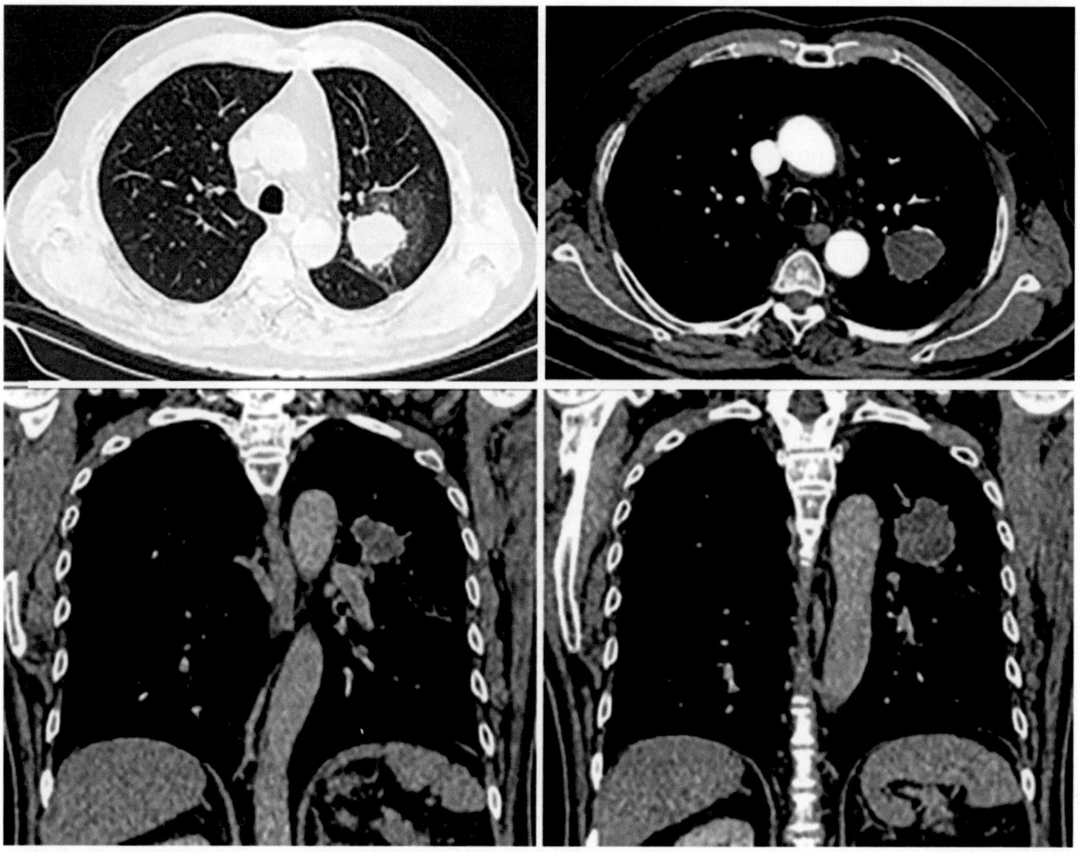

Fig. 7 Chest CT (March 30, 2016)

Chest CT (March 30, 2016): The lesion was significantly enlarged, with a size of 3.4 × 3.5 cm (Fig. 7).

[Diagnosis] Large cell carcinoma.

[Diagnosis Basis] The CT scan shows a nodule in the left upper lobe with obvious ground-glass opacity around it. Combined with the history of hemoptysis, the ground-glass opacity may be caused by bleeding. The lesion has an overlying vessel sign (red arrow); however, the enhancement pattern and degree of necrosis in this case do not support the diagnosis of sclerosing pneumocytoma. The lesions increased significantly in a short period of time, with remarkable lobulation (green arrow), supporting the diagnosis of lung cancer, especially SCLC and LCC. SCLC mostly has mediastinal lymph node metastasis in the early stage. Although the lesion is significantly enlarged in this case, the lymph node changes are not obvious, so this diagnosis of SCLC is not considered. LCC mostly occurs in elderly men, located in the periphery of the lung, mainly in the upper lobe, with necrosis and rapid proliferation. These characteristics are completely consistent with this case. The patient's postoperative pathology and immunohistochemistry were consistent with LCC.

[Analysis] Essentially, LCC is a diagnosis of exclusion, meaning non-adenomatous, non-squamous, and non-small cell lung cancer. Some studies confirmed that LCC mainly occurs in the elderly and is closely related to cigarette smoking. LCC is considered as a rapidly growing tumor. Kanashiki et al. [4] found that the mean volume doubling times (VDTs) in the patients with LCC were 134 days (median, 89 days; range, 32–361 days). In another study by

Henschke et al. [5], the median VDTs in the patients with large cell or neuroendocrine cancers were 82 days. According to the 2015 WHO classification criteria of lung tumor, the VDTs of LCC should be shorter.

Liu et al. [6] investigated the clinicopathological characteristics and genetic mutation statuses of Chinese LCC patients. Twenty-four surgically resected LCC patients previously diagnosed under the 2004 WHO criteria were reclassified under the 2015 WHO criteria. Eight patients were re-defined as LCCs, and sixteen patients were defined as non-LCCs under the refined criteria. All LCC patients were male, and seven patients were smokers. No significant differences were found in age, gender, smoking status, primary site, TNM staging, and overall survival between the LCC and non-LCC patients. 50% (4/8) of LCC patients presented TP53 mutations, and no somatic mutations were detected in the other four LCCs patients. For the 16 non-LCCs, not only TP53 and KRAS but also EGFR, PIK3CA, KIT, PTEN, IDH1, APC, ATM, and BRAF mutations were observed. In addition, LCCs without TP53 mutations did not exhibit any gene mutations under the 2004 or 2015 WHO criteria. Importantly, the patients with TP53 mutation presented a trend with a worse survival outcome at the time of follow-up. The new WHO diagnosis criteria have superior performance in precise molecular classification for LCC patients.

Xiaochuan et al. [7] retrospective analyzed 3197 LCC patients. There was a worse overall survival (OS) from LCC compared with other NSCLCs. LCC was more common in males, over age 60 and in the upper lobe. The proportion of stage III/IV in LCC was the highest, reaching 73.6%. The median OS of stage I-IV patients was 42, 22, 11, and 3 months, respectively. The elderly, males, later stage, and main bronchus location, or overlapping lesions were risk factors for survival prognosis. In stage I-III patients, treatment including surgery could significantly reduce the risk of death by 60% at least compared with no therapy. Surgery was still beneficial for stage IV patients if surgical resection involved more than one lobe. Surgery-based comprehensive treatments are effective for LCC.

References

1. Chan AW, Chau SL, Tong JH, et al. The landscape of actionable molecular alterations in immunomarker defined large-cell carcinoma of the lung. J Thorac Oncol. 2019;14:1213–22.
2. Ooi R, Tobino K, Sakabe M, et al. A case of large-cell lung carcinoma successfully treated with pembrolizumab but complicated with cholangitis. Respir Med Case Rep. 2020;31:101197.
3. Okabe N, Mine H, Takagi H, et al. Pulmonary large cell carcinoma, highly positive for PD-L1, shows marked response to pembrolizumab: A case report. Thorac Cancer. 2021:1141–4.
4. Kanashiki M, Tomizawa T, Yamaguchi I, et al. Volume doubling time of lung cancers detected in a chest radiograph mass screening program: comparison with CT screening. Oncol Lett. 2012;4:513–6.
5. Henschke CI, Yankelevitz DF, Yip R, et al. Lung cancers diagnosed at annual CT screening: volume doubling times. Radiology. 2012;263:578–83.
6. Liu R, Liu J, Shi T, et al. Clinicopathological and genetic characteristics of pulmonary large cell carcinoma under 2015 WHO classification: a pilot study. Oncotarget. 2017;8:100,754–63.
7. Xiaochuan L, Jiangyong Y, Ping Z, et al. Clinical characteristics and prognosis of pulmonary large cell carcinoma: a population-based retrospective study using SEER data. Thorac Cancer. 2020;11:1522–32.

Adenosquamous Carcinoma

Song Zhang

Adenosquamous carcinoma (ASC) is a mixed glandular and squamous cell carcinoma, accounting for a small proportion of cases of NSCLC.

1 Classification

Researchers have reached a consensus on the presence of defined components of adenocarcinomas (ADC) and squamous cell carcinoma (SCC) in ASC, but they have always disagreed on the cutoffs for the proportions of each component. In 1978, the first diagnostic criterion for ASC was published by the Japan Lung Cancer Society, ASC was defined as a tumor composed of at least 20% of each of SCC and ADC components. In the second edition of the WHO classification of lung tumors published in 1981, the proportion and differentiation between the two components of ASCs are not specified. In 1985, Fitzgibbons and Kern [1] retrospectively studied 1125 cases of lung carcinoma. Of the 21 patients initially diagnosed with ASC, only 7 patients (0.6%) were identified as ASC by strict application of histological diagnostic criteria. Five patients had died of the disease within 2 years of diagnosis, and two were short-term survivors. Another large retrospective study by Naunheim et al. [2] in 1987 showed a slightly higher incidence of ASC of 2.3% (20/873). The diagnostic criteria for the two series were similar. A major difference between the two series was the former consisted almost entirely of excised specimens, whereas the latter diagnosed on small biopsies. Takamori et al. [3] reported an incidence of 2.6% (56/2160) of ASC in a large series resection specimens of lung carcinoma. None of these studies relies on the application of ancillary research for diagnosis, particularly immunohistochemistry. In the 1999 WHO classification, the criteria for ASC were clearly defined for the first time, that is, it was considered a carcinoma containing components of both SCC and ADC, with each component comprising at least 10% of the tumor. Although this definition was still valid in the 2015 WHO classification, the biological and histogenetic properties of ASC further need to be clarified.

2 Pathology

In general, ASC should be determined by H&E staining or immunohistochemistry, and the diagnostic accuracy of cytology or tissue puncture is low. Damadoğlu et al. [4] retrospectively evaluated 13 patients with ASC confirmed by pathology. Preoperative pathological diagnosis was SCC in eight patients, adenocarcinoma in one

S. Zhang (✉)
Department of Respiratory and Critical Care Medicine, Shandong Provincial Hospital Affiliated to Shandong First Medical University,
Jinan, Shandong, China

S. Zhang (ed.), *Diagnostic Imaging of Lung Cancers*, https://doi.org/10.1007/978-981-99-6815-2_7

patient, and ASC in only four patients. Shimoji et al. [5] divided 21 postoperative ASCs into four subgroups based on the results of immunohistochemical staining for TTF-1 and p63: TTF-1+ and p63+ (10 cases), TTF-1- and p63+ (six cases), TTF-1+ and p63- (three cases), and TTF-1- and p63- (two cases). The study supported that ASC is a heterogeneous tumor.

Some studies confirmed that primary and metastatic sites showing one or the other histologic component, and even thorough sampling has failed to confirm biphasic histology. Shelton et al. [6] reported a solitary lung carcinoma case evaluated by bronchial brush and lavage cytology, bronchial biopsy, and pleural fluid cytology. Cytological evaluation of the pleural fluid demonstrated NSCLC and immunohistochemical staining confirmed a metastatic lung adenocarcinoma. The bronchial brush and lavage specimens, however, revealed the cytomorphological features of squamous cell carcinoma, which was confirmed by the bronchial biopsy. Although the dual population of malignant cells were not demonstrated in the same specimen in this case, this does not necessarily exclude the diagnosis of ASC. Burkart et al. [7] reported a young "light" ex-smoker (1-pack-year history of smoking) with a localized ASC bearing an epidermal growth factor receptor (EGFR) sensitizing mutation. CT scan showed a left upper lobe mass. Surgical pathology demonstrated an adenosquamous carcinoma with EGFR Exon 19 in-frame (18 bp) deletion. Six months after completion of adjuvant chemotherapy, he first recurred within the brain with a pure squamous histology and the same EGFR mutation. Surgical resection and postoperative focal radiotherapy rendered him disease-free. Eighteen months later, subsequent isolated recurrence within the lung was a pure adenocarcinoma, again with the same identified EGFR mutation with exon 19del type. Histologic changes (from adenosquamous to pure squamous to pure adenocarcinoma) have been described in some studies; however, EGFR tyrosine kinase inhibitor (TKI) was not used during the treatment, which eliminated the possibility of histological-type changes induced by small-molecule TKIs.

ASC contains different pathological subtypes, adding to the difficulty of diagnosis. Yamatani et al. [8] studied 30 ASC cases, 8 cases contained varying degrees of the mucoepidermoid carcinoma (MEC)-like component, and basal immunohistochemical examination showed p63-positive and TTF-1-negative. FISH analysis revealed no MAML2 gene rearrangement in the 8 cases. These unique ASCs may be either a novel ASC subtype originating from bronchial epithelium or variant-type MEC.

According to different proportions of the two components, Gawrychowski et al. [9] subdivided ASC into three groups: ADC-predominant (60%–90%) group, SCC-predominant (60%–90%) group, and a structure-balanced (the proportion of ADC and SCC is between 40% and 60%) group. Gawrychowski et al. [9] and Zhao et al. [10] have found that structure-balanced ASC was associated with better prognosis.

3 Molecular Features

ASC is not a simple mixture of ADC and SCC, but is a more complex carcinoma with distinct molecular phenotype.

Several studies have confirmed that ASC patients present EGFR and KRAS mutations in both components. Tochigi et al. [11] analyzed EGFR and KRAS mutations in 23 ASC cases. 3 cases (13%) expressed EGFR mutations, with 2 having identical mutation in the glandular and squamous elements. KRAS mutations were found in 3 cases (13%) in both histologic elements. EGFR mutations occur in ASC in the same percentages as in conventional adenocarcinoma in the Western population. KRAS mutations are less common.

Some studies found that biopsy of pure SCC (SCC without a detectable adenocarcinoma component) lacked the EGFR mutations. A study by Ohtsuka et al. [12] found that EGFR tyrosine kinase domain (TKD) mutations were detected in 1 of 7 (14%) SCCs with an adenocarcinoma component and 2 of 4 (50%) ASCs. In contrast, EGFR TKD mutations were not identified in 24 pure SCCs, 7 large-cell carcinomas, or 6 NSCLC cell lines excluding adenocarcinoma. The detection of EGFR mutations in small samples diagnosed as SCC could be a result of incomplete sampling of ASC.

Bastide et al. [13] performed a comparative transcriptome analysis on a series of nine ASC, five ADC, and five SCC induced in rats by radon exposure. The expression of some genes of ASC was similar to that of ADC or SCC. ASC could be considered as a mix of ADC and SCC, both in various proportions. However, ASC also exhibited a unique expression of some tumor-related genes, especially neuroendocrine differentiation and ERK-related pathway genes.

Shu et al. [14] retrospectively investigated the thymidylate synthase (TS) expression by immunohistochemistry in surgically resected cases. They found that the expression of TS in ASC roughly parallel that of SCC, but significantly exceeded that of ADC, instead of falling in between SCC and ADC. Furthermore, there was no prominent difference in TS expression between squamous and glandular components in ASC samples. Given high expression of TS in tumors makes the tumor resistant to pemetrexed, they extrapolated that pemetrexed may also have inferior clinical activity in ASC.

Lin et al. [15] evaluated 1021 cancer-related genes in 28 surgically resected ASCs by next-generation sequencing. The most frequent alterations included EGFR (79%), TP53 (68%), MAP3K1 (14%) mutations, EGFR amplifications (32%), and MDM2 amplifications (18%). 27 patients (96%) had shared variations between ADC and SCC, and pure SCC metastases were not found. The genomic ASC profiles by targeted sequencing looked more similar to classic ADC than SCC.

4 Histogenesis

There are currently three theories hypothesizing the origin of ASC: "collision" between ADC and SCC, "common precursors" theory, and transition between ADC and SCC.

The collision theory considers that ASC is the product of collision between separate independent foci of ADC and SCC. One study in hamster lung cancer model by Hammond et al. [16] suggested that ADC and SCC can be spatially separated into small nodules (<3.0 mm) but can collide and form larger lesions of both components. Yazawa et al. [17] reported an extremely rare case of primary collision lung cancer with two closely linked nodules. The tumor showed a tiny ground-glass opaque shadow suggesting atypical adenomatous hyperplasia 18 months prior to the operation. However, the tumor grew rapidly, and the resected tumor consisted of two closely located nodules. The tumor comprised three histological elements. The larger nodule consisted of well-differentiated adenocarcinomatous and moderately to poorly differentiated squamous cell carcinomatous elements, while the smaller nodule was composed of a large-cell neuroendocrine carcinomatous element with partial squamoid differentiation having focal continuity with the adenocarcinomatous element. Both the adenocarcinomatous and squamous cell carcinomatous elements revealed transitional features and loss of heterozygosity (LOH) of human androgen receptor (AR) and phosphoglycerate kinase (PGK-1) genes, while the large cell neuroendocrine carcinomatous element showed a monoclonal pattern but had both alleles for AR and PGK-1. The histological morphology of the two nodules was very different, and LOH detection further confirmed that the two nodules were not single cloned sources.

The common precursors theory is that ASC originated from common precursors, but differentiated into different tissue forms in the course of disease. Some studies supported this theory through the analysis of chromosome linkage polymorphism markers, LOH detection, or EGFR/RAS mutation characteristics. Niho et al. [18] analyzed the clonality of ASC from four female patients based on an X-chromosome-linked polymorphic marker, the human androgen receptor gene. SCC and ADC components showed identical monoclonal patterns in all four patients. The results suggested that the two components originated from the same precursor. ASC contains a mixture of cells with squamous (cytokeratin 5+) and adenocarcinoma (cytokeratin 7+)

phenotypes. Mather et al. [19] isolated the ASC specific cancer stem-like cells (CSLC) co-expressing CK5+CK7+ and cultured them in vitro, and grafted these cells into immune-deficient mice. These cells could successfully differentiate into SCC- and ADC-like components in mice, and had the potential to differentiate into tracheal, alveolar, or neuroendocrine cells. Therefore, ASC may originate from a primitive lung stem cell, and not from the bronchial-alveolar or basal stem cells. Vassella et al. [20] assessed the mutational profile in each component among 16 Caucasian ASC samples by next-generation sequencing (NGS), fluorescence in situ hybridization (FISH), and laser capture microdissection (LCM). The results showed that several molecular mutant phenotypes were similar between the two components. Driver mutations were predominantly in the trunk, suggesting a monoclonal origin of ASC.

The transition theory suggested that ASC is a transitional stage between ADC and SCC. Tsuhako et al. [21] found human papillomavirus (HPV) DNA expression in a high proportion (78.3%) of surgically resected ASC samples in Okinawa. The adenocarcinoma cells adjacent to the squamous cell carcinoma component were enlarged and positive for HPV, high molecular weight cytokeratin (HMC), and involucrin, indicating the transition from ADC to SCC. Kanazawa et al. [22] compared the distinct components of 12 lung ASCs by genetic alterations of p53 and K-ras, chromosomal abnormalities at 9p21 and 9q31–32, and immunohistochemical reactions. They found overexpression of p53 gene in both components of ASC and in the transitional areas. Moreover, chromosome abnormalities at 9p21 and 9q31–32 also existed in the two components. Higher expression of SCC-related antigen and lower expression of Mucin 1(an antigen predominantly expressed in ADC) were found in ADC component. These results suggested monoclonal transition from SCC to ADC in lung ASC. Han et al. [23] demonstrated that Lkb1-deficient ADC can progressively transdifferentiate into SCC in mouse models, suggesting that ASC is an intermediate step for the process of lung ADC to SCC. Krause et al. [24] first applied whole-exome sequencing (WES) to evaluate the clonal evolution of ASC. Identified truncal mutations included the pan-cancer tumor-suppressor gene TP53, as well as EGFR, BRAF, and MET, which are characteristic for ADC but uncommon in SCC. No truncated mutations were found for classical SCC driver mutations. Truncal chromosomal copy number aberrations shared by all of ASCs included losses of 3p, 15q, and 19p, and an amplified region in 5p. Furthermore, they detected loss of STK11 and SOX2 amplification in ASC, which has previously been confirmed to drive transdifferentiation from ADC to SCC in preclinical mouse models. This study provided strong evidence that the two components of ASC share a common origin and that the ADC component appears to transform to SCC.

5 Clinical Features

ASC is a relatively rare subtype of lung carcinoma, accounting for 0.4%–4% of all lung cancers. It usually occurs at an age over 60 years and displays male predominance and those with smoking history.

Studies found that central ASC usually had main components of SCC, and may resemble to central SCC, while peripheral ASC generally had main components of ADC and may behave like peripheral ADC. Its clinical and biological behaviors may also depend on the predominant histologic component.

6 Radiographic Features

Imaging of ASC lacks specificity. Lesion is more common in the periphery. Ground-glass opacity, lobulation, spiculation, and pleural tail sign are similar to those of lung adenocarcinoma (Fig. 1). Calcification occurs occasionally. Cavitation and intratumoral necrosis are common (Fig. 2). Regional lymph nodes and distant metastases can occur (Fig. 3).

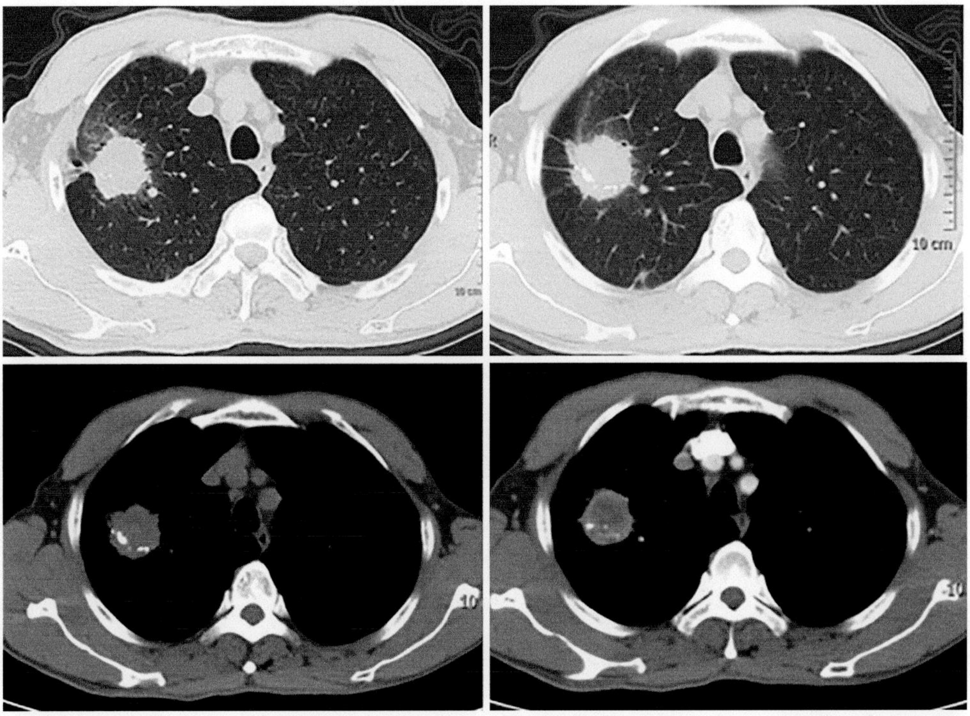

Fig. 1 Peripheral ASC in a 62-year-old man. Contrast-enhanced CT scan shows a soft-tissue mass in the right upper lung with ground-glass opacity, lobulation, spiculation, pleural tail, calcification, and necrosis

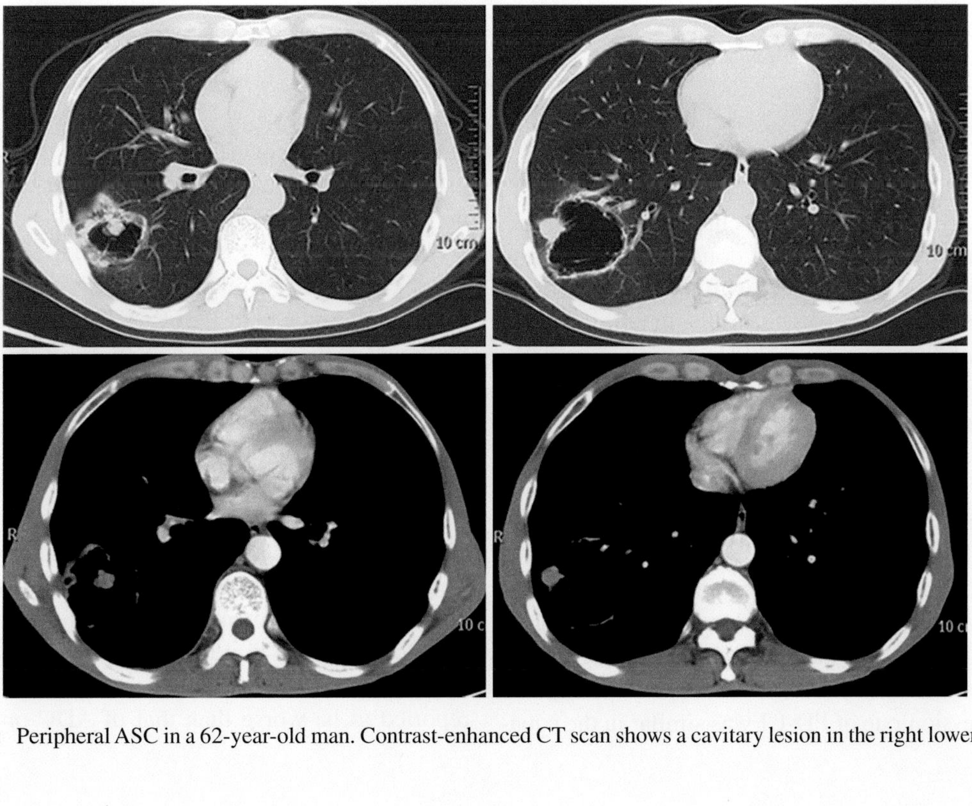

Fig. 2 Peripheral ASC in a 62-year-old man. Contrast-enhanced CT scan shows a cavitary lesion in the right lower lung

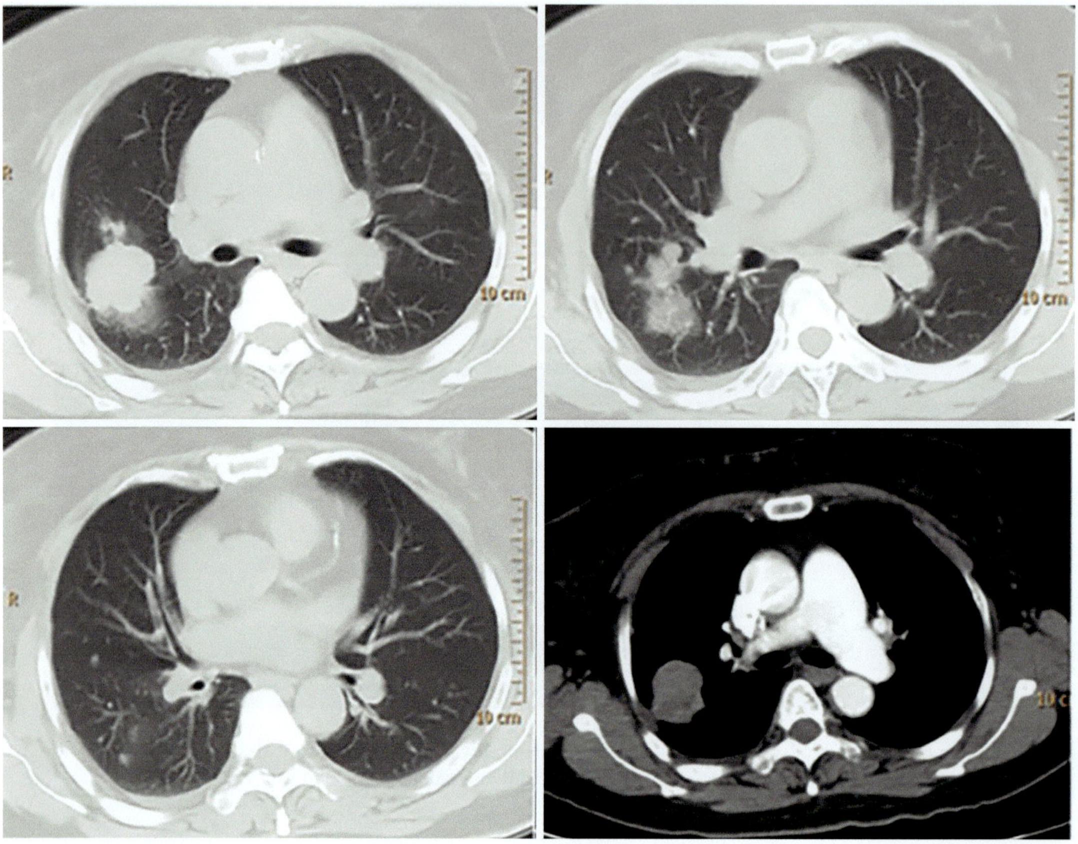

Fig. 3 Peripheral ASC with pleural and intrapulmonary metastasis in a 57-year-old woman. The pathology of metastatic carcinoma is adenocarcinoma

7 Treatment

Surgery is the mainstay in curing ASC, and postoperative platinum-based doublet chemotherapy is preferred for patients with stages IA–IIIB in order to improve patient survival and reduce the risk of distant metastases. There is no specific or standard chemotherapy regimen for ASC, and current treatment options rely on the NSCLC guidelines. Targeted treatments can be considered as first-line therapy for advanced EGFR-mutant or ALK-rearranged ASC. Immune checkpoint blockade therapy has provided a new means for the treatment of malignant tumors in recent years. Shi et al. [25] evaluated the expression of PD-L1 in patients with ASC using immunohistochemistry and in situ hybridization. The expression rate of PD-L1 was similar in the squamous cell component of ASCs and lung SCC (38.89% vs. 28.92%), so does the adenocarcinoma component of ASCs and lung adenocarcinomas (11.11% vs 13.53%). PD-L1 expression was significantly correlated with lymphovascular invasion, but not with EGFR, KRAS, and ALK mutations in lung ASCs. It may be feasible to recommend PD-L1 testing in ASC patients.

8 Prognosis

The prognosis of ASC is related to pathological staining, surgical treatment, choice of adjuvant chemotherapy regimen, and the basic condition of patients. ASC is rapidly developing and highly aggressive, and the prognosis of ASC has been reported to be worse than that of ADC or SCC alone, with 5-year survival for all stages ranging from 6% to 33%, regardless of their treatments.

Cooke et al. [26] reported that the 5-year survival of patients with stage I and II ASC after lobectomy was 59.4%. Filosso et al. [27] retrospectively analyzed 48 ASC patients at all stages. The 3- and 5-year survival rates of patients with ASC undergoing complete tumor resection were only 25% and 15%, respectively. Overall survival of ASC was worse than ADC or SCC. 3- and 5-year survival rates of ASC stage I were similar to those of stage IIIA ADC or SCC. More than half of the ASC patients developed distant metastases (MTS) or local recurrences. The presence of distant metastases, tumor perineural invasion, and tumor stage were factors associated with poor prognosis. Maeda et al. [28] retrospectively analyzed 4668 postoperative cases in Japan, including 114 cases of ASC (2.4%), 2993 cases of ADC (64.2%), and 1369 cases of SCC (29.3%). The results showed that the 5-year survival rate was 23.3% for ASC patients, 58% for ADC patients, and 40.8% for SCC patients. They found that sex, age, performance status, histology, tumor size, p-stage, operative method, and neoadjuvant/adjuvant therapy were independent prognostic factors. Liang et al. [29] retrospectively analyzed 4600 ASC patients in China. They found that age, sex, primary site of tumor, histological grade, TNM stage of the tumor, surgery to the primary site of tumors, and chemotherapy were independent risk factors for ASC patients.

In the future, more research is needed to improve the therapeutic effect and prognosis of ASC.

9 Case Analysis

9.1 Case

A 71-year-old man complained of hemoptysis for 1 week.

Chest CT: A irregular mass in right upper lobe (Fig. 4).

[Diagnosis] Peripheral adenosquamous carcinoma.

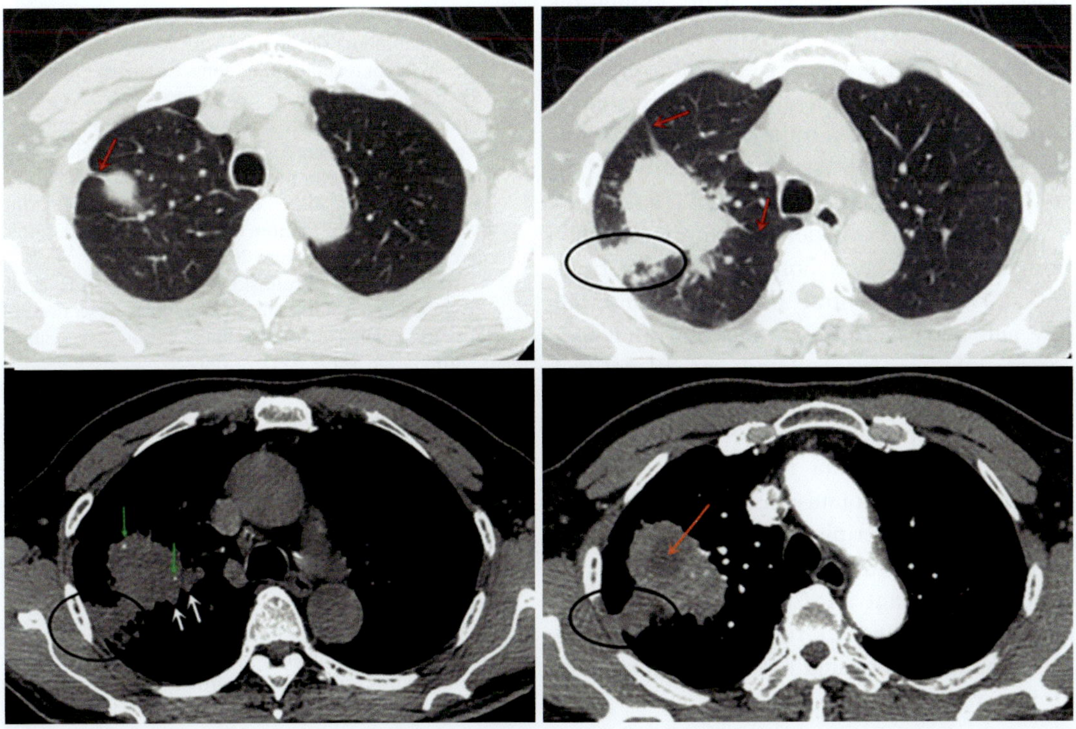

Fig. 4 Chest CT

[Diagnosis Basis] An elderly male has a history of hemoptysis. The lesion is a large irregular mass with punctate calcification (green arrow), heterogeneous enhancement, central necrosis (orange arrow), and obstructive pneumonia (black circle), which are consistent with the CT features of squamous cell carcinoma. The lesions also have ground-glass opacity, lobulation, burrs, spinous processes (white arrows), and pleural indentation (red arrows), which are in line with the characteristics of adenocarcinoma, so the possibility of lung squamous cell carcinoma or adenosquamous carcinoma is considered. The postoperative pathology of the patient was adenosquamous carcinoma (about 20% with adenocarcinoma and 80% with squamous cell carcinoma), invading the bronchus, visceral pleura, and mediastinal lymph nodes.

[Analysis] Chest CT scan shows that ASC is more likely to appear peripheral rather than central. Yu et al. [30] evaluated the correlation between CT morphological and histopathological features. The tumor was peripheral in 21 (72%) and central in 8 (28%) cases. The most common CT features were lobulation (93%), pleural tail (76%), spiculation (59%), necrosis (52%), and vessel convergence (45%). The peripheral tumor manifested a higher proportion of intratumoral necrosis and heterogeneous soft-tissue attenuation. Lee et al. [31] evaluated CT and FDG PET features of 26 patients who underwent surgical resection of ASC. ASC was more commonly peripheral (80%) than central and showed internal low and heterogeneous attenuation and possesses lobulated, spiculated, or ill-defined margin on CT. Watanabe et al. [32] found that ASC patients presented with centrally located obstructive pneumonia typical of SCC and with peripheral ground-glass opacity typical of lepidic ADC. Peripheral ground-glass opacity could be one of the predictive markers of ADC-predominant ASC. Tumor size that exceeded 5 cm and CT findings of inflammatory changes surrounding the tumor were strong predictors of poor prognosis.

In summary, the imaging findings of ASC can suggest some characteristics, but no obvious features were found to differentiate it from ADC and SCC.

References

1. Fitzgibbons PL, Kern WH. Adenosquamous carcinoma of the lung: a clinical and pathologic study of seven cases. Hum Pathol. 1985;16:463–6.
2. Naunheim KS, Taylor JR, Skosey C, et al. Adenosquamous lung carcinoma: clinical characteristics, treatment, and prognosis. Ann Thorac Surg. 1987;44:462–6.
3. Takamori S, Noguchi M, Morinaga S, et al. Clinicopathologic characteristics of adenosquamous carcinoma of the lung. Cancer. 1991;67:649–54.
4. Damadoğlu E, Aybatli A, Yalçinsoy M, et al. Adenosquamous carcinoma of the lung (an analysis of 13 cases). Tuberk Toraks. 2005;53:161–6.
5. Shimoji M, Nakajima T, Yamatani C, et al. A clinicopathological and immunohistological re-evaluation of adenosquamous carcinoma of the lung. Pathol Int. 2011;61:717–22.
6. Shelton DA, Rana DN, Holbrook M, et al. Adenosquamous carcinoma of the lung diagnosed by cytology? A diagnostic dilemma. Diagn Cytopathol. 2012;40:830–3.
7. Burkart J, Shilo K, Zhao W, et al. Metastatic squamous cell carcinoma component from an adenosquamous carcinoma of the lung with identical epidermal growth factor receptor mutations. Case Rep Pulmonol. 2015;2015:283,875.
8. Yamatani C, Abe M, Shimoji M, et al. Pulmonary adenosquamous carcinoma with mucoepidermoid carcinoma-like component with characteristic p63 staining pattern: either a novel subtype originating from bronchial epithelium or variant mucoepidermoid carcinoma. Lung Cancer. 2014;84:45–50.
9. Gawrychowski J, Brulinski K, Malinowski E, et al. Prognosis and survival after radical resection of primary adenosquamous lung carcinoma. Eur J Cardiothorac Surg. 2005;27:686–92.
10. Zhao H, Yang H, Yao F, et al. Improved survival associated with a balanced structure between adenomatous and squamous components in patients with adenosquamous carcinoma of the lung. Eur J Surg Oncol. 2016;42(11):1699–706.
11. Tochigi N, Dacic S, Nikiforova M, et al. Adenosquamous carcinoma of the lung: a microdissection study of KRAS and EGFR mutational and amplification status in a western patient population. Am J Clin Pathol. 2011;135:783–9.
12. Ohtsuka K, Ohnishi H, Fujiwara M, et al. Abnormalities of epidermal growth factor receptor in lung squamous-cell carcinomas, adenosquamous car-

cinomas, and large-cell carcinomas: tyrosine kinase domain mutations are not rare in tumors with an adenocarcinoma component. Cancer. 2007;109:741–50.
13. Bastide K, Ugolin N, Levalois C, et al. Are adenosquamous lung carcinomas a simple mix of adenocarcinomas and squamous cell carcinomas, or more complex at the molecular level? Lung Cancer. 2010;68:1–9.
14. Shu C, Cheng H, Wang A, et al. Thymidylate synthase expression and molecular alterations in adenosquamous carcinoma of the lung. Mod Pathol. 2013;26:239–46.
15. Lin G, Li C, Li PS, et al. Genomic origin and EGFR-TKI treatments of pulmonary adenosquamous carcinoma. Ann Oncol. 2020;31:517–24.
16. Hammond WG, Tesluk H, Benfield JR. Histogenesis of adenosquamous bronchogenic carcinoma. Cancer Lett. 1995;96:163–8.
17. Yazawa T, Ishii H, Ito T, et al. Colliding primary lung cancers of adenosquamous carcinoma and large cell neuroendocrine carcinoma. Pathol Int. 2003;53:58–65.
18. Niho S, Yokose T, Kodama T, et al. Clonal analysis of adenosquamous carcinoma of the lung. Jpn J Cancer Res. 1999;90:1244–7.
19. Mather JP, Roberts PE, Pan Z, et al. Isolation of cancer stem like cells from human adenosquamous carcinoma of the lung supports a monoclonal origin from a multipotential tissue stem cell. PLoS One. 2013;8:e79456.
20. Vassella E, Langsch S, Dettmer MS, et al. Molecular profiling of lung adenosquamous carcinoma: hybrid or genuine type? Oncotarget. 2015;6:23905–16.
21. Tsuhako K, Nakazato I, Hirayasu T, et al. Human papillomavirus DNA in adenosquamous carcinoma of the lung. J Clin Pathol. 1998;51:741–9.
22. Kanazawa H, Ebina M, Ino-Oka N, et al. Transition from squamous cell carcinoma to adenocarcinoma in adenosquamous carcinoma of the lung. Am J Pathol. 2000;156:1289–98.
23. Han X, Li F, Fang Z, et al. Transdifferentiation of lung adenocarcinoma in mice with Lkb1 deficiency to squamous cell carcinoma. Nat Commun. 2014;5:3261.
24. Krause A, Roma L, Lorber T, et al. Deciphering the clonal relationship between glandular and squamous components in adenosquamous carcinoma of the lung using whole exome sequencing. Lung Cancer. 2020;150:132–8.
25. Shi X, Wu S, Sun J, et al. PD-L1 expression in lung adenosquamous carcinomas compared with the more common variants of non-small cell lung cancer. Sci Rep. 2017;7:46,209.
26. Cooke DT, Nguyen DV, Yang Y, et al. Survival comparison of adenosquamous, squamous cell, and adenocarcinoma of the lung after lobectomy. Ann Thorac Surg. 2010;9:943–8.
27. Filosso PL, Ruffini E, Asioli S, et al. Adenosquamous lung carcinomas: a histologic subtype with poor prognosis. Lung Cancer. 2011;74:25–9.
28. Maeda H, Matsumura A, Kawabata T, et al. Adenosquamous carcinoma of the lung: surgical results as compared with squamous cell and adenocarcinoma cases. Eur J Cardiothorac Surg. 2012;41:357–61.
29. Liang J, Sui Q, Zheng Y, et al. A nomogram to predict prognosis of patients with lung adenosquamous carcinoma: a population-based study. J Thorac Dis. 2020;12:2288–303.
30. Yu JQ, Yang ZG, Austin JH, et al. Adenosquamous carcinoma of the lung: CT-pathological correlation. Clin Radiol. 2005;60:364–9.
31. Lee Y, Chung JH, Kim SE, et al. Adenosquamous carcinoma of the lung: CT, FDG PET, and clinicopathologic findings. Clin Nucl Med. 2014;39:107–12.
32. Watanabe Y, Tsuta K, Kusumoto M, et al. Clinicopathologic features and computed tomographic findings of 52 surgically resected adenosquamous carcinomas of the lung. Ann Thorac Surg. 2014;97:245–51.

Sarcomatoid Carcinoma

Song Zhang

Pulmonary sarcomatoid carcinoma (PSC) is a heterogeneous category of malignant neoplasm accounting for less than 1% of all primary lung cancers. It may contain both carcinomatous and sarcomatous components and recognizes 5 types: pleomorphic carcinoma, spindle cell carcinoma, giant cell carcinoma, carcinosarcoma, and pulmonary blastoma.

1 Classification

The term giant cell carcinoma was proposed by Nash and Stout in 1958 [1], who described 5 autopsy cases. The 1981 WHO classification of lung tumors regarded these tumors showing a prevalence of spindle or giant cells as morphologic variants of squamous cell carcinomas and large cell carcinomas, respectively, and defined carcinosarcomas as biphasic tumors comprising an intimate admixtures of carcinoma and sarcoma.

In 1994, the term pleomorphic (spindle/giant cell) carcinoma was first introduced by Fishback et al. [2] to indicate a specific tumor category and not simply a bizarre cell-containing tumor, including unusual variants previously defined inflammatory sarcomatoid carcinoma and pseudoangiosarcomatous carcinoma (so-called pseudovascular adenoid squamous cell carcinoma). They studied 78 cases of pleomorphic (spindle and/or giant cell) carcinoma of the lung by light microscopy and immunohistochemistry to establish clinical, gross, and histologic parameters. Histologically, foci of squamous cell carcinoma were present in 8% of the tumors, large cell carcinoma in 25%, and adenocarcinoma in 45%. Only 22% of tumors were completely spindle and/or giant cell carcinomas. Both spindle cell carcinoma and giant cell carcinoma were found in 38% of patients. The presence of nodal metastases was the most significant single prognostic factor, whereas the presence of squamous or adenocarcinomatous differentiation did not have an impact on length of survival. So spindle and giant cell carcinomas are best regarded as one type of lung cancer called pleomorphic carcinoma.

The 1999 WHO classification of lung and pleural tumors declared that there existed "a group of poorly differentiated NSCLC containing a component of sarcoma or sarcoma-like elements" encompassing 5 different histological subtypes: carcinomas with spindle and/or giant cells (pleomorphic carcinoma, spindle cell carcinoma, and giant cell carcinoma), carcinosarcomas, and pulmonary blastomas.

In the 2004 WHO classification of lung tumors, the more generic designation of sarcomatoid carcinoma was adopted and it was defined as

S. Zhang (✉)
Department of Respiratory and Critical Care Medicine, Shandong Provincial Hospital Affiliated to Shandong First Medical University, Jinan, Shandong, China

S. Zhang (ed.), *Diagnostic Imaging of Lung Cancers*, https://doi.org/10.1007/978-981-99-6815-2_8

poorly differentiated NSCLC that has a histological appearance in dating mesenchymal differentiation, including five main variants, namely pleomorphic carcinoma, spindle cell carcinoma, giant cell carcinoma, carcinosarcoma, and pulmonary blastoma.

The diagnostic criteria/terminology for PSCs had no changes in the 2015 WHO classification of lung tumors, but recommended molecular testing with histological findings.

According to this criteria, the occurrence of SCLC or LCNEC with sarcoma or sarcoma-like component is considered a combined variant into the category of neuroendocrine neoplasms rather than PSC showing small cell and/or large cell neuroendocrine components.

2 Pathology

Determining the tissue of origin and pathological subtype of PSC is challenging. The diagnosis of PSC requires a surgical specimen, which can be supplemented with immunohistochemistry and electron microscopy. In some cases of PSC, areas typical of NSCLC can be identified, revealing the true epithelial nature of the tumor. Most sarcomatoid carcinoma cases also retain some degree of cytokeratin expression by immunohistochemistry, which aids in the differential diagnosis from true sarcoma. Differentiated and even sarcomatoid areas may also retain expression of immunohistochemical markers typical of lung adenocarcinoma or squamous cell carcinoma, such as TTF-1 or p40.

Pleomorphic carcinoma is defined as a poorly differentiated NSCC, namely adenocarcinoma, squamous cell carcinoma, or undifferentiated NSCC that contains at least 10% spindle and/or giant cells or a carcinoma consisting only of spindle and giant cells. The spindle cells are generally arranged haphazardly in a fascicular or storiform pattern. Adenocarcinoma represents the most frequent finding, up to 73% of the cases.

Spindle cell carcinoma and giant cell carcinoma are almost entirely composed of spindle-shaped and pleomorphic, multi- and/or mononucleated giant cells, respectively, with no differentiated carcinomatous elements. The spindle cells frequently form irregular fascicles and cohesive nests with nuclear hyperchromasia and may also be associated with prominent inflammatory stroma. Vascular invasion is common in spindle cell carcinoma. The giant cells are discohesive and have distinct nucleoli compared with spindle cell carcinoma. These giant cells have abundant eosinophilic cytoplasm, frequently with leukocyte emperipolesis and can also have a significant inflammatory component.

Carcinosarcoma is a mixture of NSCLC and true sarcomatous elements (rhabdomyosarcoma, osteosarcoma, chondrosarcoma, leiomyosarcoma, liposarcoma, angiosarcoma, or combinations of these elements). Carcinosarcoma differs from pleomorphic carcinoma based on these heterologous components. The most common type of epithelial cell histology is squamous cell carcinoma, followed by adenocarcinoma and adenosquamous carcinoma, whereas rhabdomyosarcoma is the most frequently mesenchymal component, followed by osteosarcoma and chondrosarcoma.

Pulmonary blastoma is defined as a biphasic tumor that consists of fetal adenocarcinoma (low grade/well differentiated) and primitive mesenchymal stroma, which occasionally has foci of differentiated sarcoma (osteosarcoma, chondrosarcoma, or rhabdomyosarcoma).

3 Molecular Features

Some studies have evidenced that PSC shown a mutational profile similar to high grade pulmonary adenocarcinomas, including a high rate of TP53 and KRAS mutations, along with occasional mutations in NRAS, STK11, PIK3CA, and NOTCH1, and rare mutations in ALK and EGFR. In 2015, Fallet et al. [3] first used mass spectrometry to test 114 surgical biopsies from 81 patients with PSC for 214 mutations affecting 26 oncogenes and tumor suppressor genes. They reported mutations in KRAS (27.2%), EGFR (22.2%), TP53 (22.2%), STK11 (7.4%), NOTCH1 (4.9%), NRAS (4.9%), and PI3KCA (4.9%). Pe'cuchet et al. [4] carried out whole-exome sequencing in 15 PSC patients with a history of smoking. They classified these patients into two distinct groups based on mutational signatures: one with tobacco-associated mutations including RAS/MAP2K1 mutations and strong PD-L1 expression, and one with APOBEC enzyme and homologous recombination deficiency, associated with not only MET yet also EGFR, BRCA1/BRCA2, and IDH1 alterations. The patients with the tobacco-associated signature also had a poorer overall survival. Zhou et al. [5] investigated the genomic and immunologic profiles of pure PSC in the Chinese population. 45% of patients with pure PSC harbored at least one actionable alteration. TP53 was the most frequent mutation (74.1%), followed by KRAS (24%), SMARCA4 (14%), MET (12%), EGFR (10%), MLL4 (10%), NF1 (10%), NOTCH4 (10%), and TERT (10%). More than 60% of patients (65.5%, 38/58) had either PD-L1-positive, MSI-H, or high-TMB tumors, 26 patients (45%) had PD-L1-positive tumors (≥1%), and 14 (24%) had high PD-L1 expression (≥50%), and these might derive survival benefits from immune checkpoint inhibitors. The study by Yang et al. [6] also showed that TP53 was the most frequently mutated gene (78.6%), followed by CDKN2A (28.6%) and MYC (25.0%). The pan-cancer analysis reveals high tumor mutation burden and leukocyte fraction of PSC. Schrock et al. [7] performed a deep sequencing approach to map whole-exome mutations in a cohort of 125 PSCs. TP53 genomic alterations were identified in 73.6% of cases, followed by KRAS (34.4%), MET (13.6%), EGFR (8.8%), BRAF (7.2%), HER2 (1.6%), and RET (0.8%). MET alterations were most frequent in exon 14 skipping mutations (15 cases, including one with concurrent MET amplification), MET amplification alone (one case), and H1094L (one case). MET exon 14 alterations were enriched in PSC (12%, 15/125) compared with non-PSC NSCLCs (3%) and were more prevalent in PSC cases with an adenocarcinoma component. In summary, the gene mutation pattern in PSC is different from that in NSCLC. The observed mutations are mainly MET exon 14, while EGFR and ALK mutations are less common.

Previous studies have suggested that most of the tumors containing carcinoma and sarcomatous or sarcomatoid elements are considered monoclonal growths (divergent hypothesis) rather than collision tumors (convergent hypothesis). PSC may be an epithelial neoplasm derived from a single clonal tissue. Biphasic PSCs are potentially derived from epithelial-mesenchymal transition (EMT), particularly tumors composed of spindle and giant cells. EMT is a process that epithelial cells acquire a spindle cell morphology because of the loss of their cell-cell adhesion and polarity. Arshi et al. [8] first reported a case of histopathologic sarcomatoid transformation of lung squamous cell carcinoma after neoadjuvant therapy, which verified the EMT process.

More than half of specimens of PSC patients express PD-L1. Shimoji et al. [9] found that PD-L1 expression was associated with high proliferative activity and the EMT phenotype in pulmonary adenocarcinoma but not in squamous cell carcinoma. PD-L1 expression was a significant poor prognostic factor in lung adenocarcinoma patients. Vieira et al. [10] found that the presence of KRAS mutations, blood vessel invasion, and tumor CD163+ macrophage infiltration was associated with PD-L1 expression in PSC. The association between PD-L1 expression and KRAS mutation could be explained by heavier smoking in PSC patients. On multivariate analysis, only blood vessel invasion and CD163+ macrophages were associated with tumoral PD-L1 expression. High levels of tumor-infiltrating lymphocytes (CD3+ or CD4+ and not CD8+) constituted a factor of good prognosis on survival. A possible explanation is that PD-L1 expression is associated with the exhaustion of lymphocytes and that PD-L1 activation is an adaptive method of tumor resistance to cytokine producing tumor-infiltrating lymphocytes rather than an aberrant cell signaling. PD-L1 expression was higher in PSC than in NSCLC as well as immune-cell infiltration by macrophages and TCD3 cells. Dix et al. [11] found that patients with past history of smoking were more likely to express PD-L1 in tumor cells and less likely to have PD-L1 positive intratumoral immune cells than those who never smoked.

4 Clinical Features

Except for pediatric pulmonary blastoma, most patients were male over 60 years, and had a history of moderate to heavy smoking. Exposure to asbestos is also a significant risk factor for PSC. Their ratio male-to-female is approximately 4:1. Some studies have shown that the disease occurs more frequently in Caucasians than in other ethnicities. Patients often present with non-specific symptoms, including coughing, chest discomfort, chest pain, and hemoptysis.

5 Radiographic Features

PSCs are mostly peripheral and located in the upper lobes (Fig. 1). Most tumors are larger than 3 cm with extensive necrosis and hemorrhage. Irregular thick-walled cavities within the areas of necrosis can also occur (Fig. 2). Small-sized PSCs (2–3 cm or less) are less common. Tumors are usually round or quasi-circular, with well-defined boundaries. Lobulated lesions may occur because of an unbalanced tumor growth rate. Burr sign and

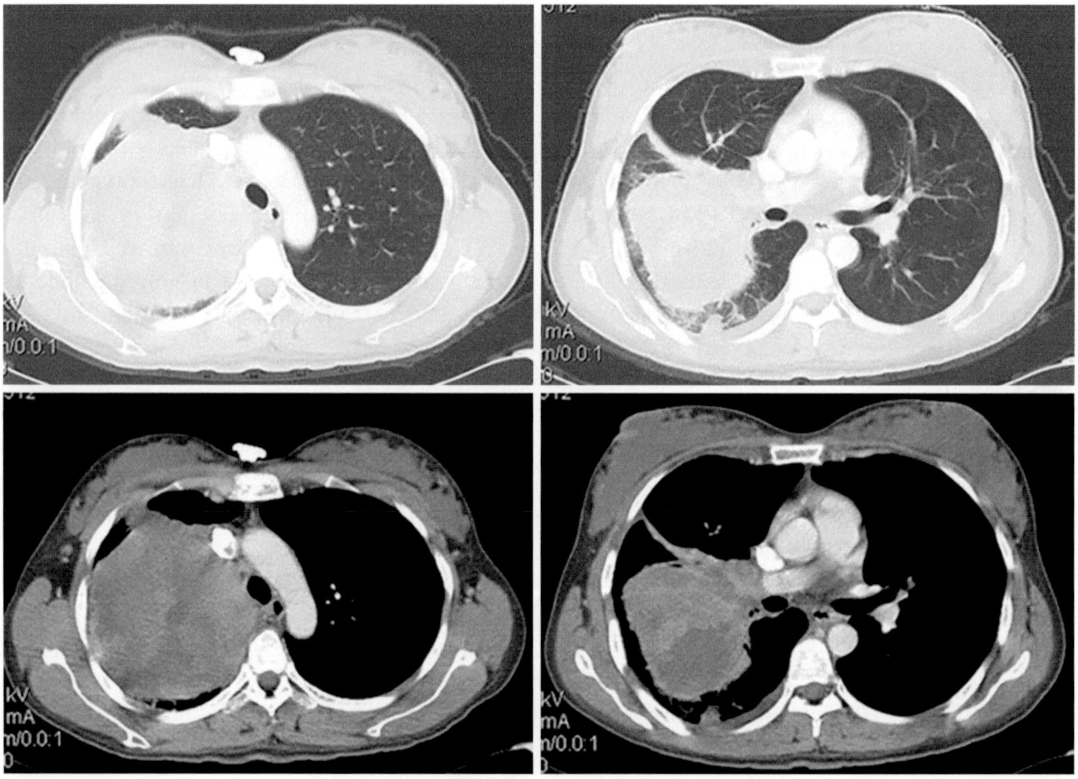

Fig. 1 Peripheral PSC in a 33-year-old woman. CT scan shows a soft-tissue mass in the right upper lung lobe with necrosis

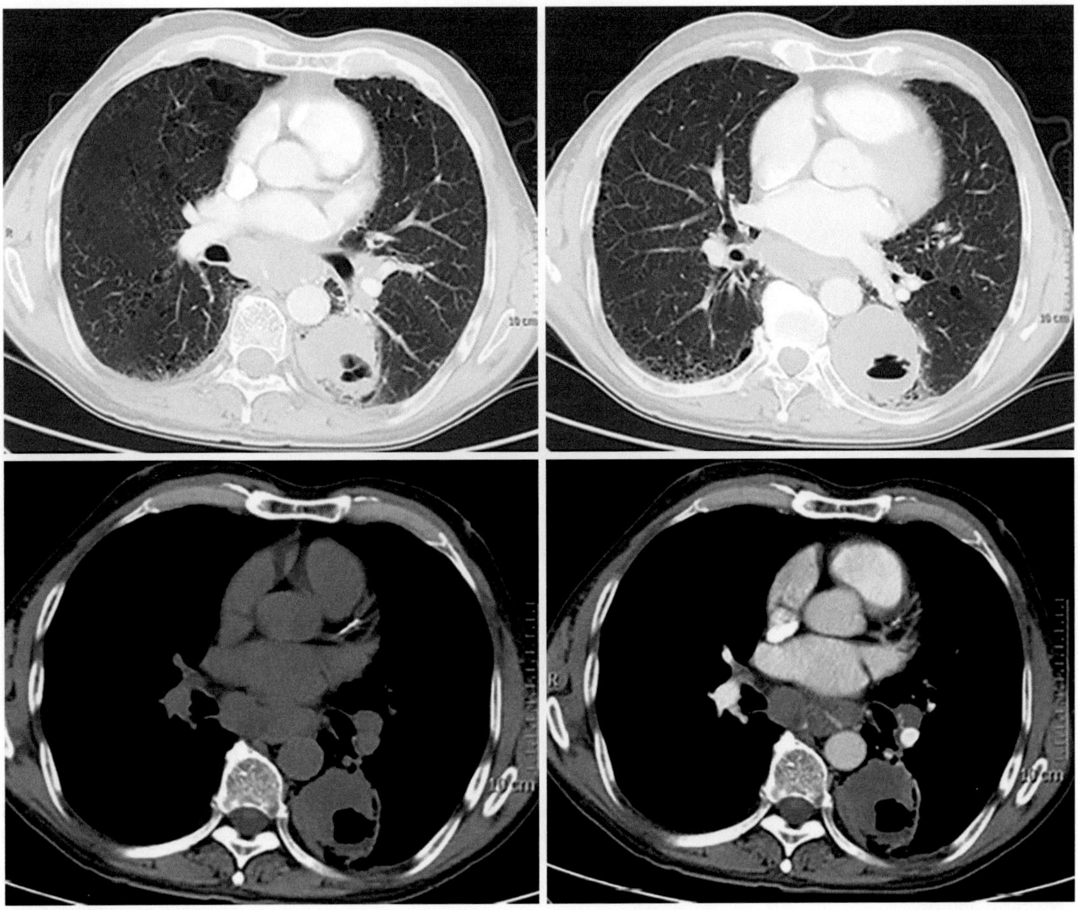

Fig. 2 Peripheral PSC in a 62-year-old man. CT scan shows a soft-tissue mass in the left lower lung lobe with cavitation and mediastinal lymphadenopathy

intratumoral calcification are rare. On contrast-enhanced CT, most masses show ring-shaped or uneven enhancement. About one half of the patients presented with a locally advanced tumor, invading the bronchial tree, the pulmonary parenchyma, and the adjacent anatomical structures such as mediastinum and chest wall (Fig. 3).

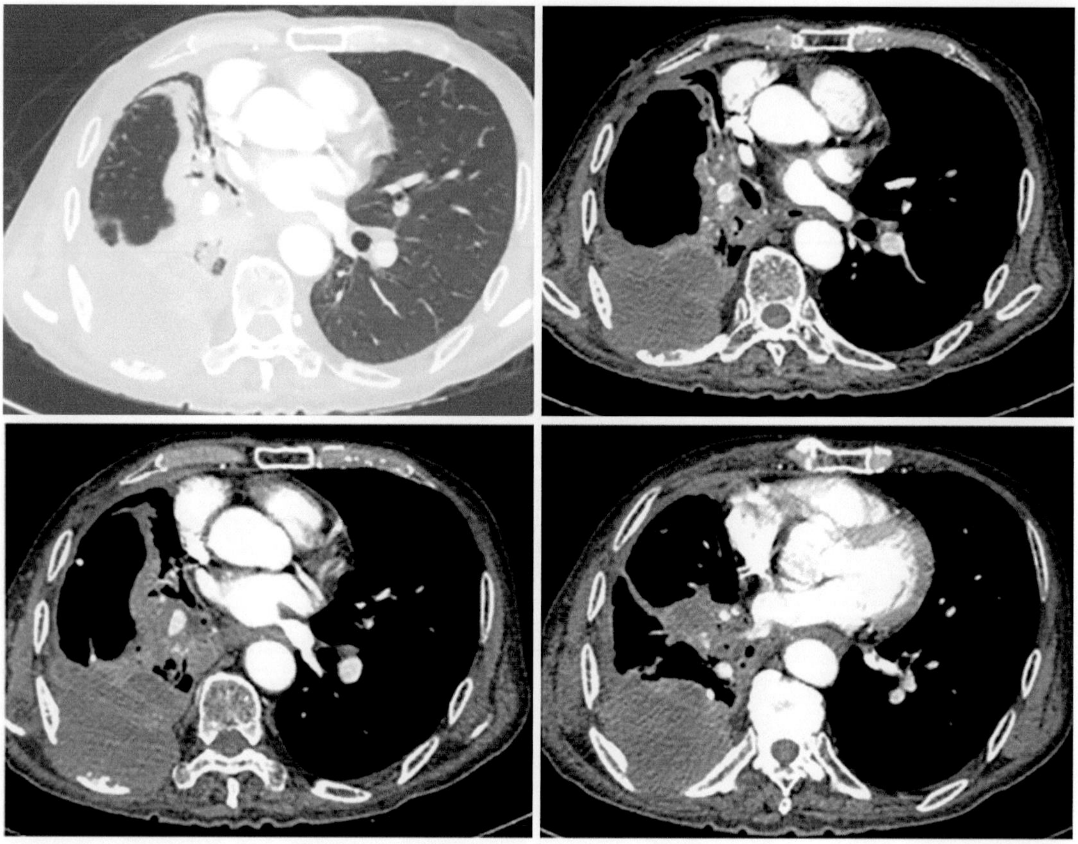

Fig. 3 Peripheral PSC in a 77-year-old man. CT scan shows a soft-tissue mass in the right lower lung lobe invading chest wall and rib

6 Treatment

For PSC, the high recurrence rate and low survival rate after surgical treatment suggested that surgical resection should only be performed on those with early stages. Surgery remains an independent favorable prognostic factor for survival. PSC is resistant to chemotherapy and radiotherapy, and the efficacy of both therapies is controversial. Abdallah et al. [12] performed a retrospective cohort study by querying the National Cancer Database for patients with a diagnosis of PSC between 2004 and 2015, including 1497 PSC patients who received complete anatomical resection with or without adjuvant chemotherapy. Adjuvant chemotherapy for PSC appears to be associated with improved survival in stage II and stage III, but not stage I patients. Neoadjuvant or adjuvant chemotherapy may be beneficial for PSC patients who can undergo surgical resection.

The rarity of these tumors and chemoresistance makes it difficult to determine appropriate chemotherapy, and reported response rates of chemotherapy range from 0% to 17%. Patients with metastatic PSC are mostly chemotherapy resistant. Several studies have shown benefits to patients with advanced PSC. Platinum-based doublet chemotherapy regimens are much better than other chemotherapeutic strategies in advanced PSC patients.

Currently, targeted therapy and immunotherapy are new research fields in PSC. The most frequently mutated genes in advanced PSC are TP53, KRAS, and CDKN2A, and the classic EGFR mutations were rarely found. Most patients are not likely to benefit from anti-EGFR therapies because of this mutational feature of PSC. MET is a receptor for hepatocyte growth factor and is involved in the growth, invasion, and metastasis of cancer cells, thus leading to poor prognosis. MET mutations specifically MET exon 14 are frequent events in PSC. Several studies have demonstrated that MET exon 14 mutation may be a promising targetable gene mutation for advanced PSC, and may benefit from a targeted therapy, including crizotinib, capmatinib, savolitinib, and tepotinib. PSC may generally be associated with a higher PD-L1 expression and a higher tumor mutational burden (TMB) compared with other lung cancers, which indicates that some PSC patients may experience a better outcome treated with immune checkpoint inhibitors (ICIs). Kim et al. [13] estimated the safety and efficacy of durvalumab (a PD-L1 inhibitor) plus tremelimumab (an anti-CTLA4 antibody) for the treatment of advanced PSC by a nonrandomized, open-label, phase II study. The PFS, OS, ORR, and DCR were 5.9 months, 15.4 months, 26.7% and 60%, respectively. The use of PD-L1/PD-1 inhibitors may prolong the OS of patients with this histological subtype.

At present, the treatment of PSC should continue to follow the NSCLC treatment model, with appropriately targeted drugs and immunosuppressive agents based on the patient's driver mutation status. In view of vascular invasion is a feature of PSC, the early use of antiangiogenic therapies (such as apatinib and anlotinib) may improve the patient's response to treatment.

7 Prognosis

The prognosis of PSC is poorer than other forms of NSCLC. The overall 5-year survival rate of PSC is approximately 11%–25% compared with 46% for other types of NSCLC. The study by Steuer et al. [14] found that PSC patients had a median age of 70 years, 59% were men, and 89% were white. 18% had stage I disease, 10% stage II, 24% stage III, and 48% stage IV. The median OS for stage I-II PSC was 16.9 months, 5.8 months for stage III, and 5.4 months for stage IV. Maneenil et al. [15] in a series of 127 PSC reported a median survival time for 9.9 months. The 1, 2, and 5 year survival rates were 42%, 23%, and 15%, respectively. Multivariate analysis showed that T stage, M stage, and treatment with surgery plus neoadjuvant chemotherapy or surgery plus adjuvant therapy were independent prognostic factors. The outcome of PSC is significantly worse than that of squamous cell carcinoma and adenocarcinoma.

8 Case Analysis

8.1 Case 1

A 66-year-old woman found a lung mass for 5 days on physical examination.

Chest CT: A mass in the right middle lobe with clear borders and extensive necrosis (Fig. 4).

[Diagnosis] Pleomorphic carcinoma.

[Diagnosis Basis] The patient performed a right middle lobe pneumonectomy and lymph node dissection. Macroscopically, the lesion was a well-circumscribed tumor of 4 × 4 × 3 cm in size with a yellow-tan cut surface with necrosis. Histologically, the tumor was composed of compact cells arranged in cords. The tumor cells were pleomorphic and spindle-like. No lymph node metastasis was observed. Immunohistochemically, the tumor cells were positive for TTF-1, CK, and vimentin. The histologic and immunohistochemical findings supported the diagnosis of pleomorphic carcinoma.

[Analysis] Pulmonary pleomorphic carcinoma (PPC) is the most common subtype of PSC (>50%) because of the pathologic definition of pleomorphic carcinoma which encompasses the widest range of cellular components.

Several studies have shown that pleomorphic carcinoma, spindle cell carcinoma, and giant cell carcinoma consist of poorly or dedifferentiated cells of epithelial origin. The immunohistochemical and molecular features related to these three subgroups are similar to

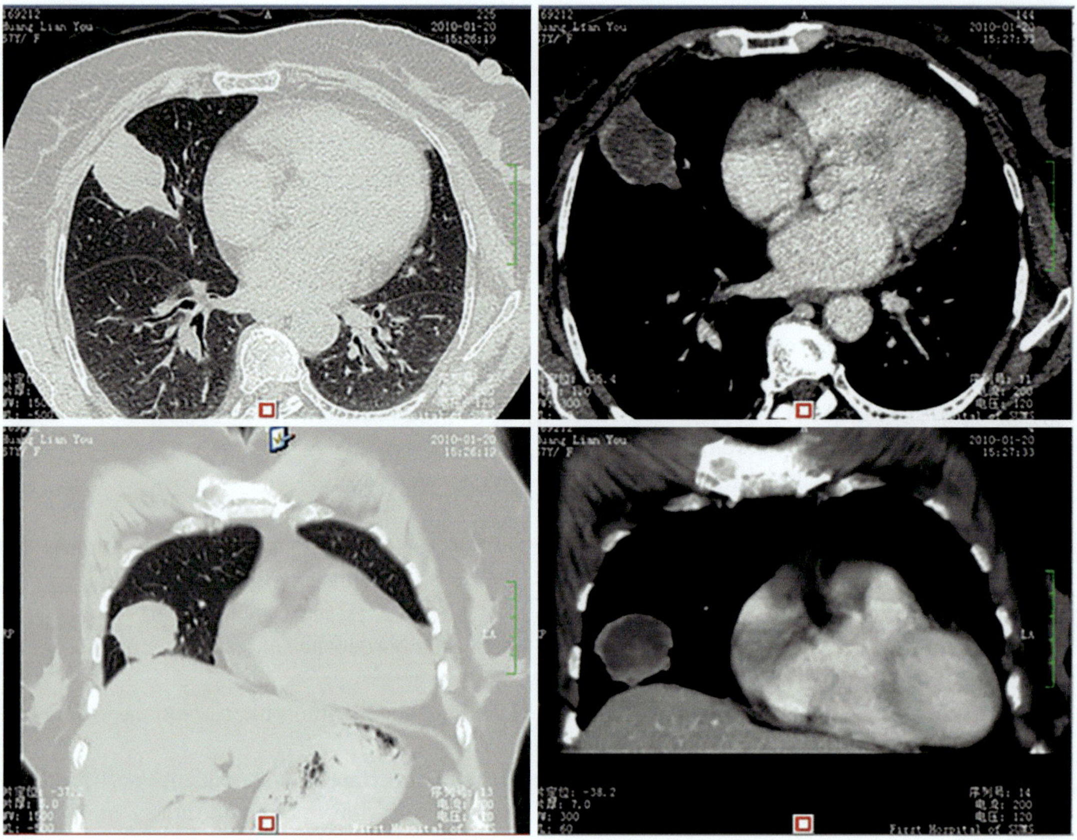

Fig. 4 Chest CT

those for epithelial NSCLC. In contrast, carcinosarcoma and pulmonary blastoma have an immunophenotypically and genetically unique origin. EMT is another explanation of tumoral development because of epithelial and mesenchymal components of PSC. Nagano et al. [16] first performed next generation sequencing analysis of the molecular profiles of PPCs. The most common driver mutations were KRAS mutations (27%), followed by EGFR (8%), and MET (8%) mutations. Epithelial and sarcomatoid components shared activating driver mutations. PD-L1 was highly expressed in the sarcomatoid component compared with the epithelial component.

Some studies have confirmed the association between the EMT status and PD-L1 expression in various types of cancer, including lung adenocarcinoma. Hisakane et al. [17] evaluated the expression of PD-L1 and EMT markers by immunohistochemistry in 16 patients with PPC who underwent surgical resection. They found that the expression of PD-L1 varied between carcinomatous and sarcomatous areas. High PD-L1 and ZEB-1 expression in sarcomatous areas predicted poor survival. There was no correlation observed between c-Met and PD-L1 expression in this study.

PD-1/PD-L1 inhibitors in combination with targeting EMT-related molecules should be a new direction for the treatment of patients with various malignant tumors.

9 Case Analysis

9.1 Case 2

A 57-year-old man found a lung mass on physical examination.

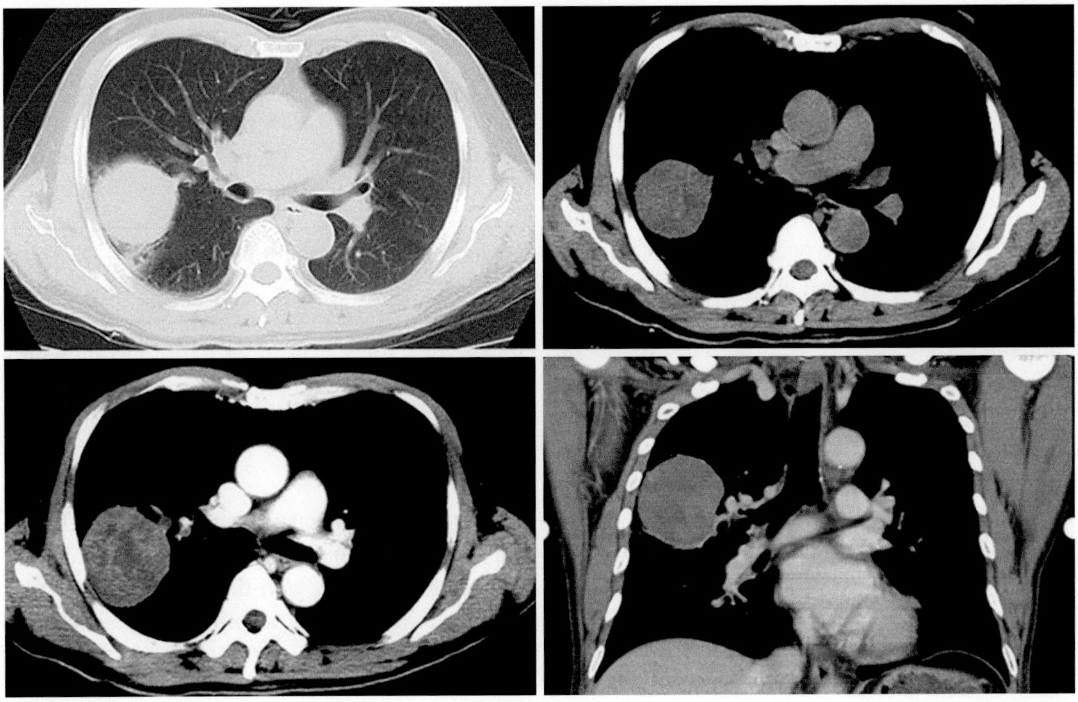

Fig. 5 Chest CT

Chest CT: A mass in the right upper lobe with clear borders and necrosis (Fig. 5).

[Diagnosis] Carcinosarcoma.

[Diagnosis Basis] The patient underwent right upper lobectomy. The lobectomy specimen revealed a well-circumscribed, firm mass measuring 9 × 9 cm. The microscopic examination revealed a malignant neoplasm with carcinoma and sarcomatous elements. Foci of spindle cells have marked atypia and conspicuous mitosis. The margins, pleura, and lymph nodes were negative for malignancy. Immunohistochemically, the tumor cells were positive for EMA and vimentin. The findings were consistent with pulmonary carcinosarcoma.

[Analysis] In 1908, Kika et al. [18] first defined pulmonary carcinosarcoma (PCS) as a poorly differentiated NSCLC containing a component of sarcoma or sarcoma-like features. The origin of PCS is controversial in light of the presence of divergent cell lineages and the clonal nature of malignancy. Several studies have demonstrated that PCS is a monoclonal tumor that can turn normal cells cancerous and then develop through sarcomatoid change in cancer. Spagnoli et al. [19] reported a metastatic PCS patient with 37 months overall survival and performed next generation sequencing to analyze the squamous and sarcomatoid component. They found that 51% of somatic mutations are shared between carcinomatous and sarcomatous elements. Specifically, in all the samples, they detected common mutations affecting PIK3CA, ERBB2, TP53, and MSH6. Among somatic mutations that were specific to either sarcomatoid or carcinomatous elements, sarcomatoid component showed mutations in CDH1, KIT, HRAS, PTEN, ATM, and IDH2, whereas the epithelial one was characterized by EGFR mutations. The result provided strong evidence that these elements originate from a common clonal ancestor through a process of dedifferentiation from the preexisting carcinomatous component. During evolution, the sarcomatoid component branches very early from the well-differentiated epithelial component and independently accumulates mutations, establishing a profound difference with the original lesion, possibly as a consequence of the EMT.

PCS often presents as large, necrotic, and locally invasive tumors. Clinically, PCS includes two major subtypes: peripheral invasive type and central endobronchial type. Sarcomas with adenocarcinoma components are usually peripheral, whereas sarcomas with squamous cell carcinoma components are usually central. The peripheral tumors tend to be associated with a poorer prognosis as they metastasize early and widely. The endobronchial lesions are usually slowly growing and have a better prognosis as they cause symptoms earlier. On the whole, PCS has a worse prognosis compared with conventional NSCLC, particularly when the sarcomatous component is predominant.

Surgery is the mainstay for the treatment of PCS since neoadjuvant/adjuvant chemoradiotherapy has limited effects on the tumor progression. Relapses occur mostly within 1 year after surgery. Immunotherapy has been shown to improve the survival of patients. About 40% of patients at the time of diagnosis present local aggressiveness and distant metastases. Prognosis is usually poor, with a median survival of about 6 months and a survival rate of 6%–21% at 5 years follow-up.

9.2 Case 3

A 69-year-old man complained of chest tightness and chest pain for half a year.

Chest CT:A mass in the left upper lobe with clear borders and extensive necrosis (Fig. 6).

[Diagnosis] Pulmonary blastoma.

[Diagnosis Basis] The patient underwent right upper lobectomy. The microscopic examination demonstrated mixed epithelial and mesenchymal malignancies which were consistent with pulmonary blastoma.

[Analysis] Pulmonary blastoma (PB) is a biphasic tumor containing a primitive epithelial component resembling a well-differentiated fetal-type adenocarcinoma and a primary mesenchymal stromal component, occasionally with foci of osteosarcoma, chondrosarcoma, or rhabdomyosarcoma.

In 1945, Barrett and Barnard first described the tumor as "embryoma" based on the histological resemblance of the tumor to fetal lung tissue. Spencer defined it as "blastoma" because of its histologic resemblance to the fetal lung at the 10–16-week stage of development (paraadenomal stage of lung development) in 1961. In 1991, Koss et al. [20] further classified it into

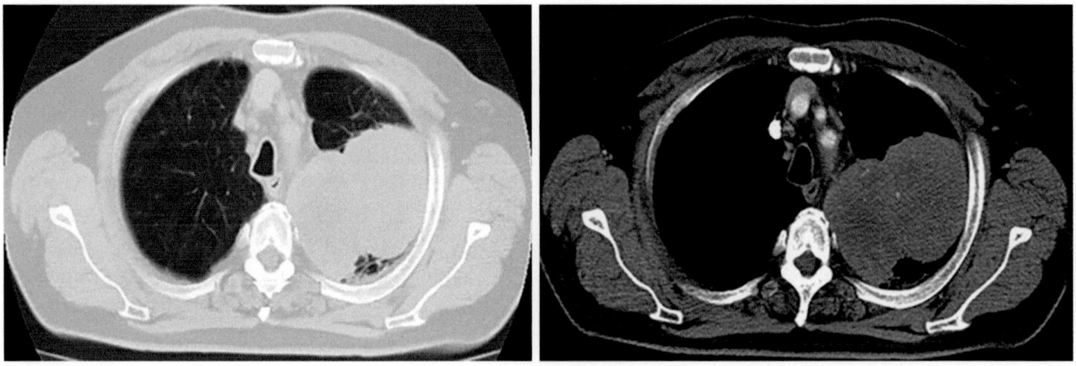

Fig. 6 Chest CT

three different subtypes: classic biphasic pulmonary blastoma (CBPB), monophasic pleuropulmonary blastoma (PPB), and well-differentiated fetal adenocarcinoma (WDFA). The 1999 and 2004 WHO classifications grouped PPB under mesenchymal tumors, WDFA was classified as an adenocarcinoma variant. PB is separated from PPB and WDFA, categorized as a type of sarcomatoid carcinoma. In latest 2021 WHO classification, PB is recognized as a rare variant of sarcomatoid NSCLC with a biphasic pattern.

Approximately 80% of PB occur in adults and has a positive association with smoking. The average age at diagnosis is 40 years. Nearly 40% of patients are asymptomatic and found during incidental imaging.

PB is frequently associated with missense mutations in CTNNB1, responsible for activation of the Wnt pathway through aberrant nuclear/cytoplasmic localization of β-catenin protein. Beta-catenin mutations are rare among lung tumors, which helps in distinguishing PB from carcinosarcoma immunophenotypically. TP53 mutation and both p53 and MDM2 protein accumulation are occasionally found. In addition, Zhao et al. [21] detected 9 mutations in the 56 genes profiled, including BRCA2, ERBB4, ALK, MET, BRAF, RAF1, PTEN, EGFR, and PIK3CA.

PB has a very poor prognosis in previous reports, with a 5- and 10-year survival rate of only 16% 25% and 8%, respectively. However, Bu et al. [22] analyzed the Surveillance, Epidemiology and End Results (SEER) database of the US population and identified 177 PB patients with a median survival of 108 months. The 5 and 10-year survival rates were 58.2 and 48.5%. No sex or race disparities in incidence and prognosis was observed. The death risk of PB was significantly associated with age at diagnosis, clinical stage, histologic subtype, and surgery treatment.

References

1. Nash AD, Stout AP. Giant cell carcinoma of the lung; report of 5 cases. Cancer. 1958;11:369–76.
2. Fishback NF, Travis WD, Moran CA, et al. Pleomorphic (spindle/giant cell) carcinoma of the lung. A clinicopathologic correlation of 78 cases. Cancer. 1994;73:2936–45.
3. Fallet V, Saffroy R, Girard N, et al. High-throughput somatic mutation profiling in pulmonary sarcomatoid carcinomas using the LungCarta TM panel: exploring therapeutic targets. Ann Oncol. 2015;26:1748–53.
4. Pécuchet N, Vieira T, Rabbe N, et al. Molecular classification of pulmonary sarcomatoid carcinomas suggests new therapeutic opportunities. Ann Oncol. 2017;28:1597–604.
5. Zhou F, Huang Y, Cai W, et al. The genomic and immunologic profiles of pure pulmonary sarcomatoid carcinoma in Chinese patients. Lung Cancer. 2021;153:66–72.
6. Yang Z, Xu J, Li L, et al. Integrated molecular characterization reveals potential therapeutic strategies for pulmonary sarcomatoid carcinoma. Nat Commun. 2020;11:4878.
7. Schrock AB, Li SD, Frampton GM, et al. Pulmonary sarcomatoid carcinomas commonly harbor either potentially targetable genomic alterations or high tumor mutational burden as observed by comprehensive genomic profiling. J Thorac Oncol. 2017;12:932–42.
8. Arshi J, Sauer M, Yin F. Rapid sarcomatoid transformation of lung squamous cell carcinoma after neoadjuvant therapy: a case report. Anticancer Res. 2020;40:1625–9.
9. Shimoji M, Shimizu S, Sato K, et al. Clinical and pathologic features of lung cancer expressing programmed cell death ligand 1 (PD-L1). Lung Cancer. 2016;98:69–75.
10. Vieira T, Antoine M, Hamard C, et al. Sarcomatoid lung carcinomas show high levels of programmed death ligand-1 (PD-L1) and strong immune-cell infiltration by TCD3 cells and macrophages. Lung Cancer. 2016;98:51–8.
11. Dix Junqueira Pinto G, de Souza VL, et al. Evaluation of PD-L1 expression in tumor tissue of patients with lung carcinoma and correlation with clinical and demographic data. J Immunol Res. 2016;2016:9839685.
12. Abdallah HM, Martinez-Meehan D, Lutfi W, et al. Adjuvant chemotherapy for pulmonary sarcomatoid carcinoma: a retrospective analysis of the National Cancer Database. J Thorac Cardiovasc Surg. 2022;163:1669–81.
13. Kim M, Keam B, Ock C-Y, et al. Phase II study of durvalumab and tremelimumab in pulmonary sarcomatoid carcinoma:KCSG-LU16-07. Thorac Cancer. 2020;11:3482–9.
14. Steuer CE, Behera M, Liu Y, et al. Pulmonary sarcomatoid carcinoma: an analysis of the National Cancer Data Base. Clin Lung Cancer. 2017;18:286–92.
15. Maneenil K, Xue Z, Liu M, et al. Sarcomatoid carcinoma of the lung: the Mayo clinic experience in 127 patients. Clin Lung Cancer. 2017;19:e323–e33.
16. Nagano M, Kohsaka S, Hayashi T, et al. Comprehensive molecular profiling of pulmonary pleomorphic carcinoma. NPJ Precis Oncologia. 2021;5:57.
17. Hisakane K, Seike M, Sugano T, et al. PD-L1 expression status predicting survival in pulmonary pleomorphic carcinoma. Anticancer Res. 2021;41:2501–9.

18. Kika G. Pathologie des Krebses Ergeb Allg Pathol Anat. 1912;16:p. 1.
19. Spagnoli L, Petrelli F, Fratini G, et al. A look towards the clonal origin of metastatic pulmonary carcinosarcoma: report of a patient with an unexpected long-term survival. Tumori. 2022;108:NP5–NP10.
20. Koss M, Hochholzer L, O'Leary T. Pulmonary blastomas. Cancer. 1991;67:2368–81.
21. Zhao YY, Liu L, Zhou T, et al. A retrospective analysis of the clinicopathological and molecular characteristics of pulmonary blastoma. Onco Targets Ther. 2016;9:6915–20.
22. Bu X, Liu J, Wei L, et al. Epidemiological features and survival outcomes in patients with malignant pulmonary blastoma: a US population-based analysis. BMC Cancer. 2020;20:811.

Lymphoepithelioma-Like Carcinoma

Song Zhang

Lymphoepithelioma-like carcinoma (LELC) is an uncommon epithelial tumor, most of which originated from the nasopharynx and few from foregut-derived organs including salivary glands, lung, stomach, thymus, etc. Primary pulmonary lymphoepithelioma-like carcinoma (PPLELC) accounts for around 0.9% of non-small cell lung cancer (NSCLC).

1 Classification

Lymphoepithelioma was first reported in the 1920s by Regaud and Schmincke in the head and neck region of Asian individuals. PPLELC was first described by Begin et al. [1] in 1987 in a 40-year-old non-smoking southeast Asian woman, considered as an epithelial carcinoma associated with Epstein-bar virus (EBV) infection. The 2004 WHO classification of lung tumors classified it into large cell lung cancer, then removed from the group of large cell carcinoma to "other and unclassified carcinomas" in the 2015 WHO classification. The 2021 WHO classification of thoracic tumors renamed it as lymphoepithelial carcinoma and classified as a type of squamous cell carcinoma.

S. Zhang (✉)
Department of Respiratory and Critical Care Medicine, Shandong Provincial Hospital Affiliated to Shandong First Medical University, Jinan, Shandong, China

2 EBV Examination

PPLELC is a rare EBV-associated carcinoma. Nearly all Asian patients have positive EBV results, while most non-Asian patients are EBV negative. Han et al. [2] investigated 32 cases of PPLELC in southern China and showed that the positive rate of EBV-encoded small nonpolyadenylated RNA (EBER) was 94% (30/32). Castro et al. [3] retrospectively studied 6 Western PPLELC patients. All 6 cases were negative for EBV, suggesting no association between EBV and LELC in the Western population. Chen et al. [4] revealed that the positive proportion of EBER in tumor tissue was 78.6%, suggesting that there might be alternative mechanisms engaged in the development of LELC beyond EBV driving.

Kobayashi et al. [5] reported a case of a 67-year-old Japanese woman with synchronous primary lung cancers of LELC and papillary adenocarcinoma. EBV genome was detected in malignant epithelial cells of LELC but not in the papillary adenocarcinoma by in situ hybridization. Predominantly CD8+ and T cell intracytoplasmic antigen (TIA-1) + cytotoxic T cells with closely associated with HLA-DR-positive LELC cells constituted the majority of tumor-infiltrating lymphocytes in LELC. The exaggerated lymphoid infiltration in and around the EBV-infected carcinoma cells may represent an enhancement of tumor immunity, suggesting a better prognostic indicator. The circulating serum EBV-DNA

S. Zhang (ed.), *Diagnostic Imaging of Lung Cancers*, https://doi.org/10.1007/978-981-99-6815-2_9

can serve as a potential marker for disease and therapy monitoring, particularly among Asian patients.

3 Pathology

PPLELC is histologically characterized by poorly differentiated tumor cells with large vesicular nuclei and prominent nucleoli showing syncytial growth patterns with heavy lymphocytic infiltration that is indistinguishable from undifferentiated nasopharyngeal carcinomas (NPC) (Fig. 1a, b). PPLELC can also display nonclassic morphology and lack significant lymphocytic infiltration. Yeh et al. [6] conducted a comprehensive clinicopathologic analysis of 61 PPLELC patients. They demonstrated that PPLELCs show a morphologically diverse spectrum, ranging from classic poorly differentiated tumors with intense lymphocytic infiltration to nonclassic morphology with little lymphocytic infiltration. Tumors with fewer lymphocytic infiltration can closely resemble nonkeratinizing squamous cell carcinoma and tend to have larger tumor sizes, and exhibit shorter times to recurrence than those with high lymphocytic infiltration. They found several distinct morphologic features in PPLELCs, including granulomatous inflammation, focal keratinization, spread through alveolar spaces, and lepidic spreading pattern. As many of these "LELCs" are different from undifferentiated nasopharyngeal carcinoma or lymphoepithelioma, they suggested using an alternative term, EBV-associated pulmonary carcinoma, to encompass the entire morphologic spectrum of this distinct disease entity.

Immunohistochemically, the tumor cells typically express CK5/6, p63, and p40, suggesting that PPLELC may be essentially more similar to squamous cell carcinoma.

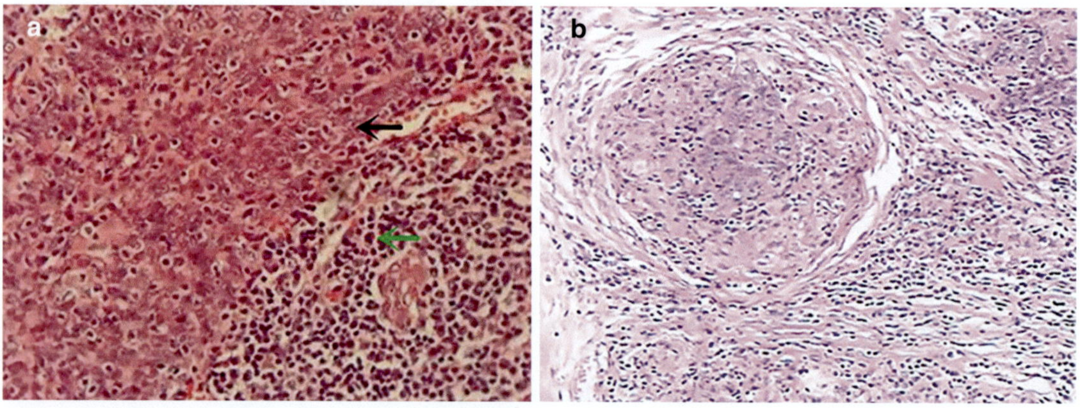

Fig. 1 (**a**) Carcinoma cells are arranged in syncytial sheets and nests (black arrow). The tumor cell nuclei are round, or elongated with mildly irregular nuclear outline, vesicular chromatin, and distinct nucleoli. The tumor cells are surrounded by abundant lymphoplasmacytic cells in the stroma (green arrow), and many lymphocytes scattered in the cancer nests. (**b**) The structure of cancer nests is clear, surrounded by a large number of lymphocytes and plasma cells

4 Molecular Features

There are few reports of mutations in PPLELC tumor driver genes, such as p53, EGFR, KRAS, ALK, BRAF, ROS1, and MET. Chang et al. [7] identified 46 PLELCs to evaluate p53 and EGFR aberrations. p53 mutations were identified in three patients (6.5%), which all occurred in exon 8. EGFR mutations were detected in 8 of 46 cases (17.4%) with a majority of exon 21 mutations but without L858R. Only one case had the classical EGFR mutation (deletion in exon 19). Notably, EGFR mutations were more commonly found in patients with tumor size ≤3 cm. p53 and EGFR mutations are uncommon in LELCs, indicating that these genes are not the important events in carcinogenesis for this tumor subtype. No KRAS, BRAF, ALK, or ROS1 aberrations could be detected in another study by Chang et al. [8]. Ose et al. [9] reported the first case of PLELC with ALK rearrangement in postoperative specimens of a 76-year-old woman with no history of smoking in Japan. Yin et al. [10] retrospectively reviewed the genetic profiles and treatment course of 330 PLELC patients at the Guangdong Lung Cancer Institute (GLCI). They found that the mutation rates of EGFR and ALK were 2.9% and 2.1%, respectively. They searched and analyzed 15 related literature, and 1071 PLELC cases mentioned the driver mutations. EGFR mutation and ALK rearrangement were detected in 15 patients and 1 patient, respectively. Four EGFR/ALK mutant PLELC patients received targeted therapy as palliative treatment. However, after 1 month of using TKIs, all cases showed disease progression.

In 2015, two case series by Fang et al. [11] and Chang et al. [8] found that the frequency of PD-L1 over-expression in PLELC was 74.3% and 75.8%, respectively. Xie et al. [12] investigated the genomic profiles and expression of PD-L1 of 29 Chinese PLELC patients at various disease stages. Except for detecting ERBB2 amplification and KRAS mutation in two patients, no other classic lung cancer driver mutations were found. 78% (21/27) of the patients had mutations in epigenetic regulators and 69% (20/29) had positive expression of PD-L1. Three patients received and benefited from a PD-1 inhibitor. The detection of high expression of PD-L1 and lack of any canonical druggable driver mutations raises the potential of checkpoint immunotherapy for PLELC.

Hong et al. [13] first reported the genomic landscape of 91 PLELC patients by targeted deep sequencing and whole-exome sequencing. They found that the frequent loss of type I interferon genes and excessive activity of the AID/APOBEC family genes were prevalent in PLELC. The excessive activity of APOBEC family genes may be induced in response to EBV infection and participate in the tumorigenesis of PLELC. Critical pathways including JAK/STAT, NF-κB, and cell cycle were also altered. They also confirmed a low degree of typical driver mutations including EGFR, KRAS, and BRAF. Although MET missense mutations were detected in two patients, they did not belong to the canonical MET exon 14 skipping mutations.

Chau et al. [14] studied tumor cells from 57 EBV-positive PLELCs and revealed a unique genomic landscape of low TP53 mutation (11%), low incidence of known drivers in the RTK/RAS/RAF (11%), and PI3K/AKT/mTOR pathways (7%), but enriched for loss-of-function mutations in multiple negative regulators of the NF-κB pathway. 47% and 79% of the cases show positive PD-L1 immunoreactivity at ≥50% and ≥1% tumor proportion score, respectively. A subgroup of patients with actionable fibroblast growth factor receptor 3 (FGFR3) aberrations (4%) and mismatch repair deficiency (4%) were potentially eligible for precision medicine.

In summary, PLELC showed a distinct genomic landscape, distinct from major NSCLC subtypes but similar to EBV-associated nasopharyngeal carcinoma.

5 Epidemiology

The incidence of PLELC has specific ethnic and regional preference. Most reported cases are distributed in East Asia, with nearly two-thirds arising from Southern China including Guangdong, Hong Kong, and Taiwan. PLELC mainly affects younger patients (51–55 years) and non-smokers, with no obvious sex predilection. Tay et al. [15] evaluated clinical characteristics, diagnosis, treatment, and prognosis of PPLELC in Singapore. All 28 patients were Chinese, 67.9% were female, and the median age was 58 years (range 37–76 years). Majority (89.3%) were never smokers. There are only few cases which have been reported in the western patients and the epidemiological characteristics in Western population may be different from those of Asian patients. He et al. [16] analyzed 62 patients with PLELC based on the data of the Surveillance, Epidemiology, and End Results database (SEER) in US. The median age at diagnosis was 65 years (ranging from 15 to 86), which was older than the Asian patients. The majority was male (64.4%,36/62), with a gender ratio of 1.33:1. The proportion of white patients is the highest (64.4%), which was consistent with the racial distribution of the Western population.

6 Clinical Features

The majority of the patients with PPLELC do not have obvious clinical manifestations at diagnosis. The most common clinical performance is cough, hemoptysis, and chest pain. Other clinical presentations include slight fever, weight loss, exertional dyspnea, night sweats, joint pain, and pleural effusion.

7 Radiographic Features

Imaging of PPLELC lacks specificity. Most PPLELCs are located in the right middle and lower lungs. Tumors in the center are larger than those in the periphery. PPLELCs consist of well-defined border (Fig. 2), lobulation, spiculation, vascular or bronchial encasement (Fig. 3), obstructive pneumonia (Fig. 4), air bronchogram, and pleura retraction. Cavities (Fig. 5) and calcifications (Fig. 6) occur occasionally. Necrosis also can occur, most

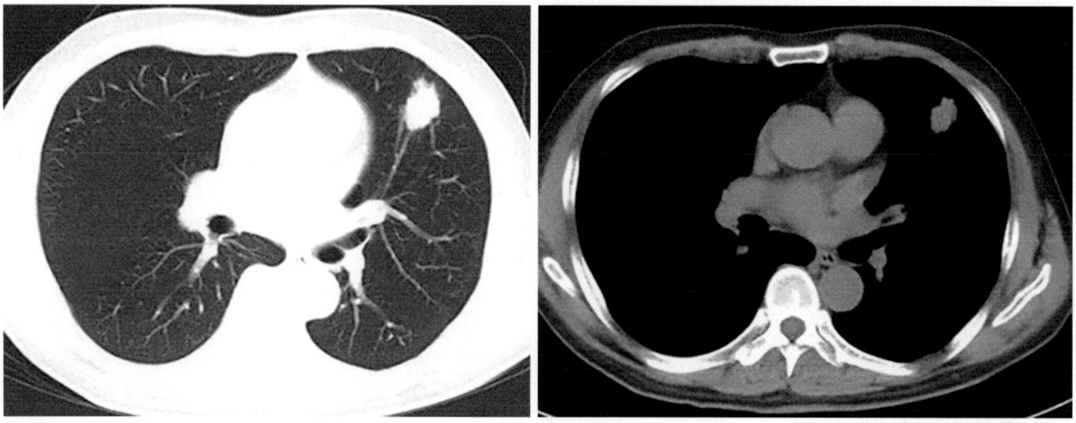

Fig. 2 PPLELC in a 55-year-old man. CT scan shows a lesion in the left upper lobe with well-defined border and lobulation

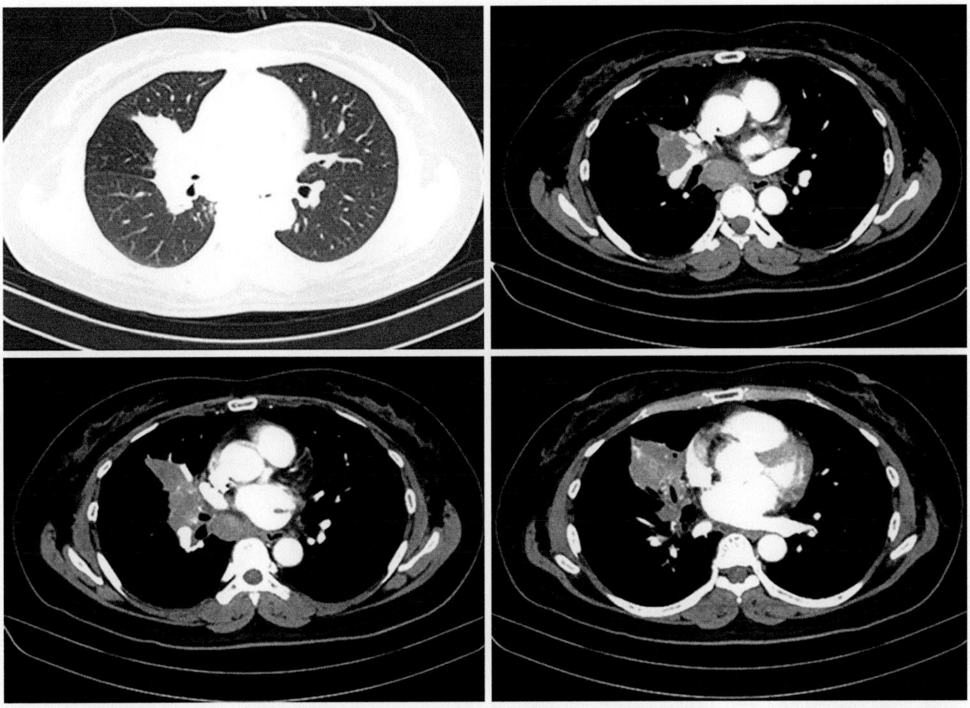

Fig. 3 PPLELC in a 47-year-old woman. Contrast-enhanced CT scan shows a mass in the right middle lobe with vascular encasement and lymph node involvement

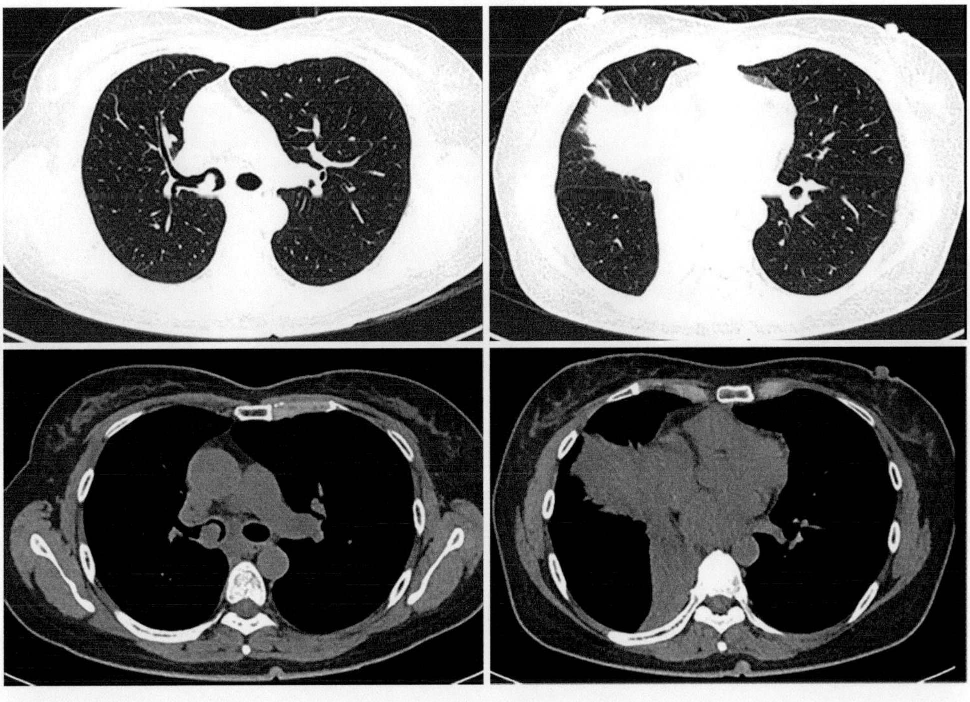

Fig. 4 PPLELC in a 54-year-old woman. CT scan shows a soft-tissue lesion in the right main bronchus with obstructive pneumonia and atelectasis

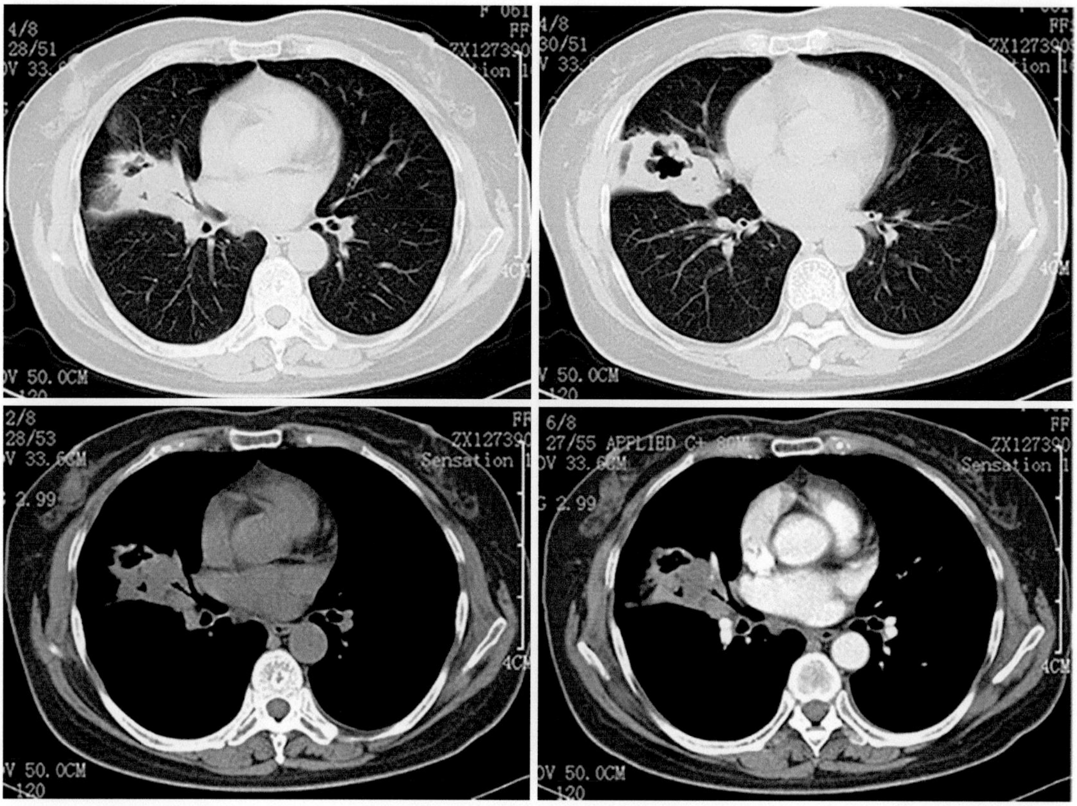

Fig. 5 PPLELC in a 61-year-old woman. Contrast-enhanced CT scan shows a mass in the right middle lobe with air bronchogram and cavities

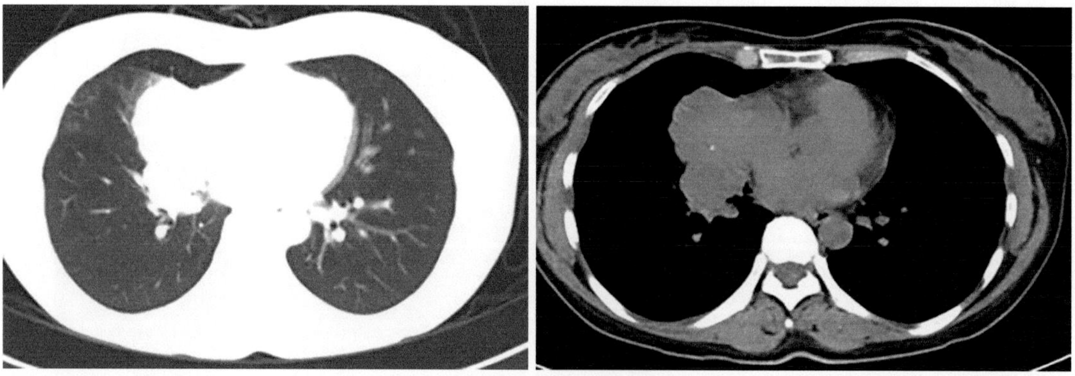

Fig. 6 PPLELC in a 47-year-old woman. CT scan shows a soft-tissue mass in the right middle lobe with lobulation and calcification

often in masses >5 cm. Contrast-enhanced CT scan reveals mild to moderate enhancement and usually delayed enhancement. Inhomogeneously enhanced tumors are significantly larger than homogeneously enhanced tumors (Fig. 7). Lymph node involvement is frequent.

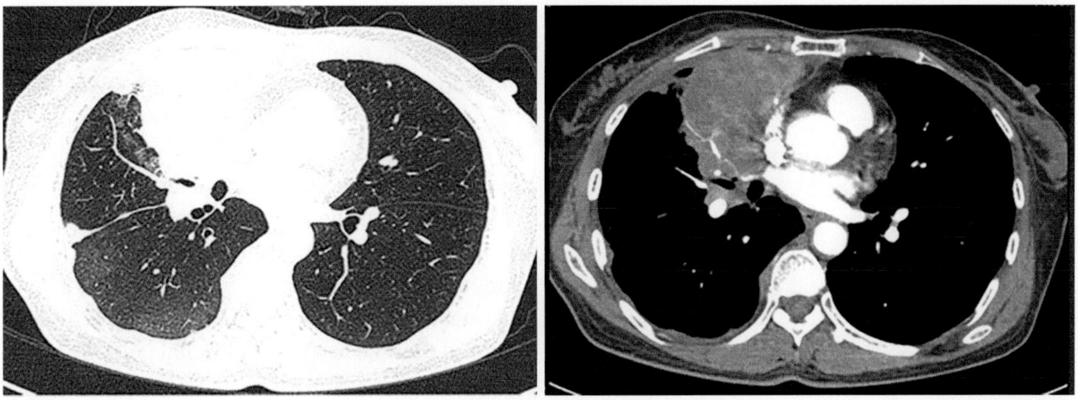

Fig. 7 PPLELC in a 53-year-old woman. Contrast-enhanced CT scan shows a mass in the right middle lobe, with uneven enhancement and neovascularization visible inside the mass

8 Treatment

Surgical resection with curative intent is the preferred approach for early and resectable stage PPLELC. Unresectable patients often undergo multimodal therapy, including chemotherapy and radiotherapy. PPLELC is sensitive to chemotherapy, and platinum-based regimens are the first choice for advanced PPLELC. Lin et al. [17] found that gemcitabine-based chemotherapy achieved the highest response rate and the longest progression-free survival compared with taxanes plus platinum and pemetrexed plus platinum in patients with advanced PPLELC.

Advanced PPLELC patients are less likely to benefit from targeted therapy due to lacking EGFR, ALK, and KRAS mutations. Owing to the positive rate of PD-L1 in PPLELC patients, immunotherapy has become a hot topic in PPLELC therapy. Kumar et al. [18] reported two cases of advanced stage LELC that progressed despite multiple lines of chemotherapy but responded favorably to a PD-1 inhibitor, nivolumab. Xiao et al. [19] investigated the efficacy and safety of different treatment regimens for 68 patients with advanced PLELC from two centers in China. The results show that the median PFS was 6.9 months in the chemotherapy group, 11.0 months in the immunotherapy group, and 11.8 months in the chemoimmunotherapy group. Chemoimmunotherapy had the highest 2-year PFS and may be the best first-line treatment for patients with advanced PLELC.

9 Prognosis

The prognosis for PLELC patients is more favorable compared with other types of lung cancer. Jiang et al. [20] found that the 2- and 5-year overall survival (OS) rates of LELC patients were 90% and 74%, respectively; the disease-free survival (DFS) rates were 87% and 47%, respectively. Patients with large tumor, accompanied with lymph nodes metastasis or at the advanced stage had the worst OS, and patients with lymph nodes metastasis or at the advanced stage had the worst DFS. Wu et al. [21] found that patients in the early stages (stage I and II) had higher progression-free survival rates and those with tumors containing obvious stroma fibrosis had worse prognosis. Only stage was the independent prognostic factor. Tang et al. [22] reviewed 13 retrospective studies with a total of 1294 patients. The incidence of PD-L1 expression in PPLELC varied from 63.3% to 75.8%. Compared with negative PD-L1 expression, positive PD-L1 expression was more likely to be observed in patients under 60 years old and was associated with worse disease-free survival (DFS). Stage was the prognostic factor for both overall survival (OS) and DFS.

10 Case Analysis

10.1 Case

A 39-year-old woman complained of cough and expectoration for 1 week.

Chest CT: A mass in the right middle lobe (Fig. 8).

[Diagnosis] Primary pulmonary lymphoepithelioma-like carcinoma.

[Diagnosis Basis] A young woman with a mass in the medial segment of the right middle lobe, adjacent to the horizontal fissure and mediastinum. Contrast-enhanced CT scan shows heterogeneous enhancement, and thick accompanying blood vessel (green arrows) is seen on the outside of the lesion, suggesting sclerosing pneumocytoma as differential diagnosis. However, sclerosing pneumocytoma is mostly round or quasi-round, with typical air crescent sign, generally without pleural traction (red arrow), and intratumoral vascular (orange arrow). The mass has well-defined border, shallow lobulation, obvious interlobar pleural traction (red arrow), vascular encasement (orange arrow), and obvious emphysema around the lesion (black arrow), which supports the diagnosis of PLELC. The patient underwent surgical resection. The size of the mass was 5.3 × 4.5 × 3.1 cm. Histopathology showed that the atypical epithelial cells were distributed in sheets with marked lymphoid tissue hyperplasia. Granuloma formation was seen in focal areas. Immunohistochemically, the tumor cells typically express CK5/6, p40, and CyclinD1, and Ki-67 positive index is about 40%. In situ hybridization showed EBER positive. According to histopathology, immunohistochemistry, and in situ hybridization, it was considered to be pulmonary lymphoepithelioma-like carcinoma. Lymph node metastasis was found in groups 3A, 9, 7,

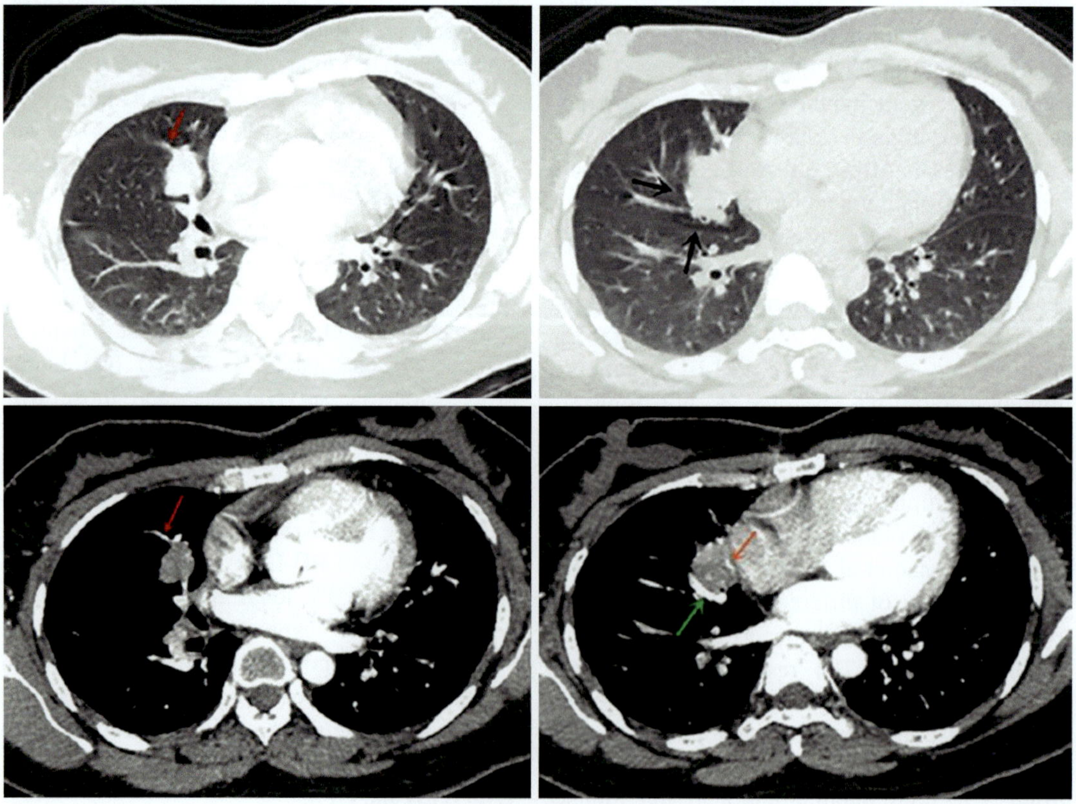

Fig. 8 Chest CT

and 10 (1/2, 2/2, 4/4, 2/3). The final clinical diagnosis was PPLELC (T2N2M0 stage IIIA).

[Analysis] Lei et al. [23] retrospectively analyzed the imaging of 215 patients with PLELC. EBER was positive in all 215 cases. The PLELC was demonstrated as a solitary nodule/mass in 188 cases (87%), multiple nodules/masses in 12 cases (6%), and lobar or segmental consolidation in 15 cases (7%). The tumor showed well-defined margin (80%), lobular sign (82%), enlarged hilar or mediastinal lymph nodes (74%), involvement of the bronchus (72%), and spicule sign (42%). Vascular encasement is one of the imaging features of PPLELC. The incidence of this sign was approximately 66% (105/158) in this study. The embedded blood vessels can be either pulmonary vessels or neovascularization of the tumor itself. The former is shown as continuous vascular shadows with clear boundaries, while the latter is shown as discontinuous small vessels. Histopathology showed that tumor cells grew around vascular shadows, and CD34 staining was high expression, which confirmed that these discontinuous vascular shadows might be immature new vessels in the tumor, rather than simply embedded pulmonary vessels. The progressive enhancement of the tumor was also closely related to the abundance of neovascularization in the tumors. When a large, lobulate, well-defined lesion with homogeneous density and vascular encasement is found, PLELC should be suspected.

Chen et al. [4] compared the characteristic and prognosis of 42 PPLELC and 134 squamous carcinomas. PLELC was more common in women with a younger median age and less smokers in comparison to squamous carcinoma. LELC seemed to be smaller in diameter on CT scans than squamous carcinoma, with few signs of spiculation and vascular convergence. Epstein–Barr virus-encoded RNA (EBER) was detected in 33 LELC cases by in situ hybridization, among whom 27 cases were positive in serum EBV-DNA examination. The median progression-free survival (PFS) of LELC patients was much longer than that of squamous cell carcinoma. Positive serum EBV-DNA, distant lymph node invasion, advanced clinical stage and receiving radiotherapy in LELC patients were correlated with the shorter PFS. However, only positive serum EBV-DNA was an independent PFS predictor.

Lee et al. [24] retrospectively investigated and compared the initial CT features and subsequent survival outcomes of LELC and small-cell lung cancer (SCLC). LELC tumors exhibited a significantly higher percentage of attenuation on contrast-enhanced CT scans. The prevalence of vascular or bronchial encasement, background emphysematous changes, and tumors located in upper lobes was significantly lower in the LELC group. Female gender, younger age, and without a history of smoking were most common factors in the LELC group. The LELC patients had a better prognosis with significantly longer median survival compared with the SCLC patients (23.4 months vs 17.3 months).

The main differential diagnosis is metastatic undifferentiated nasopharyngeal carcinoma. Therefore, examination of the nasopharynx should be performed to exclude metastatic disease.

References

1. Begin LR, Eskandari J, Joncas J, et al. Epstein-Barr virus related lymphoepithelioma-like carcinoma of lung. J Surg Oncol. 1987;36:280–3.
2. Han AJ, Xiong M, Zong YS, et al. Association of Epstein-Barr virus with lymphoepithelioma-like carcinoma of the lung in southern China. Am J Clin Pathol. 2000;114:220–6.
3. Castro CY, Ostrowski ML, Barrios R, et al. Relationship between Epstein-Barr virus and lymphoepithelioma-like carcinoma of the lung: a clinicopathologic study of 6 cases and review of the literature. Hum Pathol. 2001;32:863–72.
4. Chen B, Chen X, Zhou P, et al. Primary pulmonary lymphoepithelioma-like carcinoma: a rare type of lung cancer with a favorable outcome in comparison to squamous carcinoma. Respir Res. 2019;20:262.
5. Kobayashi M, Ito M, Sano K, et al. Pulmonary lymphoepithelioma-like carcinoma: predominant infiltration of tumor-associated cytotoxic T lymphocytes might represent the enhanced tumor immunity. Int Med. 2004;43:323–6.
6. Yeh YC, Kao HL, Lee KL, et al. Epstein-Barr virus-associated pulmonary carcinoma proposing an alter-

native term and expanding the histologic spectrum of lymphoepithelioma-like carcinoma of the lung. Am J Surg Pathol. 2019;43:211–9.
7. Chang YL, Wu CT, Shih JY, et al. Unique p53 and epidermal growth factor receptor gene mutation status in 46 pulmonary lymphoepithelioma-like carcinomas. Cancer Sci. 2011;102:282–7.
8. Chang YL, Yang CY, Lin MW, et al. PD-L1 is highly expressed in lung lymphoepithelioma-like carcinoma: a potential rationale for immunotherapy. Lung Cancer. 2015;88:254–9.
9. Ose N, Kawai T, Ishida D, et al. Pulmonary lymphoepithelioma-like carcinoma with echinoderm microtubule-associated protein-like 4-anaplastic lymphoma kinase (EML4-ALK) fusion gene. Respirol Case Rep. 2016;4:e00200.
10. Yin K, Feng HB, Li LL, et al. Low frequency of mutation of epidermal growth factor receptor (EGFR) and arrangement of anaplastic lymphoma kinase (ALK) in primary pulmonary lymphoepithelioma-like carcinoma. Thorac Cancer. 2020;11:346–52.
11. Fang W, Hong S, Chen N, et al. PD-L1 is remarkably over-expressed in EBV-associated pulmonary lymphoepithelioma-like carcinoma and related to poor disease-free survival. Oncotarget. 2015;6:33019–32.
12. Xie Z, Liu L, Lin X, et al. A multicenter analysis of genomic profiles and PD-L1 expression of primary lymphoepithelioma-like carcinoma of the lung. Mod Pathol. 2020;33:626–38.
13. Hong S, Liu D, Luo S, et al. The genomic landscape of Epstein-Barr virus-associated pulmonary lymphoepithelioma-like carcinoma. Nat Commun. 2019;10:3108.
14. Chau SL, Tong JH, Chow C, et al. Distinct molecular landscape of Epstein-Barr virus associated pulmonary Lymphoepithelioma-like carcinoma revealed by genomic sequencing. Cancers (Basel). 2020;12:2065.
15. Tay CK, Chua YC, Takano A, et al. Primary pulmonary lymphoepithelioma-like carcinoma in Singapore. Ann Thorac Med. 2018:1330–5.
16. He J, Shen J, Pan H, et al. Pulmonary lymphoepithelioma-like carcinoma: a surveillance, epidemiology, and end results database analysis. J Thorac Dis. 2015;7:2330–8.
17. Lin Z, Fu S, Zhou Y, et al. First-line platinum-based chemotherapy and survival outcomes in locally advanced or metastatic pulmonary lymphoepithelioma-like carcinoma. Lung Cancer. 2019;137:100–7.
18. Kumar V, Dave V, Harris J, et al. Response of advanced stage recurrent lymphoepithelioma-like carcinoma to nivolumab. Immunotherapy. 2017;9:955–61.
19. Xiao Y, He J, Luo S, et al. Comparison of immunotherapy, chemotherapy, and chemoimmunotherapy in advanced pulmonary lymphoepithelioma-like carcinoma: a retrospective study. Front Oncol. 2022;12:820302.
20. Jiang WY, Wang R, Pan XF, et al. Clinicopathological features and prognosis of primary pulmonary lymphoepithelioma-like carcinoma. J Thorac Dis. 2016;8:2610–6.
21. Wu Q, Wang W, Zhou P, et al. Primary pulmonary lymphoepithelioma-like carcinoma is characterized by high PD-L1 expression, but low tumor mutation burden. Pathol Res Pract. 2020;216:153043.
22. Tang L, Chen N, He W, et al. The clinicopathological features and prognosis of primary pulmonary lymphoepithelioma-like carcinoma: a systematic review and meta-analysis. PLoS One. 2020;15:e0240729.
23. Lei Y, Zhou J, Liu J, et al. The CT and PET/CT findings in primary pulmonary lymphoepithelioma-like carcinoma with pathological correlation: a study of 215 cases. Clin Radiol. 2022;77:e201–7.
24. Lee KL, Wu MH, Jhang YY, et al. Computed tomography-based differentiation of primary pulmonary lymphoepithelioma-like carcinoma and small-cell lung cancer. J Chin Med Assoc. 2020;83:936–42.

NUT Carcinoma

Song Zhang

Nuclear protein in testis (NUT) carcinoma (NC) is a rare, aggressive undifferentiated tumor with varying degrees of squamous differentiation. NC is characterized by a chromosomal rearrangement involving the NUT midline carcinoma family member 1 (NUTM1) gene (also known as NUT gene) located on chromosome 15q14 with different partners from the bromodomain-containing protein (BRD) gene family or other genes.

1 Classification

In 1991, this entity was described in two independent case reports characterized by the t(15;19) translocation. Kubonishi et al. [1] first reported a thymic carcinoma harboring a chromosome translocation t(15;19)(q15;p13) in a 22-year-old female in Japan. Kees et al. [2] reported an intrathoracic undifferentiated carcinoma in an 11-year-old girl. The cytogenetic analysis found a translocation t(15;19)(p12;q13). In 2003, French et al. [3] found that the occurrence of t(15; 19)(q13; p13.1) translocation caused the formation of a 6.4-kb bromodomain and extraterminal domain (BET) protein 4 (BRD4)-NUT fusion oncogene. In 2004, French et al. [4] further studied NUT and BRD4 rearrangements using dual-color fluorescence in situ hybridization in 98 young carcinoma patients. They found that eleven tumors had NUT gene rearrangements, including eight with BRD4-NUT fusions and three with novel rearrangements, which were designated as NUT variant. All NUT-rearranged carcinomas (NRCs) originated from midline epithelial structures. They defined such carcinomas (whether having BRD4-NUT or NUT variant rearrangements) as midline carcinoma with NUT rearrangement. In the 2004 WHO classification, this tumor was recognized in the thymus as a carcinoma with t(15;19) translocation, and it is also referred to as NUT midline carcinoma. However, more and more studies confirmed that the tumor arose not only in midline structures but also in other organs or soft tissues. Therefore, the word "midline" was removed from the name of this tumor and redefined it as NUT carcinoma and classified into "other and unclassified cancer" in the 2015 WHO classification.

2 Pathology

Pathologically, NC consists of nests and sheets of small-sized to intermediate-sized undifferentiated cells with a monomorphic appearance. The nuclei have irregular contours, with vesicular chromatin and distinct nucleoli, lacking

S. Zhang (✉)
Department of Respiratory and Critical Care Medicine, Shandong Provincial Hospital Affiliated to Shandong First Medical University, Jinan, Shandong, China

S. Zhang (ed.), *Diagnostic Imaging of Lung Cancers*, https://doi.org/10.1007/978-981-99-6815-2_10

the pleomorphism typically encountered in high-grade carcinomas. The presence of keratinization in the form of large cells with intercellular bridges, focal squamous "pearls" or frank abrupt keratinization (i.e., poorly differentiated cells immediately adjacent to well differentiated squamous cells) can be found in approximately 30% of cases and can also be observed in HPV-associated basaloid squamous cell carcinomas.

Immunohistochemically, most NC cases are positive for cytokeratin (AE1-AE3, CAM5.2, CK7, CK20), P63, P40, and NUT. TTF-1 and neuroendocrine markers are often negative. EMA and C-MYC are positive in some cases.

Misdiagnosis is often caused by the histopathological features of NC that overlap with other poorly differentiated/undifferentiated tumors or resemble several common pathologies. Demonstration of NUT rearrangement by fluorescence in situ hybridization (FISH), reverse-transcription PCR, cytogenetics, or next-generation sequencing (NGS) or immunostaining by NUT-specific antibodies (more than 50% positivity in tumor nuclei is considered to be diagnostic, as some germ cell tumors can be focally positive) are effective diagnostic methods for NC.

3 Molecular Features

The oncogene of NC includes the rearrangement of the NUT gene with a set of partner genes, mainly fused to the paralogous genes encoding bromodomain and extraterminal domain proteins (BET proteins), including BRD2, BRD3, BDR4, and BRDT. NUT gene is fused to BRD4 resulting in BRD4-NUT fusion gene in 70%–88% cases, followed by 15%–30% BRD3, and 6% other rarer NUT fusion variants including the nuclear receptor binding SET domain protein 3 (NSD3) gene, the zinc-finger-containing protein encoding genes ZNF532 and ZNF592, and other unknown genes. BRD3-NUT fusion behaves similarly to BRD4-NUT at the functional level, and the other NUT fusion partners NSD3, ZNF532, and ZNF592 form a chromatin-binding complex with BRD4/3.

NGS supports the cytogenetic findings that NC likely contains a single driving the NUT fusion gene mutation, with few additional oncogenic mutations. The pathogenesis of NC is related to translocation-associated fusion oncoproteins that block cell differentiation and promote cellular growth. Native NUT protein expression has been identified in germ cells of the testis and ovary, ciliary body, germ cell tumors, and NUT-rearranged tumors. NUT encodes a polypeptide to recruit and activate the histone acetyltransferase p300. Chromatin-binding BET protein BRD4 is able to bind to acetylated lysine residues on histones. The normal function of the NUT protein is related to spermatogenesis; however, overexpression of NUT fusion genes leads to nuclear entrapment of the NUT protein, and then, these fusion genes promote cell growth and block cell differentiation through aberrant histone acetylation and activation of MYC, SOX2, and TP63, leading to proliferation and P63 dependent-cellular differentiation blockade, inducing aggressive tumor growth.

4 Epidemiology

Though NCs typically originate from midline structures of the head, neck, and thorax, the definitive anatomical site of origin is still not known. Many cases have been reported arising outside the midline, including lung, salivary gland, bladder, kidney, pancreas, adrenal gland, and various soft tissue and bone locations. It can affect people of all ages (0–81.7 years) and predominantly in young patients or adolescents, with a median age of 16–24 years. Chau et al. [5] found that the median age at diagnosis was 23.6 years in 141 patients. Thoracic origin was 51%, followed by 41% head and neck, 6% bone or soft tissue, 1% other.

No obvious sex predilection and environmental factors are identified. Viral infections, such as human papilloma virus and Epstein–Barr virus, are not discovered to be related to NC.

5 Radiographic Features

On CT scan, NT of the lung often presents as a large heterogeneous mass, with poorly defined borders and signs of invasion of adjacent structures (Fig. 1). Calcifications and necrosis can be found within the mass. Hilar and mediastinal lymphadenopathy, pleural effusion with or without pleural nodules are often present. The distant metastatic sites were predominantly bones, liver, adrenal gland, soft tissue, etc.

6 Treatment

Currently, there is no effective treatment strategy for NC. Multimodal therapy including surgery, radiation therapy, and chemotherapy is recommended. Therapeutic success is limited to individual cases. NC is often refractory to conventional chemotherapy. Several regimens have been suggested including alkylating agents, platinum and anthracycline based-chemotherapy, or combination of cisplatin, gemcitabine, and

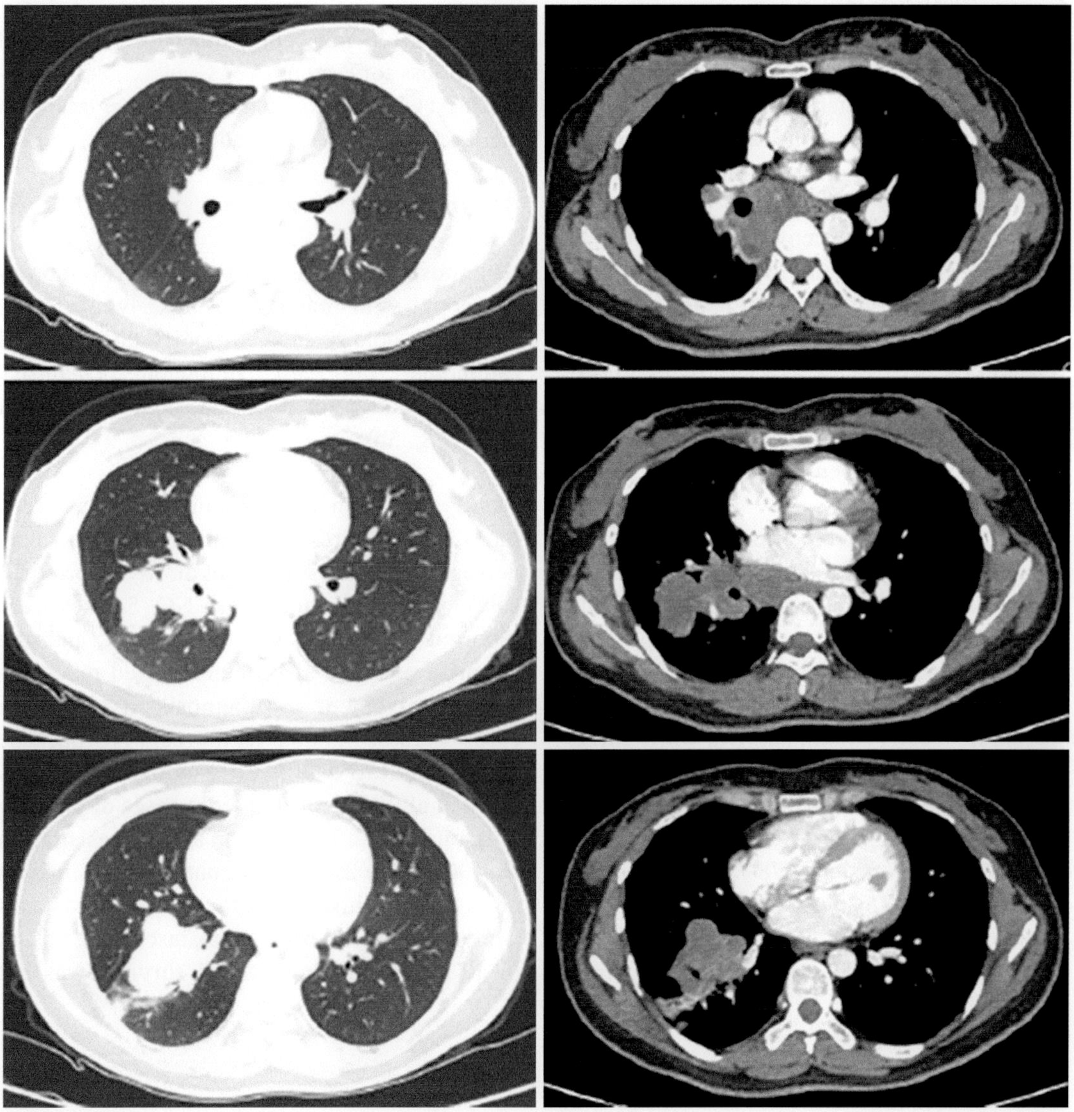

Fig. 1 NC in a 33-year-old woman. CT scan shows a soft tissue mass in the right hilum and right middle and lower lobe with mediastinal lymphadenopathy

docetaxel with or without radiotherapy. In recent years, antiangiogenic therapy, targeted therapy, and immunotherapy have also been reported. Novel targeted drugs such as BET inhibitors and histone deacetylase (HDAC) inhibitors are expected. Both of them were demonstrated to abrogate dysregulated growth and induce squamous differentiation of NC, which are translated into clinical activities. Dual HDAC/PI3K inhibitors are also considered as potential treatment.

7 Prognosis

NC has extremely poor prognosis, about 70% of patients presented distant metastases at diagnosis (lymph nodes, pleura, bone, and bone marrow), and most patients died within a year after diagnosis.

In 2012, a retrospective study of 63 NC patients by Bauer et al. [6] revealed that the median overall survival (OS) of patients with NC was 6.7 months, the 1-year OS was 30% and 2-year OS was 19%. The 2-year progression-free survival (PFS) was 9%. Multivariate analysis confirmed that extent of surgical resection and initial radiotherapy were independent predictors of PFS and OS.

Giridhar et al. [7] retrieved 119 patients from 64 publications for statistical analysis. The median OS was only 5 months, and the 1- and 5-year OS were 24.99% and 7.09%, respectively. On univariate analysis, radiotherapy and chemotherapy inclusion in primary treatment had a significant impact on overall survival while surgery had no significant impact on survival.

Chau et al. [5] showed that the median OS was 6.5 months in 141 patients. Most patients had the BRD4-NUTM1 fusion (78%), followed by BRD3-NUTM1 (15%) and NSD3-NUTM1 (6%). Nonthoracic primary BRD3- or NSD3-NUT fusion conferred the best prognosis presenting a median OS of 36 months and a 2-year OS of 64%, followed by nonthoracic primary tumors with BRD4-NUT fusion with a median OS of 10 months and a 2-year OS of 28%. Thoracic NC patients (54%), regardless of the NUT fusion have the worst survival, with a median OS of 4.4 months and a 2-year OS of 5%.

8 Case Analysis

8.1 Case

A 35-year-old man complained of fatigue and weight loss for 8 months.

Chest CT: A lesion in the right upper lobe with mediastinal lymphadenopathy (Fig. 2).

[Diagnosis] NUT carcinoma.

[Diagnosis Basis] The patient underwent bronchoscopy with mediastinal 4R lymph node biopsy. Pathology showed poorly differentiated carcinoma (Fig. 3a). Immunohistochemistry showed positive for p40, p53, p63, PD-L1, and NUT (Fig. 3b).

[Analysis] Primary pulmonary NC is very rare that often presents with a large tumor burden and metastases. Dutta et al. [8] reported 10 cases of primary pulmonary NC. 5 cases were reported occurring near the hilum, and the majority of cases also demonstrated mediastinum involvement at diagnosis. Thus, these cases were designated as thoracic NC because it is difficult to decide the exact site of origin. Sholl et al. [9] identified eight cases of primary pulmonary NC. The median age at presentation was 30 (range 21–68). Six patients had little or no smoking history. Lytic bone metastases were common but brain metastases were absent in all cases. Median overall survival was 2.2

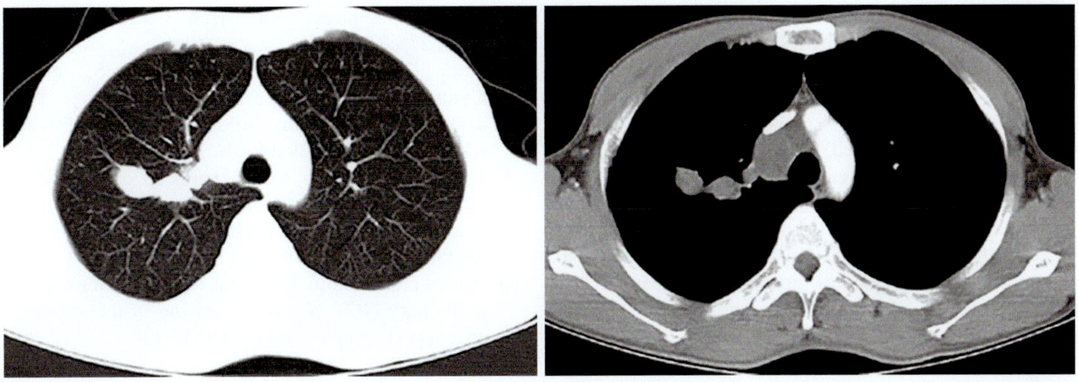

Fig. 2 Chest CT

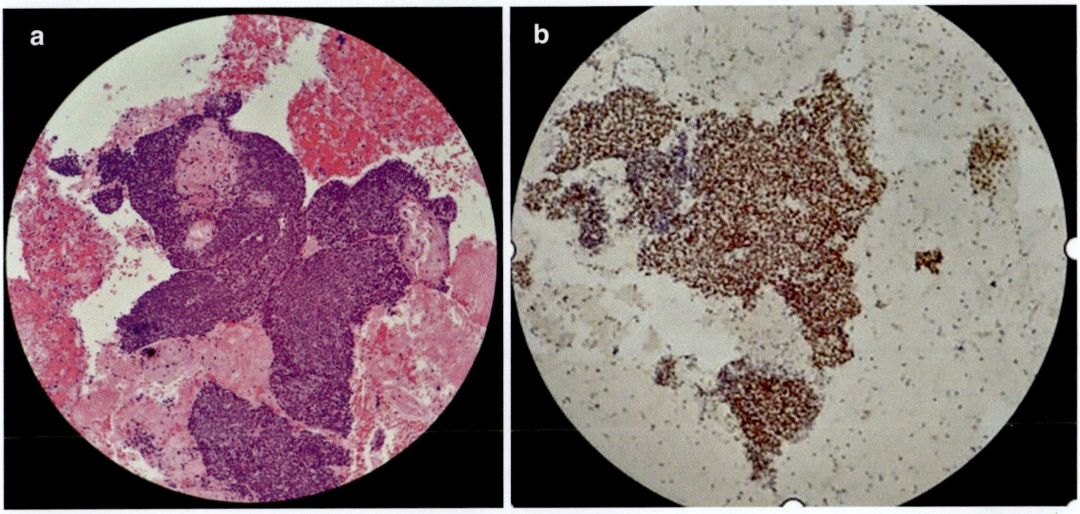

Fig. 3 (**a**) Hematoxylin-eosin-stained slide at 10×. (**b**) Positive expressions of NUT

months. Numakura et al. [10] reported an 82-year-old man with pulmonary NC which was the first case to show negativity for p63 and was the oldest among previously reported cases.

There is no standard management for primary pulmonary NC. The 2021 National Comprehensive Cancer Network (NCCN) guidelines for NSCLC recommend conducting NUT rearrangement tests on all poorly differentiated lung cancers that lack glandular differentiation or a specific etiology, particularly in non-smokers or younger patients.

References

1. Kubonishi I, Takehara N, Iwata J, et al. Novel t(15;19)(q15;p13) chromosome abnormality in a thymic carcinoma. Cancer Res. 1991;51:3327–8.
2. Kees UR, Mulcahy MT, Willoughby ML. Intrathoracic carcinoma in an 11-year-old girl showing a translocation t(15;19). Am J Pediatr Hematol Oncol. 1991;13:459–64.
3. French CA, Miyoshi I, Kubonishi I, et al. BRD4-NUT fusion oncogene: a novel mechanism in aggressive carcinoma. Cancer Res. 2003;63:304–7.
4. French CA, Kutok JL, Faquin WC, et al. Midline carcinoma of children and young adults with NUT rearrangement. J Clin Oncol. 2004;22:4135–9.

5. Chau NG, Ma C, Danga K, et al. An anatomical site and genetic-based prognostic model for patients with nuclear protein in testis (NUT) midline carcinoma: analysis of 124 patients. JNCI Cancer Spectr. 2019;4:pkz094.
6. Bauer DE, Mitchell CM, Strait KM, et al. Clinicopathologic features and long-term outcomes of NUT midline carcinoma. Clin Cancer Res. 2012;18:5773–9.
7. Giridhar P, Mallick S, Kashyap L, et al. Patterns of care and impact of prognostic factors in the outcome of NUT midline carcinoma: a systematic review and individual patient data analysis of 119 cases. Eur Arch Otorhinolaryngol. 2018;275:815–21.
8. Dutta R, Nambirajan A, Mittal S, et al. Cytomorphology of primary pulmonary NUT carcinoma in different cytology preparations. Cancer Cytopathol. 2021;129:53–61.
9. Sholl LM, Nishino M, Pokharel S, et al. Primary pulmonary NUT midline carcinoma: clinical, radiographic, and pathologic characterizations. J Thorac Oncol. 2015;10:951–9.
10. Numakura S, Saito K, Motoi N, et al. P63-negative pulmonary NUT carcinoma arising in the elderly: a case report. Diagn Pathol. 2020;15:134.

Salivary Gland-Type Tumors

Song Zhang

Primary pulmonary salivary gland-type tumors (PSGTs) are rare tumors that comprise less than 1.0% of all lung cancers.

1 Classification

In the 2015 WHO classification of lung tumors, these tumors were divided into the following four types: mucoepidermoid carcinoma (MEC), adenoid cystic carcinoma (ACC), epithelial-myoepithelial carcinoma (EMC), and pleomorphic adenoma (PA). In the 2021 WHO classification, hyalinizing clear cell carcinoma (HCCC) was added to the group of salivary gland-type tumors.

2 Pathology

Histologically, MECs consist of mucin-secreting cells (mucocytes), squamous cells (epidermoid cells), and intermediate-type cells arranged in glandular, tubular, cystic, nested, or solid architectural patterns (Fig. 1a). The mucus-secreting cells (mucocytes) may have cuboidal, columnar, clear cell, or oncocytic features. Squamous cells are characterized by intercellular bridges but keratinization or an in situ component of the overlying epithelium is strikingly absent contrary to squamous cell carcinoma. The intermediate cells are polygonal in shape and contain centrally or eccentrically placed nuclei and abundant eosinophilic or amphophilic cytoplasm. The stroma is composed of bands of fibroconnective tissue which can amount to extensive sclerotic changes (so-called sclerosing MEC) in some cases. Based on their cellular composition and cytologic features, pulmonary MECs are divided into low-grade (>80%) and high-grade variants. Low-grade MECs are characterized by mixed cystic and solid areas, low mitotic activity, minimal cytologic atypia, lack of lung parenchyma infiltration, and absence of necrosis. High-grade MECs mainly consist of epidermoid and intermediate cells in solid growth pattern with significant nuclear atypia, an increased mitotic count (>4 mitoses/10 HPF), frequent necrosis, and lymphovascular or perineural invasion. Immunohistochemically, MECs usually show positive staining for cytokeratin 7 and cytokeratin 5/6, P63 and p40, and negative staining for CK20, TTF-1, and Napsin A.

Primary pulmonary ACCs have 3 main architectural growth patterns (Fig. 1b). The cribriform or cylindromatous pattern is the most common pattern, characterized by nests and islands of tumor cells with well-defined luminal spaces containing mucinous or basement membrane-like material. The tubular pattern is composed of cells

S. Zhang (✉)
Department of Respiratory and Critical Care Medicine, Shandong Provincial Hospital Affiliated to Shandong First Medical University, Jinan, Shandong, China

S. Zhang (ed.), *Diagnostic Imaging of Lung Cancers*, https://doi.org/10.1007/978-981-99-6815-2_11

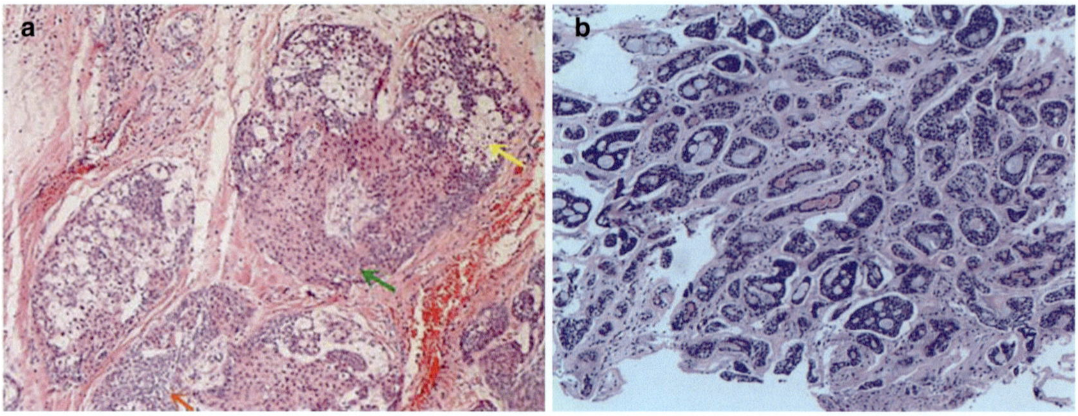

Fig. 1 (**a**) MEC shows sheets of mixed mucus cells (yellow arrow), squamous cells (green arrow), and intermediate cells (orange arrow). (**b**) ACC shows epithelial proliferation arranged in a cribriform pattern and contains myxoid hyaline material

forming small scattered gland-like spaces with wide lumina lined by 2 to 3 layers of cuboidal cells. The solid variant consists of nests of cells with only rare intercellular spaces, absence of cystic areas, and a limited stromal matrix. Cytologically, the tumor cells are composed of bland cells with round nuclei, dense chromatin, and scant eosinophilic or amphophilic cytoplasm. There is no significant pleomorphism or mitotic activity, and areas of necrosis or hemorrhage are rare. ACCs show positive staining for pan-cytokeratin, cytokeratin 7, and p63, variably reactive with smooth muscle actin (SMA) and S100, and negative for synaptophysin and TTF-1. CD117 (c-kit protein) and myeloblastosis (MYB) are also positive, which can help ACC to differentiate from other basaloid neoplasms.

EMCs have a striking biphasic appearance with duct-like structures that are formed by an inner layer of epithelial cells and a surrounding outer layer of myoepithelial cells. The epithelial cells are flat, cuboidal, or columnar-shaped and contain eosinophilic cytoplasm and round to oval nuclei. The myoepithelial layer consists of polygonal cells with eccentric nuclei, clear cytoplasm, and indistinct cell borders [1]. Immunohistochemically, the epithelial cells are positive for pan-cytokeratin and negative for SMA, S100, HMB45, CD117, glial fibrillary acidic protein (GFAP), and TTF-1. The outer myoepithelial cells express S100 and SMA, focally positive for cytokeratin, CD117, and GFAP, and negative for TTF-1 and HMB45.

Primary pulmonary PAs show a biphasic cellular composition with epithelial tubules or ducts and nests embedded in or merging with a myxoid or chondromyxoid stroma. Solid sheets of myoepithelial cells with clear cell, spindle cell, or plasmacytoid appearance also are common finding and may be the most prominent feature in some tumors. Areas of squamous metaplasia may also be seen in these lesions. These tumors are variably positive for pan-cytokeratin, S100, SMA, GFAP, calponin, and SMA [1].

Pulmonary HCCCs show tumor cells arranged in nests, cords, and trabeculae that are embedded in a dense hyalinized stroma. The tumor cells are small to medium sized and have oval nuclei with irregular nuclear contours and ample clear cytoplasm. Focal mucin pools may be evident, and mitotic activity is low. Tumors are often surrounded by a lymphocytic infiltrate. The neoplastic cells are positive for pan-cytokeratin, CK7, p63, and p40, and negative for myoepithelial markers, neuroendocrine markers, TTF-1, and Napsin A. HCCC is characterized by an Ewing sarcoma breakpoint region 1-activating transcription factor 1 (EWSR1-ATF1) gene fusions.

3 Molecular Features

Distinctive molecular events of SGTs have gradually been discovered, such as MYB-NFIB fusion in ACC and 8q12 abnormalities, pleomorphic adenoma gene 1 (PLAG1) rearrangement, and high-mobility group A2 (HMGA) amplification in PA. Several articles have described the presence of the CRTC1-MAML2 translocation in MEC. CRTC1-MAML2 translocation is formed because of the recurring chromosomal translocation t(11;19)(q21;p13), which results in the fusion transcript from the binding of exon 1 of the CRTC1 gene at 19p13 with exons 2 to 5 of the MAML2 gene. As a transcription factor on Notch and CREB regulatory pathways, CRTC1-MAML2 oncogene disrupts normal cell-cycle and differentiation, contributes to tumor development. Pérez-de-Oliveira et al. [2] studied 10 published articles that assessed the association between the CRTC1-MAML2 translocation and survival of MEC patients. The prevalence of the translocation varied from 33.7% to 69.7%. Seven studies observed a significant association between the presence of the CRTC1-MAML2 translocation and a favorable clinical outcome, which could improve disease-free, disease-specific, or overall survival.

Kato et al. [3] analyzed the molecular aberrations in 117 SGT patients. The most common abnormalities involved the TP53 gene (30.8%,36/117), cyclin pathway (CCND1, CDK4/6 or CDKN2A/B) (26.5%,31/117), and PI3K pathway (PIK3CA, PIK3R1, PTEN or AKT1/3) (23.9%,28/117). Significant associations were identified between aberrations in TP53 and ERBB2, the cyclin pathway and MDM2, and HRAS and the PI3K pathway.

Kang et al. [4] reported that TP53 was the most commonly mutated gene in MEC (28%), and mutations were found only in intermediate- and high-grade tumors. Tumors with TP53 mutations had more mutations overall than tumors without TP53 mutations. POU6F2 was the second most frequently mutated gene, found in three low-grade MECs with the same in-frame deletion. FISH analysis confirmed the presence of the MECT1-MAML2 translocation in 15 of 17 tumors (88%). They concluded that MECT1-MAML2 translocation and somatic TP53 and POU6F2 mutations appear to be the main drivers of MEC.

Wang et al. [5] profiled the molecular alterations of PSGTs via targeted NGS. Among the 32 patients, 25 had MEC and 7 had ACC. MAML2 and MYB rearrangements were detected in 80.0% (20/25) of the MEC and 71.4% (5/7) of the ACC patients. Among the MEC patients, 10 (40.0%) had ≥ 1 mutation, and 6 of them had 11 isolated mutations with abundance >5%, namely NFE2L2, MYOD1, INPP4B, CCND2, SNTG1, HSPD1, TGFBR1, RBM10, NOTCH4, ASXL1, and PTPRD mutations. The remaining 4 patients had 9 mutations with abundance <5%, namely KMT2A, PDCD11, FLT1, BRCA2, APC, SLX4, FOXP1, FGFR1, and HRAS mutations. No TP53 mutations were detected in this study, demonstrating that TP53 variations differed between pulmonary MEC and MEC at other sites. All the ACC patients had mutations, which were enriched in 5 pathways including the PI3K and NOTCH pathways, chromatin and cytoskeleton remodeling, and DNA damage. These results explained PSGTs harbor distinct driver features of MAML2 or MYB rearrangement, accompanied with wide mutational diversity with very low rate of somatic mutation. Several important pathways, including the NOTCH and PI3K pathways, and chromatin remodeling could be targeted to improve the survival in patients with ACC (reproduced with permission of copyright holder).

4 Epidemiology

MEC and ACC are the most common subtypes, comprising 90% of PSGTs. PSGTs tend to occur in the adult population and have a more indolent nature compared with other types of lung cancer. The gender distribution of PSGT varies with tumor subtype. ACC has male predominance, whereas MEC and EMC show an equal sex distribution.

5 Radiographic Features

PSGTs arise from bronchial submucosal glands and often present as endobronchial masses in the trachea or mainstem bronchi. On CT scan, it usually shows a well-circumscribed lesion in an endobronchial location causing bronchial wall thickening and/or intramural polypoid growth. The intraluminal component can be sessile, polypoid, or pedunculated. Endobronchial mass is often associated with obstructive pneumonia and/or atelectasis. Occasionally, PSGT may present as solitary nodule in the peripheral lung.

6 Treatment

Surgical resection is the standard therapy for PSGT. There is no evidence of efficacy or guidelines for chemotherapy for PSGT, though the combination of carboplatin and paclitaxel may be effective in some reports.

Kim BG et al. [6] investigated 181 PSGT patients including 72 patients who underwent bronchoscopy interventions. Among the 181 patients, 104 (57.5%) patients were diagnosed with ACC, followed 71(39.2%) MEC and 6(3.3%) EMC. The surgery group had the best OS and PFS. However, the OS was no significant difference between the surgery and bronchoscopic intervention groups in patients at high clinical stages. Bronchoscopic intervention may be useful as the initial treatment in patients at high clinical stage and as a bridge therapy prior to surgery.

7 Prognosis

Patients with PSGT frequently have a good long-term prognosis. Molina et al. [7] analyzed 62 PSGT patients diagnosed at the Mayo Clinic from 1972 to 2002. For surgical patients, the 3-, 5-, and 10-year survival rates were 82%, 70%, and 63%, respectively. For surgical MEC and ACC patients, the survival rates were 94%, 87%, 87%, and 73%, 57%, 45% at 3, 5, and 10 years, respectively. The survival rate for patients with ACC who did not undergo surgery was 74%, 53%, and 31% at 3, 5, and 10 years, respectively. The difference in survival between surgical and nonsurgical patients was statistically significant. Local recurrence is likely if complete surgical resection is not achieved. ACC has a higher likelihood than MEC to metastasize. Overall, patients with MEC survive better than patients with ACC.

Qin et al. [8] identified 462 PSGT patients, including 315 MEC, 139 ACC, and 8 EMC. The 1-, 5-, 10-, and 20-year OS rates of PSGT patients were 79.6%, 68.5%, 62.7%, and 56.3%, respectively. PSGT patients have a significantly better prognosis than non-SGT lung adenocarcinoma patients. Radiotherapy did not prolong OS. Older age (>58 years), larger lesions, metastases, and poor differentiation were independent prognostic factors for worse survival, while cancer-directed surgery was an independent protective factor. Patients with MEC were younger with smaller tumors, lower ratio of lymph node or distant metastases as well as earlier stage than those with ACC, and there was no significant difference in survival between MEC and ACC patients.

Garg et al. [9] systematically reviewed 5 studies including 233 patients. Mean age of PSGT patients was 41 years (range 6–80 years), and there was a male preponderance (1.3:1)0.15.2% of the patients found lymph node involvement. 21.1% of the patients (12.9% MEC and 37.5% ACC) observed disease recurrences. 3-, 5-, and 10-year weighted overall survival was 86.4%, 81.4%, and 73.6% (93.8%, 90.0%, and 85.0%, respectively, for MEC and 76.7%, 62.8%, and 50.5%, respectively, for ACC).

8 Case Analysis

8.1 Case 1

A 17-year-old woman complained of cough and expectoration for 10 days.

Chest CT: An oval lesion in the left lower lobe bronchus with finger-in-glove sign (Fig. 2).

[Diagnosis] Primary pulmonary mucoepidermoid carcinoma.

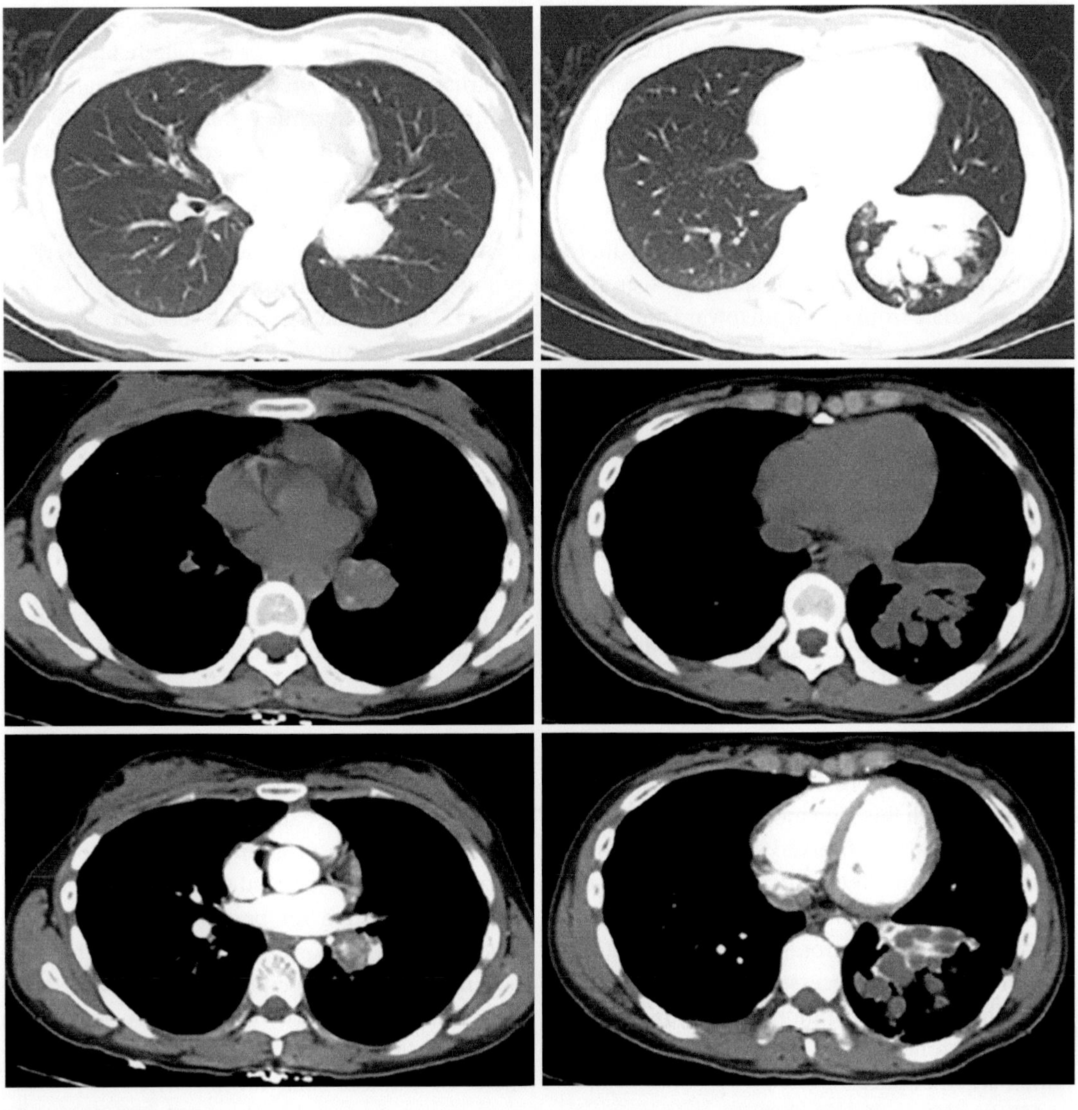

Fig. 2 Chest CT

[Diagnosis Basis] CT scan shows an oval solid endobronchial lesion with regular shape, well-defined boundary, patchy calcifications, and obvious enhancement. Bronchial finger-in-glove sign (mucus impaction) is seen. There is no evidence of lymphadenopathy. Considering that the patient is a young woman, supporting the diagnosis of pulmonary mucoepidermoid carcinoma. This case needs to be differentiated from adenoid cystic carcinoma, sclerosing pneumocytoma, and carcinoid. Adenoid cystic carcinoma occurs at an older age, tends to occur in the central airway, and infiltrates inside and outside of lumen, calcification is rare, and enhancement is not obvious. Sclerosing pneumocytoma generally does not show intrabronchial growth. In addition, finger-in-glove sign does not support the diagnosis of sclerosing pneumocytoma. Carcinoid tumor is mostly located in the bronchial tree, grows inside and outside the bronchial lumen, and may occur with atelectasis, obstructive pneumonia, and mucoid impaction. Contrast-enhanced CT scan shows specific characteristics, such as the presence of eccentric calcifications, marked enhancement, and mediastinal adenopathy. Left lower lobectomy was performed, and the postoperative pathology was low-grade mucoepidermoid carcinoma. No lymph node metastases are detected.

[Analysis] On chest X-ray or CT scan, finger-in-glove sign is described as the branching dilated airways that are filled with respiratory secretions and that radiate from the hilum toward the periphery of the lung. Both congenital and acquired abnormalities may cause mucoid impaction which often manifests as tubular opacities.

In 1951, Shaw [10] described dilated bronchi with mucoid impaction in five patients who presented with wheezing, cough, and a history of allergy. In 1978, Mintzer et al. [11] first used the term finger in glove (or gloved finger) to describe a case of ABPA. In 2008, Martinez et al. [12] classified finger-in-glove sign based both on the origin (congenital or acquired) and the nature (inflammatory, infectious, or neoplastic) of the specific disease process. Segmental bronchial atresia and cystic fibrosis are the congenital conditions in which this sign most often appears. The sign also may be observed in acquired conditions, include inflammatory and infectious diseases (allergic bronchopulmonary aspergillosis, broncholithiasis, and foreign body aspiration), benign neoplastic processes (bronchial hamartoma, lipoma, and papillomatosis), and malignancies (bronchogenic carcinoma, carcinoid tumor, and metastases).

CT is very useful in differentiating mucous impaction from other disease processes such as arteriovenous malformations, and is used to guide further diagnostic evaluation.

8.2 Case 2

A 72-year-old man complained of cough for 1 month.

Chest CT: An oval mass in the left lower lobe bronchus (Fig. 3).

[Diagnosis] Primary pulmonary mucoepidermoid carcinoma.

[Diagnosis Basis] CT scan shows an oval solid endobronchial nodule with calcifications and obstructive pneumonia. The CT attenuations of the three-phase dynamic scan are 54.9, 65.9, and 85.5 HU, respectively. Fiberoptic bronchoscopy biopsy revealed mucoepidermoid carcinoma.

[Analysis] Smetana et al. [13] first described pulmonary mucoepidermoid carcinoma (PMEC) in 1952. It originates from the submucosal glands of the tracheobronchial tree that causes approximately 0.1–0.2% of all lung malignancies. It arises more common in the lobar bronchi than in the trachea or main bronchi and rarely tumor appears as an isolated peripheral pulmonary nodule. PMEC usually occurs in younger adults with an average age of <50 years, not correlated with smoking.

PMEC may show well-circumscribed oval or lobulated mass with punctate or coarse calcification and sometimes post-obstructive pneumonia on non-enhanced CT. The incidence of calcification in PMEC is 9.1%–50%, which is much higher than in the more common forms of lung cancer. Intratumor calcifications may be caused by insufficient absorption of mucus. González-Arriagada et al. [14] found that areas of calcification were positive for periodic acid-Schiff and mucicarmine, supporting the hypothesis that they originate from the precipitation of mucous secretion. Calcification is more commonly detected in low-grade PMECs, suggesting it might be a predictor of indolent behavior in PMEC.

Some studies have evaluated the treatment and prognosis of PMEC. Hsieh et al. [15] retrospectively reviewed the prognostic factors of 41 surgical PMEC patients. Sixteen patients (39.0%) experienced tumor relapse, including 13 patients (81.3%) within 2 years. The 5-year disease-free survival rate was 57.9%. Tumor grade did not influence either disease-free survival or overall survival. Age, tumor size, and pathological factors were independent predictors of disease-free survival and overall survival. In elderly patients (>65 years), pathological T status was the only independent predictor of disease-free survival and overall survival. Qiu et al. [16] evaluated clinical characteristics and prognostic fac-

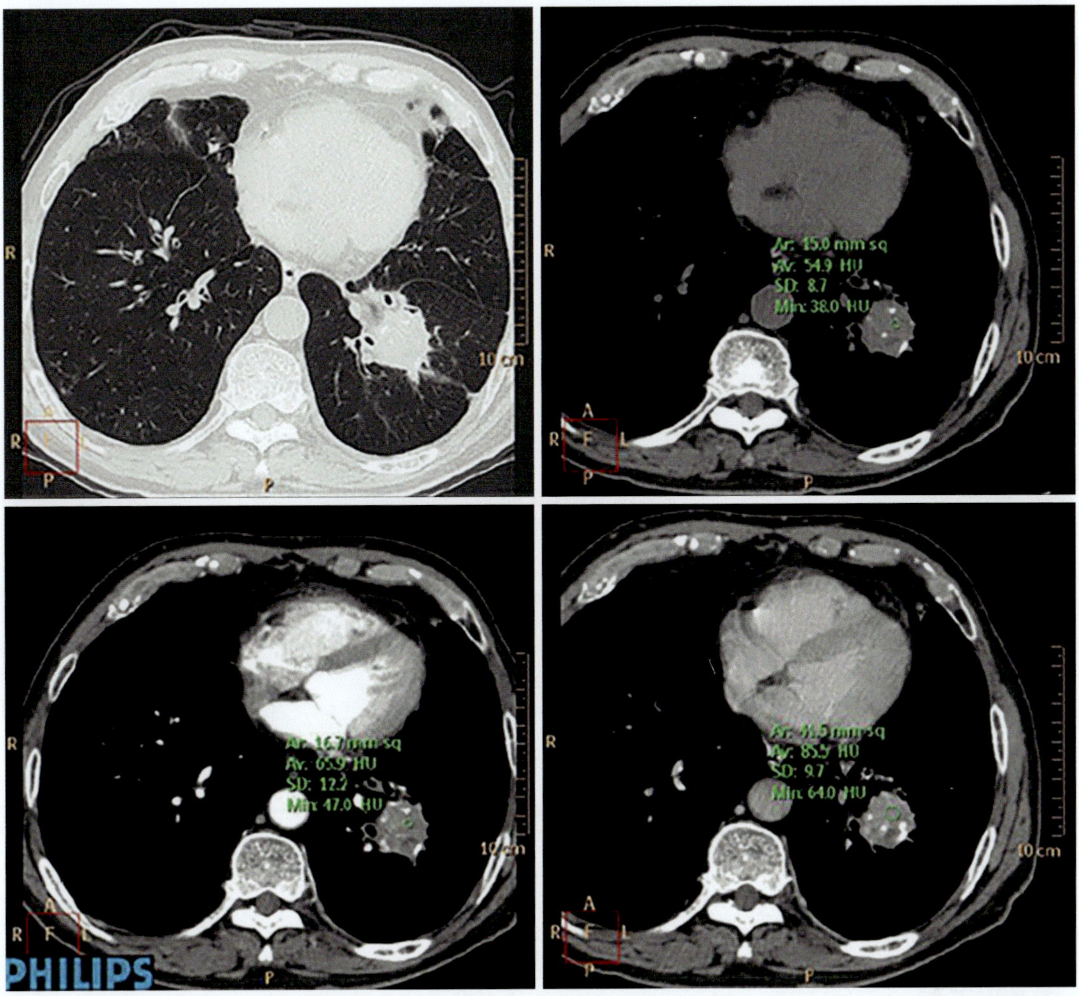

Fig. 3 Chest CT

tors of 585 PMEC patients by a SEER-based analysis. The 5- and 10-year cancer-specific survival (CSS) rates of stage I-II PMEC patients were 91.4% and 88.9%, respectively. The 1-, 3- and 5-year CSS rates of stage III-IV PMEC were 56.5%, 39.45%, and 32.1%, respectively. CSS outcomes were significantly better in patients who received surgical treatments (surgical alone, surgery plus radiation, and/or chemotherapy). Patients who received radiation and/or chemotherapy had the worst prognosis. Age, bilateral tumors, tumor size, pathological differentiation grade, lymph node metastasis, distant metastasis, TNM stage and therapy were independent prognostic factors of PMEC patients.

8.3 Case 3

A 39-year-old woman complained of cough and hemoptysis for 3 months.

Chest CT: An oval mass in the right lower lobe bronchus (Fig. 4).

[Diagnosis] Primary pulmonary mucoepidermoid carcinoma.

[Diagnosis Basis] CT scan shows an oval solid endobronchial nodule with finger-in-glove sign. Enhanced and delayed enhancement are observed. The patient underwent right lower lobectomy. The bronchus was incised, and a

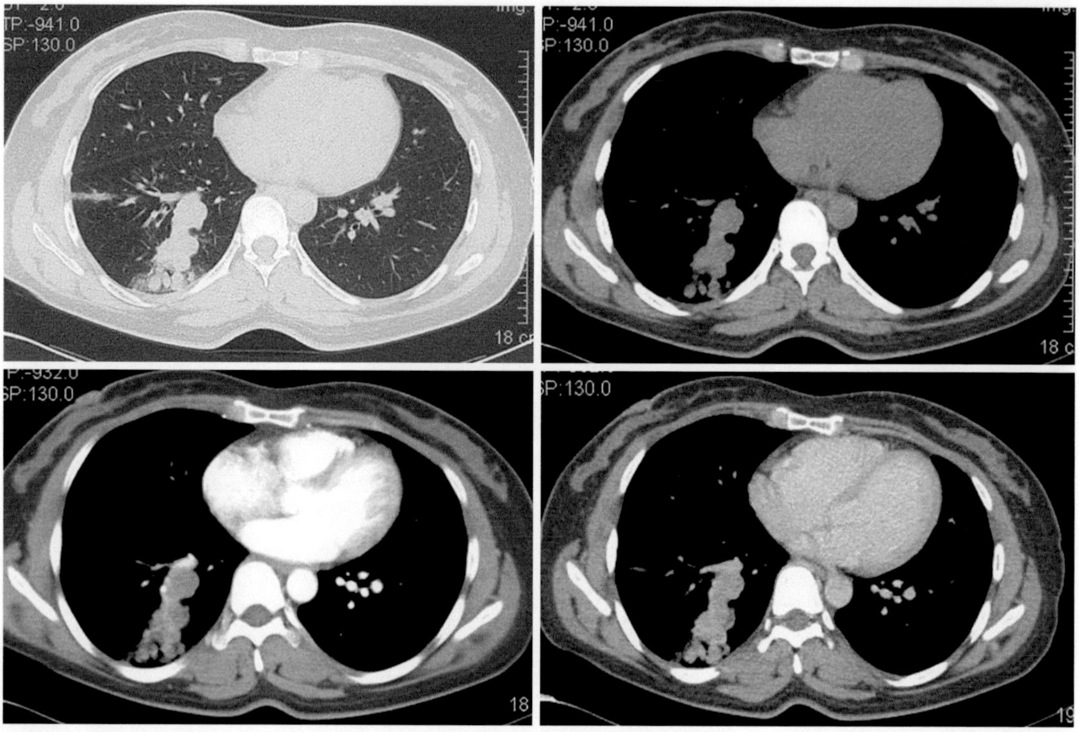

Fig. 4 Chest CT

gray-white mass with a clear boundary was found in the lumen, with a size of 5.6 × 2.8 × 3.0 cm, and part of it grew into the lung. Local lung tissue was grayish yellow. Bronchiectasis and mucus impaction were seen in the surrounding lung tissue. Pathology revealed high-grade mucoepidermoid carcinoma involving the visceral pleura. The surrounding lung tissue showed focal changes of lipoid pneumonia. No metastasis was found in the lymph nodes.

[Analysis] MEC is the most common salivary gland neoplasm, accounting for 10%–15% of all salivary neoplasms. Although the most common location of MEC was the head and neck, it can occur in many sites of the body, including the skin, breasts, lungs, and thymus.

Histologically, high-grade PMECs usually show active mitosis, nuclear pleomorphism, and necrosis. Compared with low-grade PMECs, mucus secretion is decreased because of poor differentiation, cystic lesions are less common, and necrosis is more common in high-grade PMECs. On CT, some high-grade PMECs present signs of common lung cancer, such as spiculation, pleural infiltration, lymphadenopathy, and even distant metastasis.

Wang et al. [17] characterized the CT features and clinical findings of low-grade and high-grade PMEC. High-grade PMEC tends to be peripheral, whereas low-grade PMEC tended to be central. Low-grade PMEC showed greater enhancement (46.90 ± 20.44 HU) than did high-grade PMEC (22.50 ± 8.38 HU). Cheng et al. [18] found that high-grade PMECs occurred more frequently in patients aged >40 years and were more predominant in men. Low-grade PMECs were more common in young females. MSCT revealed an oval or lobulated mass with mild enhancement, as manifested by calcification and visible mucus lakes, which may be suggestive of PMECs. High-grade PMECs tend to be peripheral and associated with lymph node metastasis. Mean survival was 59.2 months and 20.4 months for patients with low-grade PMECs and high-grade PMECs, respectively; 3-year survival rates were 55% and

14%, respectively. Pathological grade, lymph node metastasis, and TNM stage correlate with the survival of patients with PMEC.

Complete surgical resection remains the standard therapy for PMEC. Adjuvant chemotherapy may be useful for high-grade PMEC patients, especially in cases of lymph node involvement or intrathoracic invasion. PMECs with minor EGFR mutations have been reported in Asian populations, but most studies have found that EGFR mutations are absent in western population. Molecularly targeted therapy is likely to improve the prognosis of progressive high grade and recurrent MEC patients.

8.4 Case 4

A 33-year-old man complained of cough and hemoptysis for 1 week.

Chest CT: An oval mass in the left main bronchus (Fig. 5).

[Diagnosis] Primary pulmonary mucoepidermoid carcinoma.

[Diagnosis Basis] CT scan shows an oval solid nodule located in left main bronchus. The CT attenuations are 45 and 130 HU, respectively. Pathology revealed mucoepidermoid carcinoma.

[Analysis] PMECs are usually located in a lobar or segmental bronchi. Kim et al. [19] reviewed retrospectively histopathologically proved mucoepidermoid carcinomas in 12 consecutive patients. At CT, the tumors were all smoothly oval or lobulated in shape, adapting to the branching features of the airways. Punctate calcification within the tumor was seen in six patients.

PMECs usually show mild and nonuniform enhancement, but the tumor is known to be vascular, which may have contributed to the marked enhancement of PMEC. The imaging features of PMEC are sometimes similar to carcinoid tumors. 68Ga-DOTATOC PET-CT could be performed to

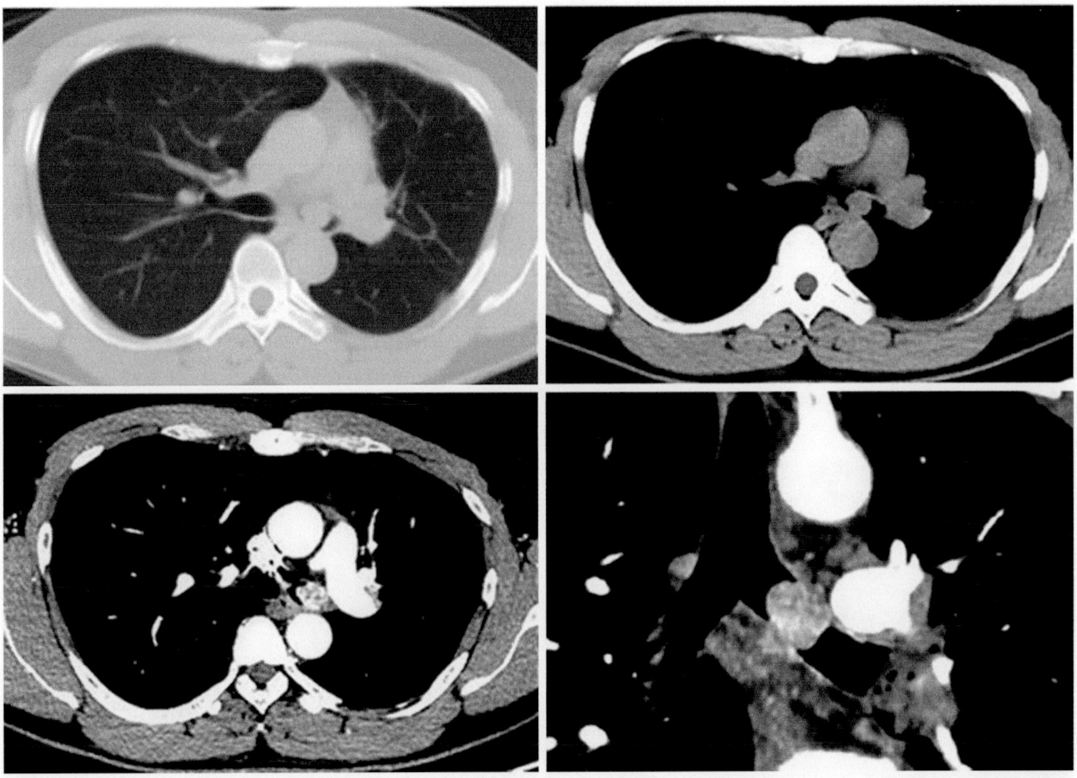

Fig. 5 Chest CT

distinguish them and is positive for typical carcinoid and negative for PMEC.

PMECs in the central airways may be difficult to distinguish from bronchogenic carcinoma. Ban et al. [20] retrospectively reviewed CT imaging features of PMEC, squamous cell carcinoma, and adenocarcinoma. The primary lung tumor with central type or hilar type, regular shape, well-defined margin, and marked enhancement indicates PMEC. Li et al. [21] compared the CT findings of PMEC and PACC. PMEC is usually the hilar type, accompanied by distal bronchial dilatation with mucoid impaction. PACC is usually the central type, with longitudinal extent greater than 3 cm and infiltration of the luminal wall more than 1/2 perimeter. Patchy areas of low density and moderate or severe enhancement are more prominent in PMEC. On the contrary, slight enhancement is more common in PACC.

8.5 Case 5

A 46-year-old man complained of suffocation and hoarseness for half a year.

Chest CT: An intratracheal nodule at the level of the upper aorta with a density of 30 HU (Fig. 6).

[Diagnosis] Primary pulmonary adenoid cystic carcinoma.

[Diagnosis Basis] Bronchoscopy showed that the tumor was located in the middle and lower segment of the trachea with a smooth surface and blocked most of the lumen. The patient underwent tracheal tumor resection. The tumor was located 2 cm above the carina, with a size of about 3.0 × 3.0 × 2.0 cm, and bulged about 1.0 cm × 1.2 cm to the outside of the trachea. The tumor surface was smooth and hard. Pathology showed adenoid cystic carcinoma, involving the tracheal wall, and no metastasis was found in the 2,4 groups and the parabronchial lymph nodes.

[Analysis] ACC is the most common salivary-type tumor of large airways and the second common primary tracheal tumor after squamous cell carcinoma, accounting for 0.04–0.2% of all primary pulmonary tumors. Patients commonly present with bronchial obstruction, resulting in cough and dyspnea.

At CT, ACC appears as a focal lesion in the trachea or main bronchi with a smooth border, peripheral or segmental localization is uncommon. ACC has a significant tendency toward submucosal extension and commonly presents with circumferential thickening or intraluminal and extraluminal extension. It may involve more than half of the airway circumference and can be differentiated from MEC based on its frequent extraluminal extension. Calcification is not observed in ACC.

FDG uptake in primary PSGT is variable on PET images, according to the grade of differentiation. Elnayal et al. [22] assessed CT features and FDG uptake of 30 consecutive patients with primary PSGT. Compared with MECs, ACCs

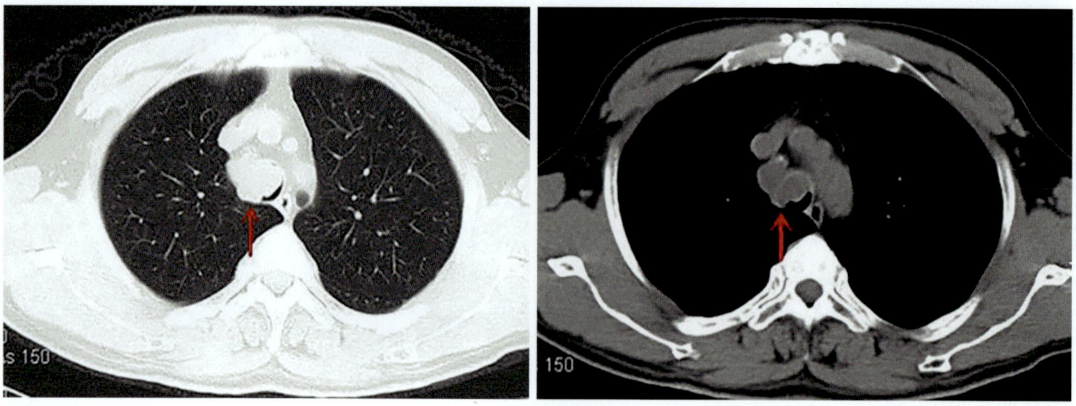

Fig. 6 Chest CT

were larger, more frequently involved the central airways (94% vs 63%), and had a higher median FDG uptake. Higher FDG uptake of the primary tumor was associated with nodal tumor involvement. The median overall survival times for patients with ACC and MEC were 7.7 and 4.0 years, respectively. Imaging features of mediastinal or hilar lymphadenopathy, suspected metastatic disease, and primary tumor heterogeneity significantly affected overall survival.

8.6 Case 6

A 33-year-old man complained of cough and hemoptysis for 1 week.

Chest CT: An oval mass in the right intermediate bronchus, the CT attenuations of the three-phase dynamic scan were 41.00, 43.50, and 60.75 HU, respectively (Fig. 7).

[Diagnosis] Primary pulmonary adenoid cystic carcinoma.

[Diagnosis Basis] Bronchoscopy of the patient showed neoplastic growth at the opening of the right intermediate bronchus, occluding 80% of the lumen. Biopsy pathology was consistent with ACC, showing neurological invasion. Immunohistochemistry was positive for CD 117 and smooth muscle actin (SMA).

[Analysis] ACC consists of ductal and modified myoepithelial cells and exhibits three predominant histological growth patterns: cribriform, tubular pattern, and solid pattern. The cribriform pattern shows a more benign behavior, and solid ACC has a more destructive clinical course and early distant metastases. Lymph node metastases and vascular emboli are uncommon, but perineural invasion has been frequently reported, which is consistent with our case.

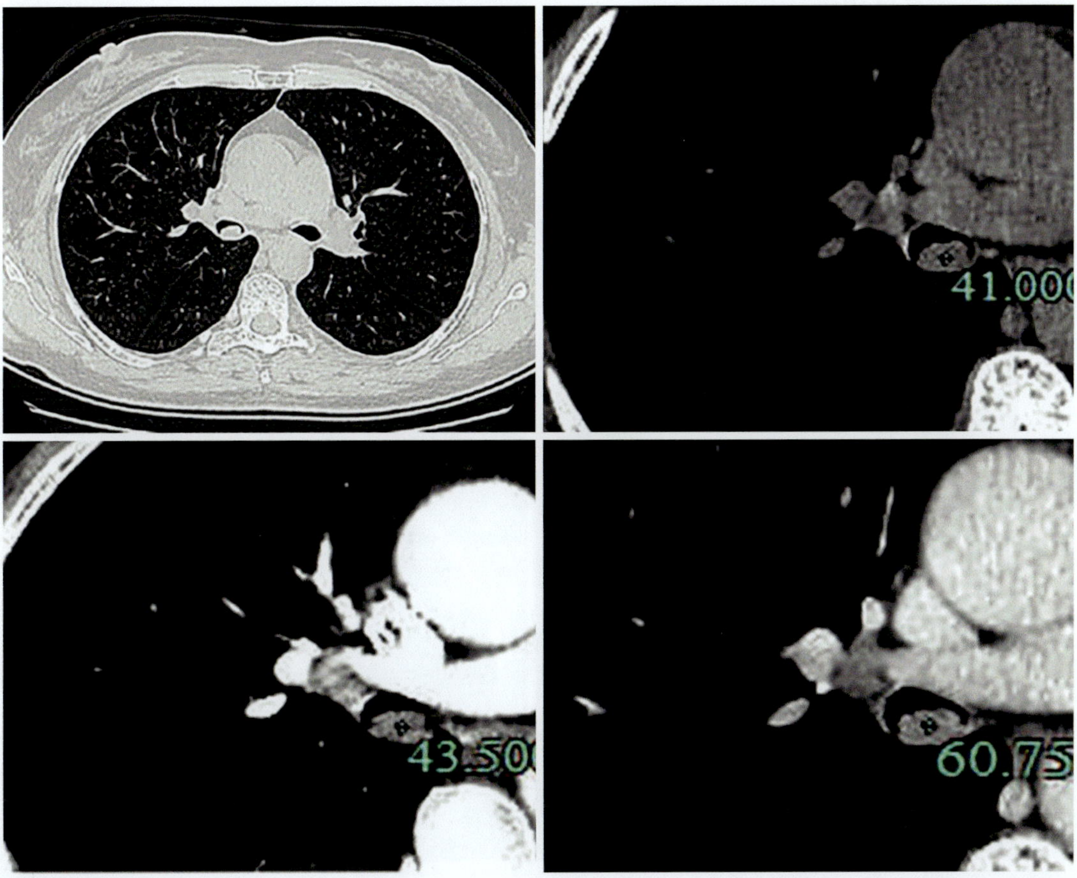

Fig. 7 Chest CT

Immunohistochemically, ductal cells are mainly positive for EMA, CEA, CK7, and CD117; myoepithelial cells are mainly positive for P63, SMA, S-100, calponin, CK5/6, and SMA. CD117 (KIT) is a type III receptor tyrosine kinase encoded by the c-kit gene. The expression of CD117 is often in ACC and EMC, but not in other types of SGT.

Surgery is the main treatment method for PACC. ACC has a prolonged clinical course with infiltrated growth and perineural invasion and tends to distant metastasis. Kumar et al. [23] analyzed demographic, clinical, and survival data from 1032 patients (546 PMEC and 486 PACC). The incidence of pulmonary PSGT is 7 cases per 10 million population in the United States and change of −32% from 1973 to 2014. The incidence of PMEC was slightly higher than PACC but there were no differences in the age and sex distribution. PACCs (55%) were significantly higher at trachea and main bronchus while PMECs were more common at peripheral lungs (85%). Compared with PMEC, significantly higher number of patients with PACC underwent radical surgery and received adjuvant radiation. The 1- and 5-year cause-specific survival were 76.6 and 62.8%, respectively. On multivariate analysis, the survival was affected by age at diagnosis, tumor stage, histological grade, period of diagnosis, and surgical resection. The histology showed that strong interaction with time and hazard ratio of patients with PACC was significantly worse than patients with PMEC only after 5 years.

8.7 Case 7

A 65-year-old man complained of cough and expectoration for 1 month.

Chest CT: An oval nodule in the right lower lung lobe, the CT attenuations of the three-phase dynamic scan were 60.2, 116.1, and 88.9HU, respectively (Fig. 8).

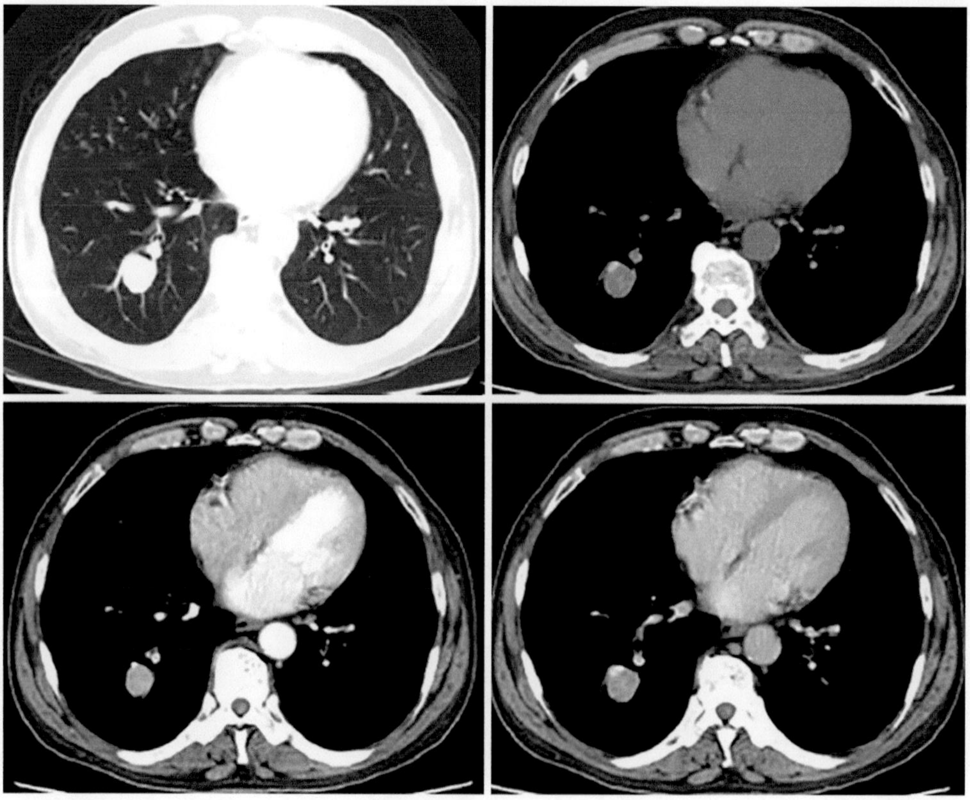

Fig. 8 Chest CT

[Diagnosis] Primary pulmonary epithelial-myoepithelial carcinoma.

[Diagnosis Basis] The patient underwent surgical resection of the lesion, and postoperative pathology showed low-grade malignant tumor with eosinophilic cytoplasm, which was considered to be epithelial-myoepithelial carcinoma (Fig. 9a, b). No vascular, lymphatic, and neural invasion was observed. Immunohistochemically, the inner layer was positive for CK7 and CK18/8, and the surrounding layer was positive for p63. Both the epithelial and myoepithelial cells were negative for TTF-1 (Fig. 10a, b). The Ki-67 labeling index was less than 10%.

[Analysis] Epithelial-myoepithelial carcinoma (EMC) was first described in 1972 in a tumor of the salivary glands by Donath et al. [24]. It accounts for 1% of all salivary gland tumors and 2% of all salivary gland malignancies. EMC typically occurs in the sixth and seventh decades of life and has an even sex distribution or a slight female predilection.

EMC is histologically characterized by biphasic tubular structures composed of inner eosinophilic ductal cells and outer clear myoepithelial cells. Of the 2 types of cells, myoepithelial cells generally outnumbered luminal ductal cells, the mean myoepithelial/epithelial cell ratio ranged from 1.8 to 4.3. EMC sometimes shows various histologic features,

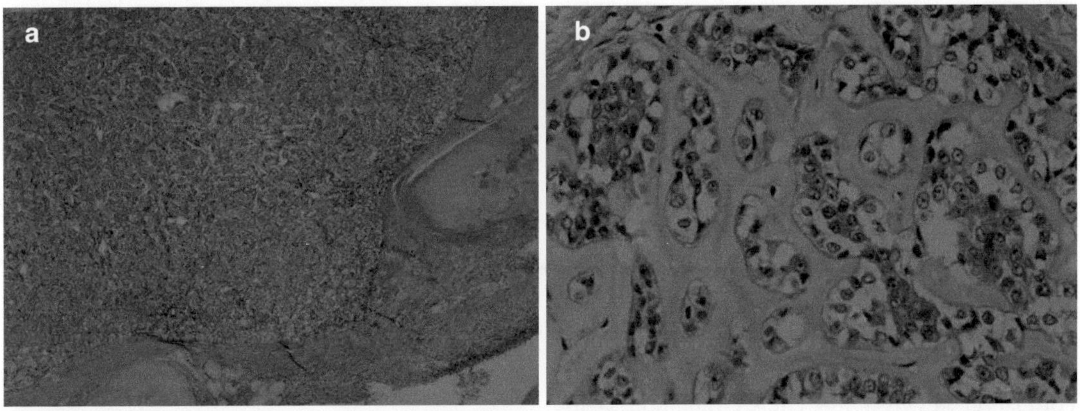

Fig. 9 (**a**) The tumor is infiltrative growth, and the bronchus is visible on the lower left side (40×). (**b**) H&E staining demonstrates the biphasic morphology, comprising an inner layer of epithelial cells with eosinophilic cytoplasm and a surrounding layer of myoepithelial cells with clear cytoplasm (400×)

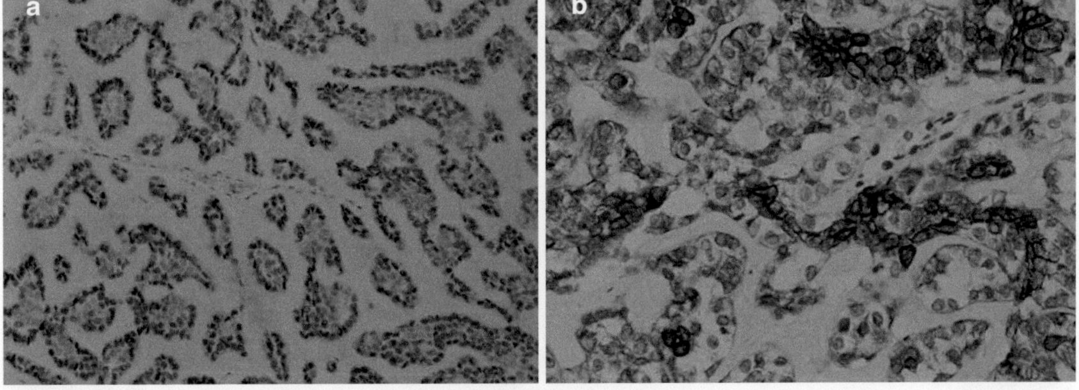

Fig. 10 (**a**) p63 expression is positive for myoepithelial cells and negative for glandular epithelium (200×). (**b**) CK18/8 expression is negative for myoepithelial cells and marked positive for glandular epithelium (400×)

including a cribriform pattern of growth, basaloid appearance, and sebaceous differentiation, etc. Immunohistochemically, epithelial cells are strongly positive for pan-cytokeratin (CK) (AE1/AE3), low-molecular-weight CK (CAM5.2), and CK7, whereas myoepithelial cells are negative to weakly positive for these markers. Among various myoepithelial markers, α-smooth muscle actin is highly sensitive and specific for myoepithelial cells, S100 protein and p63/p40 are less specific, and calponin is less sensitive. The Ki-67 labeling index varies widely among cases [1], with a mean of 16.9%–20.5%.

Several genetic mutations have been detected in EMC of the salivary glands. Urano et al. [25] investigated 87 cases of EMC arising in the major and minor salivary glands and seromucinous glands in the nasal cavity or bronchus. Classic EMC accounted for 40.2% of all cases. Other cases showed various growth patterns and cytologic features; cribriform patterns, a basaloid appearance, and sebaceous differentiation were relatively common (17.2%–18.4%), whereas oncocytic/apocrine, papillary-cystic, double-clear, squamous, psammomatous, Verocay-like, and high-grade transformation were rare. HRAS mutations were found in 82.7% of EMCs and were concentrated in codon 61. There was no significant correlation between the HRAS mutation status and histology. PIK3CA and/or AKT1 mutations were the second most frequent mutations (20.7%, 6.5%, respectively) and almost always co-occurred with HRAS mutations. The HRAS mutation was not identified in any salivary gland tumor entities manifesting EMC-like features, including adenoid cystic carcinoma, pleomorphic adenoma, basal cell adenoma/adenocarcinoma, and myoepithelial carcinoma (reproduced with permission from copyright holder).

The histologic features of EMC can overlap with various benign and malignant salivary gland tumors. PEMC needs to be differentiated from tumors with biphasic epithelial-myoepithelial cell growth, including pulmonary pleomorphic adenoma (PA) and myoepithelial carcinoma. The absence of a chondromyxoid stroma and predominance of clear myoepithelial cells helps in differentiating EMC from PA. The detection of PLAG1 and HMGA2 rearrangements can be useful for PA. EMC is distinguishing from myoepithelial carcinoma principally based on the presence or absence of true ductal formation. ACC can be distinguished by its infiltrative nature and cribriform architecture. MYB or MYBL1 rearrangement is useful for diagnosing ACC, whereas the detection of HRAS hotspot mutations can help to confirm the diagnosis of EMC.

PEMC is generally regarded as a low-grade neoplasm with a good prognosis, while distant metastases and recurrences occasionally occur.

8.8 Case 8

A 26-year-old woman complained of cough and hemoptysis for half a month.

Chest CT: An oval nodule in the left main bronchus (Fig. 11).

[Diagnosis] Primary pulmonary pleomorphic adenoma.

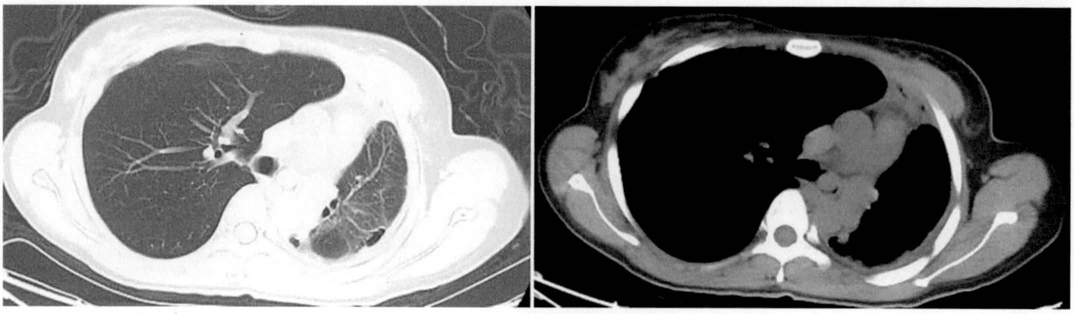

Fig. 11 Chest CT

[Diagnosis Basis] Under bronchoscopy, a spherical neoplasm was seen at the opening of the left main bronchus, which completely blocked the bronchus (Fig. 12a). Rigid bronchoscopic tumor resection was performed (Fig. 12b). Pathology showed a tumor of minor salivary gland origin in the left main bronchus, consistent with a pleomorphic adenoma (Fig. 13a, b). Immunohistochemistry showed that CK, p63, CK8/18, CK5/6, CD138, and Vimentin were positive (Figs. 14a, b and 15a, b), and Calponin, TTF-1, Napsin A, CD117, Syn, and CgA were negative. The Ki-67 labeling index was 2%.

[Analysis] Pleomorphic adenoma (PA) is the most common benign neoplasm of salivary glands and can occur in other sites, such as palate, tongue, nasopharynx, larynx, breast, skin, and soft tissue. Lung is an unusual site for PA. Primary pulmonary pleomorphic adenoma (PPPA) is extremely rare, which is more common inside the main bronchi rather than the lung parenchyma. PPPA is histologically characterized by a mixture of luminal-type ductal epithelial cells, myoepithelial tissues, and tissues that have a myxochondroid, mucoid, or chondroid appearance.

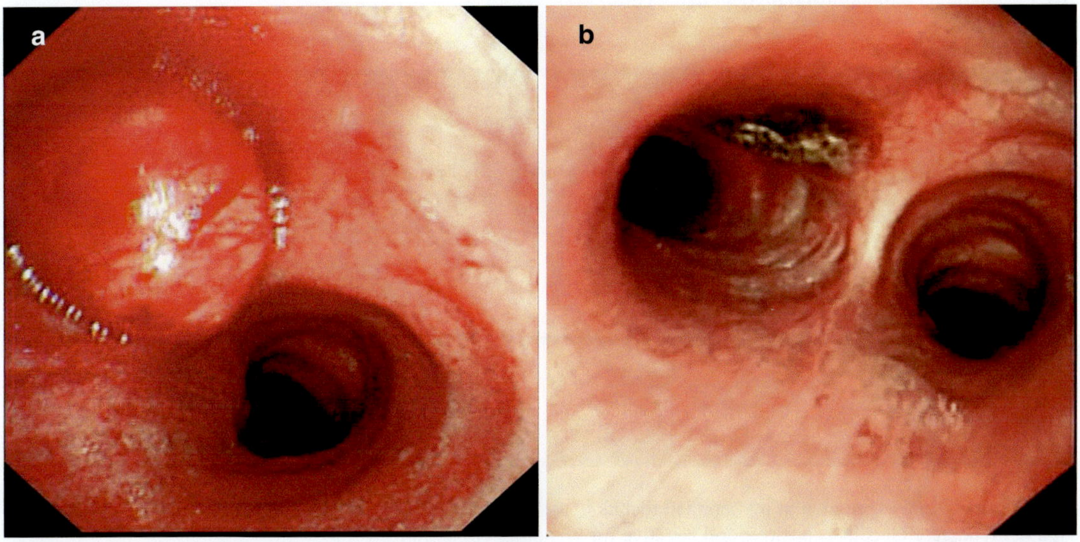

Fig. 12 (**a**) Bronchoscopic view in the left main bronchus. (**b**) Lumen after tumor resection

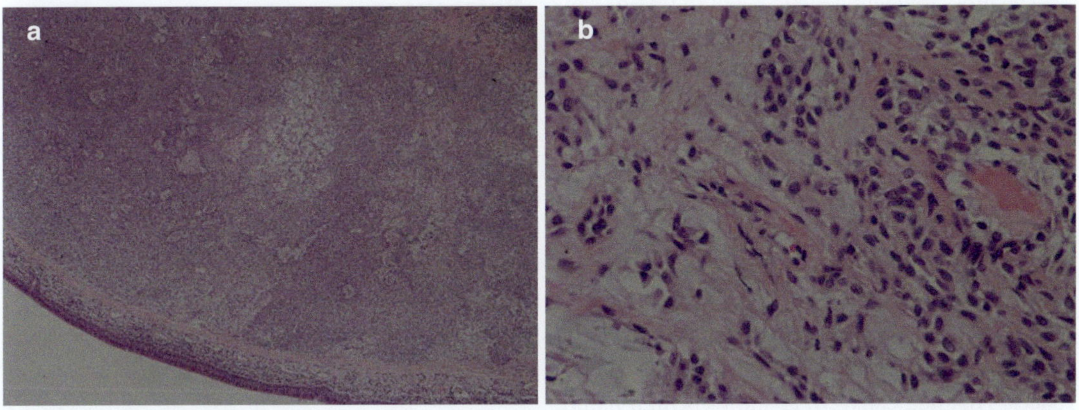

Fig. 13 (**a**) Well-circumscribed pleomorphic adenoma. (**b**) Tumors are composed of myoepithelial, glandular epithelium, and myxoid stroma

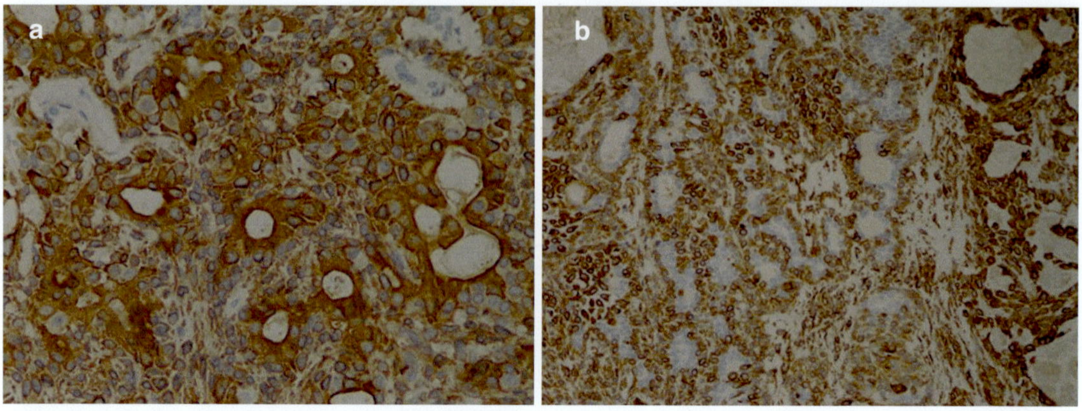

Fig. 14 (**a**) CK expression is positive in glandular epithelium and myoepithelial cells. (**b**) Vimentin expression is positive in glandular epithelium and myoepithelial cells

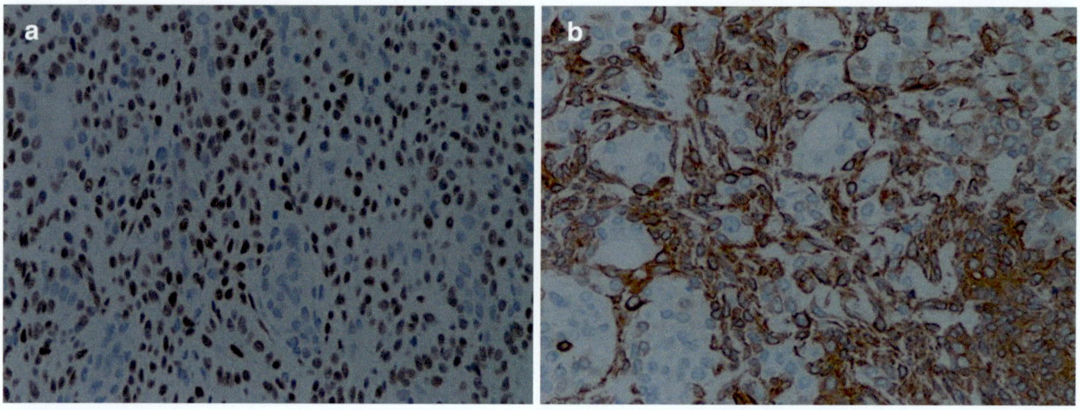

Fig. 15 (**a**) CK5/6 expression in myoepithelial cells is positive and negative for glandular epithelium. (**b**) p63 expression in myoepithelial cells is positive and negative for glandular epithelium

The most frequent genetic event in PAs of salivary glands is rearrangement of the pleomorphic adenoma gene 1 (PLAG1). Asahina et al. [26] first reported a case of pulmonary PA with CTNNB1-PLAG1 fusion and PLAG1 expression.

PPPA is slow growing, and a long-term follow-up is recommended because of the possibility of malignant behavior. PA may undergo malignant transformation to ex-pleomorphic adenoma. Metastasizing/metastasizing pleomorphic adenoma (MPA) is rare, occurs years after the initial PA, and is associated with multiple local recurrences. Histologically, MPA shows benign nature but demonstrates malignant behavior.

References

1. WHO Classification of Tumours Editorial Board. WHO classification of tumours of the lung, pleura, thymus and heart. Lyon, France: International Agency for Research on Cancer; 2015.
2. Pérez-de-Oliveira ME, Wagner VP, Araújo ALD, et al. Prognostic value of CRTC1-MAML2 translocation in salivary mucoepidermoid carcinoma: systematic review and meta-analysis. J Oral Pathol Med. 2020;49:386–94.
3. Kato S, Elkin SK, Schwaederle M, et al. Genomic landscape of salivary gland tumors. Oncotarget. 2015;6:25631–45.
4. Kang H, Tan M, Bishop JA, et al. Whole-exome sequencing of salivary gland mucoepidermoid carcinoma. Clin Cancer Res. 2017;23:283–8.

5. Wang F, Xi SY, Hao WW, et al. Mutational landscape of primary pulmonary salivary gland-type tumors through targeted next-generation sequencing. Lung Cancer. 2021;160:1–7.
6. Kim BG, Lee K, Um SW, et al. Clinical outcomes and the role of bronchoscopic intervention in patients with primary pulmonary salivary gland-type tumors. Lung Cancer. 2020;146:58–65.
7. Molina JR, Aubry MC, Lewis JE, et al. Primary salivary gland-type lung cancer: spectrum of clinical presentation, histopathologic and prognostic factors. Cancer. 2007;110:2253–9.
8. Qin BD, Jiao XD, Liu K, et al. Clinical, pathological and treatment factors associated with the survival of patients with primary pulmonary salivary gland-type tumors. Lung Cancer. 2018;126:174–81.
9. Garg PK, Sharma G, Rai S, et al. Primary salivary gland-type tumors of the lung: a systematic review and pooled analysis. Lung India. 2019;36:118–22.
10. Shaw RR. Mucoid impaction of the bronchi. J Thorac Surg. 1951;2:149–63.
11. Mintzer RA, Neiman HL, Reeder MM. Mucoid impaction of a bronchus. JAMA 1978;240:1397–8.
12. Martinez S, Heyneman LE, McAdams HP, et al. Mucoid impactions: finger-in-glove sign and other CT and radiographic features. Radiographics. 2008;28:1369–82.
13. Smetana HF, Iverson L, Swan LL. Bronchogenic carcinoma; an analysis of 100 autopsy cases. Mil Surg. 1952;111:335–51.
14. González-Arriagada WA, Santos-Silva AR, Ito FA, et al. Calcifications may be a frequent finding in mucoepidermoid carcinomas of the salivary glands: a clinicopathologic study. Oral Surg Oral Med Oral Pathol Oral Radiol Endod. 2011;111:482–5.
15. Hsieh CC, Sun YH, Lin SW, et al. Surgical outcomes of pulmonary mucoepidermoid carcinoma: a review of 41 cases. PLoS One. 2017;12:e0176918.
16. Qiu L, Song P, Chen P, et al. Clinical characteristics and prognosis of patients with pulmonary Mucoepidermoid carcinoma: a SEER-based analysis. Front Oncol. 2021;11:601185.
17. Wang YQ, Mo YX, Li S, et al. Low-grade and high-grade mucoepidermoid carcinoma of the lung: CT findings and clinical features of 17 cases. AJR Am J Roentgenol. 2015;205:1160–6.
18. Cheng DL, Hu YX, Hu PQ, et al. Clinicopathological and multisection CT features of primary pulmonary mucoepidermoid carcinoma. Clin Radiol. 2017;72:610.e1–7.
19. Kim TS, Lee KS, Han J, et al. Mucoepidermoid carcinoma of the tracheobronchial tree: radiographic and CT findings in 12 patients. Radiology. 1999;212:643–8.
20. Ban X, Shen X, Hu H, et al. Predictive CT features for the diagnosis of primary pulmonary mucoepidermoid carcinoma: comparison with squamous cell carcinomas and adenocarcinomas. Cancer Imaging. 2021;21:2.
21. Li X, Yi W, Zeng Q. CT features and differential diagnosis of primary pulmonary mucoepidermoid carcinoma and pulmonary adenoid cystic carcinoma. J Thorac Dis. 2018;10:6501–8.
22. Elnayal A, Moran CA, Fox PS, et al. Primary salivary gland-type lung cancer: imaging and clinical predictors of outcome. AJR Am J Roentgenol. 2013;201:W57–63.
23. Kumar V, Soni P, Garg M, et al. A comparative study of primary adenoid cystic and mucoepidermoid carcinoma of lung. Front Oncol. 2018;8:153.
24. Donath K, Seifert G, Schmitz R. Diagnosis and ultrastructure of the tubular carcinoma of salivary gland ducts. Epithelial–myoepithelial carcinoma of the intercalated ducts. Virchows Arch A Pathol Pathol Anat. 1972;356:16–31.
25. Urano M, Nakaguro M, Yamamoto Y, et al. Diagnostic significance of HRAS mutations in epithelial-myoepithelial carcinomas exhibiting a broad histopathologic Spectrum. Am J Surg Pathol. 2019;43:984–94.
26. Asahina M, Hayashi T, Takamochi K, et al. Identification of CTNNB1-PLAG1 gene rearrangement in a patient with pulmonary pleomorphic adenoma. Virchows Arch. 2020;477:739–42.

Papilloma

Song Zhang

Respiratory papilloma (RP) is the commonest endotracheal benign tumor accounting for less than 0.5% of all lung tumors and 7%–8% of all benign lung tumors.

Papilloma is normally classified into three separate categories: multiple papilloma, inflammatory polyp, and solitary papilloma. Multiple papilloma, representing papillomatosis, is usually related to infection with papillomavirus occurring most often in children and young adults and involving both the upper and lower respiratory tracts. Inflammatory polyp arises from chronically inflamed bronchial mucosa. Solitary papilloma predominantly affects adults.

1 Classification

The 1981 WHO classification of lung tumors subdivided it as squamous cell papilloma and "transitional cell" papilloma. In 1985, Maxwell et al. [1] expanded the classification of papillomas into four groups, including multiple papillomas (squamous), inflammatory polyps (columnar), solitary papilloma (columnar/cuboidal), and solitary papilloma (squamous).

S. Zhang (✉)
Department of Respiratory and Critical Care Medicine, Shandong Provincial Hospital Affiliated to Shandong First Medical University, Jinan, Shandong, China

In the 2015 WHO classification, papillomas were classified according to histologic features into three groups: squamous cell papilloma (exophytic; inverted), glandular papilloma, and mixed squamous and glandular papilloma. In the 2021 WHO classification, papillomas were classified as squamous cell papilloma (NOS), squamous cell papilloma (inverted), glandular papilloma, and mixed squamous and glandular papilloma.

2 Pathology

In 1998, Flieder et al. [2] classified solitary pulmonary papillomas into three histologic subtypes: squamous cell papillomas, glandular papillomas, and mixed squamous cell and glandular papillomas.

Squamous cell papilloma consists of papillary arborizing connective tissue stalks lined by keratinizing or nonkeratinizing mature squamous epithelium.

Glandular papilloma is characterized by papillary stromal cores lined by pseudostratified or single layer of ciliated or nonciliated columnar cells admixed with cuboidal cells or mucin-filled cells. The presence of ciliated cells is considered important to exclude other malignant tumors. Nuclear atypia, mitosis, and necrosis are absent.

Mixed squamous cell and glandular papilloma (MSGP) is characterized by the biphasic differentiation of both the squamous and glandular

S. Zhang (ed.), *Diagnostic Imaging of Lung Cancers*, https://doi.org/10.1007/978-981-99-6815-2_12

portions without malignant features, with at least one-third of the tumor being the glandular component.

3 Epidemiology

A retrospective study by Tryfon et al. [3] reported that solitary respiratory papilloma (SRP) had an estimated annual incidence of 3.95 cases/100,000 patients. SRP occurs more commonly in men (ratio 3:1). Squamous papillomas occur commonly during the fifth decade of life, glandular papillomas predominate in the sixth decade, and mixed type papillomas in the third to the sixth decade of life.

Squamous cell papilloma is the most common benign tumors of the airway. Glandular papilloma is most commonly found in the central tracheobronchial tree and has not been linked to human papillomavirus (HPV) infection. The characteristics of MSGP include potential association with male gender, smoking habit, preference of the central airways, and irrelevance with HPV infection.

Multiple papilloma of the upper airway often referred to recurrent respiratory papillomatosis (RRP), secondary to infection with HPV-6 and HPV-11 (low-risk). High-risk HPV infection has also been reported to cause RRP. Oh et al. [4] identified important new functions for the low-risk E6 and E7 proteins in the episomal maintenance of low-risk HPV-11 genomes and suggested that they may act in a manner similar to that observed for the high-risk proteins. Based on presentation before or after the age of 12 years, RRP is usually classified into juvenile-onset recurrent respiratory papillomatosis (JoRRP) and adult-onset recurrent respiratory papillomatosis (AoRRP). JoRRP is generally more aggressive, with higher recurrence rates. AoRRP is more indolent, although aggressive variation of the disease can occur. The estimated incidence of RRR among children is approximately 4.3 per 100,000; among adults, 1.8 per 100,000. Distribution of age of onset of RRP is generally reported to be bimodal, with peaks at approximately 5 and 30 years. San Giorgi et al. [5] studied 639 patients and concluded that RRP starts at three median ages 7, 35, and 64 years.

Some authors proposed that viral coinfections may contribute to an aggressive clinical course of RRP. A research by Chantre-Justino et al. [6] found that EBV infection has no direct effect on the invasive process of RRP. However, Formánek et al. [7] found that EBV seems to interact with HPV, enhancing cell proliferation and contributing to the pathogenesis and progression of AoRRP.

4 Radiographic Features

RP arises from the mucosal surface, and often causes airway obstruction, leading to atelectasis, air trapping, obstructive infections, and bronchiectasis. Involvement of the distal airways and parenchyma can present with multiple bilateral thin-walled cysts and nodules (Fig. 1).

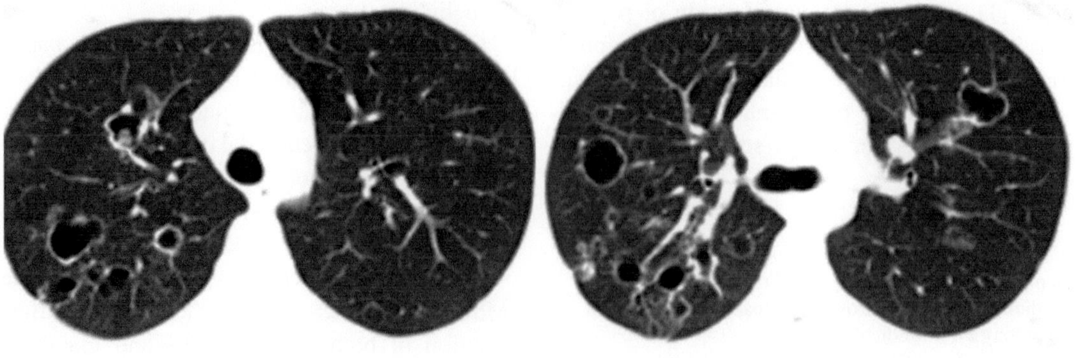

Fig. 1 A 22-year-old man with a history of laryngeal papilloma. Chest CT shows bilateral multiple thin-walled cysts and nodules

5 Treatment

Complete resection is recommended for SRP because malignant transformation of any type of pulmonary papilloma is possible. No malignant transformation has been reported in glandular papilloma and MSGP, an endobronchial resection with tissue sparing could be sufficient.

Currently, there is no cure for RRP. Surgery is the main treatment for RRP aimed at clearing the airway with preservation of normal structures. There are a variety of techniques to resect the endoluminal tumor, including argon plasma coagulation, sharp dissection, coblation, CO2 or YAG laser, microdebrider, and cold forceps. Photodynamic Therapy (PDT) is also used for RRP treatment. It stimulates gradual necrosis of diseased tissue, causing the release of HPV oncoproteins (E6 and E7), which allows the presentation of antigens and short-term immunologic viral clearance interceded by IL-10 and IFN-γ.

Even though all clinically apparent papillomas were removed, latent virus remained in adjacent tissues. Therefore, adjuvant therapy is required in about 20% cases. The role of adjuvants is limited to increasing the time interval between surgical procedures. The main indication for adjuvant therapy includes more than four surgical procedures per year, rapid regrowth of resected papilloma, or metastasis. Adjuvant therapies include the use of interferon, antiviral therapeutics (acyclovir, cidofovir, ribavirin), retinoids, and inhibitors of the cyclooxygenase-2(COX-2).

Cidofovir, a cytosine nucleotide analog that inhibits HPV replication by inhibition of DNA polymerase, is the antiviral most commonly used in medical adjuvant treatment for RRP. Gazia et al. [8] reviewed 20 reports that enrolled 185 patients with AoRRP and 85 patients with JoRRP on the use of cidofovir as adjuvant therapy in laryngeal papillomatosis. They found that intralesion use of cidofovir has a good adjuvant action in RRP increasing the complete remission of the disease. Compared to 56.5% of the JoRRP, the AoRRP response to cidofovir is better with a 74% complete response rate. Hoesli et al. [9] evaluated the safety of intralesional cidofovir. They found that adjuvant intralesional cidofovir injections did not appear to cause major complications or an increased rate of development of dysplasia and cancer.

Target gene therapy, checkpoint, and VEGF inhibitors are also being studied for RRP treatment. Wu et al. [10] found a significant increase in COX-2 levels in papillary papillomas. Overexpression of COX-2 in papillomas reflected activation of EGFR-->phosphatidylinositol 3-kinase signaling. Treatment with prostaglandin E2 (PGE2) induced COX-2 and stimulated papilloma cell growth, whereas celecoxib, a selective COX-2 inhibitor, suppressed proliferation and induced apoptosis. Because papilloma cells overexpress EGFR, together with an increased expression of COX-2 and prostaglandin E2, Rojas-Lechuga et al. [11] suggested that the combination of erlotinib and celecoxib seems plausible and could be proposed for patients with poor response to previous lines of treatment.

A study by Ahn et al. [12] found that most RRP specimens demonstrate PD-1 T-lymphocyte infiltration and PD-L1 expression on both papilloma and infiltrating immune cells. This study suggested that this checkpoint pathway may be contributing to local immunosuppression in RRP. Creelan et al. [13] first used PD-1 inhibitor(nivolumab) to treated two patients with refractory JoRRP. From on-treatment biopsy tissue, a higher amount of intraepithelial T cells and PD-L1 expression were detected in the papilloma. Nivolumab appears to have promising activity in Jo-RRP. Allen et al. [14] conducted a phase II study to investigate the clinical activity and safety of PD-L1 blockade with avelumab in patients with RRP. Twelve patients (4 JoRRP and 8 AoRRP) were treated, including 8 laryngeal disease patients, 3 pulmonary disease patients, and 1 both laryngeal and pulmonary disease patient. All laryngeal RRP patients displayed improvement in disease burden, and 5 of 9 (56%) experienced partial responses. None of the 4 patients with pulmonary RRP displayed a response. A subset of partial responders produced HPV-specific reactivity in papilloma-infiltrating T cells that correlated with reduced HPV viral load and an increased tissue inflammation signature. Avelumab demonstrated safety and clinical activity in patients with laryngeal RRP.

Bevacizumab is a recombinant monoclonal antibody that binds to vascular endothelial growth factor (VEGF). By inhibiting VEGF, bevacizumab reduces tumor angiogenesis and is also a promising adjuvant treatment for RRP. Ablanedo-Terrazas et al. [15] compared the efficacy of cidofovir versus bevacizumab used as adjuvant therapies for the control of RRP. Five children and 11 adults were enrolled in the study. The group treated with cidofovir had a significant decrease in Derkay score after 1 year. However, no significant changes were found with intralesional bevacizumab. Pogoda et al. [16] investigated the efficacy of bevacizumab as treatment option for RRP. They screened 15 studies with a total of 64 patients. In 95% of the patients treated with systemic bevacizumab, the post-bevacizumab surgical interval was significantly prolonged. Over half of them did not need any surgical intervention during mean follow-up of 21.6 months. In 62% of the patients with intralesional bevacizumab, the post-bevacizumab surgical interval (mean, 1.8 months follow-up) was extended when compared to the interval before the treatment. They concluded that systemically and intralesionally administered bevacizumab is an effective choice for the treatment of severe RRP. A systemic administration might be the preferred treatment method.

Malignant transformation of adult RRP to squamous cell carcinoma has been reported in 3%–7% cases. Therefore, a long-term follow-up is needed to monitor for disease recurrence and malignant transformation.

6 Prevention

Prevention of RRP is a challenge. HPV vaccine has been used to suppress the aggressiveness of RRP and has profound impact on the incidence of RRP. The Food and Drug Administration (FDA) in the United States has approved three prophylactic vaccines, namely Cervarix, Gardasil (quadrivalent HPV), and Gardasil-9 (nonavalent HPV), to protect against HPV infections. These vaccines are composed of virus-like particles (VLPs) derived from the major capsid protein (L1) of HPV.

Novakovic et al. [17] reported a 5-year study from Australia following the implementation of a systematic HPV vaccination program. The annual incidence rate declined from 0.16 per 100,000 in 2012 to 0.02 per 100,000 in 2016. This is the first report internationally documenting decline in JoRRP incidence in children following a quadrivalent HPV vaccination program. Matsuzaki et al. [18] reviewed the efficacy of HPV vaccination for RRP. Twenty-four RRP patients were treated with a combination therapy of surgery and three sessions of quadrivalent HPV vaccine. 52.2% (n = 12) of RRP patients who were HPV-DNA positive turned negative after the combination therapy. The mean of intersurgical interval was significantly extended from 6.85 ± 4.49 months to 30.5 ± 27.6 months. Therefore, combination therapy can postpone the recurrence and lessen the severity of RRP.

With the increasing utilization of the 9-valent and quadrivalent HPV vaccine in Australia and US, data showed that the incidence of RRP has a significant decrease. Single dose Gardasil has shown sustained immunization for at least 7 years in developing countries.

7 Case Analysis

7.1 Case 1

A 26-year-old woman complained of cough and sputum for 2 months.

Chest CT: A solitary mass in left lower lobe bronchus with obstructive pneumonia (Fig. 2).

[Diagnosis] Solitary papilloma.

[Diagnosis Basis] Bronchoscopy revealed a cauliflower-like neoplasm at the opening of the left lower lobe bronchus, completely blocking the lumen (Fig. 3a). Biopsy pathology suggested squamous papilloma (Fig. 3b).

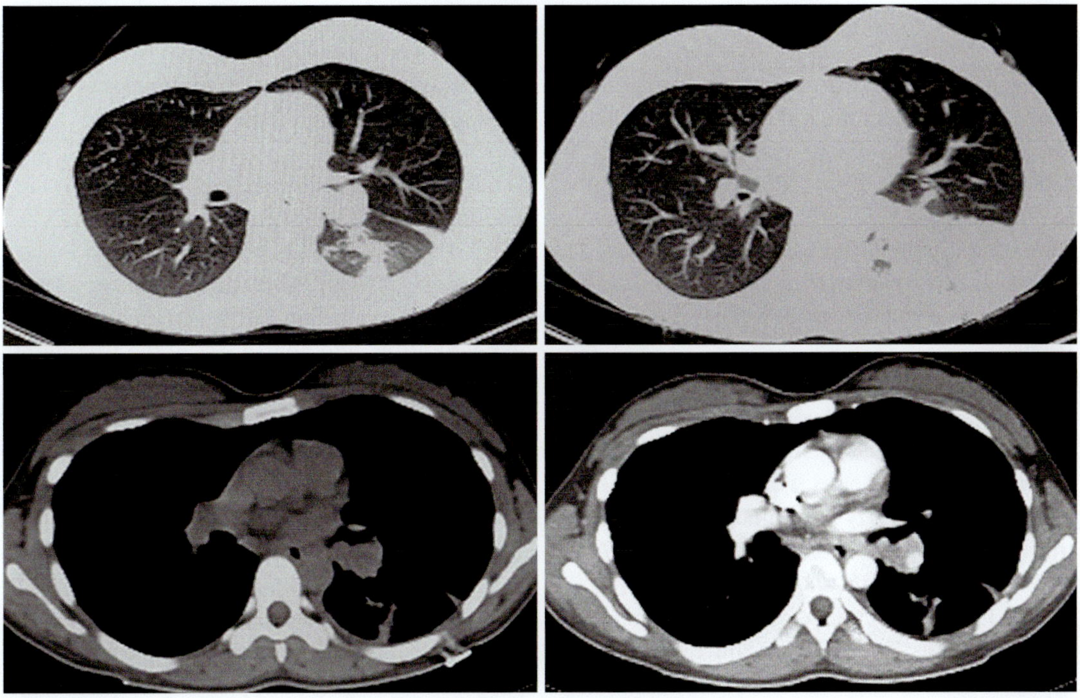

Fig. 2 Chest CT

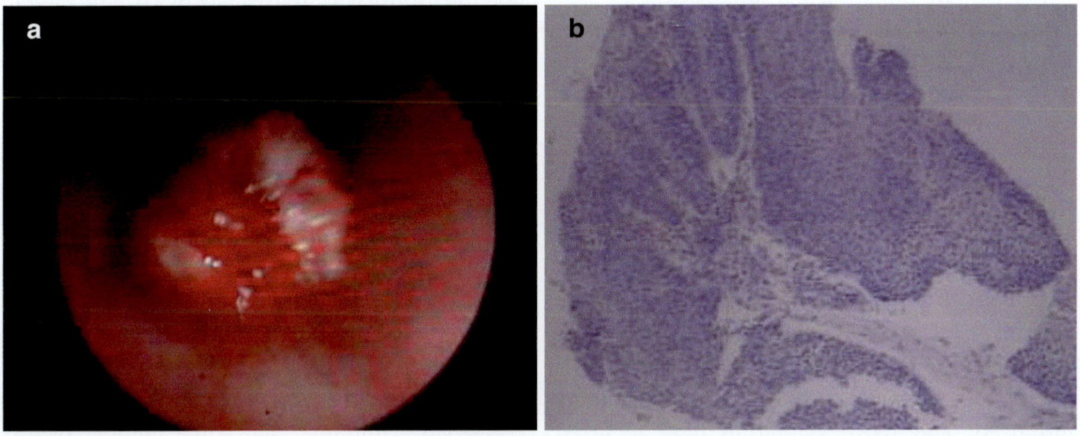

Fig. 3 (**a**) Bronchoscopic view in the left lower lobe bronchus. (**b**) A papillary structure is covered by stratified squamous epithelium

[Analysis] Solitary bronchial squamous cell papilloma (SCP) is a benign tumor originating from squamous cell epithelium cells, which was first reported in 1954. In 1993, Naka et al. [19] reported a case of solitary SCP of the trachea and reviewed 55 other previously reported cases. From the review, there seems to be no considerable difference in the prognoses between the endoscopically and surgically managed groups. In 1994, Popper et al. [20] investigated the presence of HPV-DNA in 31 solitary bronchial SCPs patients by in situ hybridization (ISH) and the polymerase chain reaction (PCR). They found that benign SCPs showed an association with HPV type 11 and rarely with type 6. Patients with SCP exhibiting HPV 16 or 18 positivity are at high risk for the development of squamous cell carcinomas (SCC). In 2013, Syrjänen et al. [21] conducted a systematic review and formal meta-analysis of the literature reporting on HPV detection in bronchial SCP. Among 89 cases of bronchial SCPs from different geographic regions, 38 (42.7%) cases tested HPV-positive. The variability in HPV detection rates reported in bronchial SCPs cannot be explained by the HPV detection method or geographic origin of the study.

Papillomatosis usually involved multiple sites along the airway from the larynx down to the pulmonary parenchyma. In 2000, Harada et al. [22] reported a rare RRP case, which was induced first by HPV 6 in early childhood and then co-transfected with HPV 16 in adolescence. After 39 years of age, a squamous papilloma appeared in the lung parenchyma. The trachea and the main bronchus were intact, and no malignant transformation was observed.

HPV infection is frequently associated with SCP, and HPV vaccines may be expected to inhibit disease initiation and progression.

8 Case Analysis

8.1 Case 2

A 10-year-old girl complained of repeated dyspnea, cough, and expectoration for 10 years, aggravated for 1 month. One month after birth, the child developed shortness of breath, hoarseness, cough, and expectoration. After anti-infection treatment, the child's symptoms improved. The above symptoms have recurred since then. One month ago, the child developed cough and yellow sticky phlegm again, and the anti-infective treatment had poor efficacy and was admitted to the hospital. The patient had a history of 1 month premature delivery. On physical examination, stridor was heard in the larynx.

Chest CT (April 2006): A lesions in the main bronchus, with multiple nodules and cavities in the right lung (Fig. 4).

Chest CT (August 2015): Multiple nodules, consolidations, cavities, and cavity shadows were seen in bilateral lungs, with obvious tree-in-bud sign in the lower right lung (Fig. 5).

[Diagnosis] Juvenile-onset recurrent respiratory papillomatosis.

[Diagnosis Basis] The child was a premature infant with symptoms such as dyspnea, cough, expectoration, and hoarseness at the first month of life. Chest CT showed a lesion in the main bronchus, and the possibility of a tracheal tumor should be considered. Juvenile respiratory papillomatosis is the second common cause of hoarseness in children, so this diagnosis should be first considered. The symptoms of the child recurred, and the lung lesions progressed significantly after 9 years, which was in line with the evolution of the disease. The child underwent video laryngoscopy, which showed that the epiglottis was not swollen, the laryngeal vestibule was covered with papillary masses, and the glottis was invisible (Fig. 6). The patient underwent thoracoscopic biopsy of the right lower lung mass, and the pathology showed papilloma carcinoma–well-differentiated squamous cell carcinoma (Fig. 7a, b).

[Analysis] Juvenile-onset recurrent respiratory papillomatosis (JoRRP) is a rare benign disease characterized by the growth of papillomas in the respiratory tract in children and is predominantly caused by HPV 6 and 11. Hoarseness is the most common symptom, and stridor is often the second clinical symptom to develop.

Genetic, immune, and some clinical factors may play an important role in the course of JoRRP. Li et al. [23] summarized the related factors affecting the disease course in patients with JoRRP. They found that mother-to-child transmission is the most important mode of disease transmission. Genetically, the presence of DRB1*0301 and HPV 6/11 E6/E7 is associated with a more severe disease. Immunologically, patients exhibit enhanced T helper 2-like

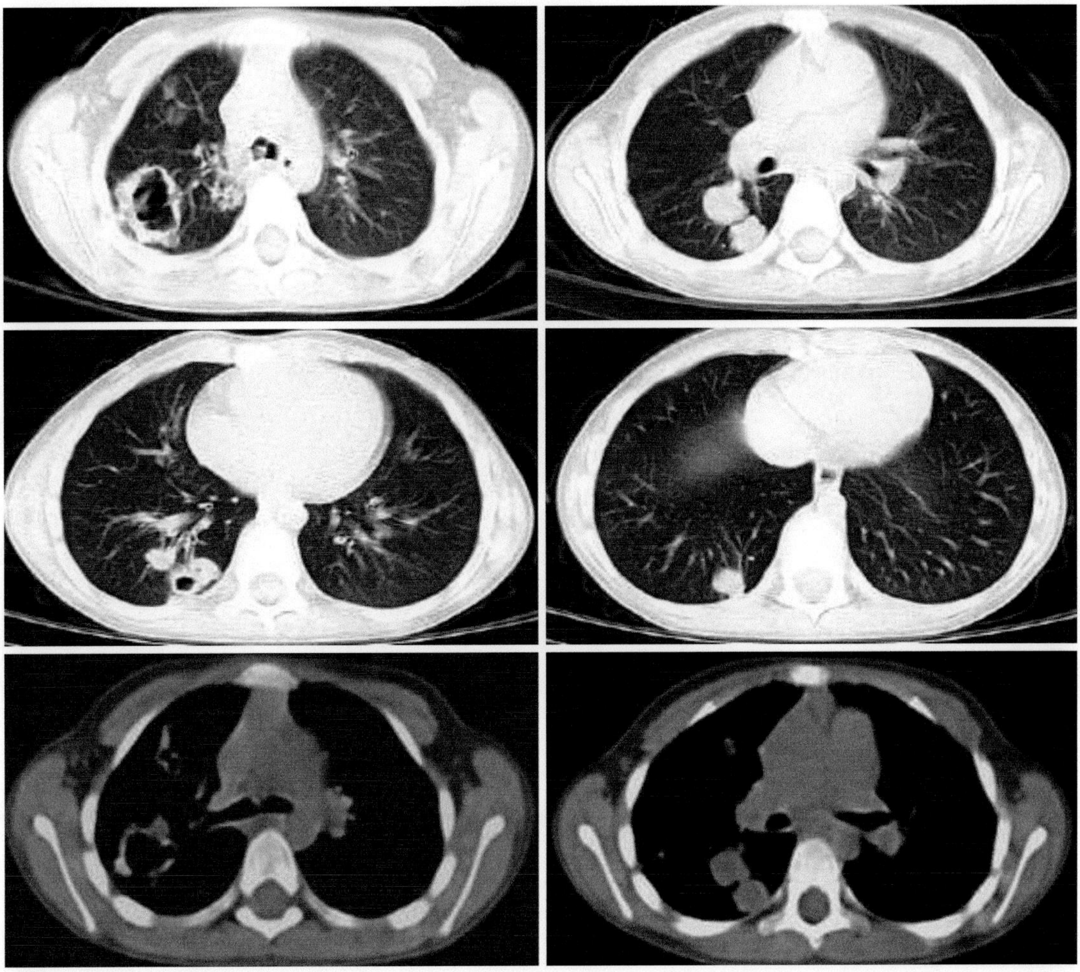

Fig. 4 Chest CT (April 2006)

response. In addition, regulatory T cells are enriched in tumors and may become one of the effective prognostic indicators. In terms of clinical characteristics, patients infected with HPV-11 have more aggressive disease. However, compared with HPV type, age at first onset is a more important factor related to the aggressiveness of JoRRP.

Amiling et al. [24] analyzed the epidemiology and HPV types in children with JoRRP. They found that children with JoRRP were commonly firstborn and vertically transmitted through the mothers infected genital tract; most of the mothers reported no HPV vaccination before delivery. Vaccine-preventable HPV was found in all specimens with detectable HPV. Increasing pre-exposure HPV vaccination could substantially reduce or eliminate JoRRP in the United States.

Armstrong et al. [25] characterized the spectrum of JoRRP in the United States. The mean number of surgical procedures per child was 4.4 per year. After adjusting for sex, race, and years of treatment, children diagnosed with RRP before age 3 years were 3.6 times more likely to have more than 4 surgical procedures per year and almost 2 times more likely to have 2 or more anatomical sites affected than were children diagnosed with RRP at later ages (≥3.0 years).

The course of JoRRP is variable. Some patients experience spontaneous remission

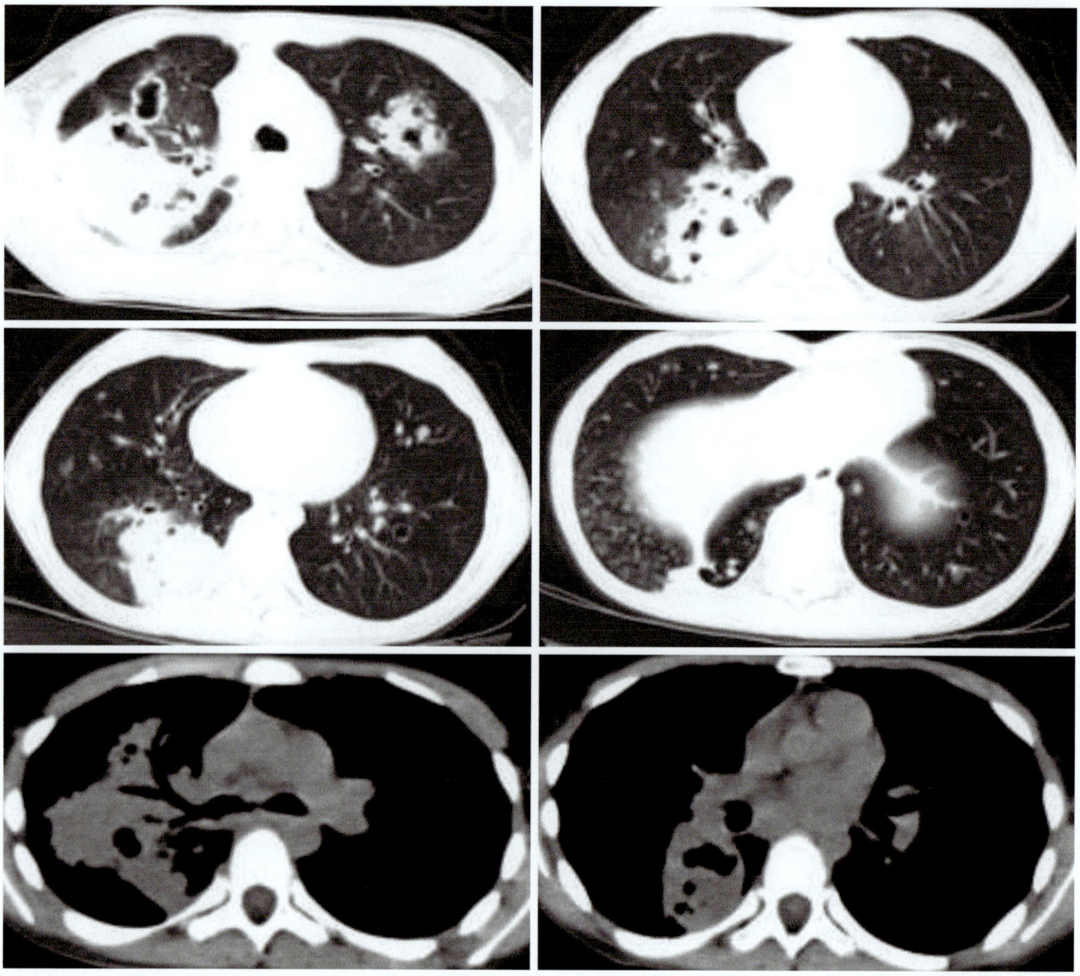

Fig. 5 Chest CT (August 2015)

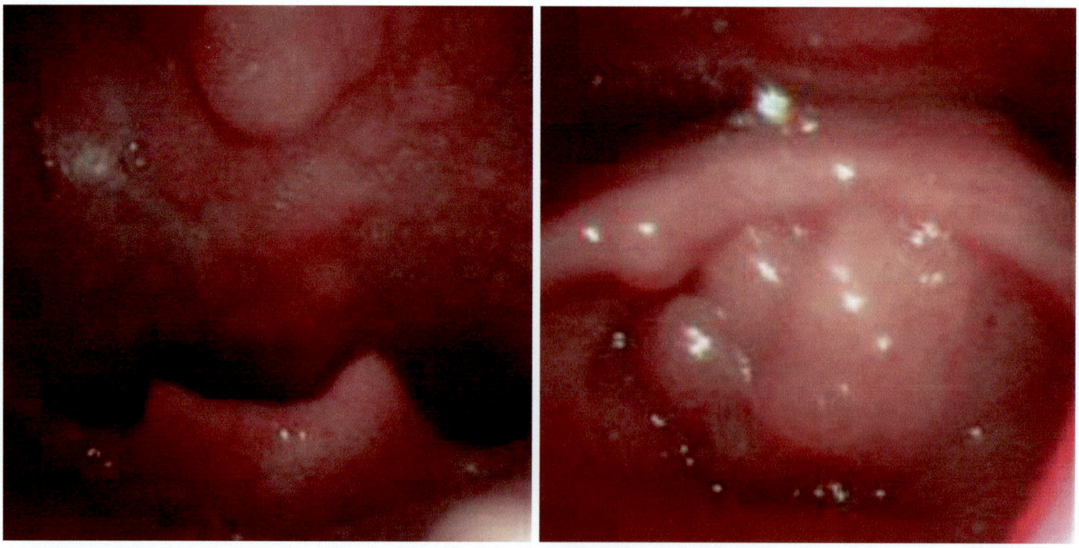

Fig. 6 Video laryngoscopy view

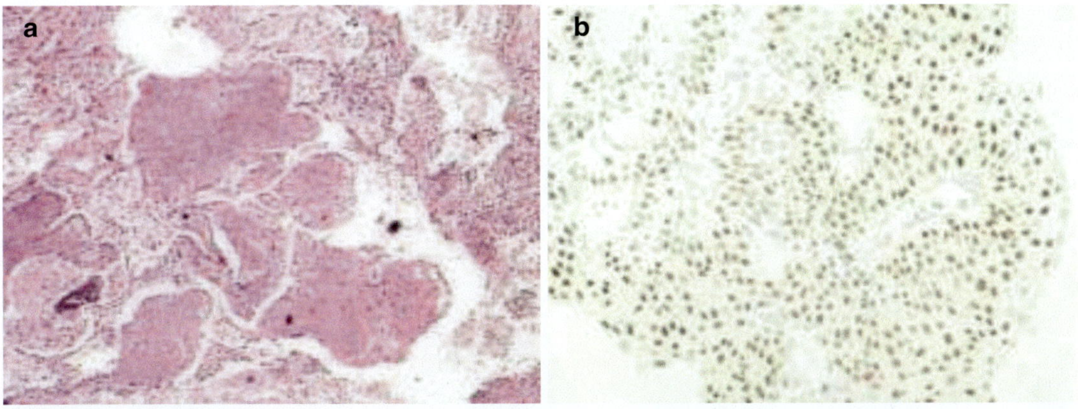

Fig. 7 (**a**) Pathology shows papillary hyperplasia of squamous epithelium. Some cells became larger in size, with hyperchromatic nuclei, obvious atypia, and malignant transformation into well-differentiated squamous cell carcinoma. (**b**) The squamous component was positive for p40

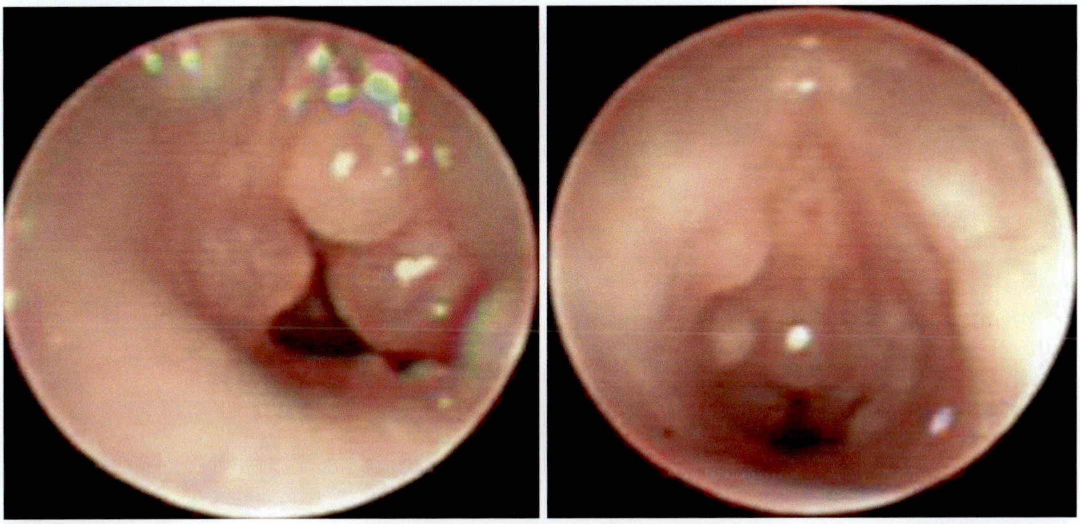

Fig. 8 A 4-month-old baby boy with JoRRP (September 2015)

(Figs. 8 and 9), others may develop aggressive papillomatous growth. New immunomodulatory approaches need to be developed to better manage RRP patients.

8.2 Case 3

A 48-year-old woman complained of cough and expectoration for 16 years, aggravated for 10 days.

Chest CT: A mass at the opening of the main bronchus, with multiple nodules, cavities and tree-in-bud sign in bilateral lungs (Fig. 10).

[Diagnosis] Malignant transformation of squamous cell papilloma.

[Diagnosis Basis] Chest CT shows a polypoid mass at the opening of the main bronchus, protruding into the lumen. Multiple cavities and tree-in-bud signs in bilateral lungs are considered to be caused by long-term tracheal obstruction. The above characteristics are consistent with the diagnosis of papilloma. Bronchoscopy was performed, and the pathology showed squamous cell papilloma malignant transformation--moderately differentiated squamous cell carcinoma (Fig. 11a, b).

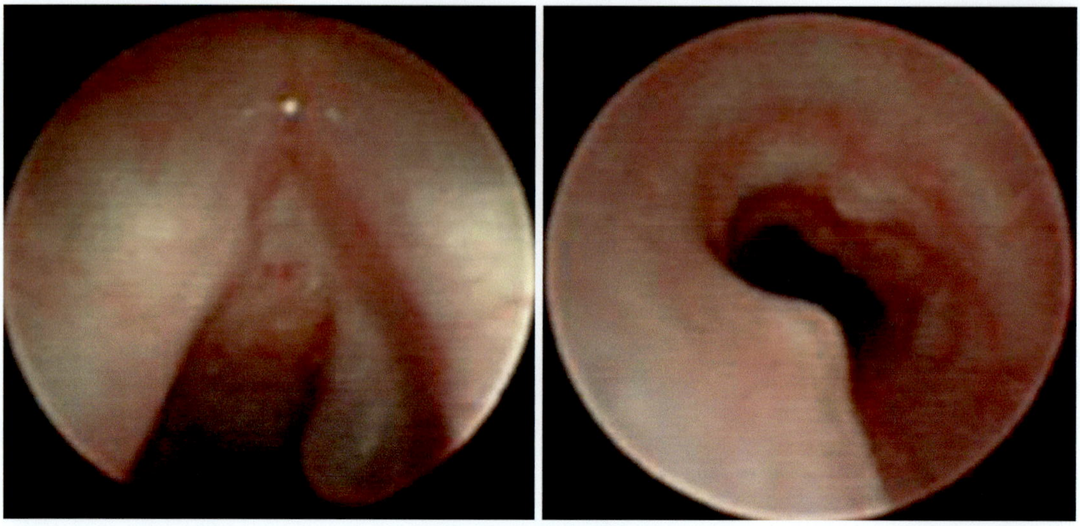

Fig. 9 Lesion regressed after 15 months (December 2016)

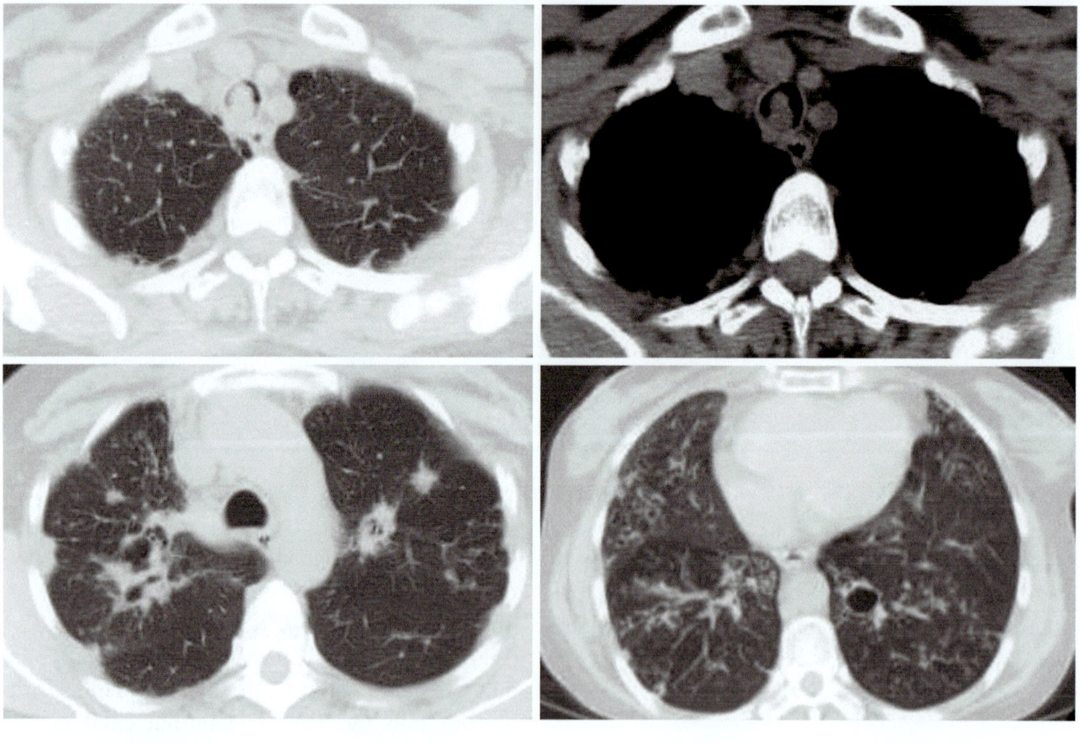

Fig. 10 Chest CT

[Analysis] Imaging findings of benign RP include formation of both cystic and solid pulmonary nodules. Small nodules are commonly seen in early disease, and enlarge and cavitate over time eventually forming cysts.

In 1978, DiMarco et al. [26] first reported about papillomas of the tracheobronchial tree with malignant degeneration. Gélinas et al. [27] reviewed 101 studies and estimated the incidence of lung involvement in RRP at 3.3%. 16% (9/55)

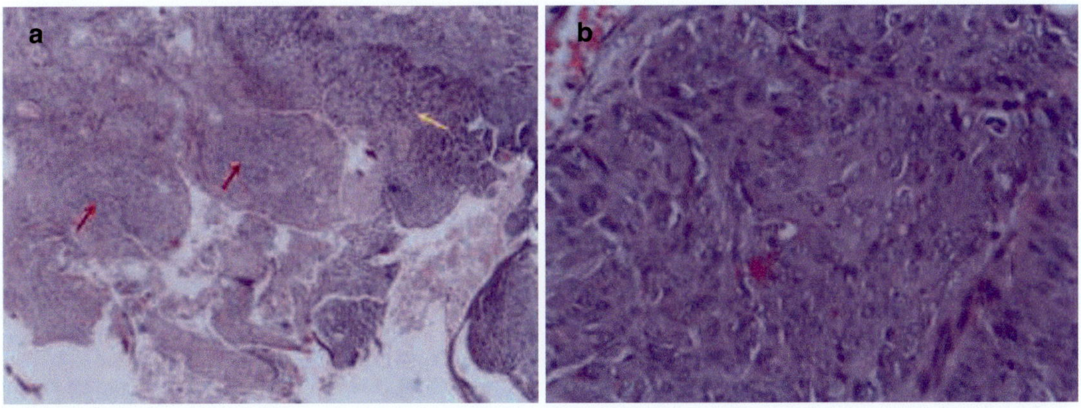

Fig. 11 (**a**) Papilloma-squamous cell carcinoma pathology. A fibrovascular axis is seen in the papilloma (red arrow) with minimal epithelial atypia; squamous epithelial atypia is prominent (yellow arrow). (**b**) Squamous cell carcinoma area

of patients with pulmonary involvement developed cancer, predominantly squamous cell carcinoma. Malignant transformation is rare and may occur at any location in the respiratory tract. However, transformation in the trachea is rarer.

The mechanism of transformation from RP to squamous cell carcinoma remains unclear. Smoking, age above 40 years, and infections with HPV 16 or 18 are risk factors for malignant transformation of benign RP. Go et al. [28] studied the histologic and molecular characteristics of 7 cases of malignant transformation of RRP to squamous cell carcinoma (SCCA). They found that spontaneous malignant transformation of RRP into squamous cell carcinoma was not characterized by a consistent temporal histological progression from squamous papilloma to severe dysplasia and then to squamous cell carcinoma. HPV 6 and 11 are the most common types of HPV associated with RRP. Transformation can result in the loss of HPV expression. HVP 16, 18, 31, 35, and 51 are rarely identified in cases of RRP and RRP-associated carcinomas. p53 expression is not considered to be a molecular marker for monitoring the transformation process and its expression is variable in papillomas and carcinomas.

RP is prone to recurrence and malignant transformation. During the treatment process, dynamic monitoring is required to be alert to the occurrence of malignant lesions.

References

1. Maxwell RJ, Gibbons JR, O'Hara MD. Solitary squamous papilloma of the bronchus. Thorax. 1985;40:68–71.
2. Flieder DB, Koss MN, Nicholson A, et al. Solitary pulmonary papillomas in adults: a clinicopathologic and in situ hybridization study of 14 cases combined with 27 cases in the literature. Am J Surg Pathol. 1998;22:1328–42.
3. Tryfon S, Dramba V, Zoglopitis F, et al. Solitary papillomas of the lower airways: epidemiological, clinical, and therapeutic data during a 22-year period and review of the literature. J Thorac Oncol. 2012;7:643–8.
4. Oh ST, Longworth MS, Laimins LA, et al. Roles of the E6 and E7 proteins in the life cycle of low-risk human papillomavirus type 11. J Virol. 2004;78:2620–6.
5. San Giorgi MR, van den Heuvel ER, Tjon Pian Gi RE, et al. Age of onset of recurrent respiratory papillomatosis: a distribution analysis. Clin Otolaryngol. 2016;41:448–53.
6. Chantre-Justino M, Figueiredo MC, Alves G, et al. Prevalence of Epstein-Barr virus infection in recurrent respiratory papillomatosis and the influence on disease severity. Diagn Microbiol Infect Dis. 2022;103:115655.
7. Formánek M, Formánková D, Hurník P, et al. Epstein-Barr virus may contribute to the pathogenesis of adult-onset recurrent respiratory papillomatosis: a preliminary study. Clin Otolaryngol. 2021;46:373–9.
8. Gazia F, Galletti B, Freni F, et al. Use of intralesional cidofovir in the recurrent respiratory papillomatosis: a review of the literature. Eur Rev Med Pharmacol Sci. 2020;24:956–62.
9. Hoesli RC, Thatcher AL, Hogikyan ND, et al. Evaluation of safety of intralesional cidofovir for

adjuvant treatment of recurrent respiratory papillomatosis. JAMA Otolaryngol Head Neck Surg. 2020;146:231–6.
10. Wu R, Abramson AL, Shikowitz MJ, et al. Epidermal growth factor-induced cyclooxygenase-2 expression is mediated through phosphatidylinositol-3 kinase, not mitogen-activated protein/extracellular signal-regulated kinase kinase, in recurrent respiratory papillomas. Clin Cancer Res. 2005;11:6155–61.
11. Rojas-Lechuga MJ, Remacha J, González-Sánchez N, et al. Juvenile recurrent respiratory papillomatosis treated with combined erlotinib and celecoxib: initial report. Int J Pediatr Otorhinolaryngol. 2020;137:110194.
12. Ahn J, Bishop JA, Roden RBS, et al. The PD-1 and PD-L1 pathway in recurrent respiratory papillomatosis. Laryngoscope. 2018;128:E27–32.
13. Creelan BC, Ahmad MU, Kaszuba FJ, et al. Clinical activity of Nivolumab for human papilloma virus-related juvenile-onset recurrent respiratory papillomatosis. Oncologist. 2019;24:829–35.
14. Allen CT, Lee S, Norberg SM, et al. Safety and clinical activity of PD-L1 blockade in patients with aggressive recurrent respiratory papillomatosis. J Immunother Cancer. 2019;7:119.
15. Ablanedo-Terrazas Y, Estrada-Camacho O, Alvarado-de la Barrera C, et al. Efficacy of cidofovir versus bevacizumab in recurrent respiratory papillomatosis: a randomized, double-blind, placebo-controlled pilot study. Acta Otorrinolaringol Esp (Engl Ed). 2022;73:82–8.
16. Pogoda L, Ziylan F, Smeeing DPJ, et al. Bevacizumab as treatment option for recurrent respiratory papillomatosis: a systematic review. Eur Arch Otorhinolaryngol. 2022;279:4229–40.
17. Novakovic D, Cheng ATL, Zurynski Y, et al. A prospective study of the incidence of juvenile-onset recurrent respiratory papillomatosis after implementation of a national HPV vaccination program. J Infect Dis. 2018;217:208–12.
18. Matsuzaki H, Makiyama K, Hasegawa H, et al. Human papillomavirus vaccination as an adjuvant therapy for recurrent respiratory papillomatosis: additional case series. J Voice. 2021; https://doi.org/10.1016/j.jvoice.2021.07.019.
19. Naka Y, Nakao K, Hamaji Y, et al. Solitary squamous cell papilloma of the trachea. Ann Thorac Surg. 1993;55:189–93.
20. Popper HH, El-Shabrawi Y, Wöckel W, et al. Prognostic importance of human papilloma virus typing in squamous cell papilloma of the bronchus: comparison of in situ hybridization and the polymerase chain reaction. Hum Pathol. 1994;25:1191–7.
21. Syrjänen K, Syrjänen S. Solitary bronchial squamous cell papilloma-another human papillomavirus (HPV)-associated benign tumor: systematic review and meta-analysis. Contemp Oncol (Pozn). 2013;17:427–34.
22. Harada H, Miura K, Tsutsui Y, et al. Solitary squamous cell papilloma of the lung in a 40-year-old woman with recurrent laryngeal papillomatosis. Pathol Int. 2000;50:431–9.
23. Li SL, Wang W, Zhao J, et al. A review of the risk factors associated with juvenile-onset recurrent respiratory papillomatosis: genetic, immune and clinical aspects. World J Pediatr. 2022;18:75–82.
24. Amiling R, Meites E, Querec TD, et al. Juvenile-onset recurrent respiratory papillomatosis in the United States, epidemiology and HPV types-2015-2020. J Pediatric Infect Dis Soc. 2021;10:774–81.
25. Armstrong LR, Derkay CS, Reeves WC. Initial results from the national registry for juvenile-onset recurrent respiratory papillomatosis. RRP task force. Arch Otolaryngol Head Neck Surg. 1999;125:743–8.
26. DiMarco AF, Montenegro H, Payne CB Jr, et al. Papillomas of the tracheobronchial tree with malignant degeneration. Chest. 1978;74:464–5.
27. Gélinas JF, Manoukian J, Côté A. Lung involvement in juvenile onset recurrent respiratory papillomatosis: a systematic review of the literature. Int J Pediatr Otorhinolaryngol. 2008;72:433–52.
28. Go C, Schwartz MR, Donovan DT. Molecular transformation of recurrent respiratory papillomatosis: viral typing and p53 overexpression. Ann Otol Rhinol Laryngol. 2003;112:298–302.

Pulmonary Sclerosing Pneumocytoma

Song Zhang

Pulmonary sclerosing pneumocytoma (PSP), formerly known as pulmonary sclerosing hemangioma, is a rare pulmonary tumor considered to originate from primitive respiratory epithelium.

1 Classification

PSP was first described by Liebow and Hubbell [1] in 1956 termed sclerosing hemangioma of the lung owing to marked sclerosis and vascularization of the tissue. It was formerly presumed to be of vascular origin, which was classified as tumor-like lesions in the 1981 WHO classification of lung tumors. In 1998, Niho et al. [2] demonstrated that sclerosing hemangioma is caused by monoclonal expansion of cells, confirming that it is a neoplasia. Therefore, it was moved to the category of miscellaneous tumors in both the 1999 and 2004 WHO classifications. However, its histological origin and differentiation were not described. In 1972, Hill and Eggleston [3] first questioned the vascular origin theory of PSP and proposed an epithelial origin by electron microscopic study. Although some theories have been proposed for its histogenesis including mesothelial, mesenchymal, epithelial, and neuroendocrine origin, most scholars considered it to be an epithelial tumor and first called it pneumocytoma in 1982 by Chan et al. [4]. This conclusion has been strongly supported by immunohistochemical studies. Devouassoux-Shisheboran et al. [5] found that more than 90% of cases expressed epithelial membrane antigen (EMA) and thyroid transcription factor-1 (TTF-1) and confirmed its origin from the respiratory epithelium. In the 2015 WHO classification, the term sclerosing hemangioma was changed to sclerosing pneumocytoma and reclassified this tumor as adenomas.

2 Pathology

PSP has four distinct histological patterns (sclerotic, hemorrhagic, solid, and papillary) and is characterized by two types of epithelial cells-cuboidal surface cells and round stromal cells (Fig. 1a, b). The sclerosis pattern is formed by hyalinized collagen tissue around the hemorrhagic areas, within the stalk of the papillae or within the solid areas. The hemorrhagic pattern is large blood-filled spaces covered with epithelial cells that can contain hemosiderin deposits, foamy macrophages, or cholesterol fissures. The hemangioma-like components are not a real vascular structure, and no normal pulmonary blood vessels and bronchial structures are found in PSP. The solid pattern is composed of sheets of uniform round cells or small tubules covered

S. Zhang (✉)
Department of Respiratory and Critical Care Medicine, Shandong Provincial Hospital Affiliated to Shandong First Medical University, Jinan, Shandong, China

S. Zhang (ed.), *Diagnostic Imaging of Lung Cancers*, https://doi.org/10.1007/978-981-99-6815-2_13

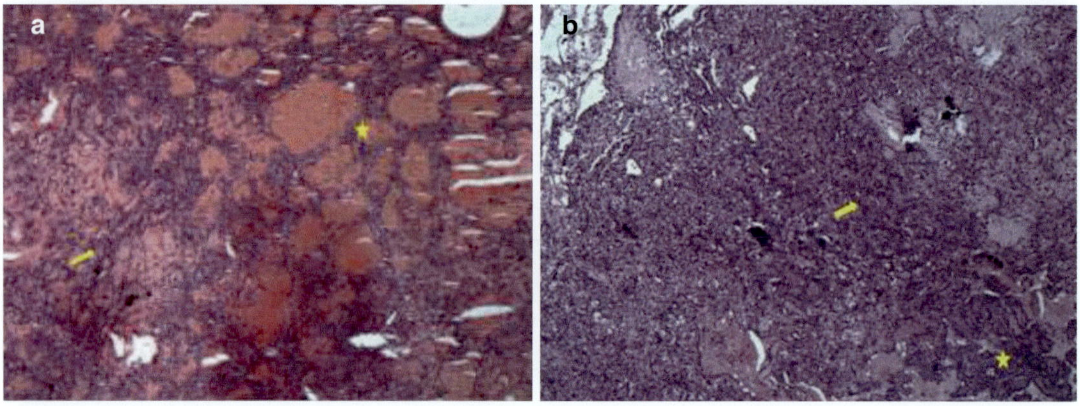

Fig. 1 (**a**) HE stain shows sclerosing (arrow) and hemorrhagic (pentagram) pattern. (**b**) HE stain shows solid (arrow) and papillary(pentagram) patterns

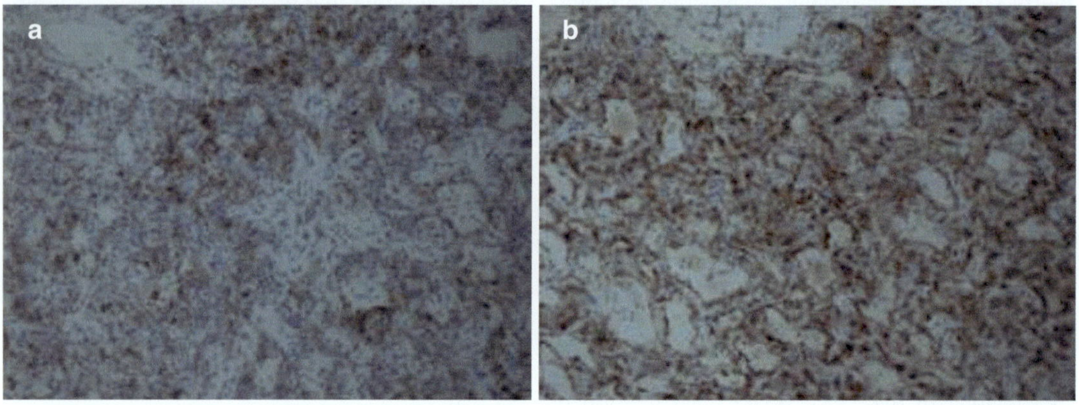

Fig. 2 (**a**) CK expression in surface cells is positive and negative for round cells. (**b**) EMA expression is positive for both surface cells and round cells

with surface cells. The papillary pattern is lined with surface cells covering a stroma of round cells. PSP usually contains of 3–4 architectural patterns in various proportions. The cuboidal cells, morphologically similar to type II pneumocytes, line the surface of the tumor and are called lining cells. The round cells, distributed in the interstitium, are uniform, oval, or polygonal-shaped cells with clear cytoplasm and fine chromatin. Both cells show little cytological atypia.

Immunohistochemically, both cells express TTF-1 and EMA. The surface cells also exhibit pancytokeratin (AE1/AE3), surfactant proteins A and B, and Clara cell antigen, indicating that they are more differentiated and originated from type II pneumocytes. The round cells lack these proteins and focally express cytokeratin-7 and CAM 5.2, suggesting that they are derived from primitive respiratory epithelium (Figs. 2a, b and 3a, b).

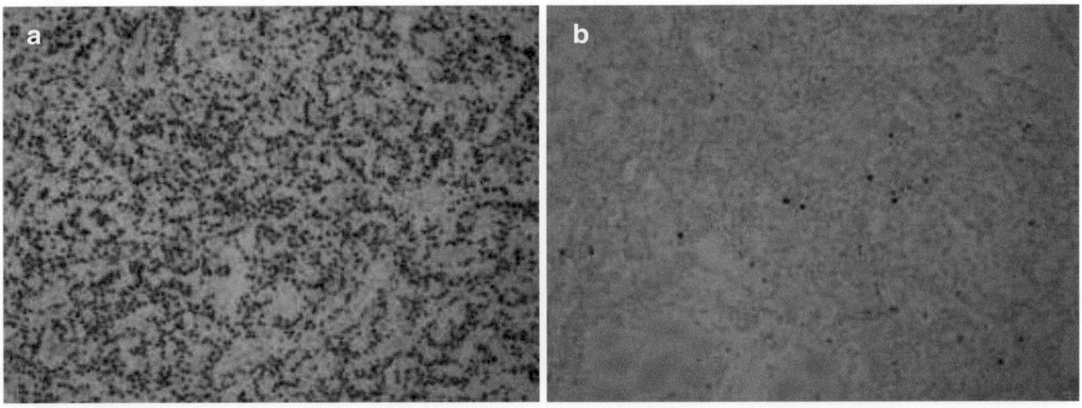

Fig. 3 (**a**) TTF-1 expression is positive for both surface cells and round cells. (**b**) Ki-67 shows low expression

3 Epidemiology

PSP typically affects Asian middle-aged women, with a female to male ratio of 5:1 or higher. The incidence of PSP is very low in western country. Lovrenski et al. [6] performed a retrospective study of 6 cases of PSP within 10 years. PSP was more frequently diagnosed in females (83.34%). The patients ranged in age from 38 to 61. Most of the patients (66.66%) were asymptomatic. The higher incidence in females suggested some relationship between this tumor and female sex hormones. Some studies have confirmed that estrogen receptors may be involved in the growth, differentiation, and surfactant production of sclerosing hemangioma. Wu et al. [7] revealed that estrogen receptor beta overexpression was found in 91.9% of PSP patients, compared with 45.8% in NSCLC. The staining pattern of the neoplastic cells of the PSP was similar to that of type II pneumocytes but quite different from NSCLC. Trabucco et al. [8] found that the cuboidal epithelial cells showed intense staining for cytokeratin-pool and TTF-1, and progesterone receptors were focal positive. Round and spindle cells were positive for vimentin, TTF-1 and focally for the progesterone receptor.

4 Clinical Features

Most of the patients are asymptomatic and detected occasionally. Symptoms such as cough, expectoration, fatigue, chest pain, dyspnea, and hemoptysis may also occur. Kuo et al. [9] retrospectively reviewed the data of 44 PSP patients (7 male and 37 female). The patient's age ranged from 16 to 72 years, with a peak at fifth decade, and 72.7% of them were asymptomatic.

5 Radiographic Features

On imaging, PSP is often solitary, well-defined, round, or oval nodule or mass (Fig. 4). Multiple lesions account for rarely 5% of cases. PSP is usually a parenchymal lesion, but it can also be juxtapleural or juxtafissural in location (Fig. 5). It often shows homogeneous enhancement and delayed enhancement. Calcification is common (Fig. 6), cystic change is rare (Fig. 7), and cavitation does not occur. Other signs include the presence of pseudocapsule (Fig. 8), overlying vessels (Fig. 9), prominent artery sign, air meniscus sign (Fig. 10), tail sign (Fig. 11), and halo sign. The marginal pseudocapsule sign is the compressed lung parenchyma adjacent to the tumor. Overlapping vessels or welt vessel signs correspond to the drainage vessels of adjacent tumors. The prominent pulmonary artery may be a result of increased arterial demand in these vascular soft-tissue tumors. The air meniscus sign is defined as a gap or crescent region without lung markings around the lesion. The tail sign is a small linear projection seen radiating out from the lesion. The halo sign presents as a lesion with surrounding GGO.

On PET/CT, some studies indicated that most PSPs showed mild to moderate FDG uptake, and

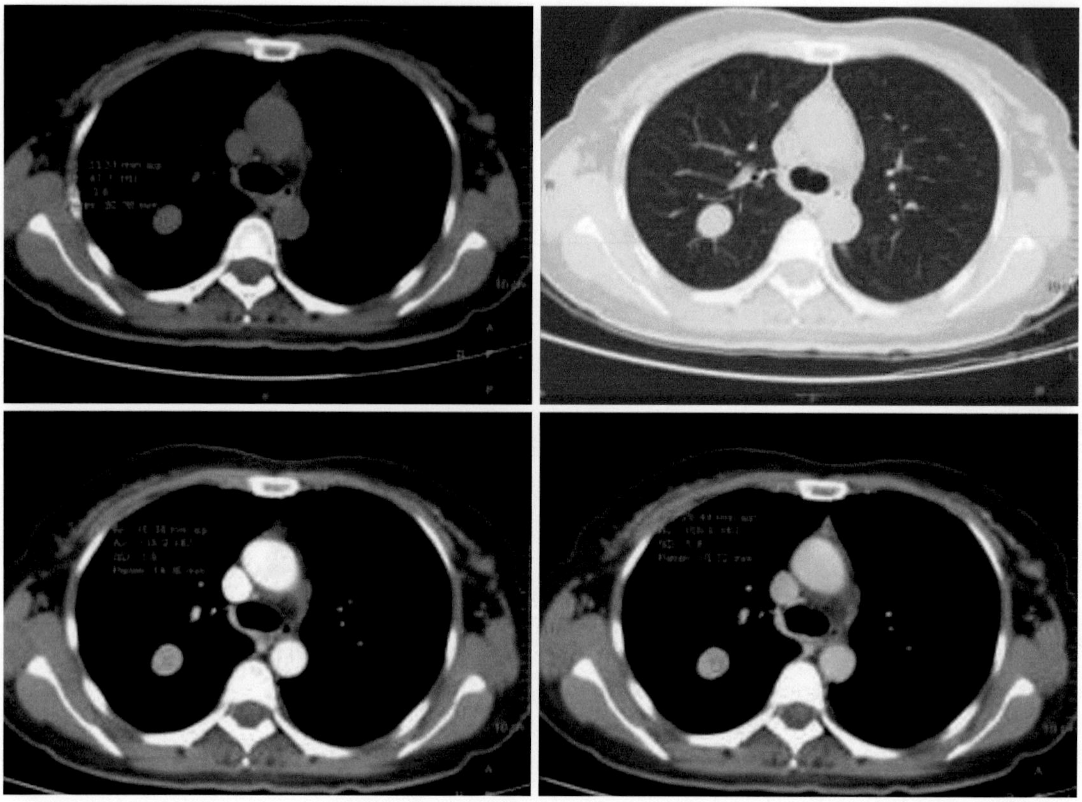

Fig. 4 A 46-year-old woman with a well-circumscribed, round nodule in the right upper lobe. The CT attenuations of the three-phase dynamic scan are 41.7, 116.9, and 109.6 HU, respectively

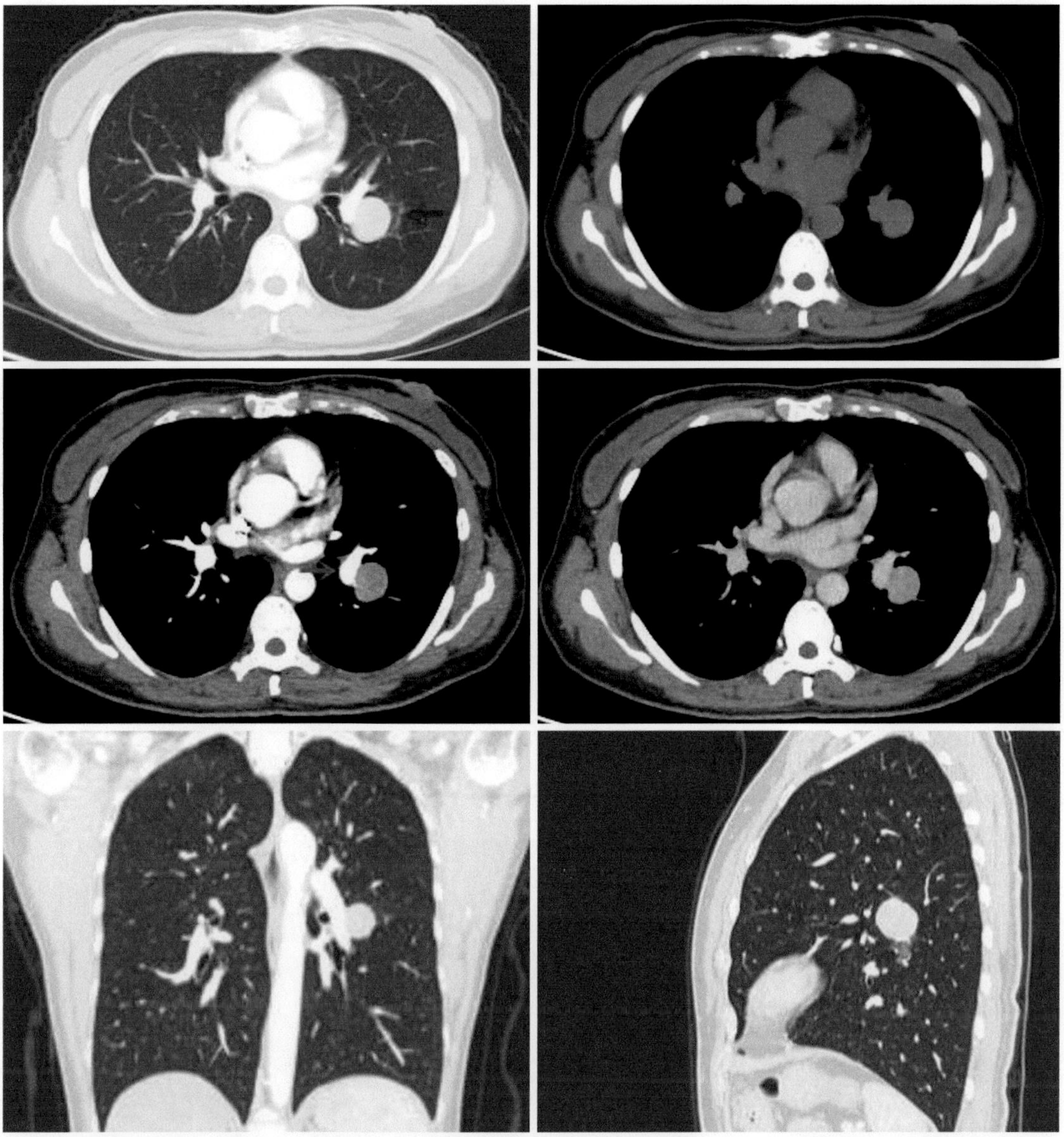

Fig. 5 A 43-year-old woman with a well-circumscribed, round nodule in the left lower lobe adjacent to interlobular fissure. Contrast-enhanced CT scan shows markedly enhanced with halo sign (red arrow) and prominent artery sign (blue arrow)

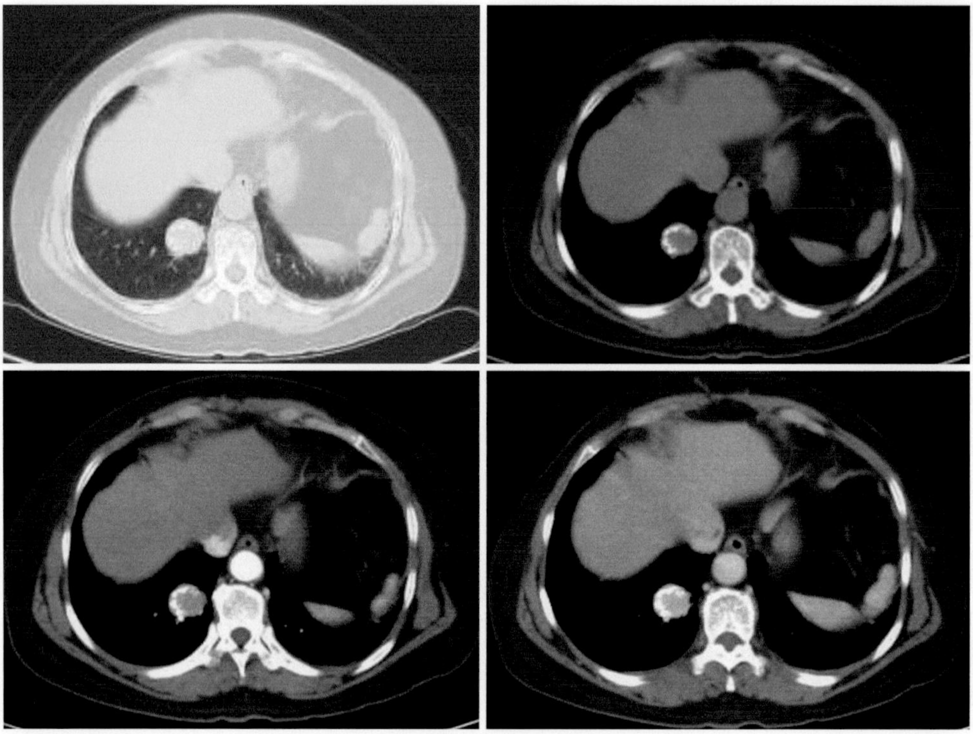

Fig. 6 A 54-year-old woman with a well-circumscribed, round mass in the right lower lobe with a diameter of 3.1 cm. Contrast-enhanced CT scan shows markedly enhanced with coarse calcifications

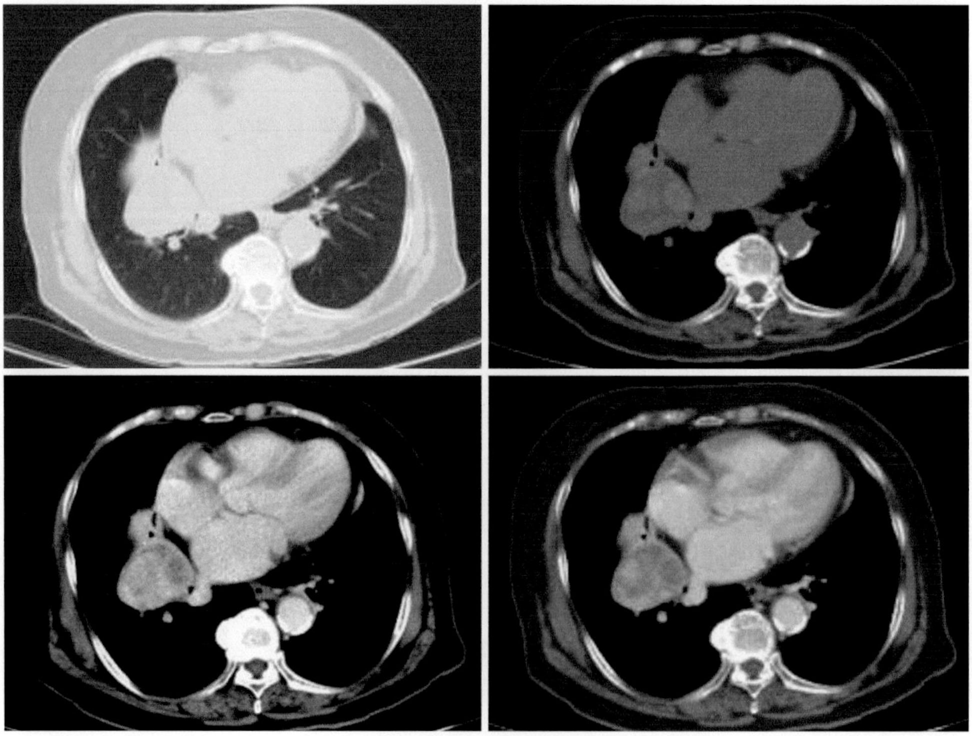

Fig. 7 A 79-year-old woman with a well-circumscribed, round mass in the right lower lobe with markedly enhanced and cystic formation

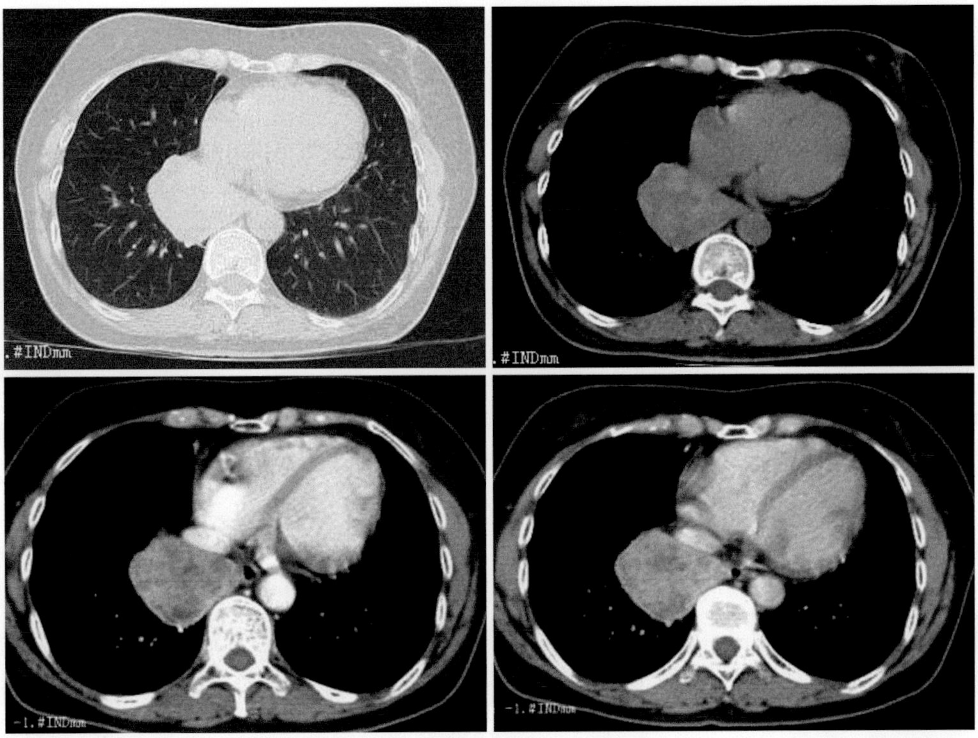

Fig. 8 A 62-year-old woman with a well-circumscribed, round mass in the right lower lobe. Contrast-enhanced CT scan shows markedly enhanced with pseudocapsule and cystic formation

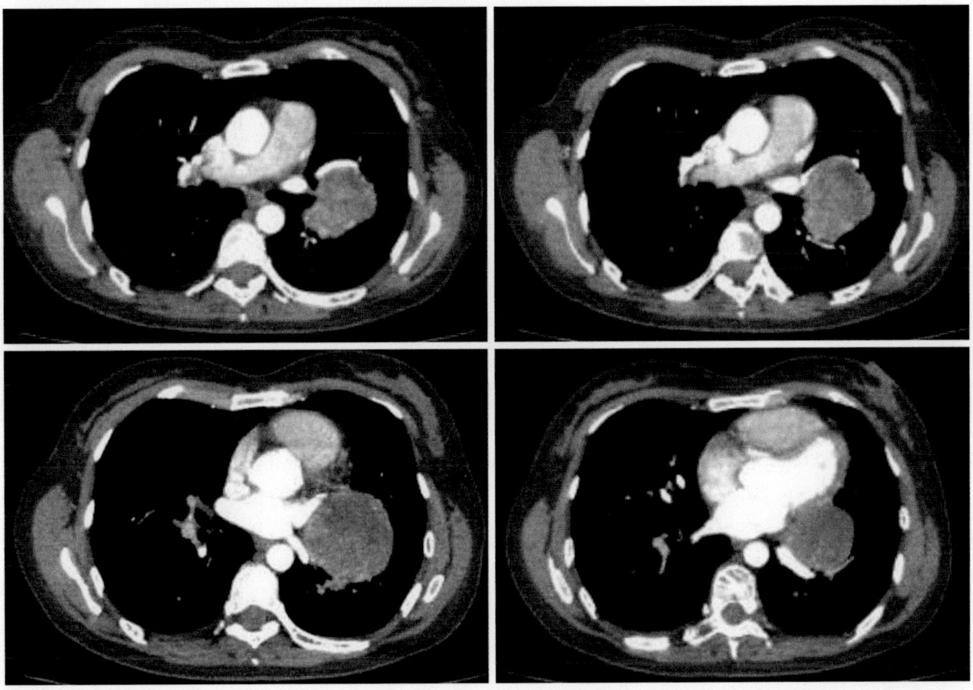

Fig. 9 A 44-year-old woman with a well-circumscribed, round mass in the left lower lobe. Contrast-enhanced CT scan shows markedly enhanced with overlying vessels, prominent artery sign, and cystic formation

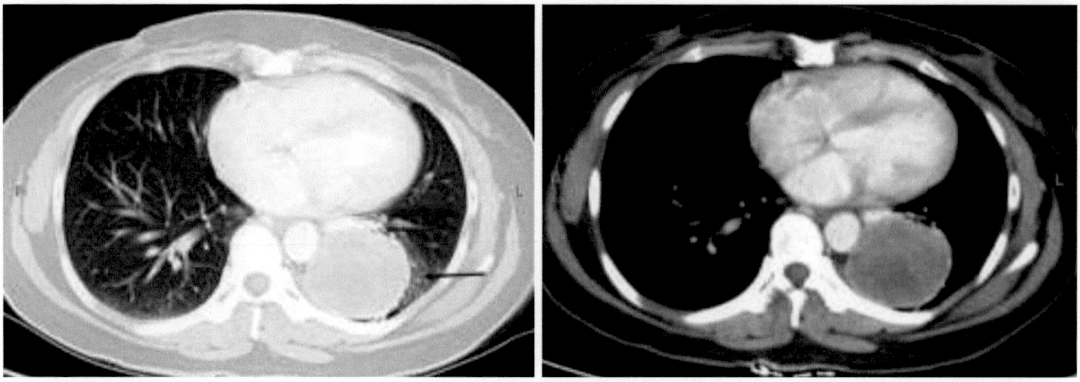

Fig. 10 A 40-year-old man with a well-circumscribed, round mass in the left lower lobe with air meniscus sign (red arrow) and halo sign (black arrow)

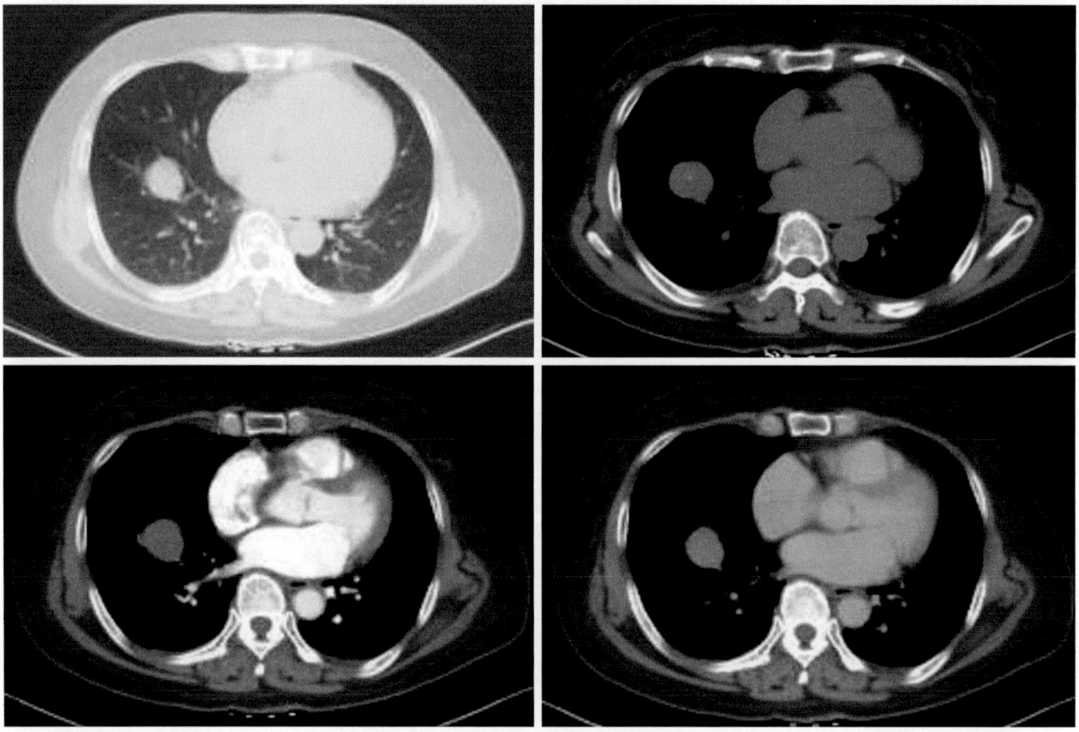

Fig. 11 A 53-year-old man with a well-circumscribed, round nodule in the right lower lobe with calcification and tail sign

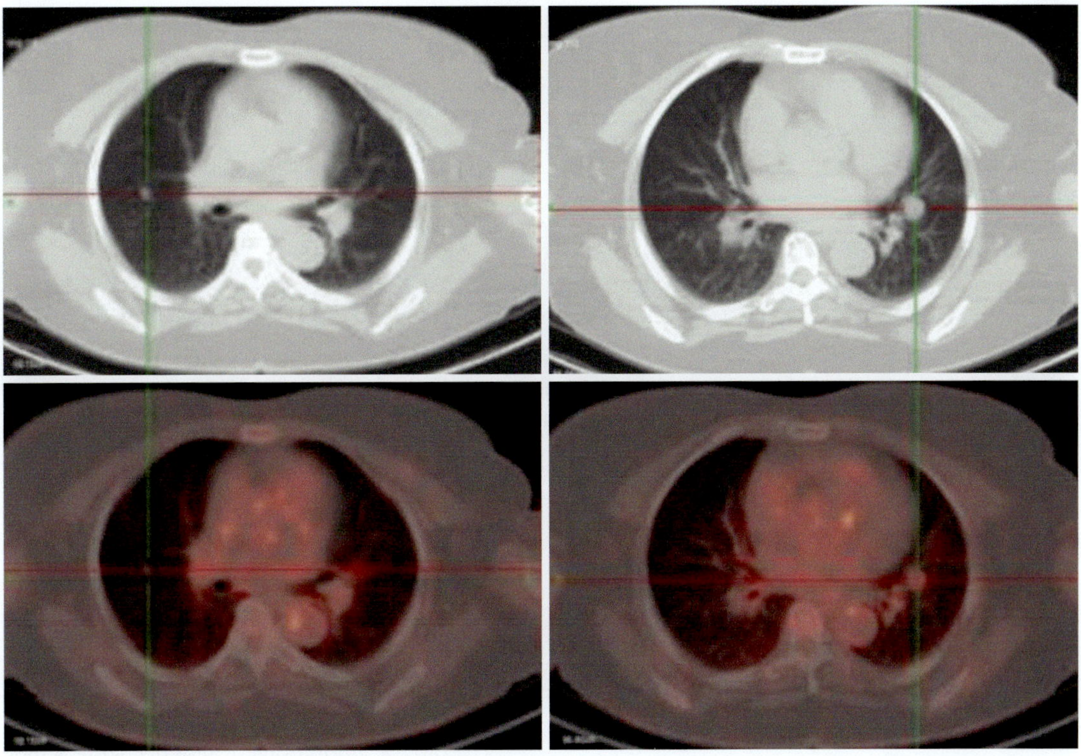

Fig. 12 A 62-year-old female with bilateral lung nodules. A round nodule in the left upper lobe with a size of about 2.0 cm × 1.5 cm, showing mild uptake with a SUVmax of 2.5. A small round nodule in the right upper lobe with a size of about 1.0 cm × 0.8 cm, showing no uptake

tumor size was positively correlated with the maximum standardized uptake value (SUVmax) (Fig. 12).

6 Treatment

PSP follows a benign course despite the rare presence of metastasis. Complete surgical excision with clear margins is the standard treatment for PSP, and there is no evidence supporting the effectiveness of adjuvant therapy.

7 Prognosis

Although some cases displayed pathologically malignant behavior, such as lymph node metastasis and necrosis, PSP is generally associated with an excellent prognosis and no tumor-related mortality has been reported in the literature.

8 Case Analysis

8.1 Case 1

A 48-year-old woman found a lung lesion on physical examination.

Chest CT: An irregular soft tissue nodule in the left lower lobe adjacent to the pericardium, the CT attenuations of the three-phase dynamic scan were 48.0, 75.4, and 95.4 HU, respectively (Fig. 13).

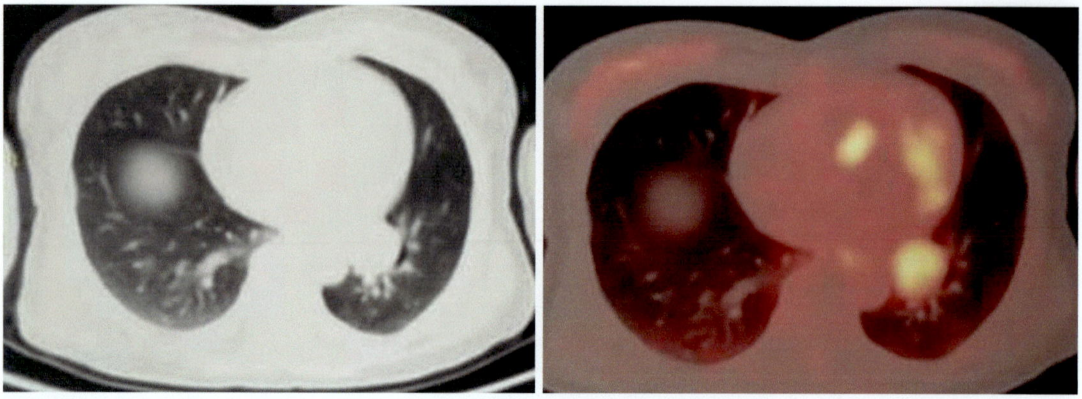

PET/CT: A relatively high uptake of FDG (SUVmax = 4.9).

[Diagnosis] Pulmonary sclerosing pneumocytoma.

[Diagnosis Basis] The patient underwent left lower lobectomy. Grossly, it was typically well-circumscribed, solid, and gray-red to brown, with a focal hemorrhage. Pathology revealed sclerosing pneumocytoma. Regional lymph nodes were chronically inflammatory changes. Immunohistochemistry, stromal components were positive for TTF-1and EMA, epithelial components were positive for CKpan, CK7, TTF-1, EMA, and Napsin A. The Ki-67 index was less than 1%.

[Analysis] PET/CT examination is useful for the differential diagnosis of benign and malignant tumors. Benign or slow-growing tumors often have low glucose metabolism. Several studies have suggested that larger PSP lesions may have more active cell proliferation or contain more cellular components, either of which may be the main reason for increased FDG uptake.

In 2011, Lin et al. [10] reported FDG PET findings of 6 cases of PSP. The mean standard uptake value was 2.45 (range, 1.8–3.93). They concluded that PSP demonstrates low to moderate uptake on FDG PET imaging. The larger PSP has higher uptake and might be misrecognized as a malignancy. Lee et al. [11] also found that PSP showed increased FDG uptakes, and the SUVmax value was significantly correlated with tumor size. PSP ≥2 cm can frequently be falsely interpreted as malignancy in FDG-PET/CT. Xu et al. [12] further found that the SUVmax value was positively correlated with tumor size in typical PSP, but not significantly correlated with tumor size in atypical PSP. A majority (90%) of atypical PSPs were found in males. They considered that morphological differences may affect the correlation between tumor size and SUV max in PSPs.

Overall, a middle-aged female with single round or ovoid soft-tissue lesion with mild to moderate FDG uptake on PET/CT images suggests a possible diagnosis of PSP.

8.2 Case 2

A 55-year-old woman found a lung lesion for 1 day on physical examination.

Chest CT: A regular soft tissue mass in the left lower lobe. (Fig. 14).

[Diagnosis] Pulmonary sclerosing pneumocytoma.

[Diagnosis Basis] A middle-aged woman has a well-circumscribed, round mass in the left lower lobe. Chest CT scan shows punctate calcifications (blue arrows), cystic changes, heterogeneous enhancement, and welt vessel sign (red arrows), consistent with PSP. The patient underwent left lower lobe resection. Grossly, the cut surface is gray-red. Pathology revealed sclerosing pneumocytoma. Immunohistochemically, epithelial components were positive for CKpan,

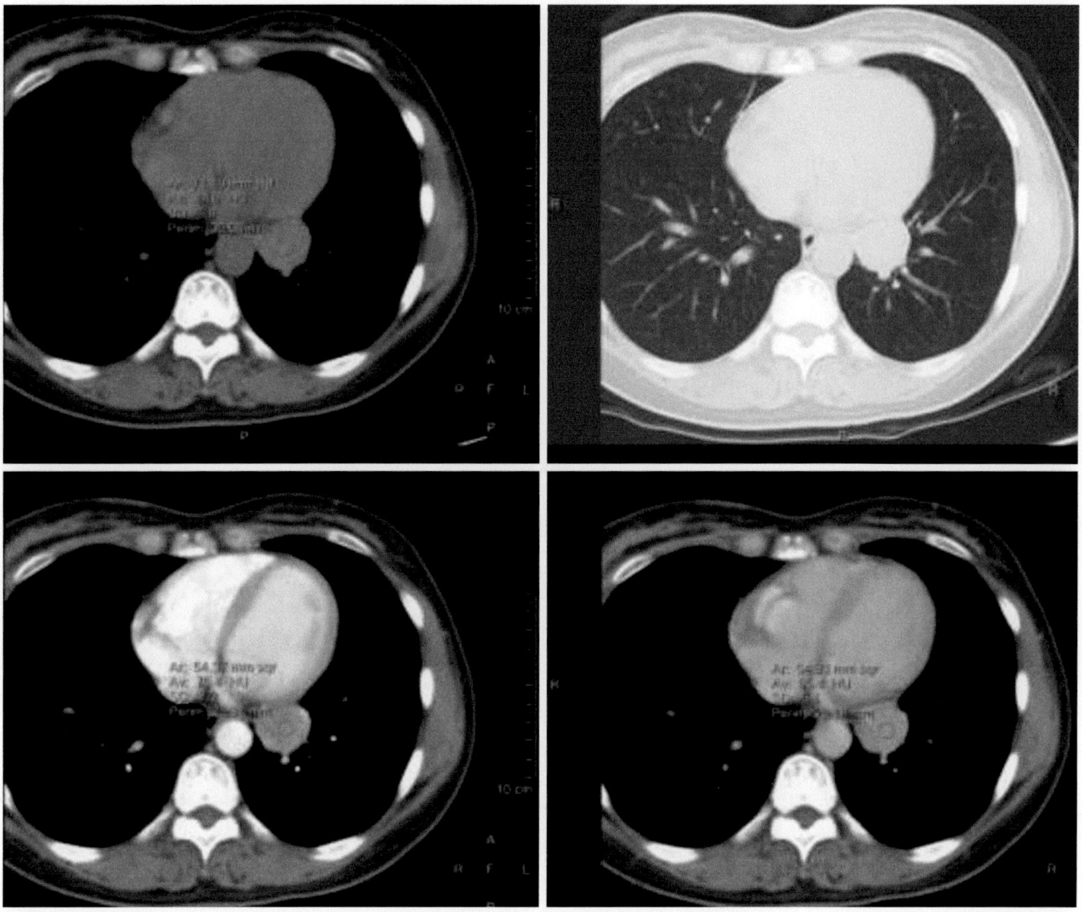

Fig. 13 Chest CT

CK7, TTF-1, EMA, and Napsin A, and stromal components were positive for TTF-1 and EMA. The Ki-67 index was less than 1%.

[Analysis] In 1994, Im et al. [13] retrospectively studied CT features of 8 PSP patients. CT findings of PSP were characterized by well-defined juxtapleural lesion with marked contrast enhancement coupled in select cases with foci of sharply marginated areas of low attenuation and calcification. Enhanced density ranged from 96 to 157 HU. On CT-pathology correlation, the higher, iso-, and lower attenuation areas corresponded with angiomatous, solid and sclerotic, and cystic areas, respectively. In 2003, Cheung et al. [14] revealed that inhomogeneous enhancement was frequently present and depended on the various compositions of the tumors, especially those in sclerotic and papillary predominant types. The presence of a tail sign, intra-tumoral cystic areas, and a prominent artery sign were the frequent features. A well-defined cystic area, corresponded to the hemorrhagic areas demonstrated on histopathological evaluation, is occasionally found in PSP and is rare in hamartomas or lung cancer. Chung et al. [15] also reported that the strong and rapid enhancement of PSP at dynamic CT attributed histopathologically to the presence of hemangiomatous or papillary components in the tumor. Wang et al. [16] retrospectively reviewed 16 pathologically confirmed PSP patients. The relatively characteristic CT findings

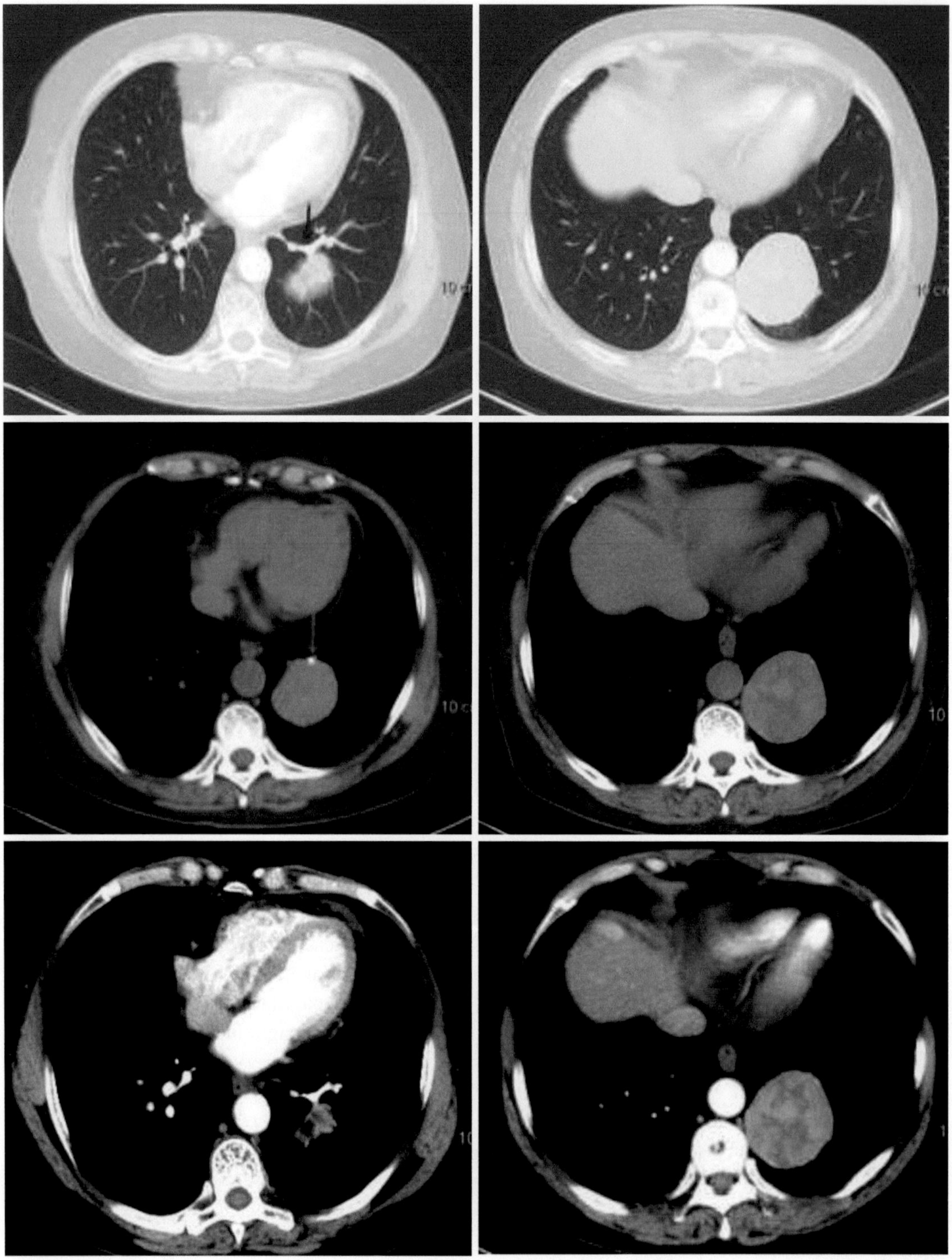

Fig. 14 Chest CT

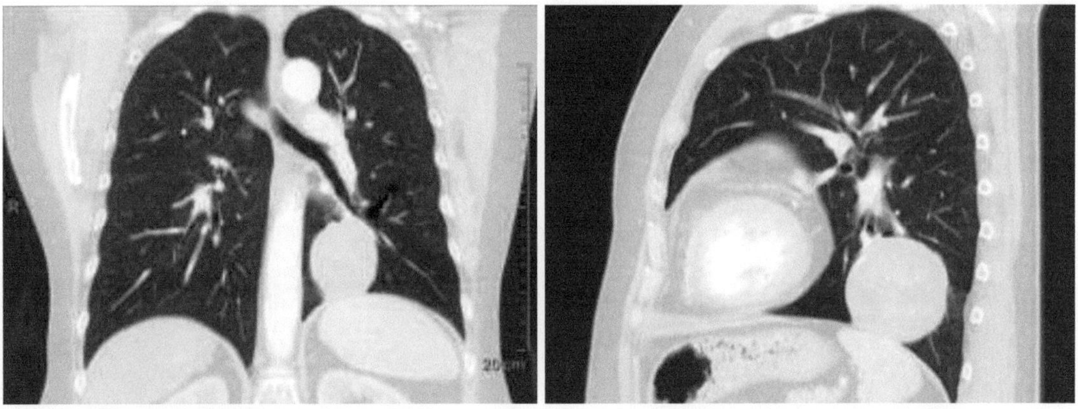

Fig. 13.14 (continued)

include a markedly contrast-enhanced juxtapleural mass with homogeneous enhancement for the smaller tumors (<3 cm) or heterogeneous enhancement for the larger tumors (>3 cm). The air crescent sign (13%), calcification (13%), and a prominent pulmonary artery (25%) were also demonstrated.

Pulmonary benign tumors in the differential diagnosis of PSP include clear cell tumor, hamartoma, and hemangioma. Clear cell tumor has a glycogen-rich abundant clear to eosinophilic granular cytoplasm with well defined cell borders and shows positive for Melan A, HMB45, and S-100. In hamartoma, mature cartilage and adipose tissue can be found in addition to the presence of bronchial epithelium. In pulmonary hemangioma, there are true vascular spaces filled with blood and lined with CD31 and CD34 positive endothelial cells.

8.3 Case 3

A 54-year-old woman complained of cough and expectoration for 1 week.

Chest CT: An irregular soft tissue mass in the right upper lobe. (Fig. 15).

[Diagnosis] Pulmonary sclerosing pneumocytoma.

[Diagnosis Basis] A middle-aged woman has irregular mass in the anterior segment of the right upper lobe, with welt vascular sign (blue arrow) and air crescent sign (red arrow), considering the diagnosis PSP. During the operation, it was seen that the right upper lobe was partially adhered to the chest wall and interlobar fissure, and the size of the mass was about 5.5 × 5 × 3 cm. Postoperative pathology was sclerosing pneumocytoma.

[Analysis] PSP is usually a solitary, well-circumscribed nodule or mass. The air crescent sign or air meniscus sign represents an air-trapping zone surrounding the tumor. The sign has also been reported in aspergilloma, hamartoma, tuberculoma, and lung carcinoma. Nam et al. [17] believed it could be of help in the confident diagnosis of PSP and in differentiating it from other benign tumors of the lung. They suggested that the air-trapping zone around PSP is possibly because of the peritumoral hemorrhage followed by clearance through air space and finally forms the peritumoral air space. Shin et al. [18] studied 76 PSP cases. Most patients had a single lesion (92.1%), smooth boundary (65.8%), and oval shape (65.8%), and the mean diameter was 2.27 cm. The CT signs included marginal pseudocapsule (50%), overlying vessel (26.3%), air gap (2.6%), and halo sign (17.1%). Xu et al. [19] analyzed 34 PSP cases. 92% of the lesions located in the right middle lobe and the lower lobe of bilateral lungs, and 46% of the lesions (16/34) were attached to the pleura. All lesions showed enhancement, with 97% (33/34) of lesions showing uneven

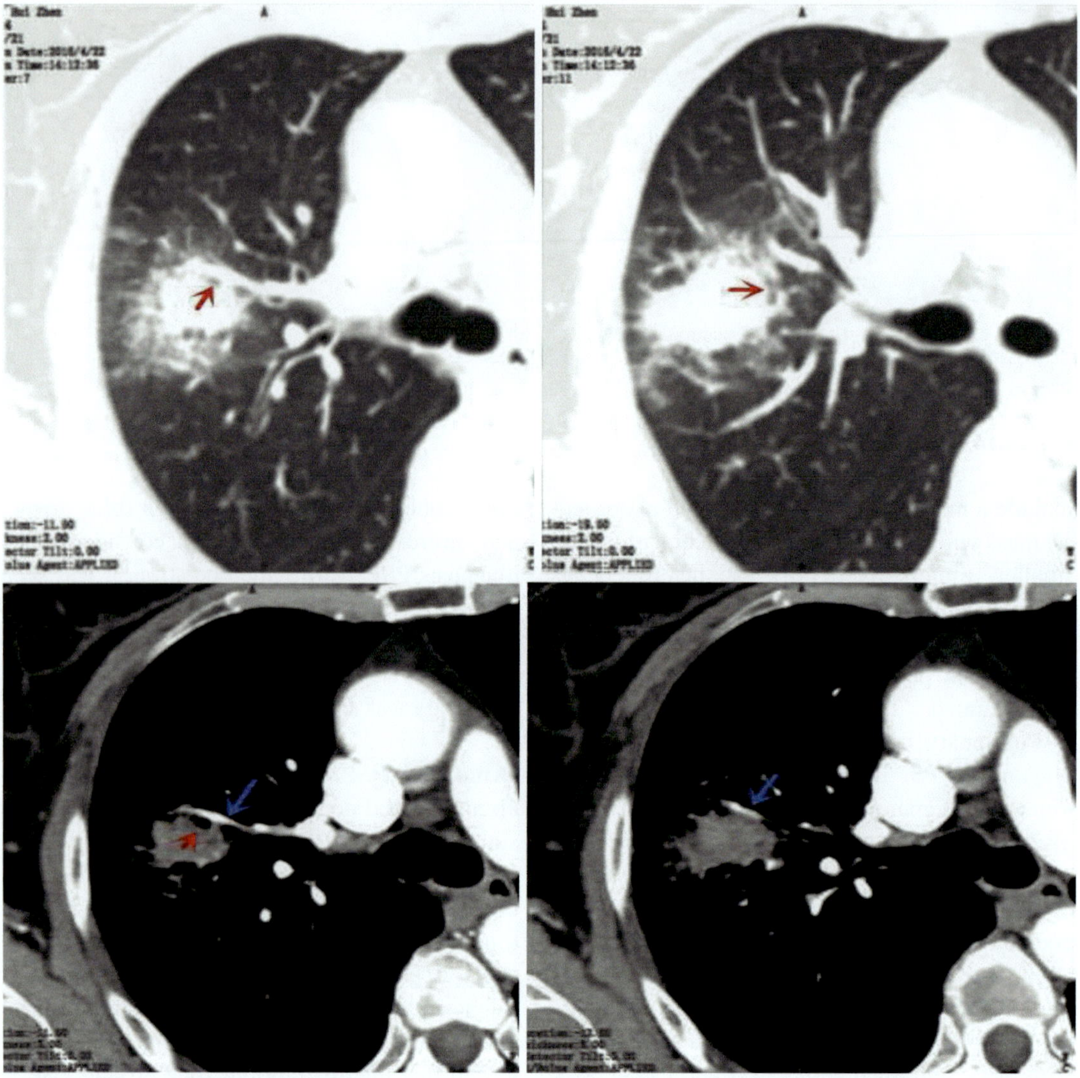

Fig. 15 Chest CT

enhancement. PSP volume was negatively correlated with the total degree of enhancement. Welt vessel sign was observed in 61.7% (21/34) of cases, and none of welt vessels entered into the lesions. There is no significant correlation between vascular-like enhancement area inside the lesion and the welt vessels outside the lesion, and no case showed entrance of bronchus into the lesion.

8.4 Case 4

A 40-year-old woman found a lung lesion on physical examination.

Chest CT: An irregular soft tissue nodule in the right lower lobe. (Fig. 16).

[Diagnosis] Pulmonary sclerosing pneumocytoma.

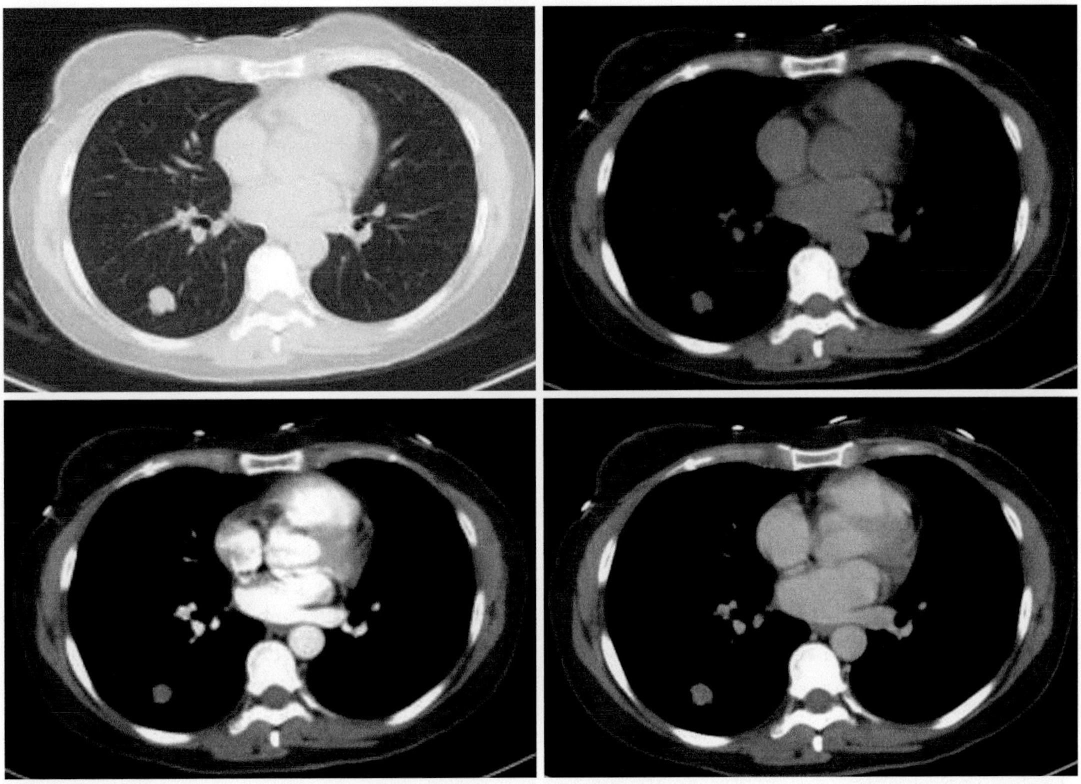

Fig. 16 Chest CT

[Diagnosis Basis] The patient underwent right lower lobe wedge resection. Grossly, the tumor size was 1.2 × 1.6 × 1.3 cm, and the cut surface was gray-white. Pathology revealed sclerosing pneumocytoma. Immunohistochemically, epithelial components were positive for CK7 and Napsin A, stromal components were positive for PR, and both cells expressed TTF-1 and EMA. The Ki-67 index was less than 2%.

[Analysis] As PSP can be treated with limited surgical resection, it is important to distinguish this tumor from other entities, especially adenocarcinoma. However, it is difficult to make a correct diagnosis of PSP, either preoperatively or intraoperatively. Kocaman et al. [20] reported a 25-year-old female patient with a 4 cm mass in the left upper lobe. Intraoperative frozen section diagnosis was adenocarcinoma, and the final diagnosis was PSP with lymph node metastasis. The key is that the papillary cores of the PSP have polygonal stromal cells rather than typical fibrovascular cores of an adenocarcinoma. Yang et al. [21] reviewed retrospectively 59 PSP cases that underwent an intraoperative frozen section examination. The rate of accurate diagnosis using frozen sections was 44.1%, the deferral rate was 15.3%, and 10 cases (16.9%) were misdiagnosed as malignant tumors. A solid-predominant pattern is misdiagnosed more frequently than other growth patterns. They proposed that the key to avoiding a misdiagnosis is to recognize the dual-cell populations in a tumor, i.e., cuboidal surface cells and stromal round cells. Maleki et al. [22] considered that there is overlap between the morphological findings of PSP and well-differentiated lung adenocarcinoma, so we should prevent a misdiagnosis and aggressive treatment.

The complicated pathological features of PSP determine the diversity of its imaging manifestations. Some PSPs have imaging signs that tend to be malignant, such as lobulation and liquefaction necrosis, which are easily confused with peripheral lung cancer. The enhancement degree of lesion can distinguish PSP from other lung cancer.

8.5 Case 5

A 25-year-old man complained of cough, expectoration, and hemoptysis for 3 days.

Chest CT: A soft tissue nodule in the left lower lobe. (Fig. 17).

[Diagnosis] Pulmonary sclerosing pneumocytoma.

[Diagnosis Basis] Chest CT shows a round nodule in the paraspinal region of the right lower lobe, with ground-glass opacity and welt vascular sign, supporting the diagnosis of sclerosing pneumocytoma. The patient underwent bronchoscopic biopsy. Pathology showed papillary and glandular-like structures covered with epithelioid cells, consistent with the diagnosis of PSP. Immunohistochemically, epithelial components were positive for TTF-1, EMA, CK7, and Napsin A. The Ki-67 index was less than 5%.

[Analysis] Some studies have reported that GGO or halo sign on CT reflects unique pathologic features of PSP. The halo sign is correlated with hemorrhage in the lung parenchyma. The difference between the tumor shrinkage rate and the pseudocapsule in PSP may cause bleeding. Hemorrhage is followed by clearance through the airspace forming the peritumoral lucent zone. Patients may manifest hemoptysis or blood-streaked sputum.

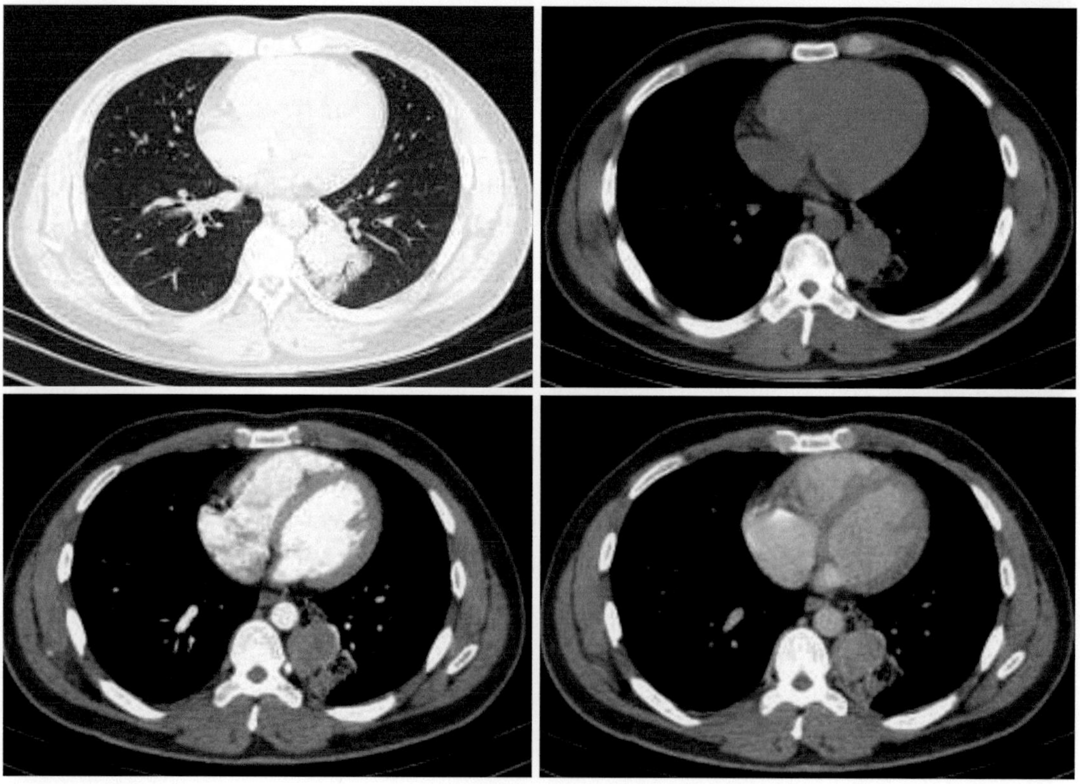

Fig. 17 Chest CT

Napsin A, a human aspartic proteinase, shows positive expression in type II pneumocytes with a granular and cytoplasmic staining pattern. It has been widely used in the diagnosis of lung adenocarcinoma along with TTF-1. Zhou et al. [23] reported an asymptomatic 33-year-old female was diagnosed to have well-differentiated adenocarcinoma with papillary features on biopsy. A lobectomy was performed. Finally, the surgical resection specimen revealed the correct diagnosis of PSP. Immunohistochemical staining demonstrated nuclear reactivity for TTF-1 in both cell types and Napsin A positivity only in surface cells.

Napsin A is useful for evaluating PSP, and that it preferentially stains cuboidal surface cells, not the stromal round cells. Tumors with immunoreactivity to both TTF-1 and Napsin A may not be lung adenocarcinoma, and PSP should be considered as a differential diagnosis, in particular, when the sample is obtained from the papillary component.

8.6 Case 6

A 58-year-old woman complained of cough and expectoration for half a year.

Chest CT: Multiple lesions in the bilateral lungs. (Fig. 18).

[Diagnosis] Pulmonary sclerosing pneumocytoma.

[Diagnosis Basis] The patient underwent lung biopsy. Pathology showed atypical glands in the fibrous interstitium, combined with immunohistochemistry, consistent with the diagnosis of PSP.

[Analysis] PSP presenting as multiple lung nodules is rare. It is unclear whether multiple PSP nodules represent lung metastases or the presence of multiple tumors. Numerous studies have showed that PSP has the potential of lymph node metastasis, extra-pulmonary metastasis, multiple lesions, and recurrence.

In 1986, Tanaka et al. [24] first reported a 22-year-old male patient diagnosed with PSP with lymph node metastasis. Wang et al. [25] reported a 26-year-old woman with surgically confirmed PSP with mediastinal and regional lymph nodes metastases. They speculated that potential mechanisms of metastasis may be related to epithelial-mesenchymal transformation. Teng et al. [26] first reported a case of malignant transformation of both cuboidal surface cells and stromal round cells. Microscopically, the cuboidal surface cells transformed to adenocarcinoma. The stromal round cells also had a malignant transformation. In addition, E-cadherin was negative in primary tumor but positive in metastatic lymph node, indicating that the mesenchymal to epithelial transition may play an important role in lymph node metastasis. Jiang et al. [27] reported gene mutation findings in a 17-year-old girl with PSP. Two mutations were identified in the tumor tissue by sanger sequencing and NGS: AKT1 E17K and BRAF (B-Raf proto-oncogene, serine/threonine kinase) V600E. Wang et al. [28] reported a 23-year-old man with cervical lymph nodes and liver metastases. PSP-specific AKT1 E17K somatic mutation accompanied with TP53 C176Y germline mutation may lead to the malignant clinical course of this tumor. Dantis et al. [29] reported a case of a massive PSP involving the right lower lobe adhering esophagus.

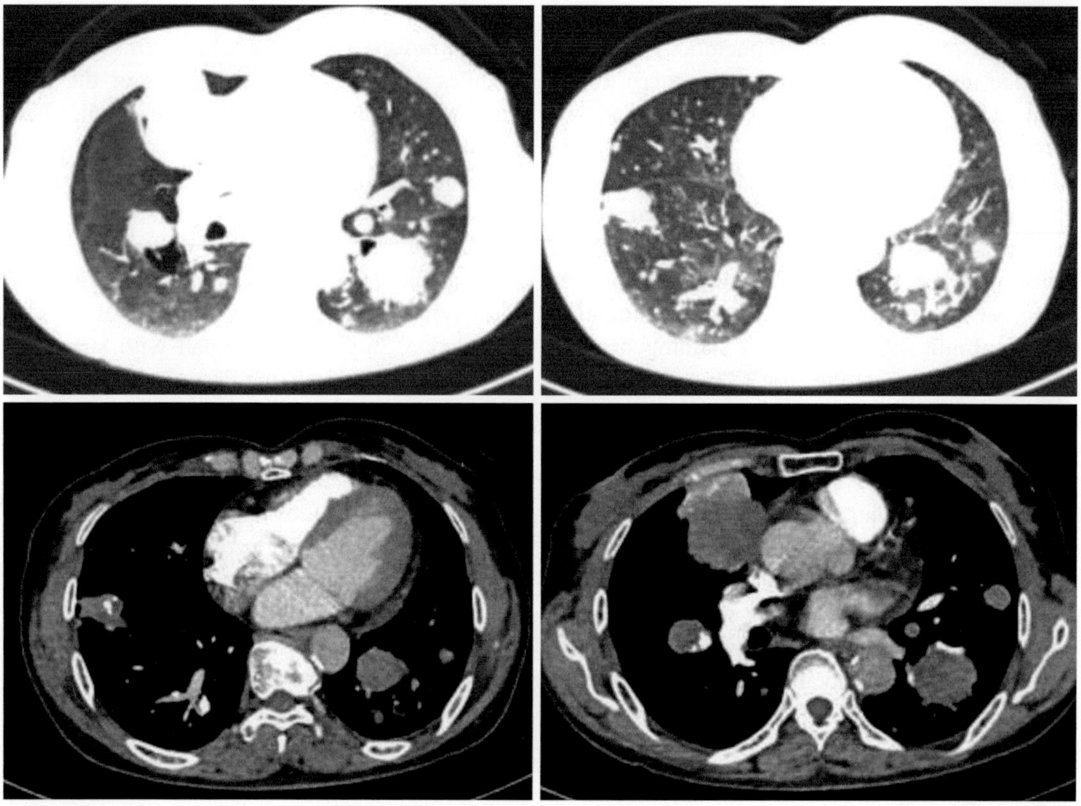

Fig. 18 Chest CT

Histopathology revealed PSP-papillary variant with concurrent mutation of BRAF V600E and PTEN genes.

The mechanism of PSP metastasis is still unclear, and further research is needed.

References

1. Liebow AA, Hubbell S. Sclerosing haemangioma (histiocytoma, xanthoma) of the lung. Cancer. 1956;9:53–75.
2. Niho S, Suzuki K, Yokose T, et al. Monoclonality of both pale cells and cuboidal cells of sclerosing hemangioma. Am J Pathol. 1998;152:1065–9.
3. Hill GS, Eggleston JC. Electron microscopic study of so-called "pulmonary sclerosing hemangioma". Report of a case suggesting epithelial origin. Cancer. 1972;30:1092–106.
4. Chan KW, Gibbs AR, Lo WS, et al. Benign sclerosing pneumocytoma of lung (sclerosing haemangioma). Thorax. 1982;37:404–12.
5. Devouassoux-Shisheboran M, Hayashi T, Linnoila RI, et al. A clinicopathologic study of 100 cases of pulmonary sclerosing hemangioma with immunohistochemical studies: TTF-1 is expressed in both round and surface cells, suggesting an origin from primitive respiratory epithelium. Am J Surg Pathol. 2000;24:906–16.
6. Lovrenski A, Vasilijević M, Panjković M, et al. Sclerosing pneumocytoma: a ten-year experience at a Western Balkan University Hospital. Medicina. 2019;55(27)
7. Wu CT, Chang YL, Lee YC. Expression of the estrogen receptor beta in 37 surgically treated pulmonary sclerosing hemangiomas in comparison with non-small cell lung carcinomas. Hum Pathol. 2005;36:1108–12.
8. Trabucco SMR, Brascia D, Cazzato G, et al. Pulmonary sclerosing pneumocytoma: a pre and intraoperative diagnostic challenge. Report of two cases and review of the literature. Medicina (Kaunas). 2021;57:524.
9. Kuo KT, Hsu WH, Wu YC, et al. Sclerosing hemangioma of the lung: an analysis of 44 cases. J Chin Med Assoc. 2003;66:33–8.

10. Lin KH, Chang CP, Liu RS, et al. F-18 FDG PET/CT in evaluation of pulmonary sclerosing hemangioma. Clin Nucl Med. 2011;36:341–3.
11. Lee E, Park CM, Kang KW, et al. 18F-FDG PET/CT features of pulmonary sclerosing hemangioma. Acta Radiol. 2013;54:24–9.
12. Xu J, Dong Y, Yin G, et al. ^{18}F-FDG PET/CT imaging: a supplementary understanding of pulmonary sclerosing pneumocytoma. Thorac Cancer. 2019;10:1552–60.
13. Im JG, Kim WH, Han MC, et al. Sclerosing haemangiomas of the lung and interlobar fissures: CT findings. J Comput Assist Tomogr. 1994;18:34–8.
14. Cheung YC, Ng SH, Chang JW, et al. Histopathological and CT features of pulmonary sclerosing haemangiomas. Clin Radiol. 2003;58:630–5.
15. Chung MJ, Lee KS, Han J, et al. Pulmonary sclerosing hemangioma presenting as solitary pulmonary nodule: dynamic CT findings and histopathologic comparisons. AJR Am J Roentgenol. 2006;187:430–7.
16. Wang QB, Chen YQ, Shen JJ, et al. Sixteen cases of pulmonary sclerosing haemangioma: CT findings are not definitive for preoperative diagnosis. Clin Radiol. 2011;66:708–14.
17. Nam JE, Ryu YH, Cho SH, et al. Air-trapping zone surrounding sclerosing hemangioma of the lung. J Comput Assist Tomogr. 2002;26:358–61.
18. Shin SY, Kim MY, Oh SY, et al. Pulmonary sclerosing pneumocytoma of the lung: CT characteristics in a large series of a tertiary referral center. Medicine (Baltimore). 2015;94:e498.
19. Xu G, Wang Z, Xiong Z, et al. Correlation between pulmonary sclerosing pneumocytoma features and MSCT imaging manifestations in 34 patients: implications for precision medicine. Front Med (Lausanne). 2021;8:650996.
20. Kocaman G, Yenigün MB, Ersöz CC, et al. Pulmonary sclerosing pneumocytoma with mediastinal lymph node metastasis: a case report. Gen Thorac Cardiovasc Surg. 2021;69:142–6.
21. Yang CH, Lee LY. Pulmonary sclerosing pneumocytoma remains a diagnostic challenge using frozen sections: a clinicopathological analysis of 59 cases. Histopathology. 2018;72:500–8.
22. Maleki Z, Muller S, Layfeld L, et al. Pulmonary sclerosing pneumocytoma: Cytomorphology and immunoprofile. Cancer Cytopathol. 2020;128:414–23.
23. Zhou J, Covinsky MH. Sclerosing Pneumocytoma: a carcinoma mimicker. A case report and literature review. Ann Clin Lab Sci. 2017;47:103–5.
24. Tanaka I, Inoue M, Matsui Y, et al. A case of pneumocytoma (so-called sclerosing hemangioma) with lymph node metastasis. Jpn J Clin Oncol. 1986;16:77–86.
25. Wang X, Zhang L, Wang Y, et al. Sclerosing pneumocytoma with metastasis to the mediastinal and regional lymph nodes. Indian J Pathol Microbiol. 2018;61:407–9.
26. Teng X, Teng X. First report of pulmonary sclerosing pneomucytoma with malignant transformation in both cuboidal surface cells and stromal round cells: a case report. BMC Cancer. 2019;19:1154.
27. Jiang G, Zhang M, Tan Q, et al. Identification of the BRAF V600E mutation in a patient with sclerosing pneumocytoma: a case report. Lung Cancer. 2019;137:52–5.
28. Wang Q, Lu C, Jiang M, et al. Case report and literature review: pulmonary sclerosing pneumocytoma with multiple metastases harboring AKT1 E17K somatic mutation and TP53 C176Y germline mutation. Front Med (Lausanne). 2021;8:655574.
29. Dantis K, Gupta AK, Kashyap NK, et al. Pulmonary sclerosing pneumocytoma masquerading adenocarcinoma with co-existing BRAF V600E and PTEN mutation. Cancer Treat Res Commun. 2021;28:100429.

Part II

Mesenchymal Tumors

Pulmonary Hamartoma

Xue-Peng Huang and Song Zhang

Hamartoma is the most common benign pulmonary neoplasm among adults, accounting for 77% of all benign lung tumors.

1 Classification

The term hamartoma derives from "hamartia" (a Greek word for "erroneous" or "faulty") and "oma" (tumor). It was originally introduced by German pathologist Eugen Albrecht [1] in 1904 that described certain tumor-like malformations resulting from an error in development of tissues normally present in the involved organ. Goldsworthy [2] defined hamartoma as a benign cartilage and adipose tissue tumors that originated in the lung in 1934.

Several synonyms have been used for pulmonary hamartoma, including hamartochondroma, chondromatous hamartoma, and mesenchymoma.

Although hamartoma in other parts of the body is generally not considered to be neoplasms, investigators have confirmed that pulmonary hamartoma represents true neoplasm rather than developmental anomaly. In the 2015 WHO classification, pulmonary hamartoma was adopted as a diagnostic term, rather than just hamartoma.

2 Pathology

Histologically, pulmonary hamartoma consists mostly of varying amounts of at least two mesenchymal elements (such as cartilage, fat, connective tissue, and smooth muscle), combined with entrapped respiratory epithelium (Figs. 1a, b and 2a, b). Hamartoma is distinguished from other benign tumors such as chondroma or lipoma by the presence of at least two mesenchymal elements, chondroma or lipoma has only one mesenchymal element, i.e., either cartilage or fat, respectively. Hamartoma can be divided into subgroups such as chondromatosis, leiomyomatous, lymphangiomyomatous, adenofibromatous, and fibroleiomyomatous based on the dominant component.

Immunohistochemically, mesenchymal markers and sex steroid receptors are positive, but immunohistochemistry is not usually necessary for diagnosis.

X.-P. Huang
Department of Respiratory and Critical Care Medicine, People's Hospital of Rizhao Lanshan, Rizhao, Shandong, China

S. Zhang (✉)
Department of Respiratory and Critical Care Medicine, Shandong Provincial Hospital Affiliated to Shandong First Medical University, Jinan, Shandong, China

S. Zhang (ed.), *Diagnostic Imaging of Lung Cancers*, https://doi.org/10.1007/978-981-99-6815-2_14

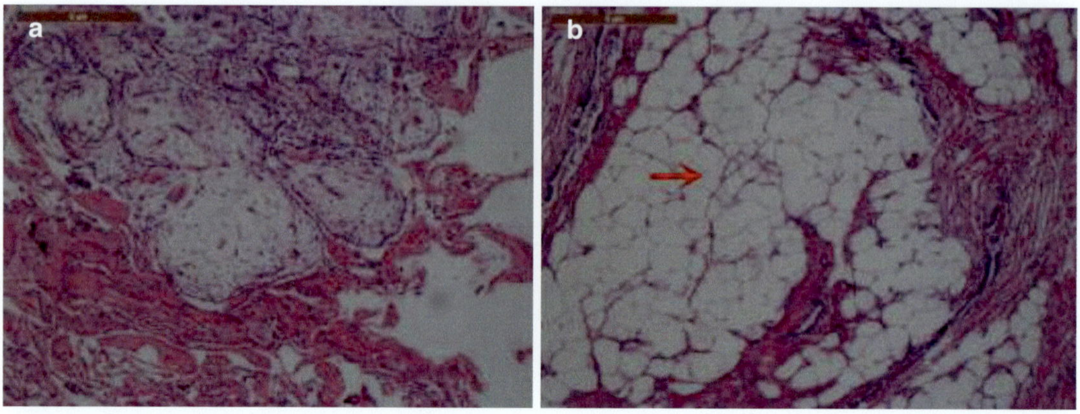

Fig. 1 (**a**) HE staining shows a clear boundary between hamartoma and lung tissue. (**b**) HE staining shows fatty components in hamartoma (red arrow)

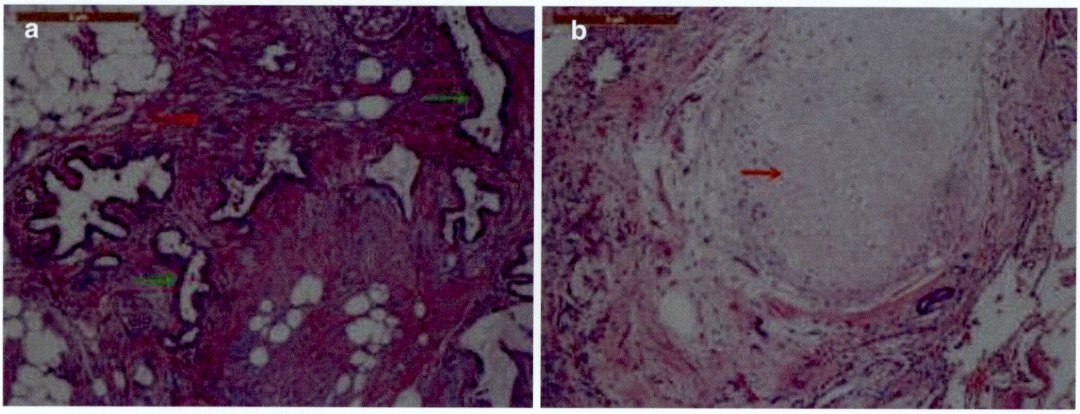

Fig. 2 (**a**) HE staining shows smooth muscle (red arrow) and bronchial mucosa (green arrow) in hamartoma. (**b**) HE staining shows cartilage in hamartoma

3 Molecular Features

The precise etiology of pulmonary hamartoma is unknown. Chromosomal aberrations involving the breakpoint region 12q14-q15 seem to be one of the most frequent chromosomal abnormalities associated with the initiation of human mesenchymal neoplasms. Some studies have identified at least two subgroups characterized by either 6p21 or 12q14-q15 abnormalities in pulmonary chondroid hamartomas (PCHs) by cytogenetic analyses. Dal Clin et al. [3] found that an inv(12)(p13q14-15) was the sole abnormality in PCH. The 12q14-15 region may be nonrandomly involved in the pathogenesis of PCH. Fletcher et al. [4] found that rearrangement of chromosome band 12q15 was most frequently, and one case was characterized by a t(12;14)(q15;q24) that was identical cytogenetically to the characteristic translocation in uterine leiomyomas. Xiao et al. [5] reported that PCHs had chromosome rearrangements located within 100 kb of HMGI(Y). HMGI(Y), a member of the high-mobility group (HMG) family of proteins which has been mapped to the short arm of chromosome 6 at 6p21. HMGI(Y) encodes DNA-binding proteins with both chromatin structural and gene regulatory roles. HMGI(Y) expression is associated with neoplastic transformation. Kazmierczak et al. [6] reported their cytogenetic and molecular cytogenetic (FISH) studies on 191 PCH cases. 70.2% of PCHs (134/191) showed abnormalities of chromosomal bands, including 6p21 (21 tumors), 12q14-15 (95 tumors), and other abnormalities (18 tumors). The most frequent translocations were t(12;14)(q15;q24) (19 cases) and t(6;14)(p21.3;q24) (18 cases). HMGI-C and HMGI(Y) protein expression as a consequence of rearrangements involving 6p21 and 12q15, respectively. High frequency of rearrangements of HMGI(Y) genes was identified in PCHs, suggesting the neoplastic nature of PCHs. Gregori-Romero et al. [7] further revealed two different 12q14-q15 rearrangements. One of them had a unique translocation t(12;14)(q14-15;q24) with presence of two normal chromosomes 12 and a der(14), but missing the der(12). Another showed a complex rearrangement between chromosomes 10 and 12 with two different derivatives.

Rearrangements of the HMGA2 gene have been found in a variety of benign tumors. Pulmonary hamartoma has a high frequency of the translocation t(3;12)(q27-28;q14-15), leading to gene fusion of the high mobility group protein gene HMGA2 and the LPP gene. The HMGA2-LPP fusion gene is typically composed of exons 1-3 of HMGA2 and exons 9-11 of LPP and seems to be expressed in all tumors with this translocation.

4 Epidemiology

In 1945, McDonald et al. [8] reported that the incidence of pulmonary hamartomas was 0.025% (2/7972) in a large autopsy series at the Mayo Clinic. In 1991, Murray et al. [9] reported that the incidence of peripheral pulmonary hamartomas was 0.32% (152/47635) in autopsy-based study from southern African miners examined between 1975 and 1988. The prevalence increased with age, from 0.8/1,000 in the third decade to 12.0/1,000 in the eighth decade. The prevalence and age distribution between white and black miners had no significant difference.

The incidence of pulmonary hamartoma is highest between the fourth and seventh decades of life, with male predilection (2-4:1).

5 Radiographic Features

The typical imaging features of pulmonary hamartoma are solitary, smooth, well-defined, round or lobulated nodule or mass with fat or calcifications (Fig. 3), and rarely near the hilar parts (Fig. 4). Tumor size is mostly 2–3 cm, rarely more than 10 cm (Fig. 5). It may increase in size,

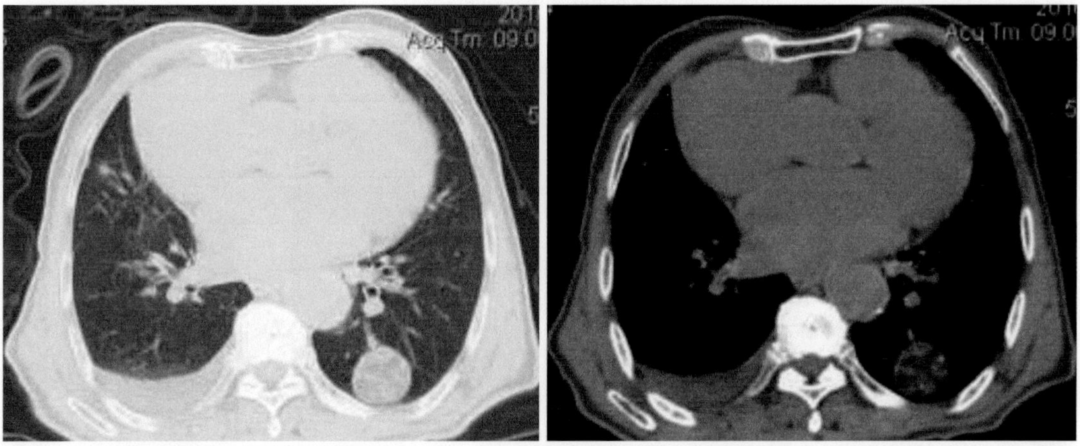

Fig. 3 A 86-year-old man with a well-circumscribed, round lesion in the left lower lobe with fat and calcifications

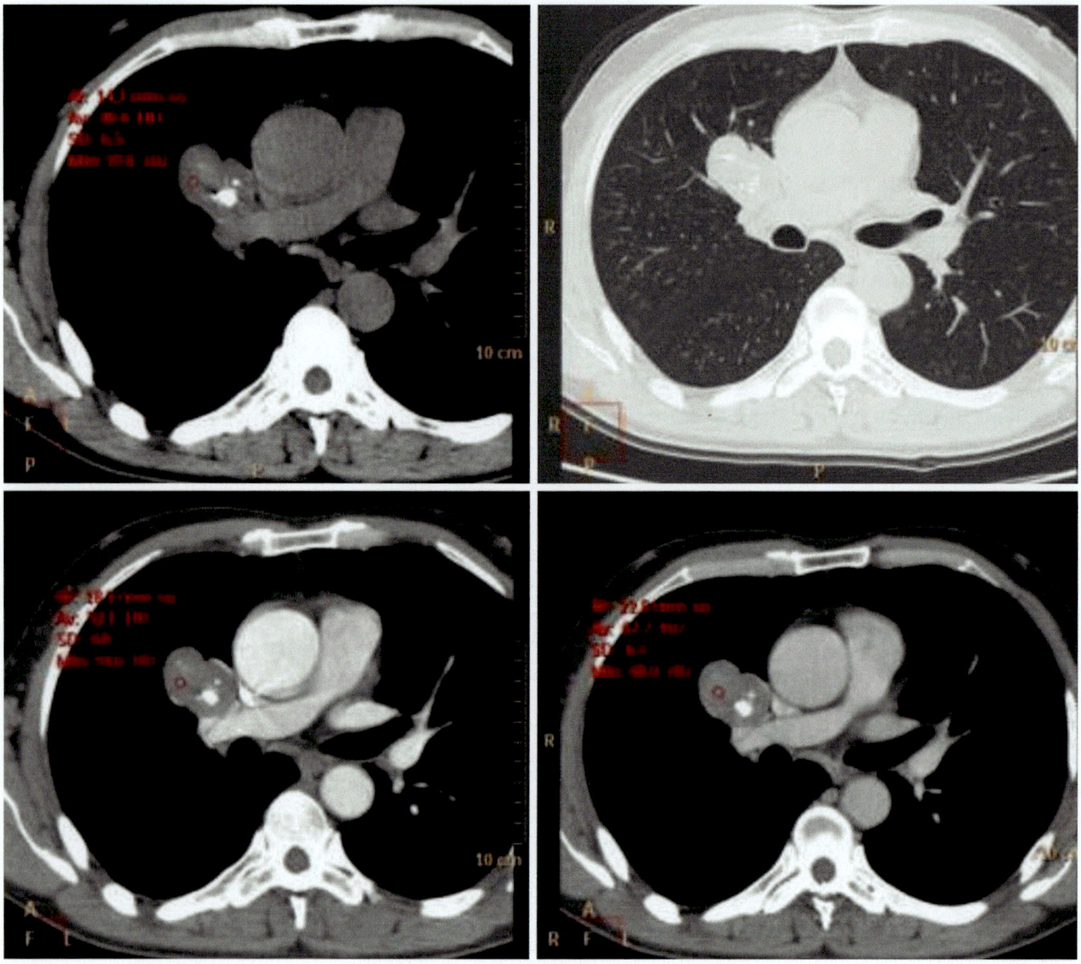

Fig. 4 A 58-year-old man with a mass near right hilum with fat and calcifications

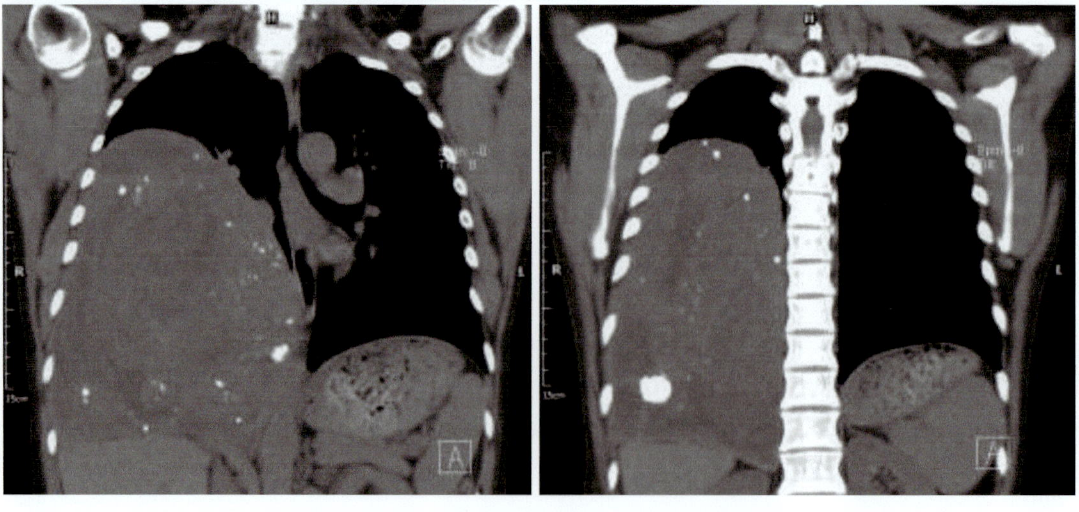

Fig. 5 A 39-year-old woman with giant hamartoma of right thoracic cavity

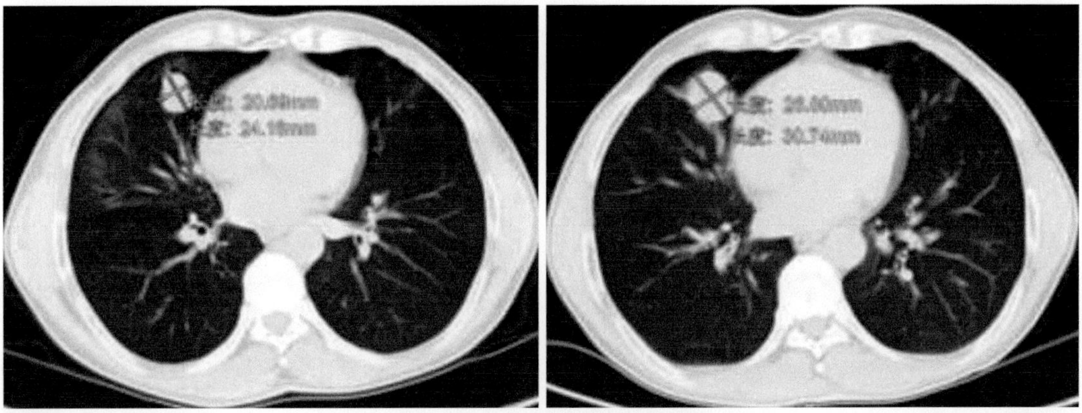

Fig. 6 A 48-year-old man with a nodule in the right middle lobe. Tumor diameter increased by 6 mm within 26 months

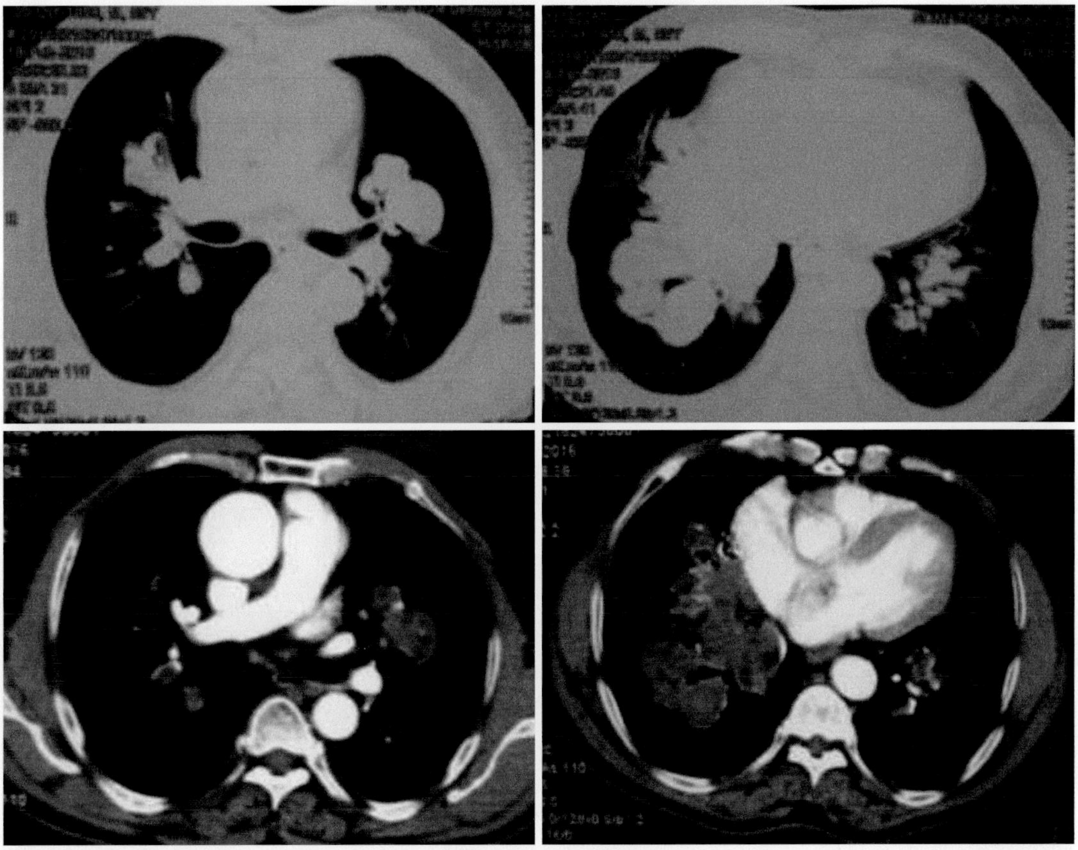

Fig. 7 A 59-year-old man with multiple hamartomas of bilateral lungs

but growth is usually slow (Fig. 6). Multiple (Fig. 7) or cystic pulmonary hamartomas (Fig. 8) have occasionally been reported. Popcorn-like or central calcifications account for 5%–50% of cases (Fig. 9). Calcification is mainly formed by the deposition of calcium salts in the cartilage. Intralesional fat was observed in approximately 60% of pulmonary hamartomas (Fig. 10). The presence of fatty components in solitary pulmonary nodules is generally only seen in hamarto-

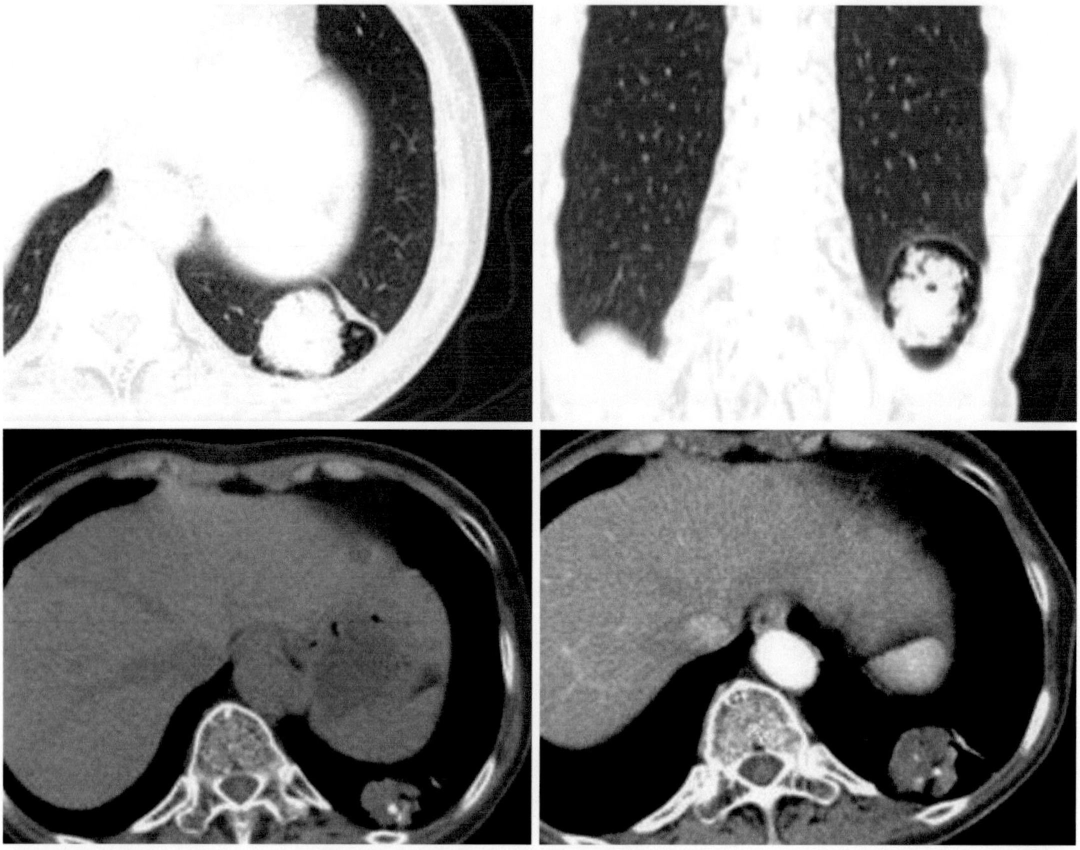

Fig. 8 A 64-year-old woman with cystic hamartoma of left lower lobe

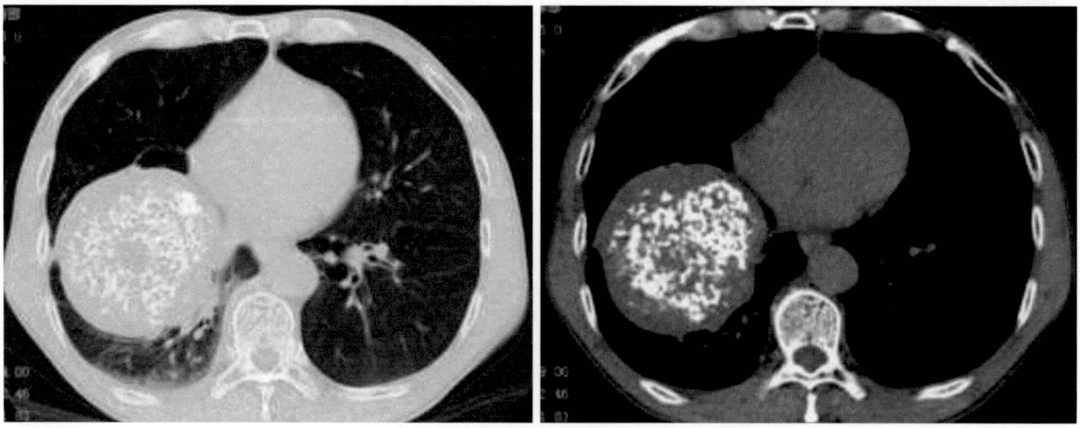

Fig. 9 A 57-year-old man with a large pulmonary hamartoma with popcorn-like calcification

mas, lipid pneumonitis, and lipomas, the latter two generally without calcification. The absence of cartilage or adipose tissue density on CT does not readily rule out the diagnosis of pulmonary hamartoma. Central or endobronchial hamartomas are less than 10% (Fig. 11).

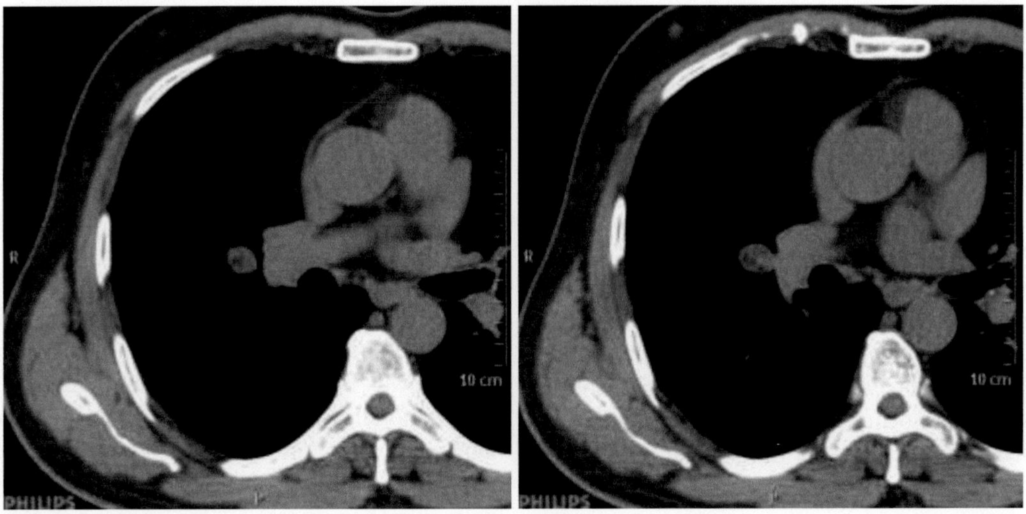

Fig. 10 A 68-year-old man with a pulmonary hamartoma with visible fat

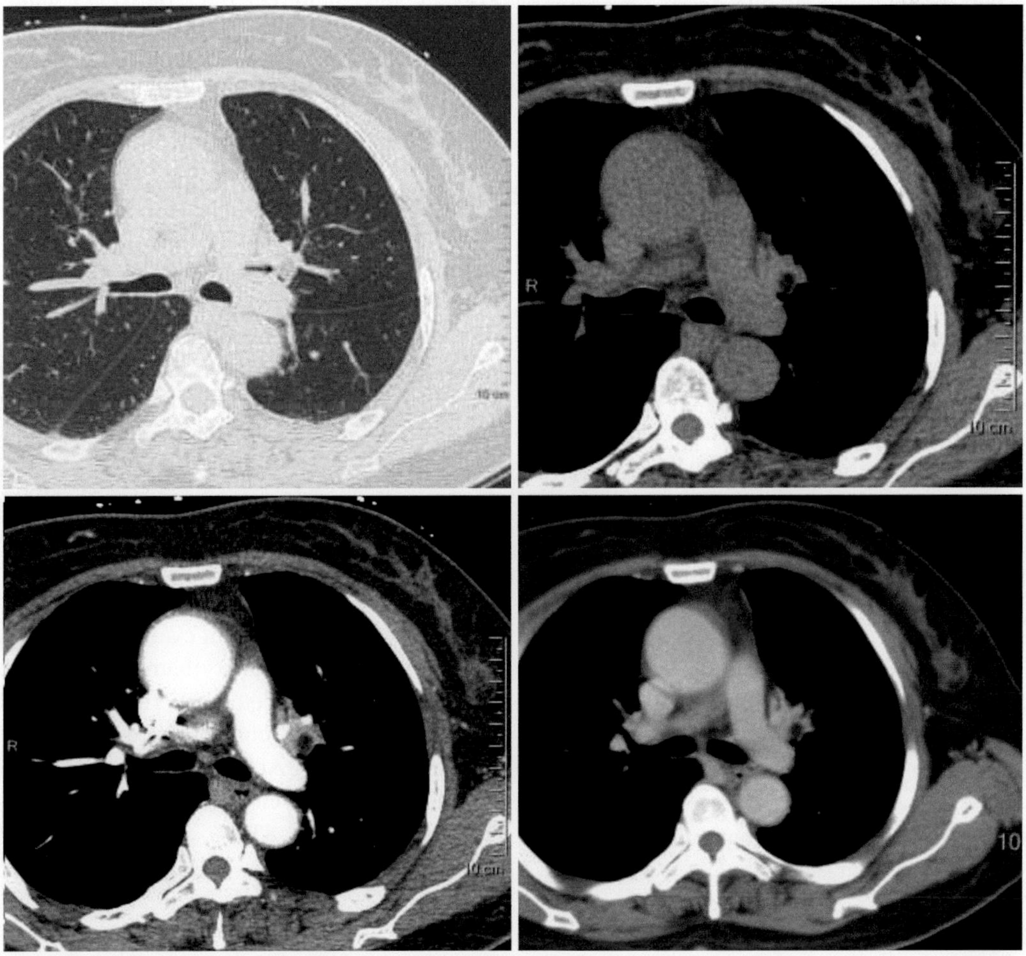

Fig. 11 A 54-year-old woman with left upper lobe endobronchial hamartoma (red arrow)

6 Treatment

Pulmonary hamartomas are benign tumor and have growth potential. The need for surgery or follow-up may be determined based on the size and location of the tumor. Guo et al. [10] reviewed a 20-year clinical history of surgical treatment for 39 patients with pulmonary hamartoma. Thirty-nine patients underwent 40 operations as follows: wedge resection (23), enucleation (10), segmentectomy (3), lobectomy (3), and pneumonectomy (1). No postoperative death was encountered. A patient was operated thrice for regional recurrence. Wang et al. [11] retrospectively enrolled 226 patients with pulmonary hamartoma who underwent surgical resection. The postoperative follow-up time was 5–22 years. They recommended tumor enucleation or wedge resection for the patients whose pulmonary hamartoma could not be confirmed preoperatively. A 10-year retrospective study by Esme et al. [12] concluded that no malignant transformation and recurrence were found during long-term follow-up. Therefore, the enucleation for pulmonary hamartoma was safe enough.

The indications of surgical removal include symptomatic rapid tumor growth, suspected primary or secondary malignant tumor, or endobronchial location of lesion with postobstructive complications. Patients with large tumors who do not choose to undergo resection may be advisable for a long-term follow-up.

7 Case Analysis

7.1 Case 1

A 66-year-old man found a lung lesion on physical examination.

Chest CT: A lesion in the left lower lobe (Fig. 12).

[Diagnosis] Pulmonary hamartoma.

[Diagnosis Basis] Chest CT shows a well-defined, lobulated mass in the left lower lobe, with calcification and fat, consistent with the diagnosis of hamartoma. The patient underwent surgical resection. The cut surface was gray-white and gray-yellow. Pathological examination revealed pulmonary hamartoma with fatty component.

[Analysis] Pulmonary hamartoma is the third most common cause of a solitary pulmonary nodule followed by granuloma and carcinoma.

Intranodular fat and calcifications are common imaging features of pulmonary hamartomas. Siegelman et al. [13] analyzed 47 patients with pulmonary hamartoma by thin-section CT. Based on the presence of fat or calcium, nodules were classified into four categories: no fat or calcium (17), fat and calcium (10), fat only (18), and calcium only (2). They identified classic CT features of pulmonary hamartomas, including size less than 2.5 cm, smooth nodule edge, at least 8 voxels reporting either fat (−40 to −120 HU) or dense calcification (>175 HU) in focal areas. They concluded that immediate surgical excision was not required in the presence of all of these findings. Gleeson et al. [14] assessed the accuracy of CT pixel analysis for fat attenuation in pulmonary hamartomas. They found that visual assessment for macroscopic fat was the most reliable method for diagnosing pulmonary hamartoma. Combining percentage of fat-attenuation pixels in the inner 2/3rds of the lesion, the specificity was increased to 100%. Mean attenuation or pixel analysis in isolation was not helpful in lesional characterization.

Hochhegger et al. [15] determined the accuracy of multidetector CT in evaluating histologically confirmed pulmonary hamartomas, with a special focus on fat detection. Histologic analyses determined fat content in 43/55 (78.2%) surgical specimens. At a density threshold of −40 HU, the accuracy, sensitivity, and specificity of fat detection were 83.7%, 100%, and 87.2%,

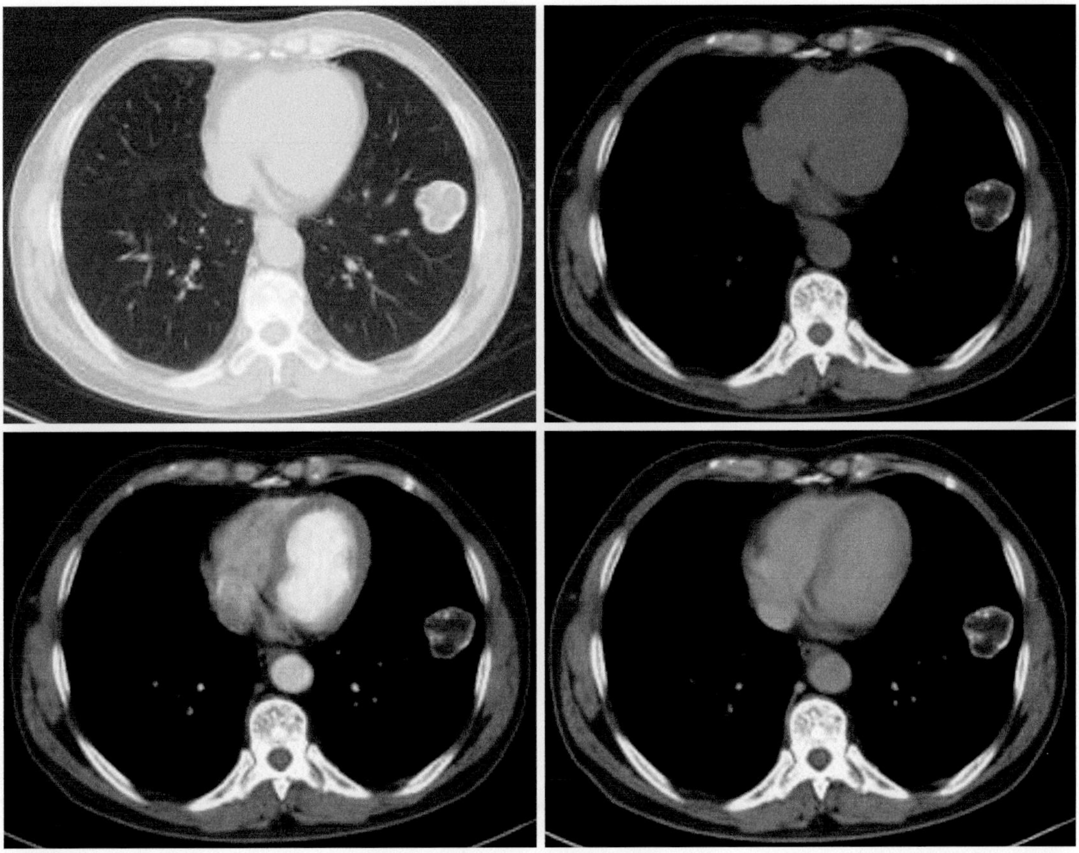

Fig. 12 Chest CT

respectively. A threshold of −33 HU resulted in better results (95.3%, 100%, and 96.3%, respectively). Popcorn-like calcifications were found in only 12/55 (21.8%) pulmonary hamartomas and were the only imaging feature suggestive of pulmonary hamartoma in 7.2% of cases. Most (66%) lesions with popcorn-like calcifications also contained fat. They concluded that the adoption of a new threshold for fat content (<−33 HU) can further improve the overall ability to detect pulmonary hamartomas by CT.

Takumi et al. [16] suggested that dual-energy CT analysis can help diagnose pulmonary hamartoma with detection of intralesional fatty tissue.

7.2 Case 2

A 54-year-old man complained of right chest pain for 2 months.

Chest CT: A lesion in the right lower lobe (Fig. 13).

[Diagnosis] Pulmonary hamartoma.

[Diagnosis Basis] Chest CT shows a well-defined, lobulated lesion in the right lower lobe, and the CT attenuations of the three-phase dynamic scan were 33.5, 39.3, and 55.0 HU, respectively. Postoperative pathology showed pulmonary hamartoma.

[Analysis] Pulmonary hamartoma results from neoplastic transformation of a primitive mesenchymal cell that differentiates along chondroid, adipose, and smooth muscle pathways.

When pulmonary hamartoma contains neither fat nor calcification, CT imaging cannot reliably diagnose pulmonary hamartoma, and also is difficult to differentiate it from primary or secondary lung cancer or tuberculoma, and excision or

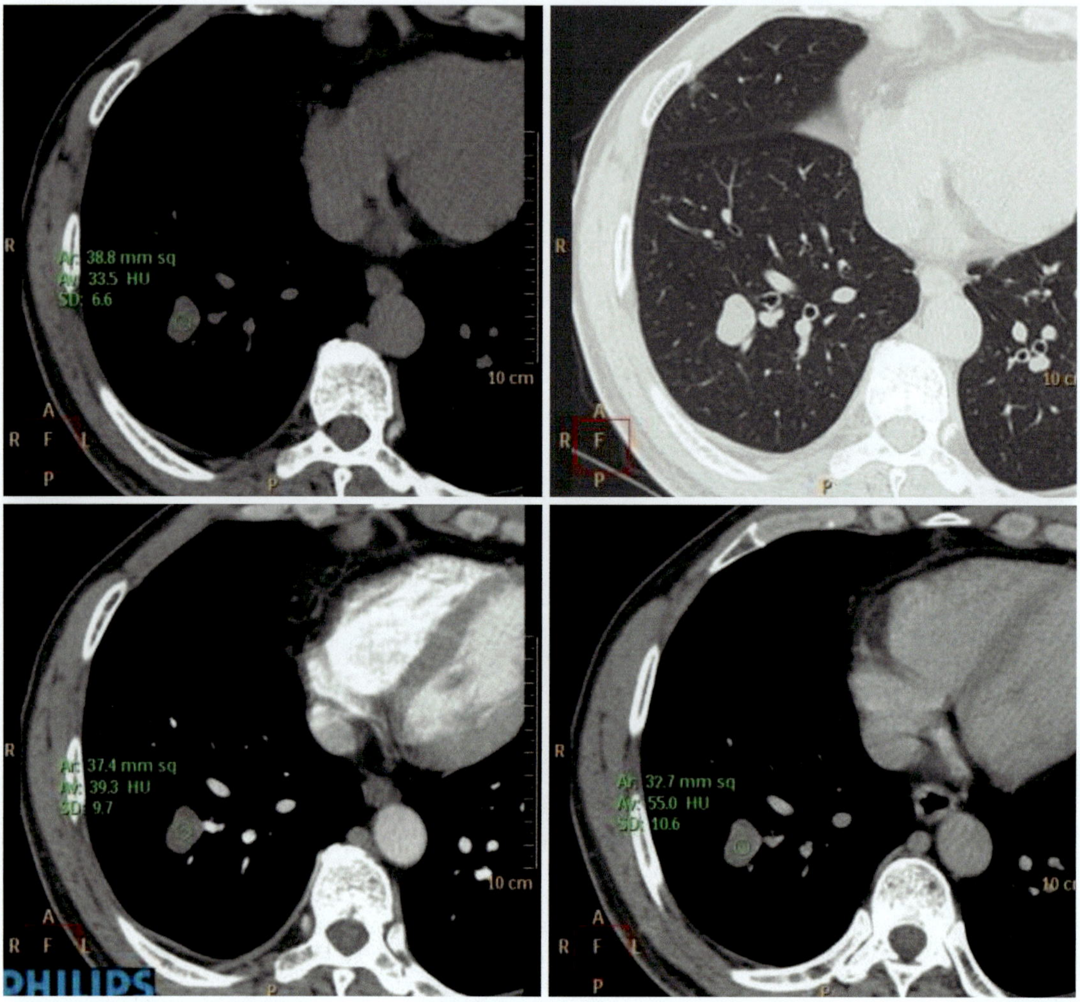

Fig. 13 Chest CT

biopsy is usually recommended. Park et al. [17] found that when a discrete pulmonary nodule shows neither fat nor calcification on CT, conventional MRI was effective in the detection of the quite typical cleft-like structure in a pulmonary hamartoma, well evident on T2WI with variable but more commonly intense T2 high signal intensity than that of main portion and variable shapes, not only peripheral linear inclusions but also curvilinear, punctate, or circular shape or intratumoral cleft-like space, which correlated with the variable mesenchymal tissue components and amount arrayed along respiratory epithelial cell-lining clefts. Furthermore, cleft-like structure enhancement with or without marginal rim enhancement proves diagnostic confidence of the pulmonary hamartoma.

Most pulmonary hamartomas are nonexpanding or slowly growing tumors. Hansen et al. [18] studied 89 cases of pulmonary hamartoma. The mean transverse diameter at diagnosis was 21.7 ± 16.2 mm. Tumor size was not related to the anatomic localization but was correlated with the age of the patients. Tumor growth was recorded in 45% (15/31) patients who had follow-up. During an average observation time of 4.1 years (1–20 years), the average expansion of transverse diameter was 3.2 ± 2.6 mm per year.

In some cases, pulmonary hamartoma may show rapid enlargement. Itoga et al. [19] reported a 65-year-old man with a lesion in the S9 area of the left lung. The nodule increased in size from 1.2 × 1.5 cm to 1.5 × 2.0 cm within 5 months. The calculated tumor doubling time (TDT) was approximately 132.2 days. A malignant tumor was strongly suspected based on the rapid growth, but postoperative pathology showed pulmonary hamartoma.

Surgical resection is an option for pulmonary nodules of unknown nature.

7.3 Case 3

A 70-year-old man found a lung mass on physical examination.

Chest CT: A mass in the left lower lung lobe (Fig. 14).

[Diagnosis] Pulmonary hamartoma.

[Diagnosis Basis] Chest CT shows a giant mass in the left lower lobe, with popcorn calcification and fat (−74.78 HU), consistent with the diagnosis of hamartoma. The patient underwent surgical resection. The tumor diameter was 10 cm, and the cut surface was gray-white and hard (Fig. 15a). Pathological examination revealed pulmonary hamartoma (Fig. 15b).

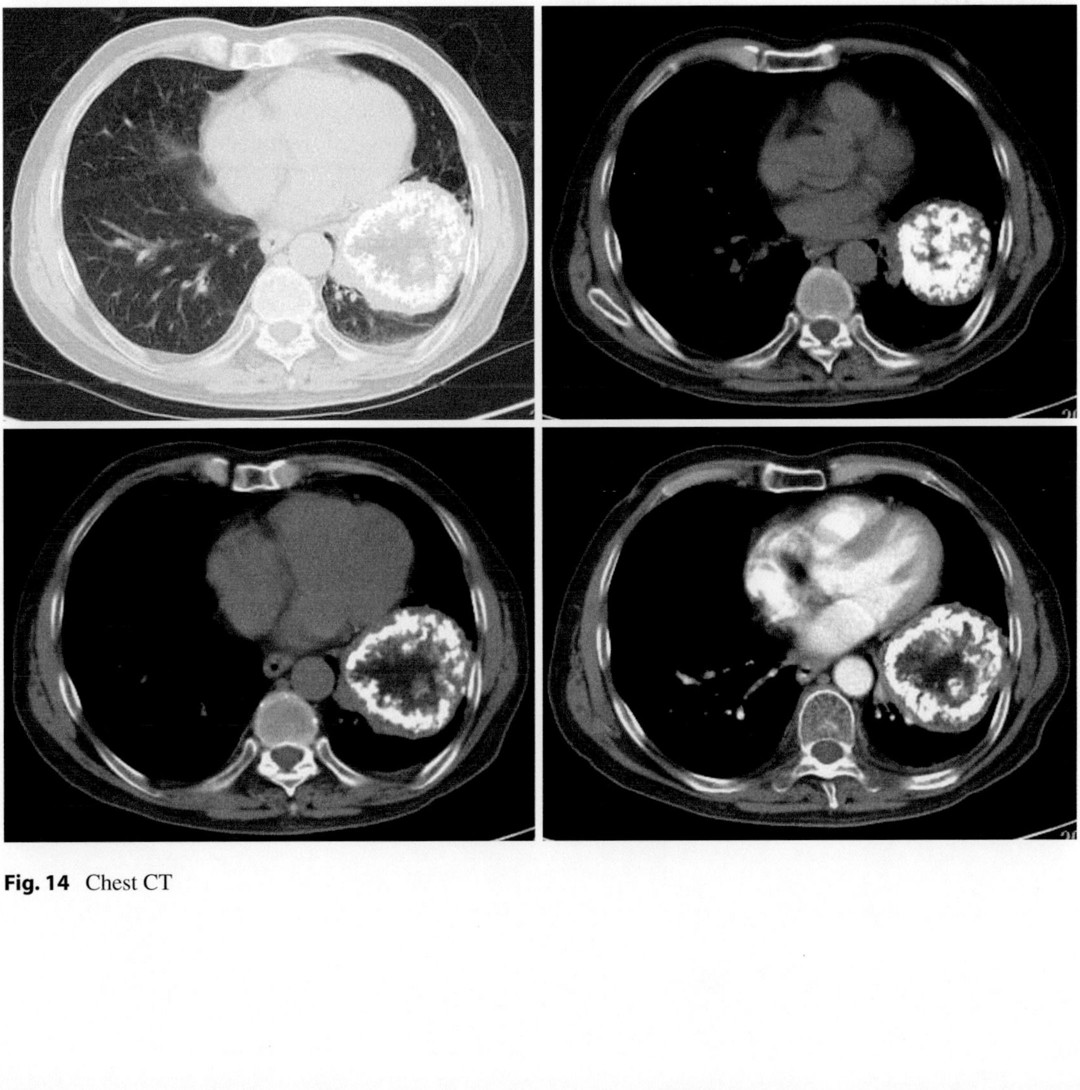

Fig. 14 Chest CT

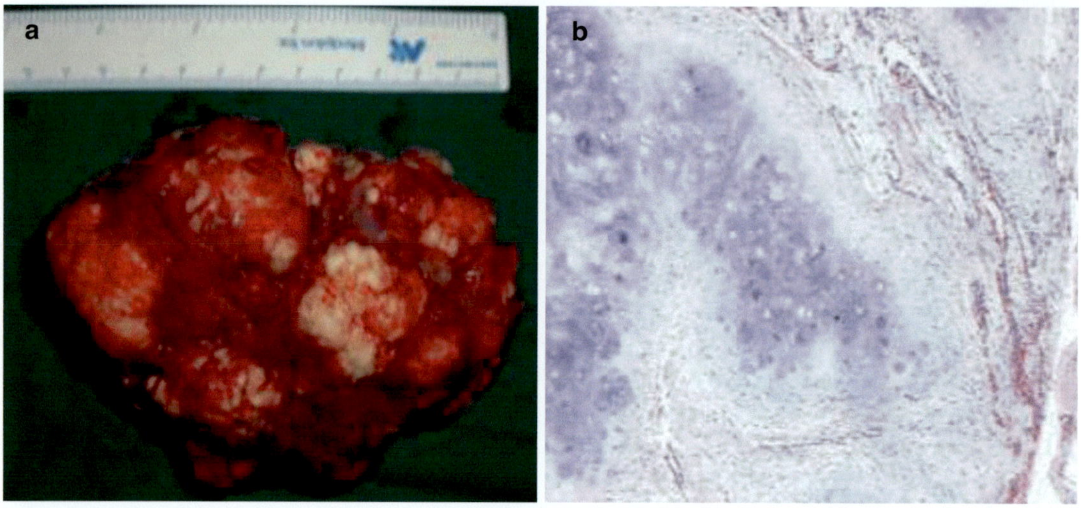

Fig. 15 (**a**) Gross specimen of hamartoma. (**b**) HE staining shows cartilage in hamartoma (400×)

[Analysis] Pulmonary hamartomas constitute 6%–8% of solitary pulmonary nodules, and 90% are located peripherally. They are mostly small with an average diameter of 2 cm and most commonly asymptomatic, incidentally discovered tumor.

Pulmonary hamartomas measuring over 8 cm are extremely rare, and sometimes symptomatic. Hutter et al. [20] reported a case of a 63-year-old woman with a giant pulmonary hamartoma, measured 26 × 25 cm and weighed 3.2 kg. Joshi et al. [21] described a case of a 59-year-old female patient with a giant chondroid hamartoma presenting with acute right heart failure. Miyaoka et al. [22] reported a unique case of giant pulmonary hamartoma with a dominant CD34 (+) smooth muscle cell component. Resected tissue contained a solid mass of 13 × 10 × 8 cm in size with a prominent unilocular cyst (8 × 6.5 × 5 cm). The tumor was composed of a dominant smooth muscle cell component with entrapped glandular respiratory epithelium. Hindaria et al. [23] reported a 33-year-old lady with a huge pulmonary hamartoma measuring 25.5 × 17.5 × 15.5 cm and weighing about 2200 g.

Surgical resection is preferred for symptomatic large pulmonary hamartomas.

7.4 Case 4

A 52-year-old man found a lung lesion on physical examination.

Chest CT: A mass in the right lung lobe, the CT attenuations of the three-phase dynamic scan were −12.2, 4.3, and −0.4 HU, respectively (Fig. 16).

[Diagnosis] Fibroleiomyomatous hamartoma.

[Diagnosis Basis] The patient underwent a wedge resection of the right upper lobe. The mass involved the posterior segment of the right upper lobe and the dorsal segment of the right lower lobe, and was firm, gray-white in color on sectioning. Histologic section revealed focal fibrous tissue, smooth muscle, and bronchiolar hyperplasia, without cellular atypia and mitotic figs. A few inflammatory cells were detected in the mesenchymal component (Fig. 17). Immunohistochemically, smooth muscle actin (SMA), HHF-35, and desmin were positive, and estrogen receptor, progesterone receptor, Melan A, and HMB-45 were negative. The final diagnosis was fibroleiomyomatous hamartoma.

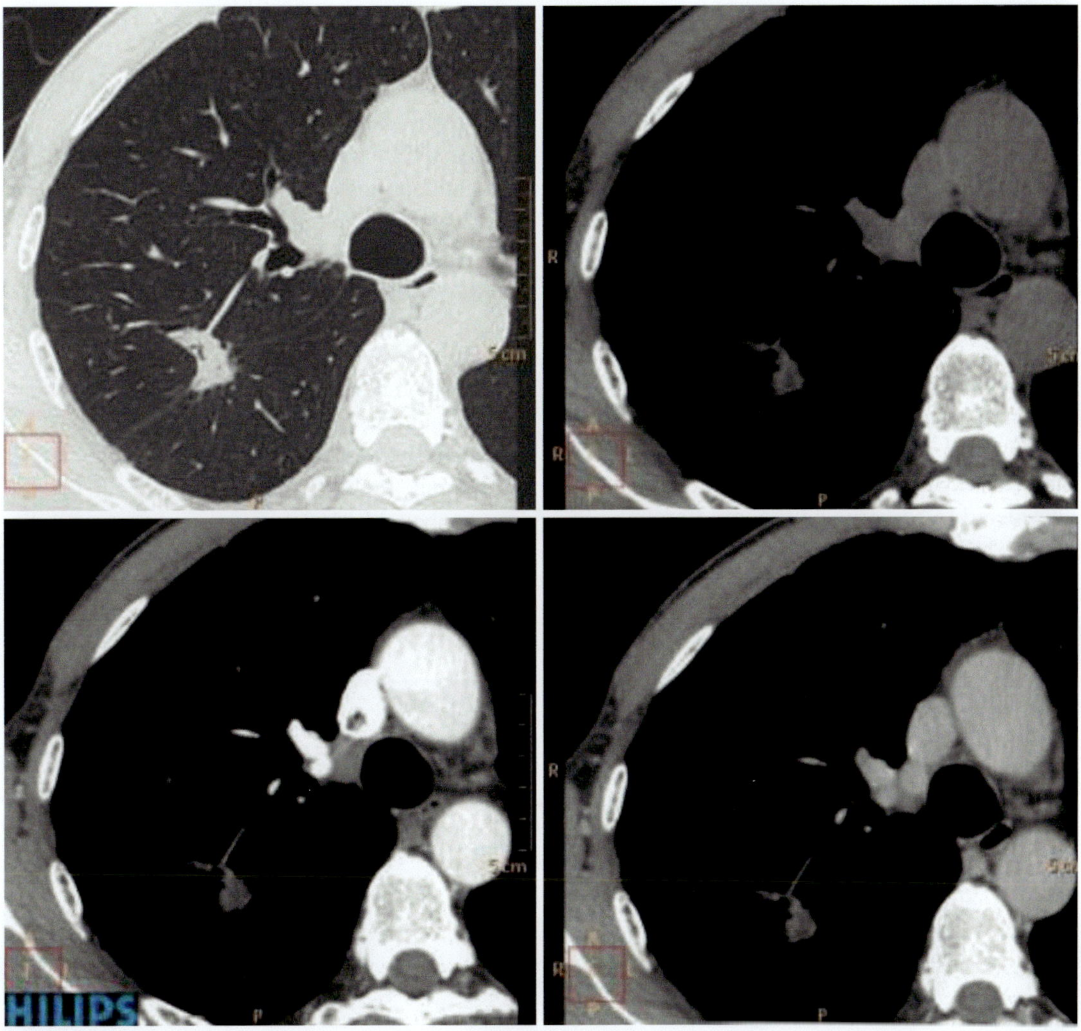

Fig. 16 Chest CT

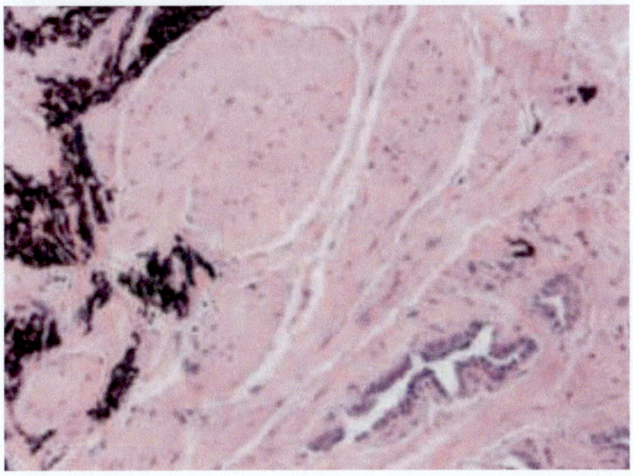

Fig. 17 Microphotograph shows the proliferation of spindle cells and tubular or cleft-like entrapped epithelial components

[Analysis] Pulmonary hamartoma has been defined as a tumor consisting of varying combinations of cartilage, fat, fibrous tissue, smooth muscle, and respiratory epithelium derived from entrapped alveoli. Pulmonary fibroleiomyomatous hamartoma was first described by Cruickshank and Harrison in 1953 [24]. It is an extremely rare tumor and may demonstrate the multinodular form, solitary coin lesion, or diffuse interstitial pattern on CT.

The pathogenesis of this tumor is controversial. Some scholars believe that it represents the metastasis from benign leiomyoma or low-grade leiomyosarcoma, most commonly from the uterus; some scholars consider that it occurs due to the implantation and proliferation of benign smooth muscle tissue, which is embolized by intravenous leiomyomatosis or by mechanical means; other scholars consider it a primary intrapulmonary smooth muscle hyperplasia, tumor, or hamartoma.

The histological characteristic of fibroleiomyomatous hamartoma is a well-circumscribed nodule composed of smooth muscle cells with numerous epithelial inclusions, and no cellular atypia or mitotic figures. Histologically, fibromyomatous hamartoma is indistinguishable from benign metastatic leiomyomas.

This case is a 52-year-old male patient without a pre-existing smooth muscle tumor, which is considered to be a true pulmonary fibroleiomyomatous hamartoma.

7.5 Case 5

A 67-year-old woman found a lung lesion for one day on physical examination.

Chest CT: A mass in the left upper lobe, the CT attenuations were 20 and 66 HU, respectively; a nodule in the left upper lobe (Fig. 18).

[Diagnosis] Adenocarcinoma; hamartoma.

[Diagnosis Basis] Chest CT shows an irregular soft tissue mass in the left upper lobe, with shallow lobulation, burrs and pleural traction, which is consistent with the CT findings of lung adenocarcinoma. Punctate nodule is seen in the left lower lobe with clear borders, and the possibility of metastasis was not excluded. The patient's

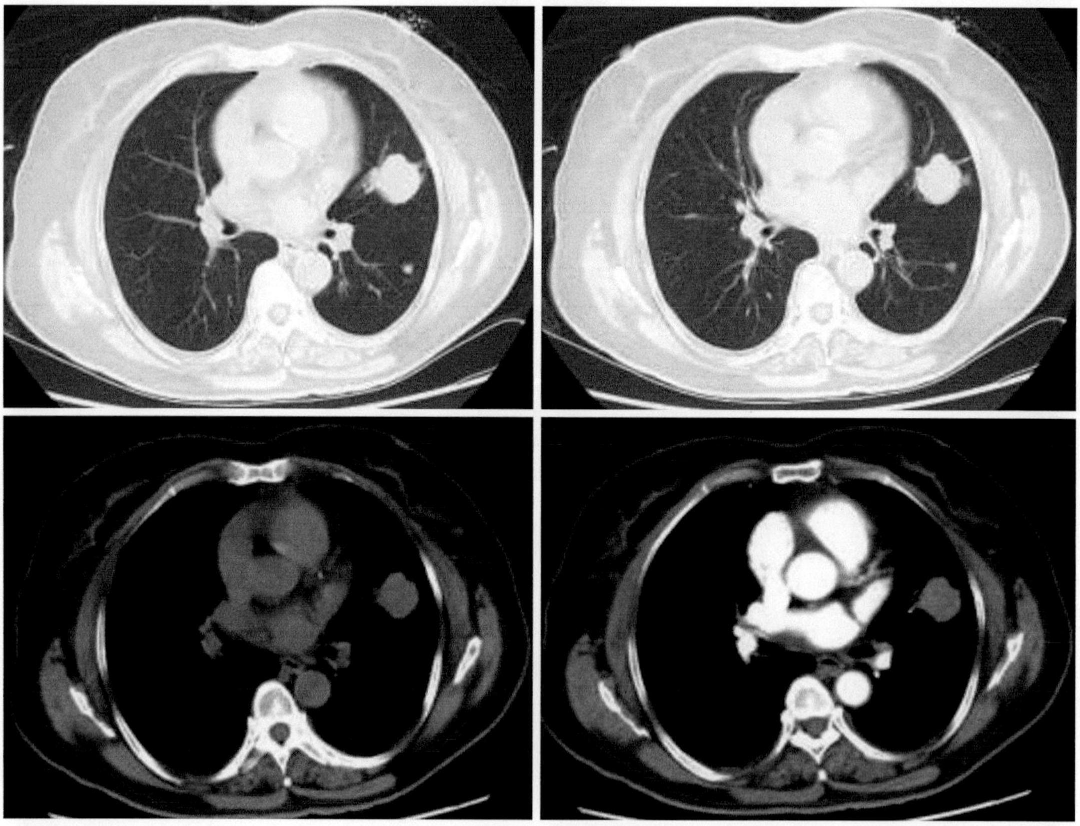

Fig. 18 Chest CT

operation revealed hypoplasia of the oblique fissure, and a nodule of about 3 cm in diameter was seen in the lingual segment of the left upper lobe. A small nodule of about 0.6 cm in diameter located in the left lower lobe. Pathology showed invasive adenocarcinoma in the left upper lobe with predominantly acinar pattern involving the visceral pleura; nodules in the left lower lobe were consistent with pulmonary hamartoma.

[Analysis] Karasik et al. [25] first studied the association of pulmonary hamartoma and bronchial carcinoma. Fifty-two patients with chondromatous hamartoma of the lung (CHL) operated on between 1960 and 1975 were followed through the end of 1976 for occurrence of malignancy. Four cases of carcinoma of the lung were observed in this group, and the risk of lung cancer in CHL patients was estimated to be 6.3 times higher than the general Israeli population. Ribet et al. [26] analyzed 65 patients operated on for pulmonary (60) or endobronchial (5) hamartoma. Eight were associated with carcinomas, and three of these were bronchial carcinomas. The risk of bronchial cancer developing in patients with hamartoma was 6.66 times higher than the general northern France population.

The higher incidence of lung cancer in patients with pulmonary hamartoma does not imply that pulmonary hamartoma is a true risk factor for the development of lung cancer. Gjevre et al. [27] retrospectively reviewed 215 patients with histologically confirmed pulmonary hamartoma. The peak incidence of occurrence was in the seventh decade of life. Sixty-three patients (29.3%) had a concurrent neoplasm (most commonly, lung carcinoma). Pulmonary hamartoma and carcinoma may be independent from each other, no evidence of either a malignant transformation or an unexplained association with other lung neoplasms was found. Fiorelli et al. [28] analyzed a 20-year historical series of patients with pulmonary hamartoma undergoing surgical resection, with the aim of evaluating the characteristics, the outcomes, and the association between hamartoma and lung cancer. The multicenter study included 540 patients,76 patients (14%) with associated lung cancer, 9 (12%) with synchronous, and 67 (88%) with metachronous. Only age >70-year-old and smokers >20 cigarettes/day were the significant risk factors for lung cancer. The presence of pulmonary hamartoma did not increase the risk of

lung cancer development, and the coexistence of the two tumors is due to exposure to the same risk factors of smoking and advanced age.

7.6 Case 6

A 60-year-old man complained of cough and hemoptysis for 20 days.

Chest CT: A intratracheal lesion with right upper lobe atelectasis (Fig. 19).

[Diagnosis] Endobronchial hamartoma.

[Diagnosis Basis] Chest CT shows discontinuous calcification in the bronchus, which can exclude a bronchial foreign body. Calcifications are located within hypodense nodule which are consistent with endobronchial pulmonary hamartoma. Fiberoptic bronchoscopy revealed a polypoid lesion in the right upper lobe (Fig. 20a) that completely obstructed the lumen. Bronchoscopy biopsy revealed a hamartoma, and the postoperative histopathology revealed cartilaginous hamartoma (Fig. 20b), with focal mild atypical hyperplasia of the bronchial mucosal epithelium.

[Analysis] Based on the invasive site, pulmonary hamartoma can be classified into the central, peripheral, or mixed types. Endobronchial hamartoma accounts for approximately 10% of all pulmonary hamartomas and often causes atypical symptoms related to endobronchial obstruction, including cough, expectoration, wheezing, dyspnea, hemoptysis, pulmonary infection, and lobar atelectasis. Liu et al. [29] reported a rare case of giant endobronchial hamartoma coexisting with lung atelectasis for more than 3 years. After flexible fiberoptic bronchoscopy examination, the lesion was removed completely using snare electrocautery combined with argon plasma coagulation.

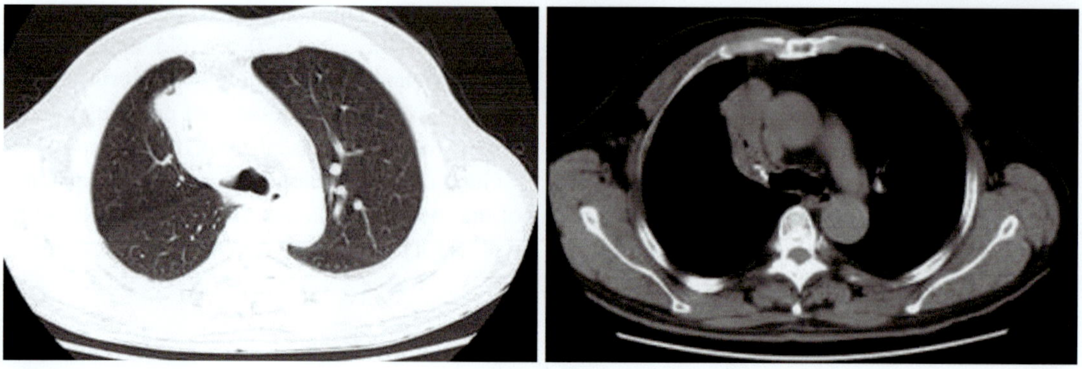

Fig. 19 Chest CT

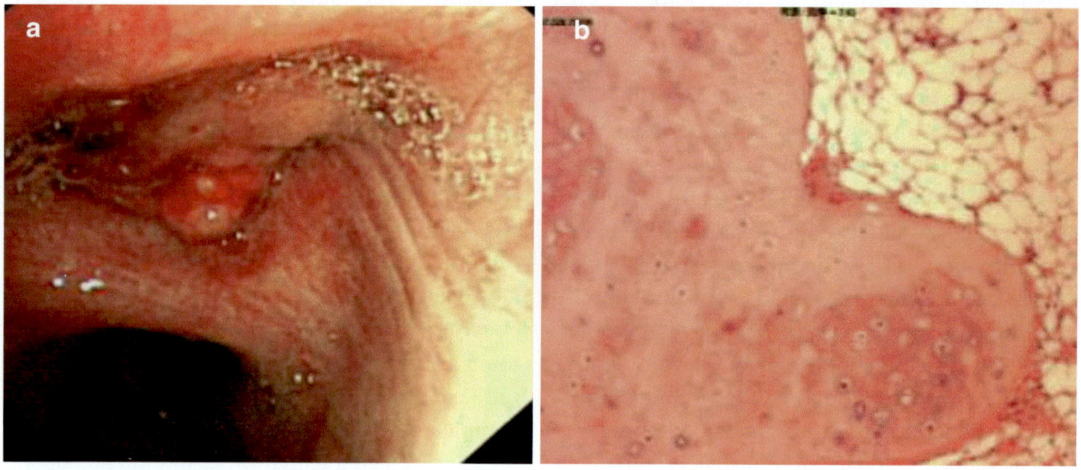

Fig. 20 (**a**) Bronchoscopic view in the right upper lobe bronchus. (**b**) Pathological section shows insular cartilage and adipose tissue

Histologically, pulmonary hamartoma contains a predominance of cartilage (chondromatous hamartoma), as well as variable amounts of fibromyxoid connective tissue, bone, fat, and smooth muscle. Fat may be more abundant in endobronchial hamartoma.

The treatment of endobronchial hamartoma depends on the size, location, and symptoms of the patient and includes endobronchial approach (mechanical resection, laser, cryotherapy and Argon plasma coagulation, etc.) and lung surgery (lobectomy, segmentectomy, bronchotomy, and pneumonectomy). Lobectomy may be necessary in cases with recurrent pneumonia. A meta-analysis by Abdel Hady et al. [30] showed that bronchoscopic treatment should be the first choice except in patients with end stage lung damage requiring surgical resection. Pneumothorax is the most common complication.

Endobronchial hamartoma has a good prognosis and low risk of relapse.

7.7 Case 7

A 56-year-old woman found a lung lesion on physical examination.

PET/CT: A mass in the left upper lobe (Fig. 21).

[Diagnosis] Pulmonary hamartoma.

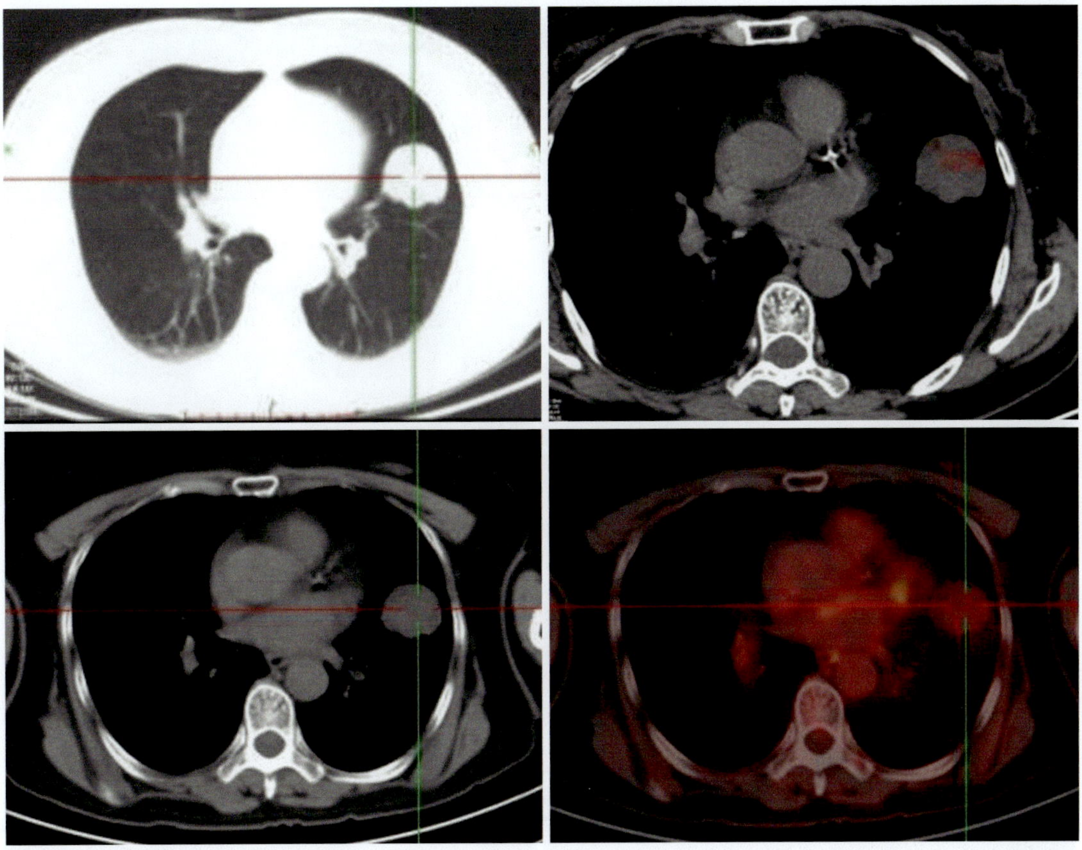

Fig. 21 PET/CT

[Diagnosis Basis] PET/CT reveals a round soft tissue mass in the upper lobe with a size of 3.8 × 3.4 cm. It shows fat density (around −20 HU) and mild radioactive uptake (SUVmax = 2.5). Postoperative pathology showed hamartoma.

[Analysis] Pulmonary hamartoma generally presents as a well-circumscribed, peripheral, solitary lung nodule or mass with calcification and fat components on CT. It needs to be distinguished from other benign or low-grade malignant nodules such as pulmonary sclerosing pneumocytoma (PSP) or carcinoid tumor. The relationship between carcinoids and small airways helps differentiate carcinoids from hamartomas.

^{18}F-FDG PET/CT has high sensitivity (81.9%) but lower specificity (62.4%) in differentiating benign from malign pulmonary nodules. Ergonul et al. [31] evaluated ^{18}F-FDG PET/CT findings of 106 patients with benign lung lesions. This study included 19(17.9%) hamartoma patients. The SUVmax of hamartomas ranged from 0 to 4.5 and was significantly lower than in the other groups.

Jiang et al. [32] retrospectively reviewed ^{18}F-FDG PET/CT characteristic findings of 12 PSP patients and 14 pulmonary hamartoma patients. The mean diameter and SUVmax of pulmonary hamartoma were 1.7 ± 0.8 cm and 1.5 ± 0.6, respectively, and there was a significant correlation between the size and SUVmax. The SUVmax of PSP (2.6 ± 1.0) was significantly higher than that of pulmonary hamartoma. When the SUVmax of 1.95 was applied as a cutoff for the diagnosis of PSP, the sensitivity and specificity for PET/CT to differentiate PSP from pulmonary hamartoma were 83.3% and 78.6%, respectively. When the SUVmax of a pulmonary nodule or

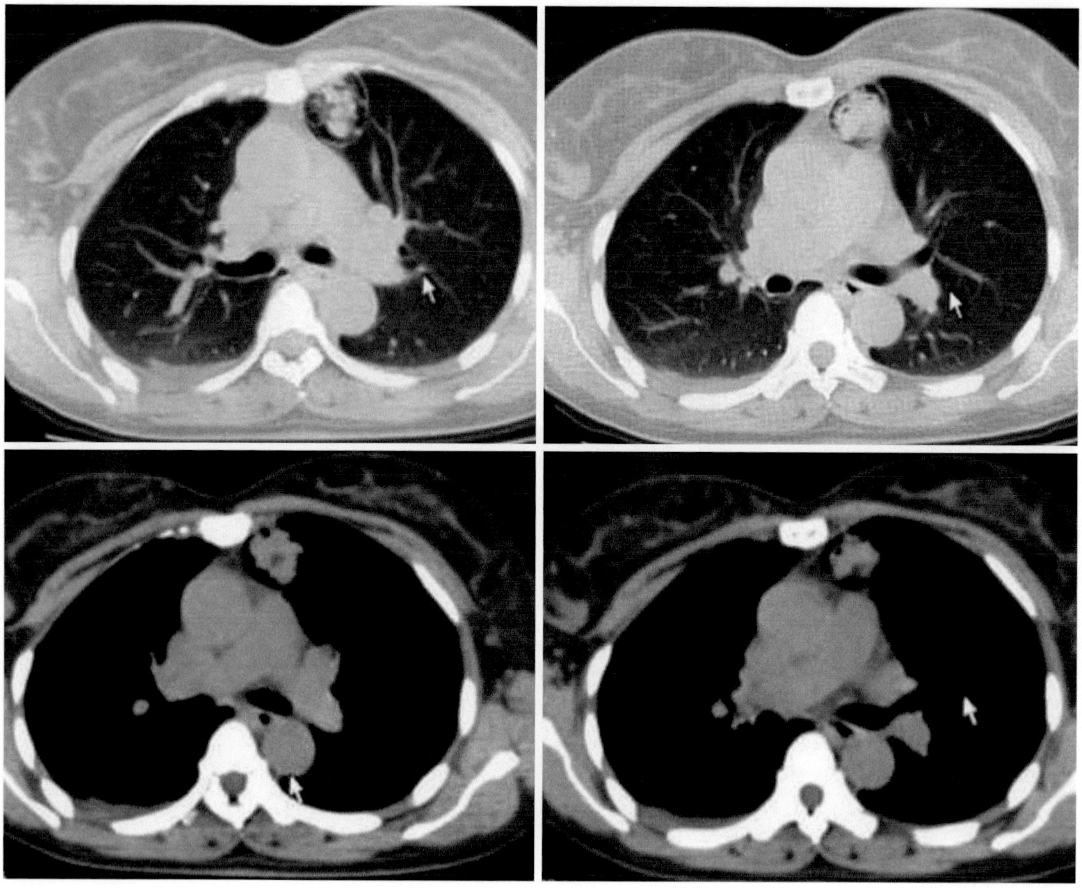

Fig. 22 Chest CT

mass exceeds 2.5, it is usually interpreted as a possible malignancy. In the study, the SUVmax of 50% of PSPs exceeded 2.5.

Uhlén et al. [33] found that the SUVmax of pulmonary carcinoids (mean, 3.9) was higher than that of hamartomas (mean, 1.4). The SUVmax of atypical and typical carcinoids was similar, 5.0 and 3.8, respectively. It was possible to differentiate the carcinoids from the hamartomas, but atypical carcinoids could not be distinguished from the typical carcinoids by PET measurements of the ^{18}F-FDG uptake. Tatcı et al. [34] found the mean SUVmax of atypical carcinoids (5.97 ± 3.7) and typical carcinoids (4.22 ± 1.7) were higher than those of hamartomas (1.65 ± 0.9).

The SUVmax of ^{18}F-FDG PET/CT may be useful in differentiating benign from malignant solitary pulmonary nodules.

7.8 Case 8

A 52-year-old woman found a lung lesion for 3 days on physical examination.

Chest CT: A cystic-solid lesion in the lingual segment of the left upper lobe (Fig. 22).

[Diagnosis] Mesenchymal cystic hamartoma.

[Diagnosis Basis] Chest CT shows a cystic-solid lesion in the upper lobe of the left lung. The solid component was located in the cystic cavity, with irregular margins and fat density. The patient underwent VATS wedge resection. Under thoracoscopy, a small amount of yellow effusion was found in the pleural cavity. The fissure was well developed, and there was no pleural adhesion. The lesion was located in the lingual segment of the left upper lobe, about 4 × 3 × 3 cm (Fig. 23a),

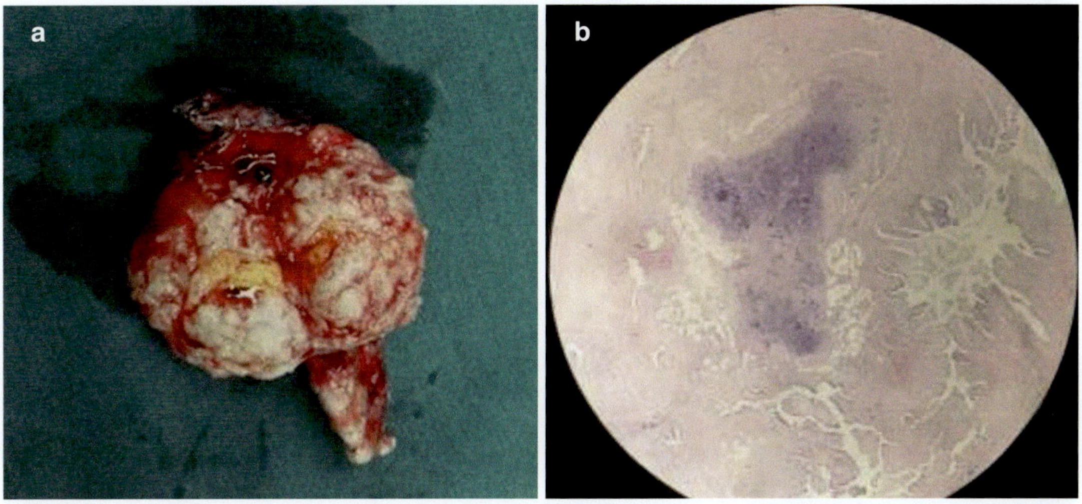

Fig. 23 (**a**) Gross specimen of hamartoma. (**b**) Tumors consist of hyperplastic smooth muscle, islands of cartilage, and fissures lining the respiratory epithelium

postoperative pathology revealed mesenchymal cystic hamartoma, the cyst wall was normal lung tissue (Fig. 23b).

[Analysis] Cystic-solid pulmonary hamartomas are unusual. The mechanism of the cyst formation is unknown. Some authors hypothesized that as hamartoma grows in size, the tendency to become cystic increases. The degenerative changes coupled with the growth result in formation of cleft-like spaces that ultimately expand into cysts. Some authors suggested that the proximity of a hamartoma to a bronchiole with air-entry and a check-valve mechanism may lead to the expansion of small epithelial-lined tubules into cysts.

Varying degrees of fluid may be observed in the cysts of cystic-solid pulmonary hamartomas. Erber et al. [35] reviewed 47 surgical lung specimens of non-epithelial neoplasms for frequency and pattern of intralesional epithelial entrapment. They found that entrapped glands frequently showed prominent regenerative and reactive changes mimicking neoplastic glands. The size and type of gland vary greatly from small acinar-type glands or microcystic spaces lined by flattened epithelial cells and containing mucoid secretion to branching leaflet-like papillary spaces. All of the factors led to differences in epithelial secretory function. Therefore, the cysts may be well inflated or partially or even completely filled with fluid in the cystic-solid pulmonary hamartomas. Through a literature review, Guo et al. [36] found that the CT image density of cystic-solid pulmonary hamartomas can vary from ground glass density to solid density depending on the proportion of the solid part.

For large mesenchymal cystic hamartoma, prompt surgical resection is the recommended treatment.

7.9 Case 9

A 52-year-old woman complaint of left back pain for half a year.

Chest CT: A mass in the cortex of the left posterior rib (Fig. 24).

[Diagnosis] Mesenchymal hamartoma of the chest wall.

[Diagnosis Basis] Chest CT shows an irregular mass along the ribs on the left side of the spine with clear borders, and intratumoral fat and calcifications are seen. The adjacent rib swells and deforms, showing cystic changes, which is con-

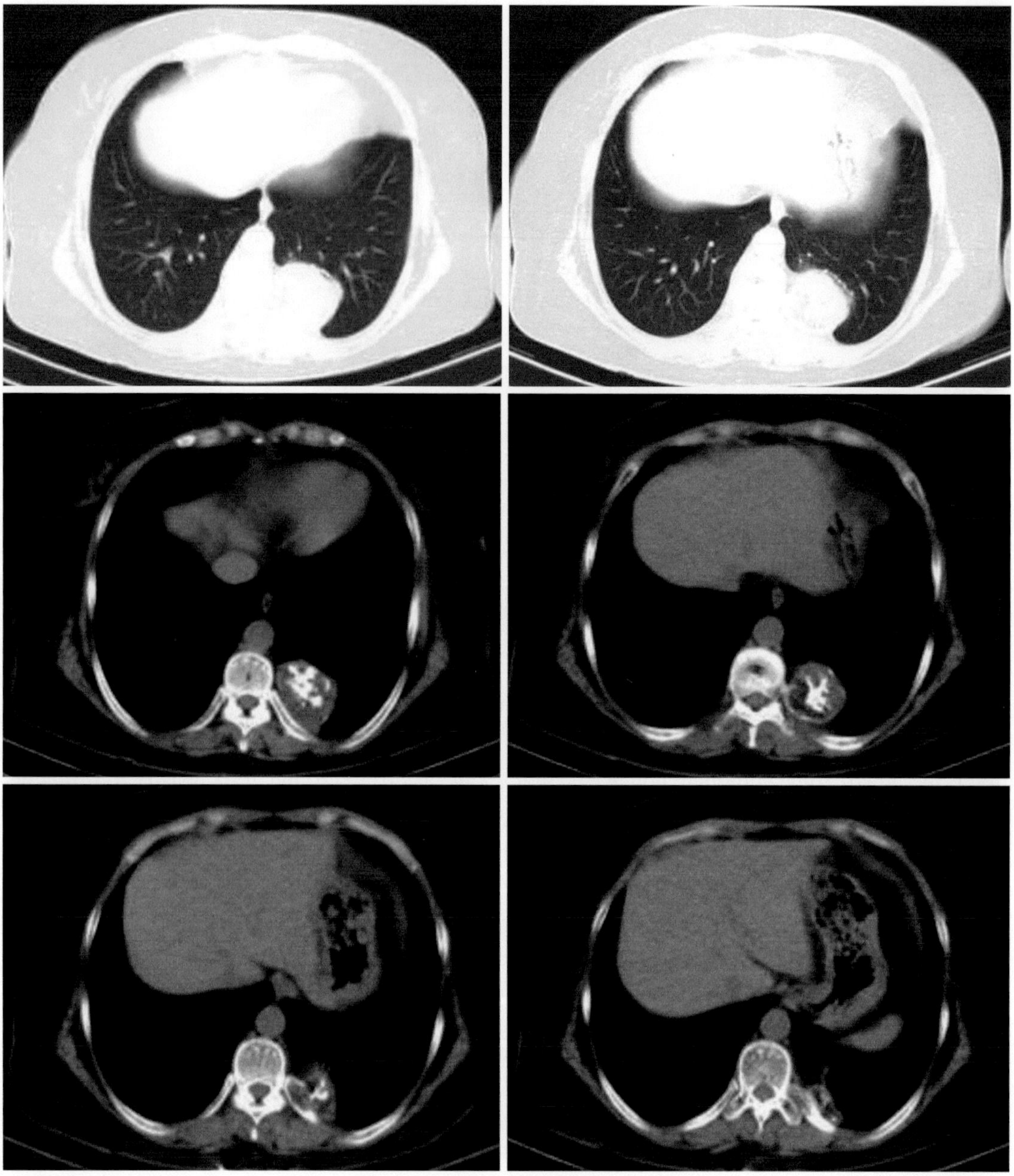

Fig. 24 Chest CT

sidered to be a mesenchymal hamartoma of the chest wall. The patient underwent surgical resection. The tumor was located in the paravertebral side of the ninth and tenth thoracic vertebrae, about 5 × 5 cm in size, and adhered to the lung tissue. The tumor originated from the paravertebral body of the tenth posterior rib near the costovertebral joint, with a diameter of about 3 cm, and the pedicle was connected to the rib. Pathology showed an intact capsule, and chondromesenchymal hamartoma was considered.

[Analysis] Mesenchymal hamartoma of the chest wall (MHCW), also known as chondromesenchymal hamartoma, is a rare benign tumor that arises from one or more ribs. In 1979, Mcleod and Dahlin [37] proposed the term MHCW, which reflects a benign overgrowth of normal skeletal elements. It typically appears in early infancy and in childhood, although a few cases have been reported in adults. MHCW generally presents as solitary and unilateral, but multiple or bilateral MHCW have been reported.

Radiologically, MHCW is characteristically a large expansile solid to cystic intrathoracic mass originating from central position of ribs with destruction of adjacent ribs and secondary changes evident in other ribs and vertebrae. Histopathologically, it is typically a solitary well-defined lesion arising from ribs with cystic areas composed of mucoid and bloody contents and solid areas comprising cartilage, collagen, and bone. Clinically, it may enlarge progressively and causes significant destruction to surrounding structures causing distortion and displacement of airways, lungs, heart, major vessels, or erode ribs.

Kim et al. [38] analyzed the radiologic and pathologic correlation of MHCW. Radiologically, MHCW was well-defined mass with solid and cystic components with multiple fluid-fluid levels in association with single or multiple rib destruction or change. CT scan revealed the typical findings of chest wall hamartoma, and the MR showed heterogeneous signal intensities of the mass on T1- and T2-weighted images. The MR also revealed more concisely a secondary aneurysmal bone cyst formation with multiple fluid-fluid levels on the T2-weighted image. Microscopically, MHCW revealed alternating areas of cartilaginous islands and primitive appearing mesenchymal proliferation, which corresponded well with the solid component on the radiologic findings.

Freeburn et al. [39] reported a case of spontaneous regression of a chest wall hamartoma in infancy, supporting recommendations for conservative management in asymptomatic children. Jozaghi et al. [40] believed that the relative tumor size peaks at birth and starts to involute thereafter. Most lesions stop growing in the first year of life. Therefore, for asymptomatic lesions, observation alone is enough; for symptomatic lesions, resection with chest wall reconstruction is indicated.

Older patients have a lower chance of spontaneous regression, surgical resection is recommended when symptoms are noted.

References

1. Albrecht D. Ueber hamartome. Verh Dtsch Ges Pathol. 1904;7:153–7.
2. Goldsworthy NE. Chondroma of lung (hamartoma chondromatosum pulmonis) with report of case. J Pathol Bacteriol. 1934;39:291–8.
3. Dal Clin P, Kools P, De Jonge I, et al. Rearrangement of 12q14-15 in pulmonary chondroid hamartoma. Genes Chromosomes Cancer. 1993;8:131–4.
4. Fletcher JA, Longtine J, Wallace K, et al. Cytogenetic and histologic findings in 17 pulmonary chondroid hamartomas: evidence for a pathogenetic relationship with lipomas and leiomyomas. Genes Chromosomes Cancer. 1995;12:220–3.
5. Xiao S, Lux ML, Reeves R, et al. HMGI(Y) activation by chromosome 6p21 rearrangements in multilineage mesenchymal cells from pulmonary hamartoma. Am J Pathol. 1997;150:901–10.
6. Kazmierczak B, Meyer-Bolte K, Tran KH, et al. A high frequency of tumors with rearrangements of genes of the HMGI(Y) family in a series of 191 pulmonary chondroid hamartomas. Genes Chromosomes Cancer. 1999;26:125–33.
7. Gregori-Romero MA, Lopez-Gines C, Cerda-Nicolas M, et al. Recombinations of chromosomal bands 10q24, 12q14-q15, and 14q24 in two cases of pulmonary chondroid hamartoma studied by fluorescence in situ hybridization. Cancer Genet Cytogenet. 2003;142:153–7.
8. McDonald JR, Harrington SW, Clagett OT. Hamartoma (often called chondroma) of the lung. J Thorac Surg. 1945;14:128–43.
9. Murray J, Kielkowski D, Leiman G. The prevalence and age distribution of peripheral pulmonary hamartomas in adult males: an autopsy-based study. S Afr Med J. 1991;79:247–9.
10. Guo W, Zhao YP, Jiang YG, et al. Surgical treatment and outcome of pulmonary hamartoma: a retrospective study of 20-year experience. J Exp Clin Cancer Res. 2008;27:8.
11. Wang T, Liu Y. Outcomes of surgical treatments of pulmonary hamartoma. J Cancer Res Ther. 2016;12(Supplement):116–9.
12. Esme H, Duran FM, Unlu Y. Surgical treatment and outcome of pulmonary hamartoma: a retrospective study of 10-year experience. Indian. J Thorac Cardiovasc Surg. 2019;35:31–5.
13. Siegelman SS, Khouri NF, Scott WW Jr, et al. Pulmonary hamartoma: CT findings. Radiology. 1986;160:313–7.
14. Gleeson T, Thiessen R, Hannigan A, et al. Pulmonary hamartomas: CT pixel analysis for fat attenua-

tion using radiologic-pathologic correlation. J Med Imaging Radiat Oncol. 2013;57:534–43.
15. Hochhegger B, Nin CS, Alves GR, et al. Multidetector computed tomography findings in pulmonary hamartomas: a new fat detection threshold. J Thorac Imaging. 2016;31:11–4.
16. Takumi K, Nagano H, Harasawa T, et al. Pulmonary hamartoma: feasibility of dual-energy CT detection of intranodular fat. Radiol Case Rep. 2021;16:1032–6.
17. Park KY, Kim SJ, Noh TW, et al. Diagnostic efficacy and characteristic feature of MRI in pulmonary hamartoma: comparison with CT, specimen MRI, and pathology. J Comput Assist Tomogr. 2008;32:919–25.
18. Hansen CP, Holtveg H, Francis D, et al. Pulmonary hamartoma. J Thorac Cardiovasc Surg. 1992;104:674–8.
19. Itoga M, Kobayashi Y, Takeda M, et al. A case of pulmonary hamartoma showing rapid growth. Case Rep Med. 2013;2013:231652.
20. Hutter J, Reich-Weinberger S, Hutarew G, et al. Giant pulmonary hamartoma—a rare presentation of a common tumor. Ann Thorac Surg. 2006;82:e5–7.
21. Joshi HM, Page RD. Giant pulmonary hamartoma causing acute right heart failure. Ann Thorac Surg. 2014;97:e21–2.
22. Miyaoka M, Ogura G, Hamanaka R, et al. Giant pulmonary hamartoma with dominant CD34- positive smooth muscle cell component. Tokai J Exp Clin Med. 2018;43:1–4.
23. Hindaria S, Garg A, Dolas A. Giant pulmonary hamartoma with placental transmogrification-a case report. Indian J Thorac Cardiovasc Surg. 2021;37:702–5.
24. Cruickshank DB, Harrison GK. Diffuse fibroleiomyomatous hamartomatosis of the lung. Thorax. 1953;8:316–8.
25. Karasik A, Modan M, Jacob CO, et al. Increased risk of lung cancer in patients with chondromatous hamartoma. J Thorac Cardiovasc Surg. 1980;80:217–20.
26. Ribet M, Jaillard-Thery S, Nuttens MC. Pulmonary hamartoma and malignancy. J Thorac Cardiovasc Surg. 1994;107:611–4.
27. Gjevre JA, Myers JL, Prakash UB. Pulmonary hamartomas. Mayo Clin Proc. 1996;71:14–20.
28. Fiorelli A, D'Andrilli A, Carlucci A, et al. Pulmonary hamartoma associated with lung cancer (PHALC study): results of a multicenter study. Lung. 2021;199:369–78.
29. Liu C, Wang JJ, Zhu YH, et al. Successful use of snare electrocautery via flexible fiberoptic bronchoscopy for removal of an endobronchial hamartoma causing chronic lung atelectasis and mimicking malignancy. Ther Adv Respir Dis. 2017;11:435–8.
30. Abdel Hady SM, Elbastawisy SE, Hassaballa AS, et al. Is surgical resection superior to bronchoscopic resection in patients with symptomatic endobronchial hamartoma? Interact Cardiovasc Thorac Surg. 2017;24:778–82.
31. Ergonul AG, Akcam TI, Özdil A, et al. Diagnostic value of 18F-FDG-PET/CT in benign lung diseases. Kardiochir Torakochirurgia Pol. 2018;15:1–4.
32. Jiang L, Huang Y, Tang Q, et al. ^{18}F-FDG PET/CT characteristics of pulmonary sclerosing hemangioma vs. pulmonary hamartoma. Oncol Lett. 2018;16:660–5.
33. Uhlén N, Grundberg O, Jacobsson H, et al. 18F-FDG PET/CT diagnosis of bronchopulmonary carcinoids versus pulmonary hamartomas. Clin Nucl Med. 2016;41:263–7.
34. Tatcı E, Özmen Ö, Öztürk A, et al. Contribution of 18F-FDG PET/CT in the differential diagnosis of pulmonary hamartomas and pulmonary carcinoids. Mol Imaging Radionucl Ther. 2021;30:101–6.
35. Erber R, Haller F, Hartmann A, et al. Prominent entrapment of respiratory epithelium in primary and metastatic intrapulmonary non-epithelial neoplasms: a frequent morphological pattern closely mimicking adenofibroma and other biphasic pulmonary lesions. Virchows Arch. 2020;477:195–205.
36. Guo XW, Jia XD, Ji AD, et al. Large cystic-solid pulmonary hamartoma: a case report. World J Clin Cases. 2022;10:2650–6.
37. McLeod RA, Dahlin DC. Hamartoma (mesenchymoma) of the chest wall in infancy. Radiology. 1979;131:657–61.
38. Kim JY, Jung WH, Yoon CS, et al. Mesenchymal hamartoma of the chest wall in infancy: radiologic and pathologic correlation. Yonsei Med J. 2000;41:615–22.
39. Freeburn AM, McAloon J. Infantile chest hamartoma—case outcome aged 11. Arch Dis Child. 2001;85:244–5.
40. Jozaghi Y, Emil S, Albuquerque P, et al. Prenatal and postnatal features of mesenchymal hamartoma of the chest wall: case report and literature review. Pediatr Surg Int. 2013;29:735–40.

Pulmonary Chondroma

Xue-Peng Huang and Song Zhang

Chondroma is a benign cartilaginous tumor that usually occurs in the short tubular bones of the hands and feet. Extraskeletal chondroma is rare, and pulmonary chondroma is very rare.

1 Etiology

The etiology of pulmonary chondroma is unknown so far, the possible reasons are as follows: (1) It originates from ectopic cartilage of lung tissue during embryonic development, (2) Chondrocytes from other parts flow into the lungs by bloodstream, (3) Connective tissues and reticulocytes develop into original direction under certain stimulate conditions, become embryonic mesenchymal tissue, and then develop into chondrocytes [1].

X.-P. Huang
Department of Respiratory and Critical Care Medicine, People's Hospital of Rizhao Lanshan, Rizhao, Shandong, China

S. Zhang (✉)
Department of Respiratory and Critical Care Medicine, Shandong Provincial Hospital Affiliated to Shandong First Medical University, Jinan, Shandong, China

2 Pathology

Pulmonary chondroma is composed of differentiation of mature cartilage tissue, wrapped around the cartilage matrix. Cartilage tissues can be elastic cartilage, hyaline cartilage, and fibrous cartilage, or diverse cartilage mixed together without other stromal and epithelial elements, adipose tissues, and abnormal mitotic. Chondrocytes may encounter calcification, ossification, and mucoid degeneration [2].

3 Clinical Features

Chondroma presents in any age-group and is highest between the fourth and fifth decades of life, with female predilection. The symptoms of pulmonary chondroma depend on the size and location of the tumor. Most of the patients are asymptomatic and detected occasionally. Symptoms such as cough, expectoration, chest pain, hemoptysis, and shortness of breath may occur.

4 Radiographic Features

The CT appearance of pulmonary chondroma is smooth, well-defined, round or oval nodule or mass with mild lobulation. Multiple pulmonary chondromas have been reported. Calcifications

S. Zhang (ed.), *Diagnostic Imaging of Lung Cancers*, https://doi.org/10.1007/978-981-99-6815-2_15

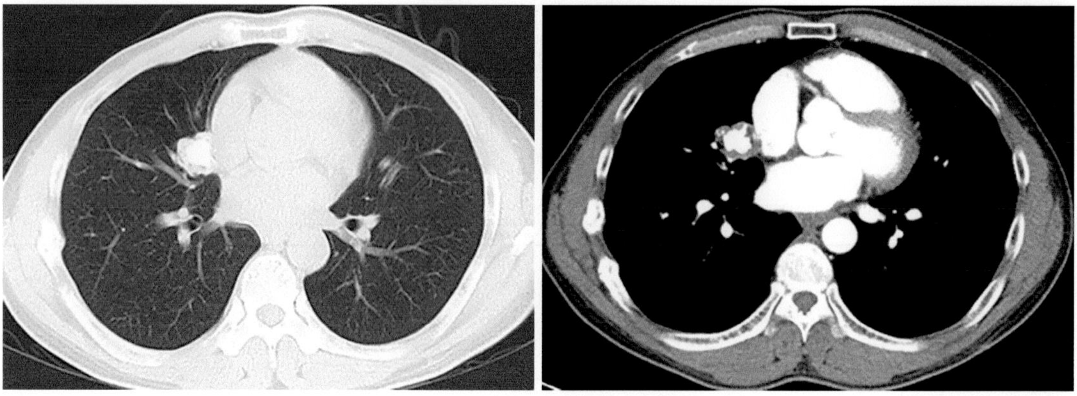

Fig. 1 A 50-year-old man with a lesion in the right middle lobe. Contrast-enhanced CT scan shows markedly central calcification

(central, popcorn, laminated, or diffuse) are common (Fig. 1). No burrs or enlarged lymph nodes at the hilus of lung or mediastinum are observed. Pulmonary chondroma can display no or slight early enhancement and delayed enhancement because of the relatively slow blood flow within the tumor.

5 Treatment

Treatment depends on the size, location, and condition of the parenchyma distal to the lesion. Surgical techniques are the main choice. The prognosis is excellent. It can recur if not completely removed, and cases of degeneration into chondrosarcoma have been reported.

6 Case Analysis

6.1 Case 1

A 67-year-old woman complained of shortness of breath for half a year.

Chest CT: A intratracheal tumor (Fig. 2, images in left).

[Diagnosis] Endobronchial chondroma.

[Diagnosis Basis] Chest CT shows a mass in the trachea with smooth edges and uniform density, which is connected to the tracheal wall with a wide base. Fiberoptic bronchoscopy (Fig. 2, images in right) showed that the tumor surface was smooth, with abundant blood supply and no obvious necrosis, which was consistent with benign tumor. Biopsy pathology showed tumor-like hyperplasia of cartilage tissue without epithelial components, which was diagnosed as a chondroma.

[Analysis] Benign lung tumors can originate from all cell types including epithelial tumors, such as papillomas and adenomas, and nonepithelial tumors like hamartoma, lipomas, leiomyomas, and chondromas. Chondroma is the second most common benign pulmonary tumors of mesenchymal origin. Based on the histogenesis of pulmonary chondroma, Bateson [3] distinguished endobronchial chondroma from pulmonary chondroma. Endobronchial chondroma accounts for fewer than 25% of all benign cartilage neoplasms of the lung.

Pulmonary chondroma differentiates from pulmonary cartilaginous hamartoma based on the presence of a thin fibrous pseudocapsule, purely cartilaginous (hyaline cartilage), frequent bone metaplasia, calcification, and also the absence of entrapped epithelium and fat.

Chondromas usually grow in bones and more frequently in the axial skeleton and can rarely appear in the larynx, trachea, and major bronchi. Endobronchial chondroma grows by invading the bronchial lumen and may cause symptoms due to airway irritation and obstruction, such as intrac-

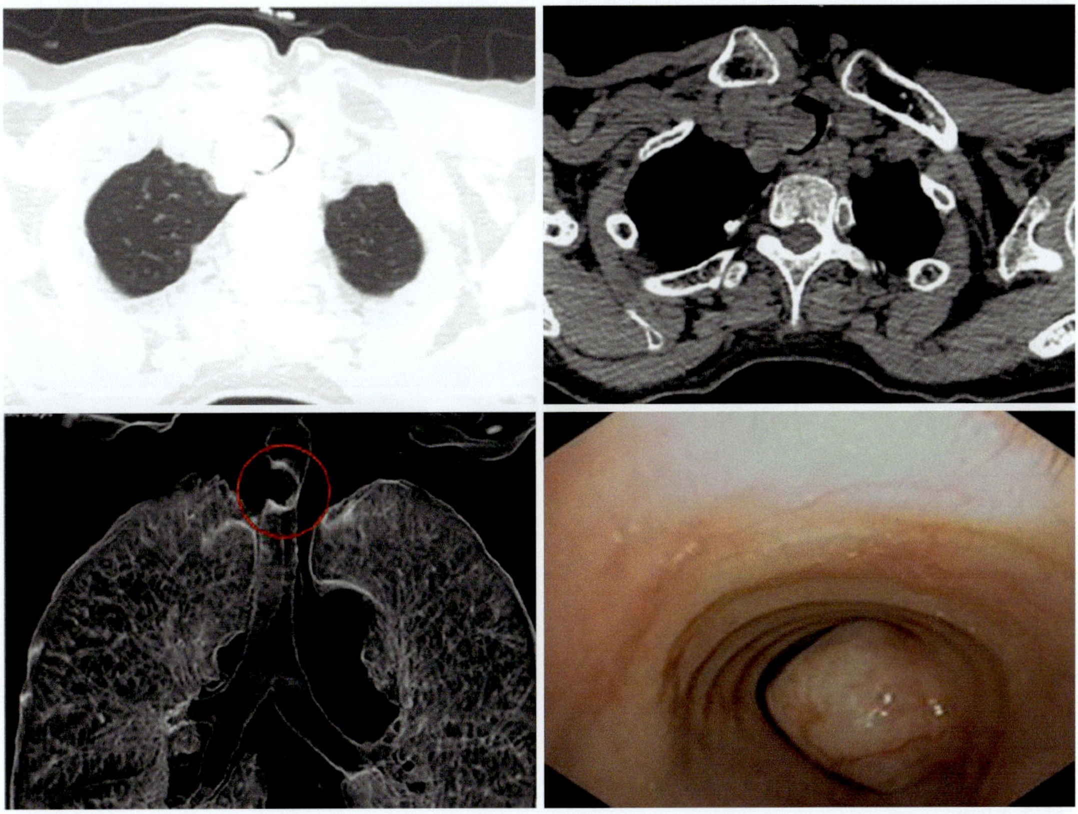

Fig. 2 (Top left, top right, and bottom left) Chest CT. (Bottom right) Fiberoptic bronchoscopy findings

table cough, asthmatic symptoms, and hemoptysis. Chest imaging reveals a solitary endobronchial lesion that may occlude a bronchus and cause complications such as pneumonia, bronchiectasis, atelectasis, and fibrosis. Endoscopically, it is exophytic tumor, little vascularized and covered with normal bronchial mucosa.

Endobronchial techniques (argon plasma coagulation, YAG laser, etc.) and surgical excision (enucleation, bronchectomy, lobectomy, or pneumonectomy) are the mainstay of treatments.

6.2 Case 2

A 16-year-old woman found lung lesions for half a year. The patient had a history of asthma and anemia. Gastric stromal tumor was diagnosed 6 months ago.

Chest CT: Multiple nodules in bilateral lungs (Fig. 3).

[Diagnosis] Pulmonary chondroma.

[Diagnosis Basis] Right lung biopsy showed cartilage tissue, tending to be chondroma.

[Analysis] Carney triad is a rare, nonhereditary syndrome in which at least 3 different tumor entities occur simultaneously or metachronous: gastric gastrointestinal stromal tumor (GIST), pulmonary chondroma, and extra-adrenal paraganglioma. Only 25%–30% cases completely present the triad. A patient who meets 2 of 3 criteria is diagnosed with incomplete Carney triad. More than 80% of affected patients being women with early onset of symptoms.

Carney's triad was first reported in 1977 as a combination of gastric leiomyosarcoma (later renamed GIST), functioning extra-adrenal paraganglioma, and pulmonary chondroma [4].

In 1999, Carney [5] investigated the natural history of the triad. Of all 79 patients (67 women

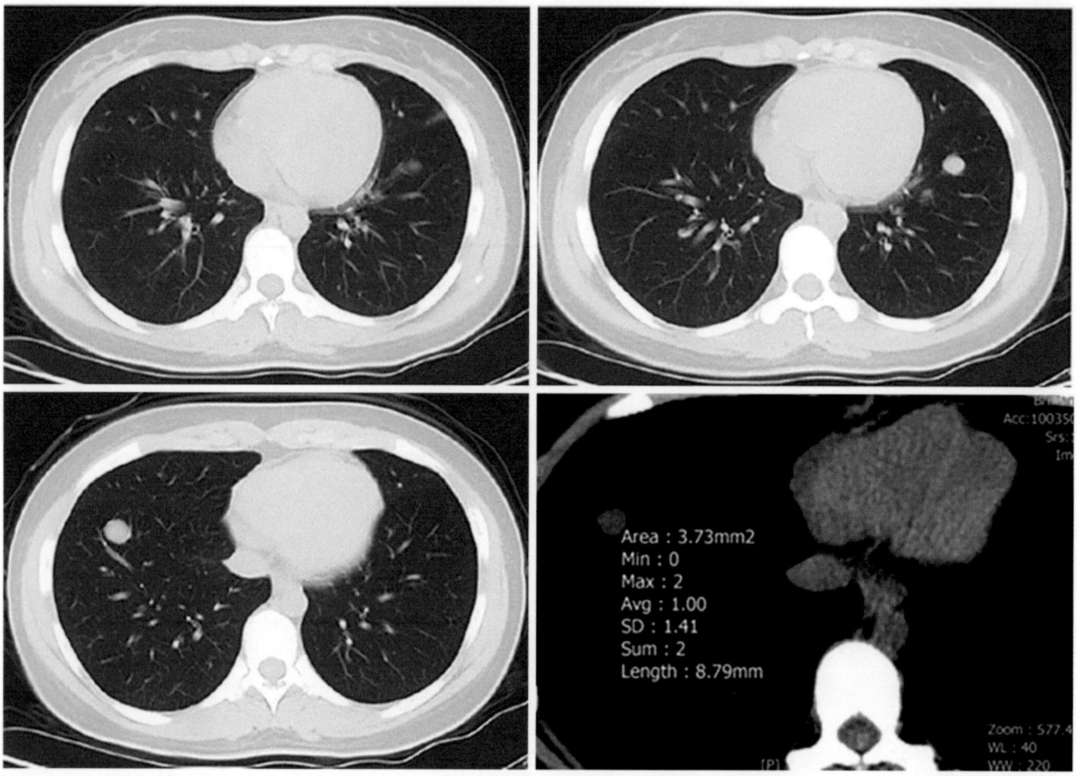

Fig. 3 Chest CT

and 12 men), 17 (22%) had 3 tumors and 62 (78%) had 2 tumors. Forty-two (53%) had stomach and lung tumors. The longest interval between detection of the first and second components was 26 years. Sixty-four patients (81%) were alive, 19 (24%) were significantly free of disease, and 45 (57%) had residual or metastatic tumors. Thirty-two patients (41%) had one or more local recurrences of gastric sarcoma; the longest interval to first recurrence was 36 years. Twenty-one survivors (27%) had liver metastatic gastric sarcoma and were followed for 1–25 years. Fifteen patients (19%) died, including 10 (13%) from the disease. Ten patients (13%) had non-functioning adrenocortical tumors. Carney concluded that the triad is a chronic, persistent, and indolent disease. Benign adrenocortical tumors are a component of the condition [5].

In 2009, Carney [6] analyzed 77 patients with Carney triad. Among 77 patients, 85% were women and 15% were men. The syndrome affects at least five organs: the stomach, lung, paraganglionic system, adrenal (cortex and medulla), and esophagus. The gastric lesion was usually the presenting tumor (75%), followed by the lung lesion (15%) and the paraganglionic tumor (10%). 20% of patients had adrenocortical adenomas, and 10% had esophageal leiomyomas. All the tumors were multifocal. One third of gastric tumors and one tenth of paraganglia tumors metastasized. The pulmonary tumors were asymptomatic and benign[].

In 2010, Zhang et al. [7] studied the clinical and pathologic characteristics of the gastric neoplasm in 104 patients with the syndrome. The majority (88%) were young women with a mean age of 22 years, and the usual presentation was gastric bleeding. Fourteen patients (13%) died of metastatic gastrointestinal stromal tumor (GIST) with a mean age of 45 years. Estimated 10- and 40-year survivals were 100% and 73%, respectively. Compared with sporadic gastric GISTs, the gastric stromal tumor in Carney triad showed distinctive features: young patient age, female predilection, epithelioid cell predominance, multifocality, frequent lymph node metastasis, serial tumor occurrence, and unpredictable behavior. Thus, the Carney triad gastric stromal tumor is different clinically, pathologically, and behaviorally from sporadic gastric GIST.

Haller et al. [8] first reported a recurrent aberrant dense DNA methylation at the gene locus of SDHC in tumors of patients with Carney triad, while this DNA methylation pattern was not present in tumors of patients with Carney-Stratakis syndrome or paraganglioma, or in sporadic GISTs with KIT mutations. Settas et al. [9] found that most cases of Carney triad show down-regulation of SDH through site-specific hypermethylation of the SDHC gene. Overall, Carney triad is characterized by a deficiency of the mitochondrial succinate dehydrogenase (SDH) enzymatic complex, which results from epigenetic silencing of the SDHC gene by its promoter hypermethylation.

Gastric GIST and paraganglioma are generally treated with surgery, while the first choice for pulmonary chondroma is conservative treatment.

References

1. Hoekstra MO, Bertus PM, Nikkels PG, et al. Multiple pulmonary chondromata. A rare cause of neonatal respiratory distress. Chest. 1994;105:301–2.
2. Rodriguez FJ, Aubry MC, Tazelaar HD, et al. Pulmonary chondroma: a tumor associated with Carney triad and different from pulmonary hamartoma. Am J Surg Pathol. 2007;31:1844–53.
3. Bateson EM. Histogenesis of intrapulmonary and endobronchial hamartomas and chondromas (cartilage-containing tumors): a hypothesis. J Pathol. 1970;101:7783.
4. Carney JA, Sheps SG, Go VL, et al. The triad of gastric leiomyosarcoma, functioning extra-adrenal paraganglioma and pulmonary chondroma. N Engl J Med. 1977;296:1517–8.
5. Carney JA. Gastric stromal sarcoma, pulmonary chondroma, and extra-adrenal paraganglioma (Carney triad): natural history, adrenocortical component, and possible familial occurrence. Mayo Clin Proc. 1999;74:543–52.
6. Carney JA. Carney triad: a syndrome featuring paraganglionic adrenocortical, and possibly other endocrine tumors. J Clin Endocrinol Metab. 2009;94:3656–62.
7. Zhang L, Smyrk TC, Young WF Jr, et al. Gastric stromal tumors in Carney triad are different clinically, pathologically, and behaviorally from sporadic gastric gastro- intestinal stromal tumors: findings in 104 cases. Am J Surg Pathol. 2010;34:53–64.
8. Haller F, Moskalev EA, Faucz FR, et al. Aberrant DNA hypermethylation of SDHC: a novel mechanism of tumor development in Carney triad. Endocr Relat Cancer. 2014;21:567–77.
9. Settas N, Faucz FR, Stratakis CA. Succinate dehydrogenase (SDH) deficiency, Carney triad and the epigenome. Mol Cell Endocrinol. 2018;469:107–11.

PEComatous Tumors

Xue-Peng Huang and Song Zhang

Perivascular epithelioid cell tumor (PEComa) is a mesenchymal neoplasm showing perivascular epithelioid cell differentiation. The PEComa family includes angiomyolipoma (AML), pulmonary clear cell sugar tumor (CCST) and lymphangioleiomyomatosis, clear cell myomelanocytic tumor of the falciform ligament/ligamentum teres, primary extrapulmonary sugar tumor, abdominopelvic sarcoma of perivascular epithelioid cells, and other tumors with similar features at various sites.

PEComas typically exhibit female preponderance with a mean onset age of around 45 years. Anatomically, the most common site of origin is the kidney, lung, and liver.

1 Classification

In 1992, Bonetti et al. [1] first introduced the term perivascular epithelioid cell (PEC) to identify a "novel" cell type described by Apitz as an "abnormal myoblast" in renal AML in 1943 [2]. In 1994, based on morphological and phenotypical similarities, Bonetti et al. [3] found that clear cell tumors of the lung and AMLs belong to the same family of lesions, characterized by the presence of PECs. In 1996, Zamboni et al. [4] first introduced the term PEComa. They reported a pancreatic tumor with overlapping features of the benign clear cell sugar tumor of the lung and named this new entity clear cell sugar tumor of the pancreas characterized by a pure proliferation of perivascular epithelioid cells (PEComa). The 2002 WHO classification of pathology and genetics of tumors of soft tissue and bone defined PEComa as "a mesenchymal tumor composed of histologically and immunohistochemically distinctive perivascular epithelioid cells" [5].

In the lung, PEComa can take several forms: a diffuse multicystic proliferation termed LAM, a benign localized mass termed a clear cell tumor or PEComa, and a diffuse proliferation with overlapping features between LAM and clear cell tumor. In the 1999 WHO classification, LAM was grouped under tumor-like lesions. In the 2004 WHO classification, it was moved to mesenchymal tumors. In both 1999 and 2004 WHO classifications, clear cell tumor was classified under miscellaneous tumors. In the 2015 WHO classification, these lesions were grouped together under the title PEComatous tumors with three groups of tumors: (1) LAM, (2) PEComa, benign including clear cell tumor, and (3) PEComa, malig-

X.-P. Huang
Department of Respiratory and Critical Care Medicine, People's Hospital of Rizhao Lanshan, Rizhao, Shandong, China

S. Zhang (✉)
Department of Respiratory and Critical Care Medicine, Shandong Provincial Hospital Affiliated to Shandong First Medical University, Jinan, Shandong, China

S. Zhang (ed.), *Diagnostic Imaging of Lung Cancers*, https://doi.org/10.1007/978-981-99-6815-2_16

nant. In the 2021 WHO classification, PEComatous tumors included LAM; PEComa, benign; and PEComa, malignant.

2 Pathology

The PEComa cells are typically arranged around blood vessels and infiltrate the smooth muscle of small- to medium-sized vessels. Periluminal cells are usually epithelioid, and peripheral cells are spindle shaped. PEC has clear to granular cytoplasm, round to oval, centrally located nucleus, and inconspicuous nucleolus. It sometimes has focally marked nuclear atypia. Prominent melanin pigmentation is rare. Fatty change can be seen, especially in the peripheral cells that can mimic lipoblasts.

Immunohistochemically, PEComa expresses myogenic markers, such as SMA, actin, calponin, muscle myosin, and sometimes h-caldesmon, and melanocytic markers, such as HMB45, HMSA-1, Melan A, and microphthalmia transcription factor (Mitf). Desmin is less commonly, although more frequently expressed in cutaneous and sclerosing PEComas.

At present, PECs do not have a known normal counterpart. Some studies speculated that they are derived from genetically modified mesenchymal stem cells of perivascular origin [6].

3 Molecular features

PEComas are related to TSC mutations and TFE3 gene rearrangements.

The mutations in TSC have been mapped to chromosomes 9q34 (TSC1) and 16p13.3 (TSC2). TSC1 and TSC2 genes encode hamartin and tuberin, respectively. Hamartin interacts with tuberin to function together as a heterodimer and affects signaling pathways related to growth and proliferation [7]. Hamartin, a growth inhibitory protein, stabilizes tuberin, resulting in the inhibition of cell growth. The tumor suppressor genes TSC1 and TSC2 play an important role in negatively regulating the Rheb/mTOR/p70S6K cascade. Tuberin has a Rheb (Ras homologue enriched in brain) GTPase-activating protein activity which inactivates Rheb. Alterations of tuberin lead to hyperactivation of Rheb, which subsequently stimulates the mTOR pathway. Activated mTORC1 drives the mTOR/p70S6K metabolic pathway, which promotes cell growth, and particularly regulates vascular smooth muscle differentiation. Activation of mTOR pathway results in elevated phospho-p706K with reduced phospho-AKT and phosphorylation of ribosomal protein subunit S6 (a target of S6Kinase).

Malfunction of the TSC1/TSC2 complex may result from somatic deletion of TSC1, inactivating mutations in TSC1 or TSC2, or missense mutations in TSC2. Kenerson et al. [8] examined the activity of Rheb/mTOR/p70S6K pathway in sporadic AMLs and PEComas using immunohistochemical and biochemical analyses. They found increased levels of phospho-p70S6K in 15 of 15 non-TSC AMLs. This was accompanied by a decrease in phospho-AKT expression, a pattern that is consistent with the disruption of TSC1/2 function. Western blot analysis confirmed mTOR activation concurrent with the loss of TSC2 and not TSC1 in sporadic AMLs. Similarly, 14 of 15 cases of extrarenal PEComas showed elevated phospho-p70S6K and reduced phospho-AKT expression. These observations suggested that mTOR activation is common to sporadic, non-TSC-related AMLs and PEComas.

Most PEComas harbor loss-of-function TSC1/TSC2 mutations, but around 20% of PEComas are positive for TFE3 nuclear staining, among which many of them carry TFE3 gene rearrangements. The DNA-binding factor TFE3 is closely related to microphthalmia-associated transcription factor (MiTF) and is involved in differentiation of melanocytes and osteoclasts. Agaram et al. [9] investigated 38 PEComas consisted of 11 soft tissue tumors and 27 visceral site tumors, including uterus, kidney, liver, lung, and bladder. 23% (n = 9) of TFE3 gene-rearranged tumors were identified, with 3 cases showing an SFPQ/PSF-TFE3 fusion and 1 case showing a novel DVL2-TFE3 gene fusion. 80% of the TFE3 fusion-negative cases tested found TSC2 mutations. 63% of the TSC2-mutated PEComas found coexistent TP53 mutations. The result revealed that TFE3-rearranged PEComas lacked coexisting TSC2 mutations, indicating alternative pathways of tumorigenesis. In addition, 3 (8%) uterine PEComas found novel RAD51B gene rearrangements, which showed a complex fusion pattern and were fused to RRAGB/OPHN1 genes in 2 cases. Other nonrecurrent gene fusions, HTR4-ST3GAL1 and RASSF1-PDZRN3, were identified in 2 cases.

TSC1/2 and TFE3 aberrations are considered mutually exclusive in PEComa, representing two different pathogenic mechanisms leading to tumorigenesis. However, Schmiester et al. [10] reported a clinically aggressive TCS1-mutated PEComa patient displaying a TFE3-altered phenotype. They believed that the TSC1/2-mTOR pathway and TFE3 overexpression can simultaneously contribute to tumorigenesis in PEComa.

4 Treatment

At present, PEComa mainly relies on surgical treatment. There is still no effective treatment for some cases with huge inoperable tumors, tumor spread, or multiple metastases. Conventional radiotherapy and chemotherapy had no obvious effect. It has been reported that postoperative use of ifosfamide and adriamycin combined with chemotherapy can prevent recurrence and malignant transformation.

The mTOR inhibitor sirolimus has potential as a targeted therapy for PEComa. It is important to recognize TFE3-rearranged PEComas because of hypothetical ineffectiveness of targeted mTOR inhibitor therapy [11]. Lin et al. [12] reported a case of ovarian TFE3 reactive PEComa that did not respond to sirolimus and developed liver recurrence. However, Purwar et al. [13] reported first case of malignant pelvic TFE3 PEComa showing response to mTOR therapy. This 45-year-old woman was started on everolimus after her diagnosis of PEComa; repeat imaging after 3 months of therapy showed complete response. Xu et al. [14] reported a case of malignant gastrointestinal PEComa with TFE3 rearrangement which responded to the targeted therapy of an anti-VEGFR tyrosine kinase inhibitor (TKI), apatinib. The tumor remained stable during apatinib treatment, with progression-free survival (PFS) lasting about 7 months. This case suggested that targeting the VEGF/VEGFR signaling pathway may be an essential new therapeutic choice for TFE3-associated malignant PEComas.

Most PEcomas have good prognosis, and there are also a few cases of postoperative recurrence.

5 Case Analysis

5.1 Case 1

A 37-year-old woman complained of cough and expectoration for 1 month.

Chest CT: A nodule in the right middle lobe with obvious enhancement (Fig. 1).

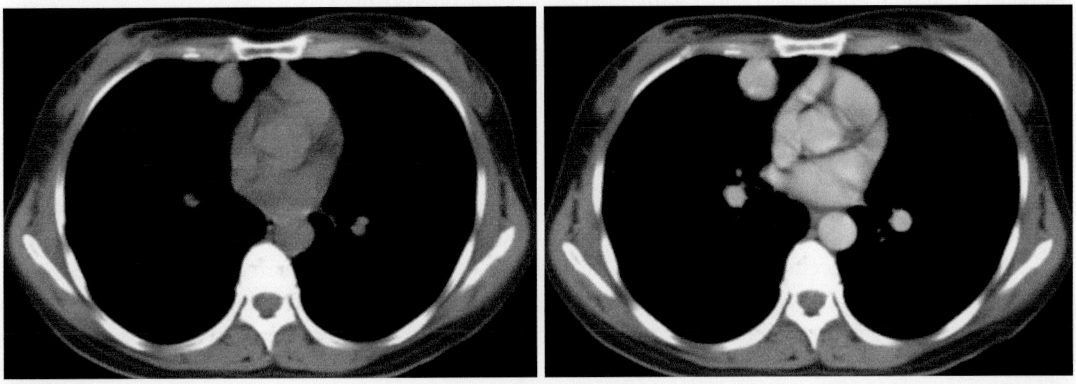

Fig. 1 Chest CT

[Diagnosis] Pulmonary clear cell tumor.

[Diagnosis Basis] The patient underwent thoracoscopic surgery. The tumor was located in the right middle lobe and adhered to the upper lobe, with a size of 2 × 2 cm. The pathological diagnosis was clear cell tumor.

[Analysis] In 1963, Liebow and Castleman [15] first described a rare tumor of the lung composed of clear cells rich in glycogen, named "sugar" tumor. They extensively reported 12 examples of the same entity in 1971 [16].

Clear cell tumor occurs in various age-groups (8–73 years), but is most often seen in the elderly, with a slight female predominance. Ntanasis-Stathopoulos et al. [17] analyzed 104 clear cell sugar tumor of the lung cases. The majority of cases were stemming from the USA (43.3%) and Asia (34.6%). The median age at diagnosis was 52 years without gender predominance. Most of the tumors were asymptomatic (60.7%) and had a benign clinical course (73.3%). This tumor also affects extrapulmonary tissues including the rectum and vulva.

Tumors are usually discovered incidentally during physical examination. Benign clear cell tumor typically presents as a smooth, well-defined, round or oval, and peripheral parenchymal nodule without evidence of cavitation or calcification. Clear cell tumors often show intense enhancement on contrast-enhanced CT scan, which appears to be related to their rich vascular stroma.

Histologically, tumor cells are composed of round to polygonal epithelioid cells, with clear or eosinophilic cytoplasm containing periodic acid-Schiff-positive glycogen, and abundant thin-walled blood vessels. Immunohistochemically, clear cell tumor is positive for HMB-45 and S-100 and is negative for cytokeratin 7 or epithelial membrane antigen (EMA). It is also positive for tyrosinase, Melan A, Mitf, and NKI/C3.

Clear cell tumor needs to be differentiated from metastasis of renal clear cell tumor and pulmonary carcinoma. These metastases also show abundant glycogen, but are positive for cytokeratin7 and EMA. Clear cell pulmonary carcinoma has abundant mitosis, necrosis, and reactivity to cytokeratin. However, benign clear cell tumor lacks evidence of reoccurrence, extensive tissue invasion, or metastasis, even after enucleation.

Clear cell tumor may co-existence with tuberous sclerosis complex (TSC) or Birt–Hogg–Dube (BHD) syndrome. The incidence of PEComas has been associated with TSC, and mutations in TSC ultimately result in aberrant cell proliferation that is primarily mediated by the mTOR signaling pathway. Gunji-Niitsu et al. [18] first reported a patient with BHD syndrome who was complicated with a clear cell "sugar" tumor of the lung. BHD syndrome is caused by germline mutation of the folliculin (FLCN) gene, a tumor suppressor gene whose protein product is involved in mechanistic target of rapamycin (mTOR) signaling pathway regulating cell growth and metabolism. The case indicated that folliculin and mTORC1 are closely associated with the tumorigenesis of this rare disease.

Clear cell tumor can be treated solely by surgical resection with no need for adjuvant chemotherapy or radiotherapy.

5.2 Case 2

A 49-year-old woman complained of chest tightness, dyspnea, dizziness, nausea, and vomiting for 2 h.

Chest CT: A mass in the left lower lobe with obvious enhancement (Fig. 2).

Brain MRI: Abnormal signal in left cerebellar hemisphere(Fig. 3).

[Diagnosis] Malignant perivascular epithelioid cell tumor.

[Diagnosis Basis] Chest CT shows a well-defined mass in dorsal segment of left lower lobe with heterogeneous enhancement. Brain MRI shows a lesion in left cerebellar hemisphere. The neoplasms in the left brain and left lung were resected. The lung tumor was adjacent to the pleura with a size of 11.0 × 6.5 × 5.5 cm. The

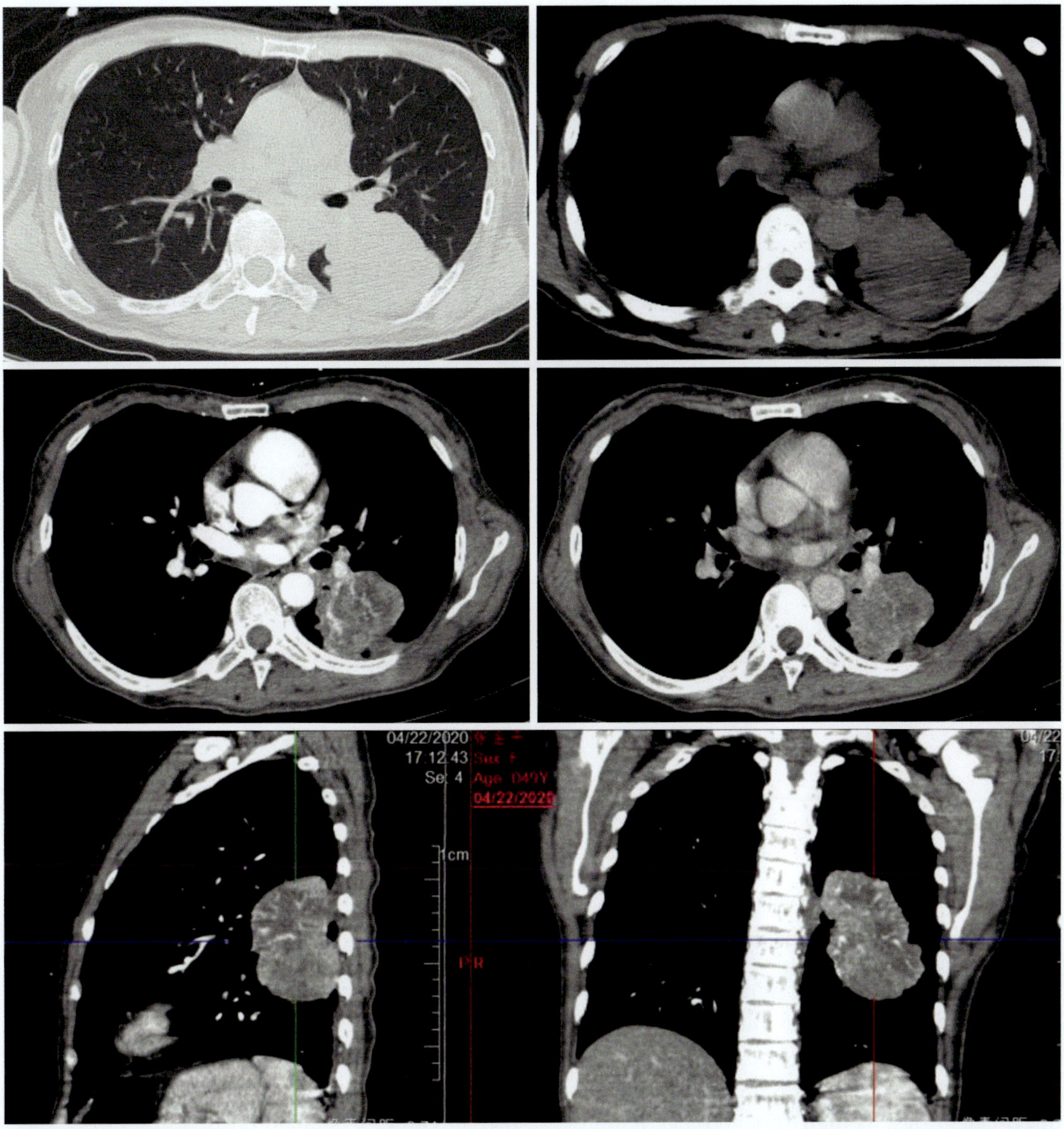

Fig 2 Chest CT

tumor cells had spindle morphology with obvious necrosis. Tumor invaded the pleura, bronchi, and vessels, but not involved the hilar and mediastinal lymph nodes. The pathological diagnosis of lung and brain tumors showed malignant perivascular epithelioid cell tumor (Fig. 4a, b). Immunohistochemistry was positive for HMB45, Melan A, TFE3, CD34, PR, Vimentin(focal), and S-100(focal), and negative for cytokeratin 7, EMA, CD10, PAX8, TTF-1, Napsin A, P40, and CK5/6. The Ki-67 index was 50%–60%.

[Analysis] Malignant PEComas arising from the lung are very rare. Although malignant PEComas have been reported in multiple sites including soft tissue, gynecology, retroperitoneum, gastrointestinal tract, and uterus, diagnostic criteria and treatment strategies for malignant pulmonary PEComa have not been established.

The 2002 WHO soft tissue and bone book stated that PEComas displaying any combination of infiltrative growth, marked hypercellularity,

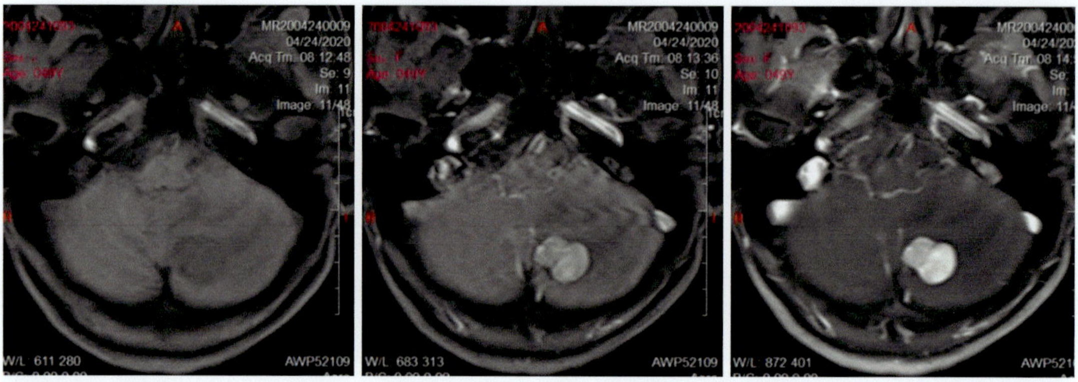

Fig. 3 Brain MRI

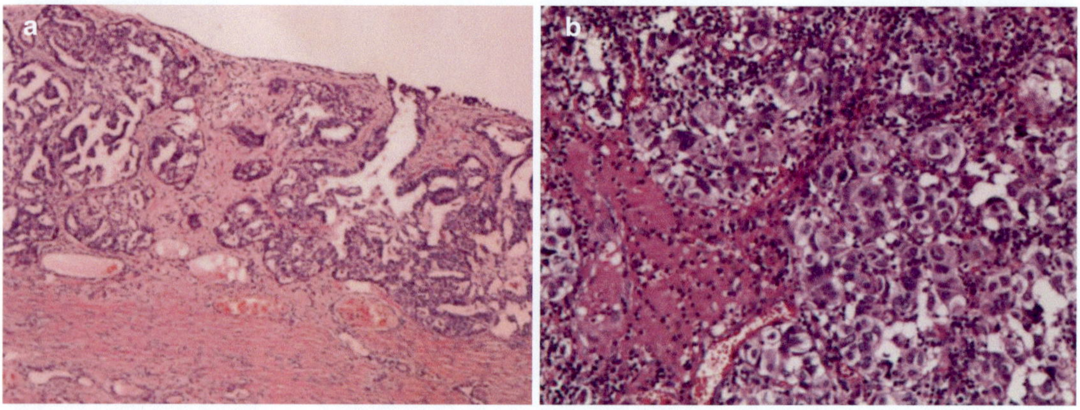

Fig. 4 (**a**) 10 Pathologic finding with malignant pulmonary PEComa. (**b**) Pathologic finding with malignant cerebellar PEComa

nuclear enlargement and hyperchromasia, high mitotic activity, atypical mitotic figures, and coagulative necrosis should be regarded as malignant. Folpe et al. [19] divided PEComas into three categories: benign (no atypical features), uncertain malignant potential (nuclear atypia or size >5 cm), and malignant by any 2 morphological and pathological criteria such as gross size (>5 cm), infiltrative growth pattern, high nuclear grade, necrosis, vascular invasion, or a mitotic rate higher than one per 50 HPF. Schoolmeester et al. [11] classified PEComas as malignant when these lesions meet four out of the five criteria including gross size ≥5 cm, high-grade nuclear features, necrosis, vascular invasion, or a mitotic rate ≥1/50 HPF. Our case meets all of the above criteria.

In this case, the lung and brain were involved, but no mediastinal lymph node metastases were found. Although single case of brain metastasis was reported [20], the cerebellar PEComa seems unlikely to metastasis from lung. We considered that malignant PEComas may have a multifocal origin. Our case stained positive for TFE3, speculating that it may be associated with a TFE3 gene rearrangement.

For malignant PEComa, surgical resection is the primary choice of treatment.

References

1. Bonetti F, Pea M, Martignoni G, et al. PEC and sugar. Am J Surg Pathol. 1992;16:307–8.
2. Apitz K. Die Geschwülste und Gewebsmissbildungen der Nierenrinde. II Midteilung. Die mesenchymalen Neubildungen. Virchows Arch. 1943;311:306–27.
3. Bonetti F, Pea M, Martignoni G, et al. Clear cell ("sugar") tumor of the lung is a lesion strictly related to angiomyolipoma--the concept of a family of lesions

characterized by the presence of the perivascular epithelioid cells (PEC). Pathology. 1994;26:230–6.
4. Zamboni G, Pea M, Martignoni G, et al. Clear cell "sugar" tumor of the pancreas. A novel member of the family of lesions characterized by the presence of perivascular epithelioid cells. Am J Surg Pathol. 1996;20:722–30.
5. Folpe AL. Neoplasms with perivascular epithelioid cell differentiation(PEComas). In: Fletcher CD, Unni KK, Epstein J, Mertens F, editors. Pathology and genetics of tumours of soft tissue and bone. Lyon, France: IARC; 2002. p. 221–2. World Health Organization Classification of Tumours.
6. Crisan M, Yap S, Casteilla L, et al. A perivascular origin for mesenchymal stem cells in multiple human organs. Cell Stem Cell. 2008;3:301–13.
7. Nellist M, van Slegtenhorst MA, Goedbloed M, et al. Characterization of the cytosolic tuberin-hamartin complex: tuberin is a cytosolic chaperone for hamartin. J Biol Chem. 1999;274:35647–52.
8. Kenerson H, Folpe AL, Takayama TK, et al. Activation of the mTOR pathway in sporadic angiomyolipomas and other perivascular epithelioid cell neoplasms. Hum Pathol. 2007;38:1361–71.
9. Agaram NP, Sung YS, Zhang L, et al. Dichotomy of genetic abnormalities in PEComas with therapeutic implications. Am J Surg Pathol. 2015;39813-25
10. Schmiester M, Dolnik A, Kornak U, et al. TFE3 activation in a TSC1-altered malignant PEComa: challenging the dichotomy of the underlying pathogenic mechanisms. J Pathol Clin Res. 2021;7:3–9.
11. Schoolmeester JK, Dao LN, Sukov WR, et al. TFE3 translocation-associated perivascular epithelioid cell neoplasm (PEComa) of the gynecologic tract: morphology, immunophenotype, differential diagnosis. Am J Surg Pathol. 2015;39:394–404.
12. Lin RJ, Melamed J, Wu J. PEComa with transcription factor E3 overexpression: a diagnostic and therapeutic challenge. Case Rep Oncol. 2017;10:531–3.
13. Purwar R, Soni K, Shukla M, et al. TFE3-associated perivascular epithelioid cell tumor with complete response to mTOR inhibitor therapy: report of first case and literature review. World J Surg Oncol. 2022;20:62.
14. Xu J, Gong XL, Wu H, et al. Case report: gastrointestinal PEComa with TFE3 rearrangement treated with anti-VEGFR TKI apatinib. Front Oncol. 2020;10:582087.
15. Liebow AA, Castleman B. Benign "clear cell tumors" of the lung. Am J Pathol. 1963;43:13a–4a.
16. Liebow AA, Castleman B. Benign clear cell ("sugar") tumor tumors of the lung. Yale J Biol Med. 1971;43:213–22.
17. Ntanasis-Stathopoulos I, Kyriazoglou A, Tsilimigras DI, et al. Clear cell sugar tumor of the lung; a systematic review for a rare entity. J BUON. 2021;26:17–32.
18. Gunji-Niitsu Y, Kumasaka T, Kitamura S, et al. Benign clear cell "sugar" tumor of the lung in a patient with Birt-Hogg-Dubé syndrome: a case report. BMC Med Genet. 2016;17:85.
19. Folpe AL, Mentzel T, Lehr HA, et al. Perivascular epithelioid cell neoplasms of soft tissue and gynecologic origin: a clinicopathologic study of 26 cases and review of the literature. Am J Surg Pathol. 2005;29:1558–75.
20. Parfitt JR, Keith JL, Megyesi JF, et al. Metastatic PEComa to the brain. Acta Neuropathol. 2006,112:349–51.

Lymphangioleiomyomatosis

Xue-Peng Huang and Song Zhang

Lymphangioleiomyomatosis (LAM) is a rare, slowly progressive, neoplastic disease characterized by infiltration and proliferation of abnormal smooth muscle-like LAM cells, leading to the destruction of lung parenchyma and formation of diffuse thin-walled cysts in lungs. Multisystem involvement can occur with formation of fluid-filled cystic structures in the axial lymphatics such as lymphangioleiomyomas and renal angiomyolipomas (AMLs).

1 Pathology

Histologically, LAM is characterized by proliferation of peculiar smooth muscle cells (LAM cells) in the bronchioles, pulmonary veins, and lymphatic vessels, leading to obstruction of the airways, thickening of the vascular walls, lymphatic disruption, venous occlusion, and hemorrhage.

There are two types of LAM cells: small, spindle-shaped cells that are centrally located in the LAM nodules and large, epithelioid cells in the periphery. Both types of cells are immunoreactive for smooth muscle antigens, such as α-actin, vimentin, and desmin. The spindle-shaped cells are positive for proliferating cell nuclear antigen (PCNA), indicating a proliferative phenotype. The epithelioid cells show reactivity to HMB-45 monoclonal antibody and estrogen and progesterone receptors [1]. Beta-catenin has been identified as another potential marker for LAM and had higher immunoreactivity to LAM cell than HMB-45, ER-α, and PR [2].

2 Molecular Features

LAM cells arise from an unknown source and deposit in the lungs via the lymphatic system or bloodstream, causing parenchymal destruction and cystic disease. Crooks et al. [3] isolated circulating LAM cells in the blood, urine, and chylous effusion from LAM patients. This study is compatible with a multisite origin for LAM cells and confirms the existence of disseminated, potentially metastatic LAM cells. To date, the source of LAM cells may be the uterus, pelvis, angiomyolipomas, the lymphatic system, and the bone marrow.

LAM may occur sporadically (S-LAM) or in association with the tuberous sclerosis complex (TSC-LAM). Mutations of the tumor suppressor genes TSC1and TSC2 can occur in both S-LAM

X.-P. Huang
Department of Respiratory and Critical Care Medicine, People's Hospital of Rizhao Lanshan, Rizhao, Shandong, China

S. Zhang (✉)
Department of Respiratory and Critical Care Medicine, Shandong Provincial Hospital Affiliated to Shandong First Medical University, Jinan, Shandong, China

S. Zhang (ed.), *Diagnostic Imaging of Lung Cancers*, https://doi.org/10.1007/978-981-99-6815-2_17

and TSC-LAM and activate the mechanistic target of rapamycin (mTOR) signaling pathway that regulates multiple cellular functions including growth, motility, and survival and ultimately leads to cell growth and proliferation. LAM cells with TSC2 loss of heterozygosity (LOH) were detected in more than 90% of blood samples. LAM cells in most S-LAM patients have a common genetic origin, consistent with a metastatic model. In some cases, however, there was evidence for genetic heterogeneity between LAM cells in different sites or within a site [4].

LAM cells also express the lymphangiogenic growth factor, vascular endothelial growth factor C and D (VEGF-C and VEGF-D), which stimulate the formation of lymphatic channels within and around LAM cells that likely facilitate access to the circulation and metastatic spread [5, 6].

Increased matrix metalloproteinases (MMPs) play an important role in the pathogenesis of LAM. MMPs can destroy the extracellular matrix, thus promoting cell migration and cystic formation in the lungs. Hayashi et al. [7] confirmed that MMP-2 and MMP-9 (both of which can degrade elastin and collagens) are responsible for the connective tissue destruction and cyst formation in LAM. Zhe et al. [8] found that tissue inhibitor of metalloproteinase (TIMP)-3, one of MMP inhibitors, is down-regulated in LAM lesions and ubiquitously presents in normal lung parenchyma. Odajima et al. [9] found that serum levels of MMP-9, but not MMP-2, were significantly elevated in LAM patients compared with controls. Lee et al. [10] concluded that TSC1/TSC2 deficiency leads to MMP-2 overproduction that is rapamycin-insensitive.

Female hormones are implicated in the pathogenesis of LAM based on the predominance of LAM in females and exacerbations of LAM during exposures to estrogen supplementation, such as pregnancy, hormonal contraception and during menstruation. LAM cells express estrogen and progesterone receptors. Estrogen is an important driver of LAM cell proliferation, migration, and metastasis. Attenuation in the rate of FEV1 decline after menopause further supports a role for estrogen in the pathogenesis of LAM [11].

3 Epidemiology

S-LAM accounts for about 85% of LAM patients and occurs almost exclusively in reproductive women, with few cases developing before puberty or after menopause. LAM can also occur in males with TSC. Ryu et al. [12] described the clinical characteristics of pulmonary LAM (PLAM). All 230 patients were women, aged 18–76 year (mean 44.5 ± 0.65 year). The average age at onset of symptoms was 38.9 ± 0.73 year and at diagnosis was 41.0 ± 0.65 year. TSC was present in 14.8% of patients.

Very few cases have been reported in men without TSC. Schiavina et al. [13] reported an unequivocal case of PLAM occurring in a 37-year-old man with no clinical or genotypic evidence of TSC. Moreover, the HMB-45-positive cells lining the cysts also showed strong reactivity for estrogen and progesterone receptor proteins. The case indicates that TSC is not a necessary condition for onset of LAM in men.

Johnson et al. [14] identified 50 cases of LAMs in the UK over a five-year period. The median age at onset was 35 years (range 22–50). Five presented when postmenopausal (four taking hormone replacement therapy). The five-year period prevalence was one per 1.1 million population in UK. Another epidemiological survey conducted in seven countries including in the USA, UK, and Switzerland found that the incidence of PLAM is approximately 3.4–7.8 per million women [15], but the true prevalence is probably higher because many patients with LAM are undiagnosed.

LAM occurs in at least 40% of women with TSC. Cudzilo et al. [16] studied 133 female patients with TSC aged $\geq$15 years. Forty-eight (47.5%, 48/101) met the criteria of TSC-LAM on the initial CT scan. The risk of LAM was age dependent, rising by about 8% per year. The prevalence of LAM was 27% in subjects $<$21 years and 81% in subjects $>$40 years. Most women with TSC ultimately develop cystic changes consistent with LAM, and TSC-LAM was associated with appreciable morbidity and mortality in this referral population.

4 Clinical Features

Recurrent pneumothorax and dyspnea are the most common presenting features, leading to progressive loss of lung function, and sometimes resulting in respiratory failure and death. About 50%–80% of patients have one or more pneumothoraces and tend to recur. Patients with larger cysts are more likely to occur pneumothorax [17]. A study confirmed that the incidence of frequent pneumothorax in LAM is 1000 times higher than in the general female population and is further increased threefold after air travel [18]. Another frequent presentation is dyspnea on exertion, which worsens with time. Cohen et al. [19] found that the main symptoms of LAM patients were dyspnea (74%), fatigue (72%), cough (47%), and chest pain (44%); younger patients (<40 years) were less likely to report dyspnea. TSC patients were less likely to report dyspnea and 76.5% reported angiomyolipoma compared with S-LAM patients. Patients with pneumothorax (63.0%) were less likely to report dyspnea or fatigue than patients without pneumothorax. A possible explanation is that the occurrence of pneumothorax prompts lung imaging studies to detect the presence of lung cysts and lead to diagnosis. Other respiratory symptoms include cough, chest pain, hemoptysis, and chyloptysis. Obstruction of pulmonary venules causes vascular congestion, pulmonary venous hypertension, and hemoptysis, and the rupture of dilated and tortuous venules leads to hemosiderosis.

Lymphatic manifestations of LAM include thoracic duct wall invasion, lymphangioleiomyoma formation, chylous fluid collections in the pleural, peritoneal, and pericardial spaces, chylous pulmonary congestion, chyloptysis, chylocolporrheal chylometrorrhea, chyle leak from the umbilicus, lymphadenopathy, and lower extremity lymphedema [20]. Avila et al. [21] analyzed 80 patients with LAM underwent chest and abdominopelvic CT and abdominopelvic ultrasonographic. Sixty-one patients (76%) had positive abdominal findings, including renal AML in 43 patients (54%), enlarged abdominal lymph nodes in 31 (39%), and lymphangiomyoma in 13 (16%), ascites in eight (10%), dilatation of the thoracic duct in seven (9%), and hepatic AML in three (4%). A significant correlation was found between enlarged abdominal lymph nodes and increased severity of lung disease.

5 Radiographic Features

On chest CT, lung cysts are essential for the diagnosis of LAM and are present in all patients. LAM cysts are thin-walled, bilateral, diffusely distributed, round, 2–5 mm in diameter but occasionally as large as 30 mm, and typically devoid of internal structure. The cysts are typically symmetrical and uniformly distributed throughout the lungs. There is normal-appearing lung parenchyma between the cystic areas (Fig. 1). The diameter of lung cysts tends to increase with dis-

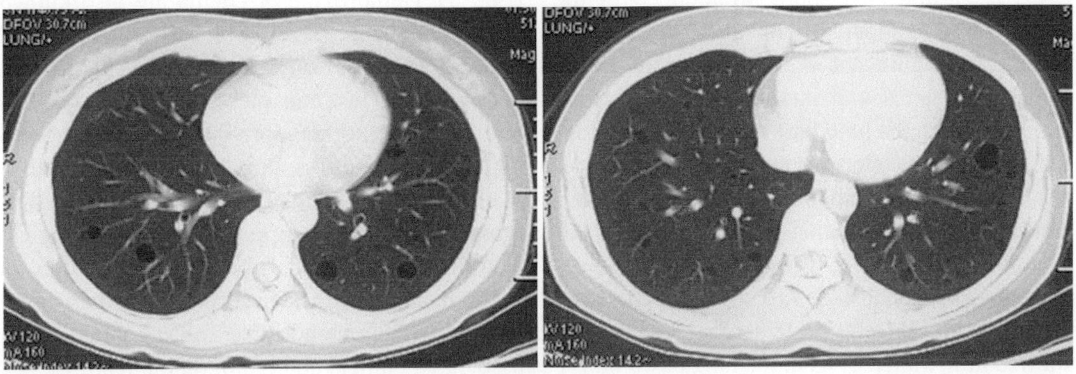

Fig. 1 HRCT in a 35-year-old woman with S-LAM demonstrates characteristic thin-walled cysts with normal intervening lung

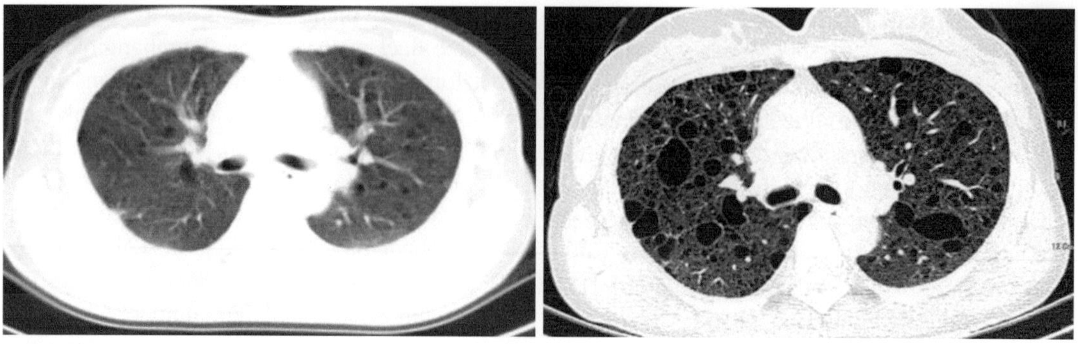

Fig. 2 HRCT in a 32-year-old woman with S-LAM demonstrates disease progression over a 4-year period with an increase in size and number of cysts

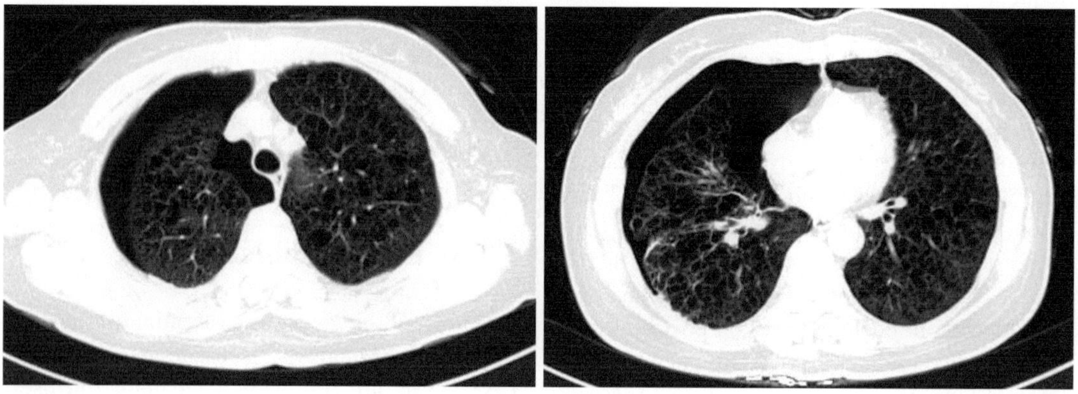

Fig. 3 HRCT in a 48-year-old woman with S-LAM demonstrates thin-walled cysts with right-sided pneumothorax

ease progression (Fig. 2). Cysts progressively replace the lung parenchyma and result in the development of pneumothoraces (Fig. 3). In severe cases, nearly all of the normal lung parenchyma is replaced (Fig. 4). Theilig et al. [22] found that the distribution of cystic lesions in LAM is significantly more pronounced in the central lung compared with peripheral areas. There is a significant predominance of cystic changes in apical and intermediate lung zones compared with the lung bases. Some studies suggested that cystic changes are prevalent in upper or lower zones. Nonetheless, segmental predominance is not clearly demonstrated.

Adriaensen et al. [23] performed a retrospective, cross-sectional study in a cohort of 206 adult TSC patients. Fifty-two (28%, 52/186) patients showed thin-walled cysts in the lung bases on CT scan. Pulmonary cysts were detected in 42% (40/95) female patients and in 13% (12/91) male patients. On the whole, cysts were larger and more numerous in women than in men.

Pneumothorax, pleural effusion, and chylothorax are common complications of LAM (Fig. 5). Hemorrhage or edema are also known complications of LAM, which result in ground glass attenuation. Kobylianskii et al. [24] reported a 40-year-old woman presenting with dyspnea and self-limiting hemoptysis. Chest CT showed diffuse ground glass opacities and small thin-walled cysts. She underwent video-assisted thoracoscopic lung biopsy. Histopathological examination revealed LAM and hemosiderosis without capillaritis, confirming a diagnosis of diffuse alveolar hemorrhage in the context of the associated clinical and radiographic features.

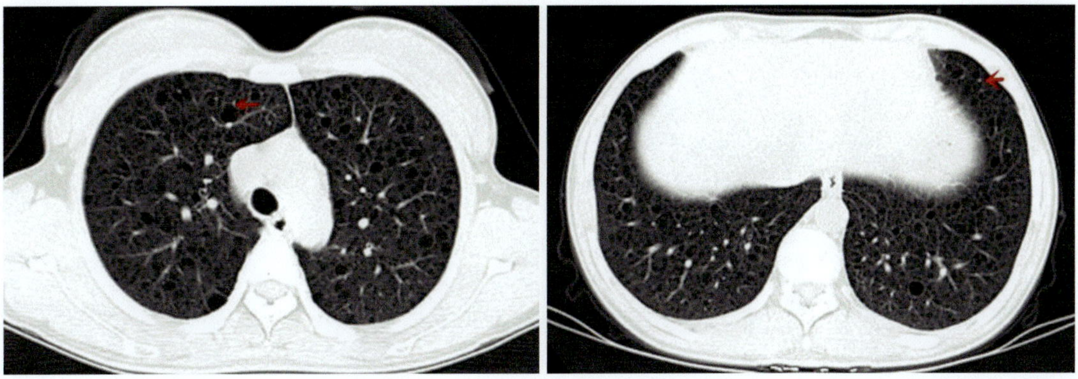

Fig. 4 HRCT in a 40-year-old woman with S-LAM demonstrates diffuse severe thin-walled cysts with eccentric vessels on the margin of cysts (red arrow)

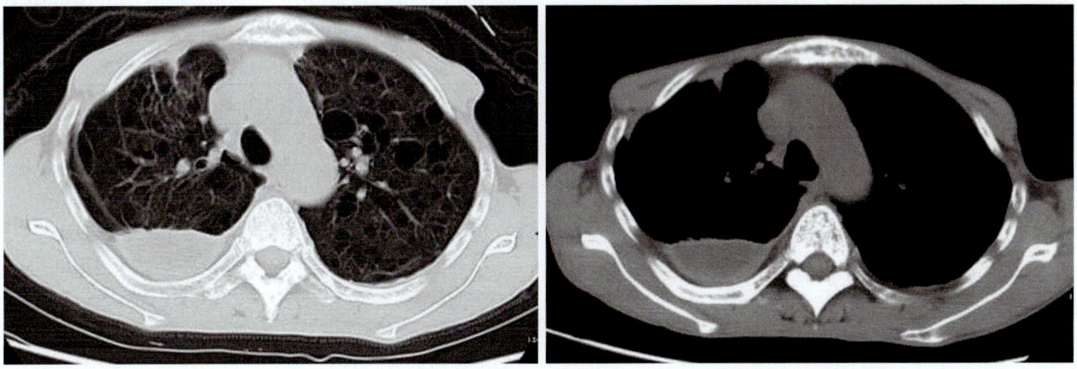

Fig. 5 HRCT in a 51-year-old woman with S-LAM demonstrates thin-walled cysts with right-sided chylothorax

Renal AML is the most frequent abdominal lesions and usually manifests as asymptomatic, small, bilateral tumors of fat attenuation in the renal cortex. AML, lymphangioleiomyomas, lymphadenopathy, and ascites may be found by CT scans, ultrasonography, or magnetic resonance imaging (Fig. 6).

Compared with TSC-LAM, S-LAM had more extensive lung involvement and lymphatic involvement, including higher frequency of lymphangioleiomyoma, thoracic duct dilatation, chylous pleural effusion, or ascites. While hepatic and renal AMLs and noncalcified lung nodules are more common in TSC-LAM [25].

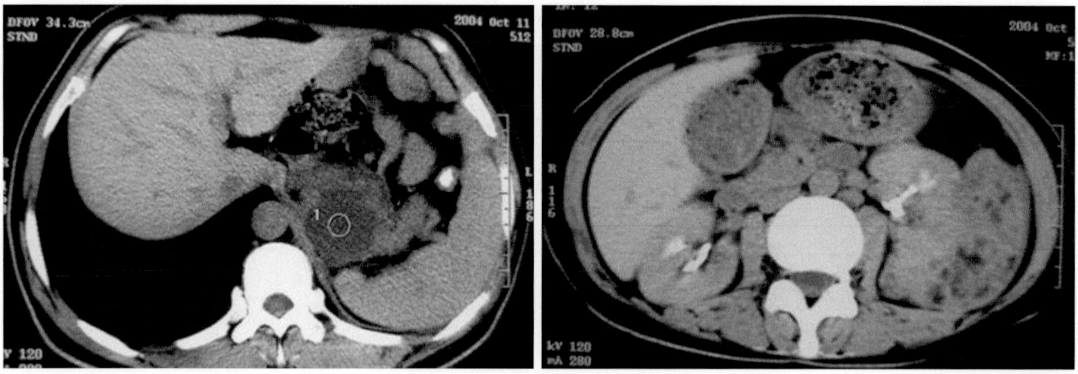

Fig. 6 HRCT in a 36-year-old woman with S-LAM demonstrates abdominal lymphadenopathy and left-sided AML

6 Diagnostic Criteria

The definitive diagnosis of LAM requires tissue or cytological confirmation, but a chest CT scan revealing diffuse, thin-walled cystic change is the key to correct diagnosis. European Respiratory Society (ERS) guidelines on LAM were published in 2010 [26], the diagnostic criteria were as follows: Definite LAM: (1) Characteristic or compatible lung HRCT, and lung biopsy fitting the pathological criteria for LAM; or (2) Characteristic lung HRCT and any of the following: angiomyolipoma (kidney); thoracic or abdominal chylous effusion; lymphangioleiomyoma or lymph-node involved by LAM; and definite or probable TSC. Probable LAM: (1) Characteristic HRCT and compatible clinical history; or (2) Compatible HRCT and any of the following: angiomyolipoma (kidney); and thoracic or abdominal chylous effusion. Possible LAM: Characteristic or compatible HRCT. The diagnosis criteria are only for females. HRCT features characteristic of LAM are multiple (>10) thin-walled round well-defined air-filled cysts with preserved or increased lung volume with no other significant pulmonary involvement specifically no interstitial lung disease with the exception of possible features of multifocal micronodular pneumocyte hyperplasia in patients with TSC. HRCT features are compatible with pulmonary LAM when only few (>2 and ≤10) cysts as described are present. Compatible clinical features include pneumothorax (especially multiple and/or bilateral) and/or altered lung function tests as in LAM. All patients with LAM or suspected LAM should have an abdominopelvic CT at diagnosis or during work-up to identify angiomyolipoma and other abdominal lesions. Patients with abdominal symptoms should be evaluated for the presence of lymphadenopathy or lymphangioleiomyomas by CT scanning (reproduced with permission of the © ERS 2023: European Respiratory Journal 35 (1) 14–26; DOI: 10.1183/09031936.00076209 Published 31 December 2009).

Official American Thoracic Society (ATS)/Japanese Respiratory Society (JRS) clinical practice guidelines on LAM were published in 2016 [27]. They recommend VEGF-D testing for patients whose CT scan shows cystic abnormalities characteristic of LAM but have no confirmatory clinical or extrapulmonary radiologic features of LAM, and that consider to proceed to diagnostic lung biopsy. Confirmatory features of LAM include TSC, AMLs, chylous pleural effusions or ascites, and cystic lymphangioleiomyomas. They recommend the higher VEGF-D threshold of 800 pg/mL.

Hirose et al. [28] found that serum VEGF-D measurements in Japan and the United States were very similar. Baseline serum VEGF-D levels effectively differentiated LAM from other diseases and healthy volunteers at a cut-off level of 645 pg/mL and were diagnostically specific at 800 pg/mL, which was consistent with the recommendations of the ATS/JRS LAM Guidelines.

Serum VEGF-D levels significantly decreased during treatment with sirolimus, but not with gonadotrophin-releasing hormone (GnRH) analogues.

7 Differential Diagnosis

The differential diagnosis of LAM includes emphysema, pulmonary Langerhans cell histiocytosis (PLCH), Birt–Hogg–Dubé syndrome (BHD), follicular bronchiolitis, lymphoid interstitial pneumonia (LIP), amyloidosis, light chain disease, allergic alveolitis, bronchiectasis, Meunier–Kuhn syndrome, sarcoidosis, pneumoconiosis, and chronic lung infectious processes.

Most of these diseases can be discriminated based on clinical, histopathological, and radiologic findings. The radiological characteristics of cysts, including distribution, wall thickness, internal structure, and relationship to other structures, can provide helpful clues. The presence of nodules, thicker cyst walls, upper lobe predominance, atypical cyst shapes, and relative sparing of the bases could indicate PLCH. Cysts with multiple, thin-walled, round or elliptical, predominant in the lower subpleural medial regions, often paramediastinal, and closely associated with pleura and blood vessels are characteristic of BHD. Follicular bronchiolitis or LIP is more variable in size, usually contains internal septae, and is bordered by eccentric vessels. Cystic lesions are rare, thin-walled and peripherally distributed in localized amyloidosis.

8 Treatment

The association between mTOR signaling and LAM pathogenesis led to the investigation of mTOR inhibitors for treatment of LAM. In 2008, an open-label, uncontrolled trial in which 25 patients with TSC or LAM were treated with escalating doses of sirolimus (also called rapamycin) for 12 months, followed by an observation period of 1 year showed that angiomyolipomas regressed somewhat during sirolimus treatment but tended to increase in volume after the treatment was stopped. Some lymphangioleiomyomatosis patients had improvement in spirometric measurements and gas trapping that persisted after treatment [29]. Sirolimus was recommended in patients with TSC-related or sporadic renal AMLs. In 2011, another two-stage trial of sirolimus involving 89 patients with LAM revealed that a 12-month treatment of sirolimus effectively stabilized the trend of a decline in forced expiratory volume in 1 s (FEV1), reduced serum VEGF-D levels, and was associated with a reduction in symptoms and improvement in quality of life [30]. Based on this study, sirolimus was approved for the treatment of LAM in Japan in 2014, and in the United States in 2015. The ATS/JRS guideline recommended sirolimus for those whose pulmonary function is reduced (FEV1 less than 70% predicted) or rapidly declining (FEV1 loss more than 90 mL per year) or who have symptomatic chylothorax/chylous ascites. Sakurai et al. [31] first reported sirolimus might effectively suppress the recurrence of pneumothoraces in LAM patients who received surgical pleural covering of entire lung (SPC). A study by Hu et al. [32] found that sirolimus therapy is effective at improving or stabilizing pulmonary function, oxygen levels, exercise capacity, and quality of life in LAM patients for up to 4 years. VEGF-D is maintained at a lower level for 4 years after therapy. Adverse events related to sirolimus were mild. Revilla-López et al. [33] retrospectively reviewed a series of 48 patients with LAM diagnosed, followed up and treated with sirolimus in a single center. After 5 years of sirolimus therapy, 59% had a positive response, 30% had a partial response, and 11% had a negative response. They concluded that sirolimus therapy had a positive long-term effect on most LAM patients.

The ATS/JRS guideline did not recommend using hormone therapy for LAM because it is known to worsen with exposure to estrogen and improves in the postmenopausal period. Hormonal therapies include progestins, GnRH agonists, selective estrogen receptor modulators like tamoxifen, and oophorectomy. Estrogen-based contraceptives are contraindicated. If patients are receiving estrogen-containing products at the time of diagnosis, this should be discontinued. Patient with advanced LAM should be advised to avoid pregnancy and to commence sirolimus rather than delay.

Proteolytic enzymes such as matrix metalloproteinases (MMPs) may degrade the extracellular matrix and contributes to cyst formation in patients with LAM. Doxycycline is a tetracycline antibiotic that effectively inhibits the production and activity of several MMPs, including MMP-2 and MMP-9. The ATS/JRS guideline did not recommend using doxycycline as treatment for LAM because no beneficial effects due to doxycycline therapy were confirmed in patients with LAM who had respiratory impairment.

Wang et al. [34] analyzed 14 prospective studies regarding five pharmacological treatments (including sirolimus, everolimus, triptorelin, doxycycline, and a combination therapy of sirolimus and hydroxychloroquine). Sirolimus and everolimus were recommended for the treatment of LAM because they may stabilize lung function and alleviate renal AML. Triptorelin(a GnRH antagonist) and doxycycline were not recommended for the treatment of LAM because no beneficial outcomes were consistently observed.

Lung transplantation is an increasingly viable option for end-stage respiratory failure in LAM. In 1984, Estenne et al. [35] reported the first case of lung transplantation for LAM. In the United States, the 1-, 5-, and 10-year survival rates for lung transplantation in LAM were 94%, 73%, and 56%, respectively. The median survival after lung transplantation in LAM is 12 years and is substantially better than in other lung diseases [36]. The use of rapamycin in patients awaiting lung transplant is controversial. A survey suggested favorable outcomes for those patients that did continue mTOR inhibitor up to time of transplant [37].

9 Prognosis

Data from the LAM Foundation indicated that the estimated median transplant-free survival time for LAM patients in the United States was 29 years after symptom onset and 23 years after diagnosis. The 10-year survival transplant free was 86%. Age at disease onset, race, smoking status, presence of TSC, occurrence of pneumothorax, and pregnancy did not demonstrate an association with survival or transplant. Greater age at diagnosis and presence of angiomyolipoma were associated with better survival [38].

Records from the National Heart, Lung, and Blood Institute (NHLBI) LAM registry suggested that the estimated 5-, 10-, 15-, and 20-year transplant-free survival rates were 94%, 85%, 75%, and 64%, respectively. The median survival in patients with LAM since diagnosis is >20 years. Menopausal status, as well as structural and physiologic markers of disease severity, significantly affects the rate of decline of FEV 1 and progression to death or lung transplantation in LAM [11]. Survival is expected to improve further with the use of mTOR inhibitor sirolimus (rapamycin) for the treatment of LAM.

Yoon et al. [39] retrospectively analyzed the clinical data of 104 patients with LAM. Among all patients, the mean age was 40.3 years. Over a median follow-up period of 7.1 years, 6.7% of all patients died and 1.9% underwent lung transplantation, while 35.9% of 92 patients with serial lung function data experienced disease progression. The 5- and 10-year survival rates were 93.0% and 90.9%, respectively. Older age, lower lung function, and poorer exercise capacity were associated with a poor prognosis in LAM patients.

Harari et al. [40] described changes in the management and natural history of LAM following the publication of the ERS and the ATS/JRS guidelines and the introduction of sirolimus. The cumulative incidence of mortality after 5 years was significantly lower in patients who entered the observation since 2011 (after publication of the MILES trial) than in patients who entered the observation before 2011.The emergence of sirolimus and the publication of international guidelines changed the natural history of LAM lowering the mortality and reducing the need of invasive diagnostic techniques.

Pregnancy in women with LAM may increase complications and worsen lung function. Taveira-DaSilva et al. [41] assessed CT scans and lung function before and after pregnancy in 16 women with LAM. Pneumothorax was frequent and mean FEV1 fell from 77% ± 19% prepregnancy to 64% ± 25% predicted and DL CO from 66 ± 26 to 57 ± 26 during the pregnancy. Women with LAM, especially with moderate or advanced disease should be consulted on adverse events and loss of lung function during the pregnancy.

10 Case Analysis

10.1 Case 1

A 31-year-old woman was hospitalized 8 times for recurrent pneumothorax.

Chest CT: Numerous thin-walled cysts with left-sided pneumothorax (Fig. 7).

[Diagnosis] Pulmonary lymphangioleiomyomatosis.

[Diagnosis Basis] The chest CT shows diffuse distribution of thin-walled cysts, unequal in size, and recurrent pneumothorax in a woman of childbearing age, which is consistent with the typical performance of PLAM. She was never a smoker, and her renal ultrasound was negative for renal angiomyolipoma. The patient underwent multiple closed thoracic drainage and chemical pleurodesis, and video-assisted thoracoscopic wedge resection. Histopathological examination confirmed the final diagnosis of PLAM (Fig. 8).

[Analysis] Patients with LAM have a greater risk of developing spontaneous pneumothoraces because of smooth muscle hyperplasia, airway narrowing, and alveolar damage.

Pleurodesis is a viable option to prevent recurrent pneumothoraces through lung re-expansion. ERS LAM guidelines recommend chemical pleurodesis for first pneumothorax. Patients who do not respond to initial therapy including pleurodesis should undergo an appropriate surgical procedure. The ATS/JTS guidelines recommend surgical intervention after an initial pneumothorax rather than postponing the procedure until the first recurrence and against

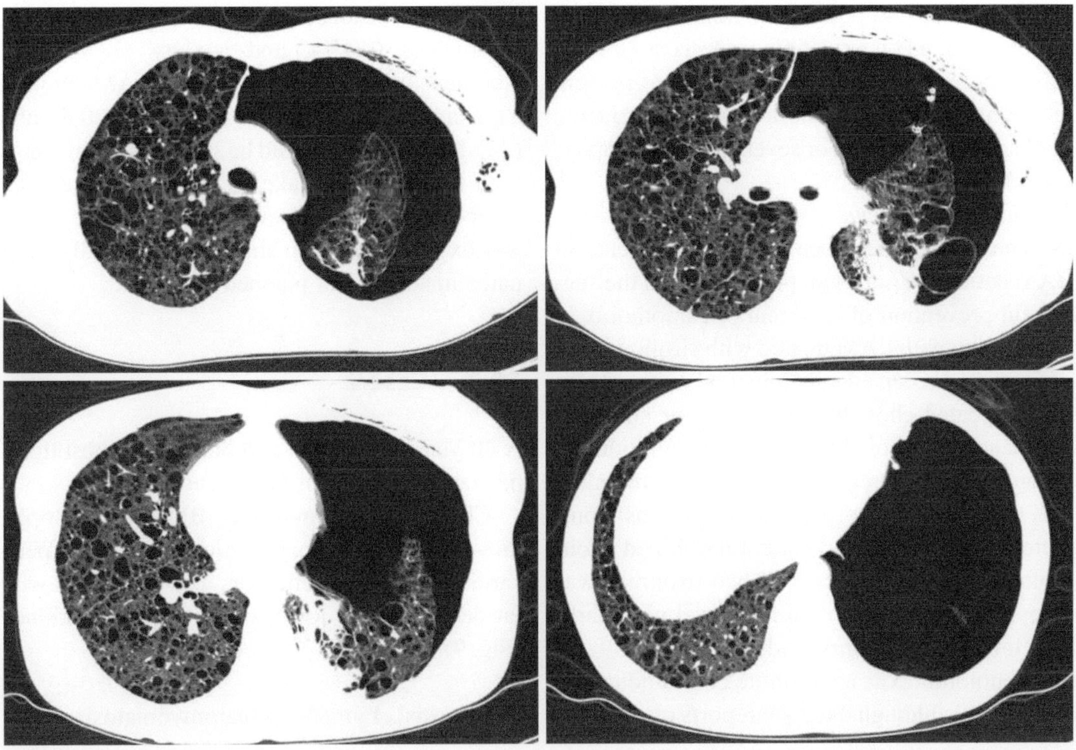

Fig. 7 Chest CT

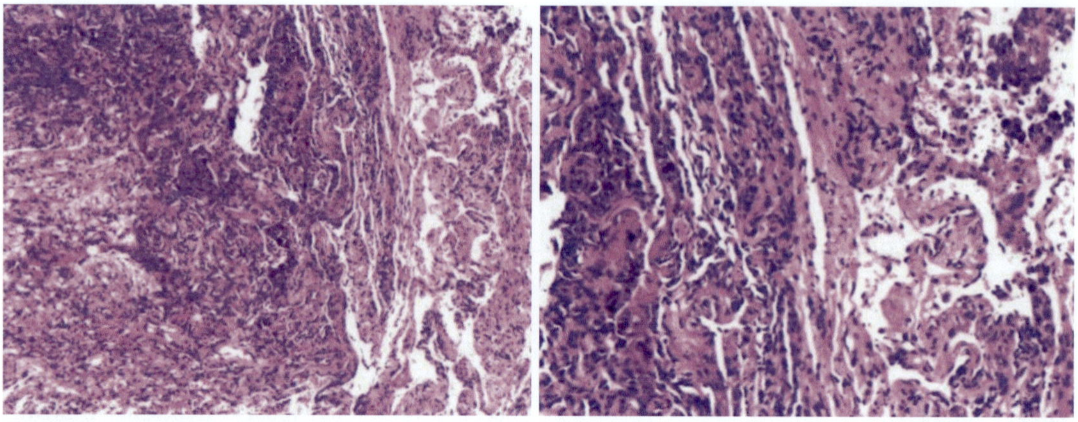

Fig. 8 Histopathology shows closely communicating lymphatic vessels and smooth muscle hyperplasia

pleurodesis being used as a reason to exclude patients from lung transplantation.

Recently, total pleural covering (TPC) and modified TPC (mTPC) were recommended as surgical treatment options for patients with LAM-associated pneumothorax. TPC is an innovative surgical procedure in which the entire visceral pleura is covered with sheets of oxidized regenerated cellulose (ORC) mesh. Suzuki et al. [42] evaluated the effects of TPC on pneumothorax recurrence and pulmonary function in LAM patients with no history of pleurodesis or thoracic surgeries. They found that TPC can prevent recurrence of pneumothorax without causing ventilatory impairment or severe pleural symphysis in LAM patients.

Some studies have confirmed that sirolimus may prevent further pneumothorax incidents in LAM patients. Zhou et al. [43] described the successful prevention of recurrent pneumothorax in five women with LAM treated with sirolimus. All patients had received supplemental oxygen support, repeated chest tube drainage, or surgeries for management of the recurrent pneumothorax before sirolimus treatment. Sirolimus treatment was used when the pneumothorax was completely resolved, and no patient developed pneumothorax during treatment. When sirolimus was stopped or the plasma sirolimus level was markedly low, pneumothorax tended to relapse.

Pneumothorax is an absolute contraindication to air travel although there are reports of uneventful air travel for those with chronic stable pneumothorax. Air travel may increase the risk of pneumothorax in patients with LAM through rupture of subpleural cysts induced by ambient barometric pressure change. A survey of 327 LAM patients reported a rate of 2.2% for pneumothorax in flight. Other reported symptoms during air travel included shortness of breath (14%), nausea or dizziness (8%), chest pain (12%), unusual fatigue (11%), oxygen desaturation (8%), headache (9%), blue hands (2%), hemoptysis (0.4%), and anxiety (22%) [44]. Another study of 281 patients with LAM reported a pneumothorax rate of 2.9% (1.1 per 100 flights) [45]. In general, it should be safe for most patients with LAM to undertake air travel. Patients with symptoms of sudden/new chest pain, dyspnea, or low oxygen saturation should be medically evaluated in advance of planned air travel.

10.2 Case 2

A 40-year-old woman complained of chest tightness and shortness of breath for 1 week.

Chest and abdomen CT: Bilateral, multiple, thin-walled pulmonary cystic lesions with pericardial, left pleural effusion, and solid mass with fat density in the lower part of the right kidney (Fig. 9).

[Diagnosis] Lymphangioleiomyomatosis.

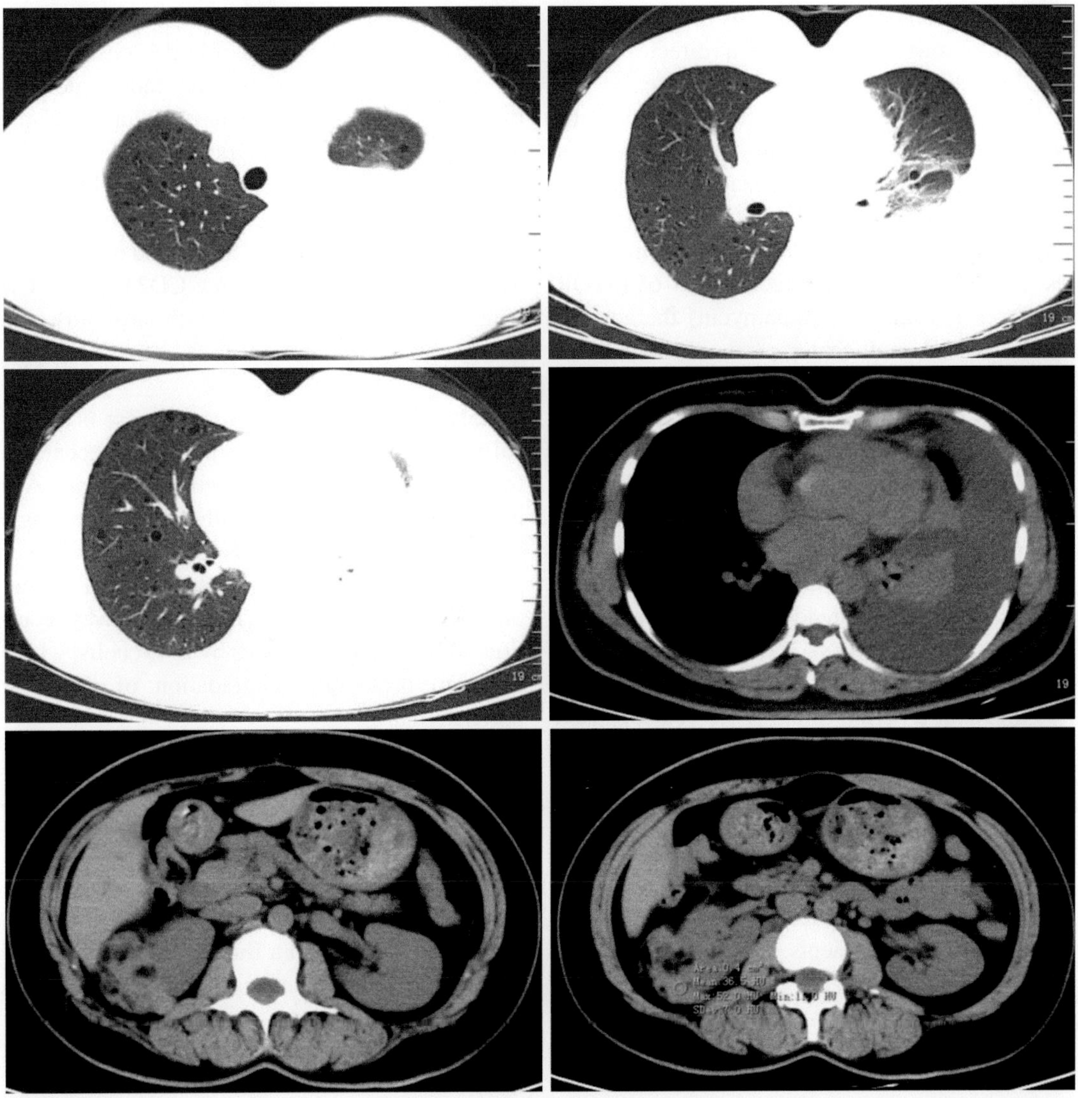

Fig. 9 Chest and abdomen CT

[Diagnosis Basis] The chest and abdomen CT reveals multiple lung cysts, pericardial effusion, pleural effusion, and renal angiomyolipoma (AML), which is consistent with the typical performance of LAM.

[Analysis] LAM is a rare disease characterized by proliferation of abnormal LAM cells resulting in cystic lung disease, lymphatic abnormalities, and abdominal tumors.

Extrapulmonary involvement of LAM includes benign mixed mesenchymal tumors called AMLs and abdominal lymphatic masses called lymphangioleiomyomas. AMLs are tumors composed of aberrantly differentiated cells that contain three dysmorphic components resembling adipocytes, smooth muscle-like cells, and vascular cells. AMLs occur primarily in the kidneys but can occur in the liver, lung, bowel, bladder wall, etc. Renal AMLs are found in approximately 30%–50% of patients with S-LAM and 90% of those with TSC-LAM. Carsillo et al. [46] demonstrated that somatic mutations in the TSC2 gene occur in the

AMLs and pulmonary LAM cells of women with S-LAM, strongly supporting a direct role of TSC2 in the pathogenesis of this disease.

Bleeding is the main risk for AMLs. On the basis of ERS guidelines, the management of renal AMLs included embolization therapy for actively bleeding patients or nephron-sparing surgery for tumors larger than 4 cm. Some studies have confirmed the effectiveness of mTOR inhibitors (sirolimus or rapamycin) therapy for renal AMLs. A multicenter, randomized, double-blind, placebo-controlled trial (EXIST-2) by Bissler et al. [47] showed that 42% of patients with TSC or S-LAM achieved a response defined as 50% reduction of tumor volume. Further research showed that a total of 58% of 112 patients who received ≥1 dose of everolimus achieved AML response during approximately 4 years. No AML-related bleeding or nephrectomies were reported [48]. Taveira-DaSilva et al. [49] found that sirolimus therapy stabilized lung function over a period of 4.5 ± 1.6 years, caused resolution of lymphatic disease, and reduced the size of AMLs and VEGF-D levels. Watanabe et al. [50] analyzed the effects of sirolimus on different components of AMLs. Their study showed that sirolimus reduces the size of AMLs by decreasing primarily their highly-vascularized and fat-poor compartments.

10.3 Case 3

A 35-year-old woman complained of abdominal distension for more than half a year and found a retroperitoneal mass for 1 day. She has a history of emphysema for 3 years.

Chest and abdomen CT: Bilateral, multiple, thin-walled pulmonary cystic lesions, and cystic masses in the retroperitoneum (Fig. 10).

[Diagnosis] Lymphangioleiomyomatosis.

[Diagnosis Basis] The chest and abdomen CT of a woman of childbearing age shows multiple thin-walled pulmonary cystic lesions and cystic masses in the retroperitoneum known as lymphangioleiomyomas. The lower boundary of the abdominal lesion reaches the pelvic cavity (red arrow). The diagnosis of LAM is established by clinical manifestations and radiologic features. The patient underwent a biopsy of the abdominal tumor. Histologically, it was considered a tumor with perivascular epithelioid cell differentiation (Fig. 11a). Immunohistochemistry was positive for HMB-45, SMA, and negative for Melan A, S-100, Desmin, CD34, and CR (Fig. 11b). She was treated with sirolimus, and her symptoms relieved partially.

[Analysis] Diffuse cystic lung disease is a typical feature of S-LAM. One possible mechanism for cyst formation is the growth of nodular LAM lesions in the lumens of small airways, creating a "ball valve" effect that leads to over-expansion of the terminal alveolar units and eventual formation of cysts. Another mechanism involves secretion of proteolytic enzymes by LAM cells, which leads to proteolytic degradation of the lung parenchyma.

Lymphatic involvement in LAM occurs in the retroperitoneum, pelvis, and posterior mediastinum and is composed of lymphangioleiomyomas, lymphadenopathy, pleural effusions, and ascites. Lymphangioleiomyomas are chyle-filled encapsulated lymphatic masses comprising an outer wall and a fluid-rich region central region and are characterized by a proliferation of LAM cells arranged in fascicular, trabecular, and papillary patterns, which are associated with slit-like vascular channels. Lymphangioleiomyomas may compress adjacent organs and cause symptoms such as back pain, bloating, abdominal pain, urinary frequency, constipation, and edema of the lower extremities. Biopsy helps to diagnose lymphangioleiomyoma and to rule out a malignant neoplasm. Lymphangioleiomyomas may exhibit diurnal variation in size, enlarging during the day and shrinking during the night, which may explain worsening of symptoms during the day [51]. Taveira-DaSilva et al. [52] found that the volume of lymphangioleiomyoma decreased during the fasting state. Conversely, a combination of food intake and decreased chyle flow through lymphatics partially obstructed by

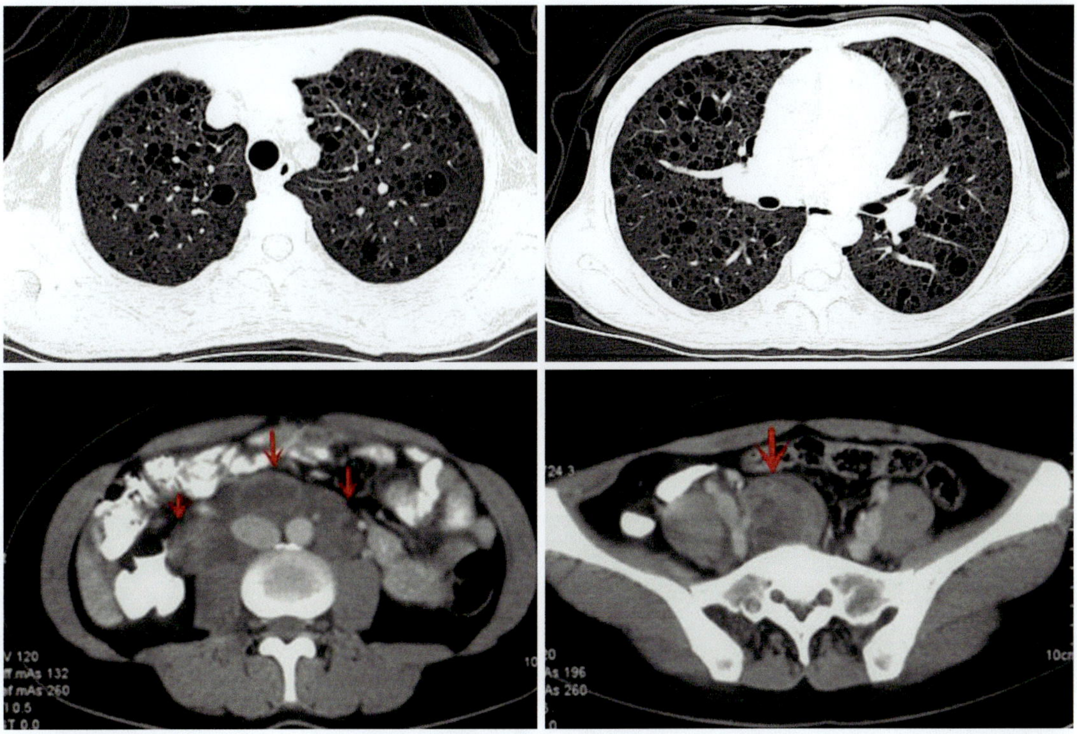

Fig. 10 Chest and abdomen CT

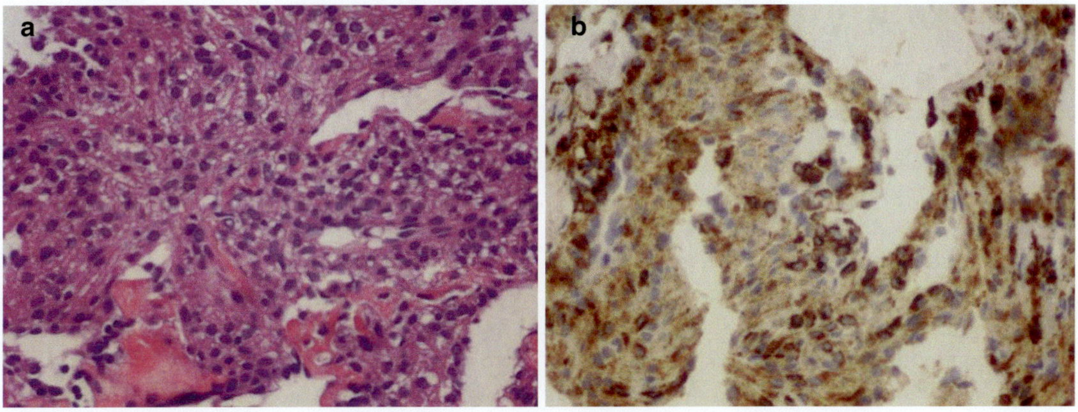

Fig. 11 (**a**) Microscopic examination reveals a proliferation of spindle-shaped to epithelioid cells with pale eosinophilic cytoplasm (hematoxylin-eosin, 200×). (**b**) The neoplastic cells are positive for HMB-45

LAM cells may be the reason for the increase in lymphangioleiomyoma size. Imaging studies performed under fasting conditions may help in differentiating whether an abdominal tumor is a result of LAM or malignancy.

10.4 Case 4

A 46-year-old woman complained of dyspnea for more than 1 month. Physical examination revealed multiple brownish papules on the face (Fig. 12a).

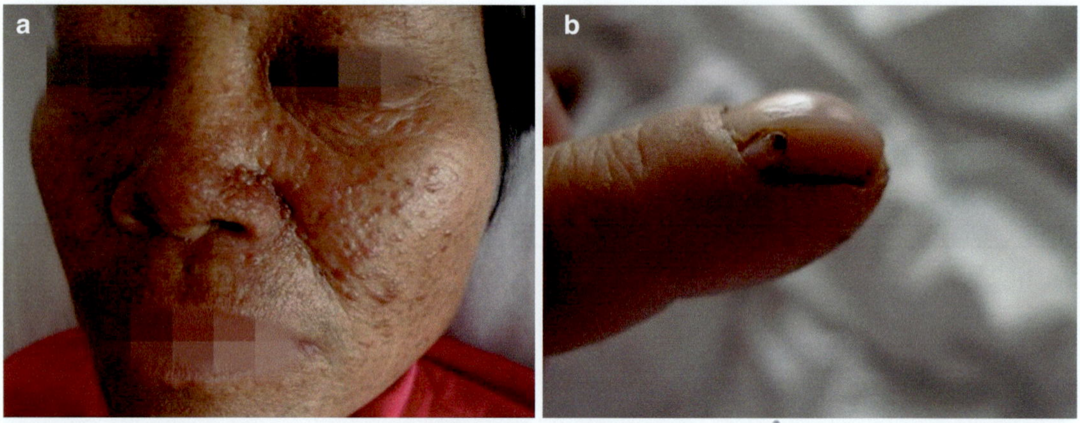

Fig. 12 (**a**) Facial angiofibromas. (**b**) Periungual fibroma

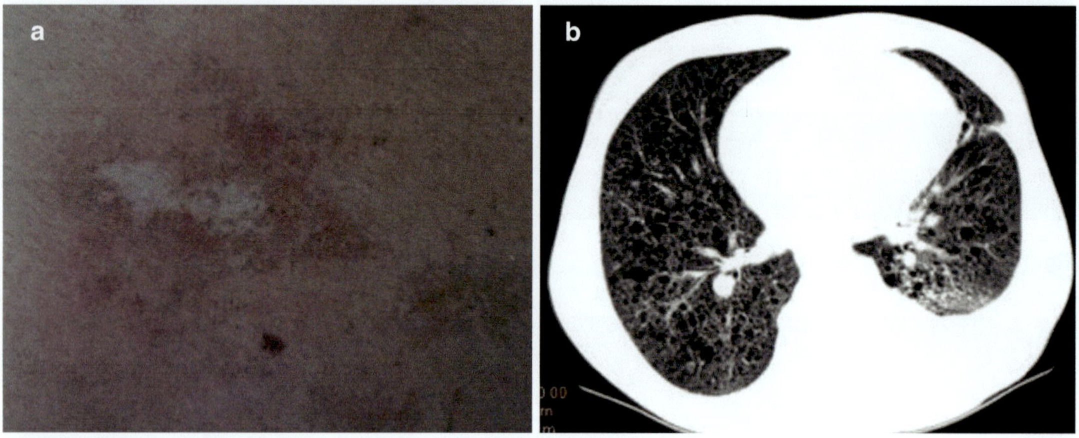

Fig. 13 (**a**) Hypomelanotic macules. (**b**) Cysts and left pleural effusion

Irregular hypomelanotic macules located on the back (Fig. 12b). Fibromas were seen on fingernails (Fig. 13a). Electroencephalogram was normal. Brain CT showed calcifications and increased periventricular density. Abdominal CT showed multiple renal tumors. Chest CT showed multiple cysts and left pleural effusion (Fig. 13b).

[Diagnosis] Tuberous sclerosis complex.

[Diagnosis Basis] A women of childbearing age has a history of dyspnea. The patient has multiple organ lesions such as facial angiofibromas, periungual fibromas, skin hypomelanotic macules, pulmonary LAM, multiple kidney tumors, and craniocerebral lesions, which meet the diagnosis of TSC.

[Analysis] Tuberous sclerosis complex (TSC), also known as epiloia or Bourneville-Pringle disease, is an autosomal dominant neurocutaneous syndrome, which affects multiple organs, including skin, central nervous system, heart, lungs, and kidney. The pathogenesis is driven by hyperactivation in the mTOR pathway because of the de novo or inherited mutations in TSC1 or TSC2 genes.

In 1835, French dermatologist Pierre François Olive Rayer described facial angiofibromas as vascular vegetations. In 1862, TSC was identified by German pathologist Friedrich Daniele von

Recklinghausen in a newborn who died shortly after birth with cardiac rhabdomyomas and cortical tubers in the brain. In 1880, TSC was recognized as an entity by French neurologist Désiré-Magloire Bourneville and hence the disease was named after him as the Bourneville disease. He used the term "tuberous sclerosis of the cerebral convolutions" to describe the brain of a child with seizures and intellectual disability, and "hard masses, one the size of a walnut,in both kidneys" to report renal angiomyolipomas. Campbell in 1905 and Vogt in 1908 established the triad for TSC as mental retardation, epilepsy, and Pringle type of sebaceous adenoma (angiofibroma). In 1942, Dr. Sylvan Moolten first used the term TSC.

In 1979, Spanish-American neurologist Manuel Rodríguez Gómez recognized that at least 1/3 of the patients have normal intelligence and established the first diagnostic criteria for TSC and since has been viewed as the father of TSC in the United States. The TSC2 and TSC1 genes were identified in 1993 and 1997, respectively, as the genetic loci mutated in TSC.

The International Tuberous Sclerosis Complex Consensus conferences updated the diagnostic criteria in 1998 and 2012. The identification of TSC1 or TSC2 pathogenic mutation in DNA from normal tissue is sufficient to make a definite diagnosis of TSC. Pathogenic mutation is defined as a mutation that explicitly inactivates the function of the TSC1 or TSC2 proteins (e.g., nonsense or out-of-frame indel mutation), prevents protein synthesis (e.g., large genomic deletion), or is a missense mutation whose effect on protein function has been established through functional assessment. Other TSC1 or TSC2 variants whose effect on function is less certain do not meet these criteria, and are not sufficient to make a definite diagnosis of TSC. Approximately 10–25% of TSC patients have no mutation identified by conventional genetic testing, and a normal result does not exclude TSC, or have any effect on the use of clinical diagnostic criteria for diagnosing TSC. Clinical diagnostic criteria include major and minor features, determining a TSC diagnosis to be categorized as definite or possible. A definite diagnosis can be made when two major features or one major feature with ≥2 minor features are fulfilled. Patients with one major feature or ≥2 minor feature meet the criteria for having a possible TSC diagnosis. Major features include hypomelanotic macules (≥3, at least 5-mm diameter), angiofibromas (≥3) or fibrous cephalic plaque, ungual fibromas (≥2), shagreen patch, multiple retinal hamartomas, cortical dysplasias, subependymal nodules, subependymal giant cell astrocytoma, cardiac rhabdomyoma, LAM, and angiomyolipomas (≥2). Minor features include "confetti" skin lesions, dental enamel pits (>3), intraoral fibromas (≥2), retinal achromic patch, multiple renal cysts, and nonrenal hamartomas [53].

Guidelines have been further revised in the 2018 World TSC Conference on July 25 and 26 in Dallas, TX, USA. They made two changes to the clinical diagnostic criteria: "multiple cortical tubers and/or radial migration lines" replaced the more general term "cortical dysplasias," and sclerotic bone lesions were reinstated as a minor criterion.

10.5 Case 5

A 37-year-old woman complained of recurrent foamy urine for more than 1 year. Serum creatinine was 600 umol/L. She was discharged after hemodialysis. Patient was admitted to the hospital due to sudden chest tightness and shortness of breath. She had a history of epilepsy for several years. She underwent right nephrectomy 14 years ago for ruptured renal hamartomas, and local surgery for left renal hamartomas 10 years ago. Laboratory tests revealed mild anemia, and her room air arterial oxygen saturation by pulse oximetry (SpO_2) was 83.5%. Her symptoms improved, and the SpO_2 increased to 95% after receiving bronchodilator drugs. A subsequently performed CT scan revealed multiple thin-walled cysts and nodules in the bilateral lungs (Fig. 14), subependymal calcifications of the brain (Fig. 15), a well-defined 2-cm-sized hypodense

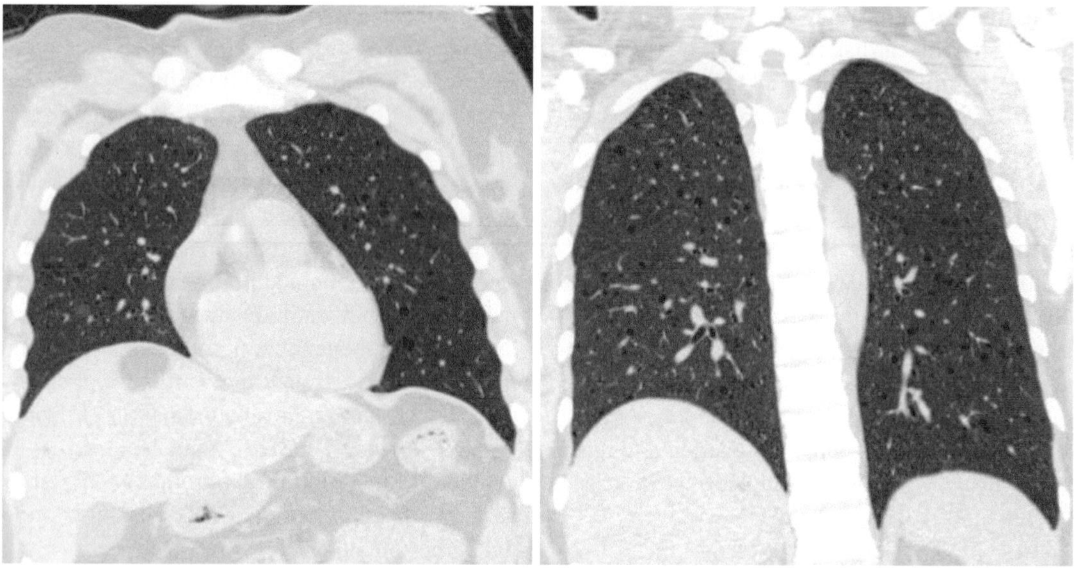

Fig. 14 Multiple cysts and nodules

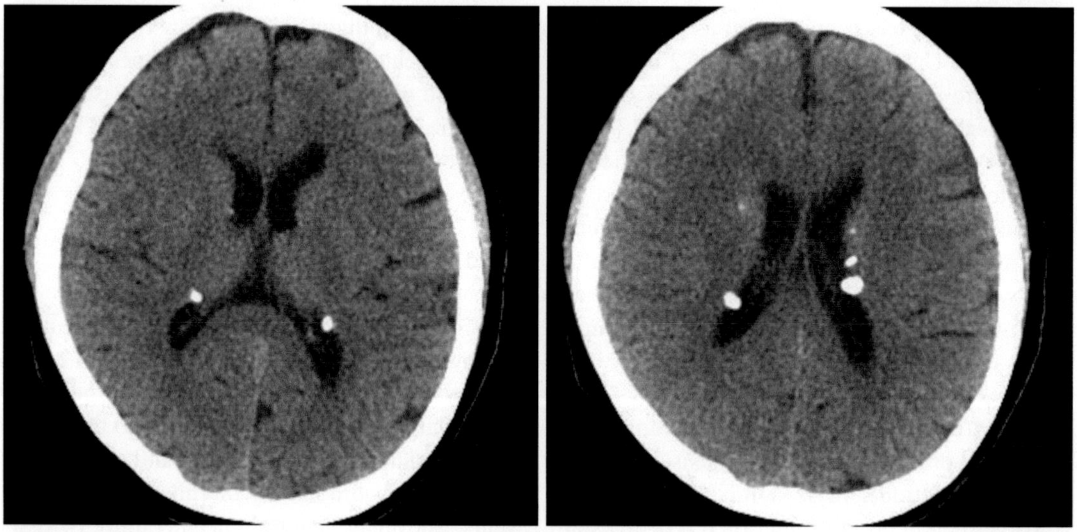

Fig. 15 Subependymal calcifications

round lesion in the liver (Fig. 16a), and extensive fat attenuating tissue in the left kidney (Fig. 16b).

[Diagnosis] Tuberous sclerosis complex.

[Diagnosis Basis] A women of childbearing age has a history of dyspnea and epilepsy. The patient has multiple organ lesions such as pulmonary LAM, subependymal calcifications, hepatic and renal angiomyolipomas, which meet the diagnosis of TSC based on the TSC diagnostic criteria.

[Analysis] Seizures or dermatologic manifestations such as hypomelanotic macules, shagreen patch, and/or facial angiofibromas are often the first overt clinical symptoms. Approximately 80%–85% of patients with TSC develop epilepsy and most develop multiple seizure types. Onset

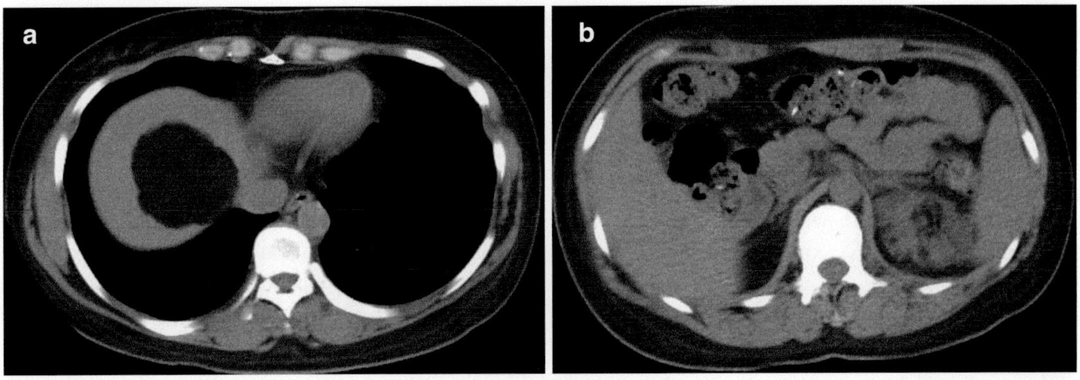

Fig. 16 (**a**) Hepatic angiomyolipoma. (**b**) Renal angiomyolipomas

typically occurs in the first year of life, but some patients may not have their first seizure until adolescence or early adulthood [54].

Pulmonary involvement in patients with TSC includes LAM and less commonly, multifocal micronodular pneumocyte hyperplasia (MMPH), occurring together or alone. MMPH is not present in patients with S-LAM. MMPH manifests as multiple solid and ground glass nodules with a random distribution on chest CT. Histologically, MMPH is composed of papillary or tubular proliferation of type II pneumocytes without nuclear atypia lining the thickened alveolar septa and lymphocyte infiltration. Immunohistochemically, cytokeratin and surfactant proteins A and B are positive in alveolar lining cells of all MMPH lesions [55].

Muzykewicz et al. [56] retrospectively reviewed chest CT images of 73 patients with TSC. MMPHs were identified in 42 (58%) of 73 patients and were independent of sex and LAM. Tanaka et al. [57] retrospective analyzed pulmonary involvement in 59 Japanese TSC patients and pulmonary function testing in TSC-LAM. One male (6.7%, 1/15) patient and 19 female (43.2%, 19/44) patients were diagnosed with LAM and 7 male and 23 female patients were diagnosed with MMPH. The incidence of renal angiomyolipoma and history of seizures in patients with multiple pulmonary nodules are higher than in patients without nodules. DLco and the number of cysts are useful predictors for the onset and progression of TSC-LAM. Other studies also confirmed that MMPH has a benign and stable nature as compared to LAM which is often relentlessly progressive with associated lung function decline [58]. Konno et al. [59] retrospectively analyzed 9 TSC patients with MMPH. Radiographic findings and pulmonary function were stable in all MMPH cases. Serum SP-A and SP-D, but not KL-6, may be useful markers for suspicion of the presence of MMPH in TSC patients.

Daccord et al. [60] reported a case of a woman with TSC and MMPH who received everolimus treatment for subependymal giant cell astrocytoma (SEGA). A remarkable decrease in density of all pulmonary MMPH lesions was observed after 3 months of therapy, without any change in size. They concluded that everolimus is active on MMPH similarly to its effects on renal AMLs, SEGA, and PLAM in TSC and indicated that the dysregulated activation of mTOR which characterizes TSC also plays a role in the pathogenesis of MMPH.

Shoji et al. [61] reported the first case of everolimus efficacy shown for histologically confirmed MMPH in genetically determined TSC patient. MMPH and AML were markedly reduced after oral administration of everolimus. Further, serum levels of SP-A and SP-D, which reflect type II pneumocyte hyperplasia, decreased to the normal range after starting treatment with everolimus.

10.6 Case 6

A 43-year-old woman was admitted to the hospital due to shortness of breath. Physical examination revealed facial angiofibromas, periungual fibroma, and hypomelanotic macules. CT scan revealed multiple thin-walled cysts in the bilateral lungs (Fig. 17a), subependymal calcifications of the brain, and extensive fat attenuating tissue in the kidney (Fig. 17b).

[Diagnosis] Tuberous sclerosis complex.

[Diagnosis basis] The generation sequencing shows TSC2 gene mutation.

[Analysis] TSC occurs in 1 in 12000–14000 children under 10 years of age in a population-based studies in UK [62] or 1 in 6000 live births [63]. Approximately 30% of TSC cases are inherited in an autosomal dominant manner, and around 70% of cases are sporadic. There are about 1500 known pathogenic variants for TSC1 and TSC2, including nonsense, deletion, and missense mutations, and all pathogenic mutations are inactivating, leading to loss of function effects on the encoded proteins TSC1 and TSC2.

Intellectual disability was significantly more frequent in TSC2 sporadic cases than in TSC1 sporadic cases [64]. Au et al. [65] identified mutations in 72% (199/257) of de novo and 77% (53/68) of familial cases, with 17% and 50% of mutations in the TSC1 and TSC2 gene, respectively. There were 4% unclassified variants and 29% with no mutation identified. This study showed that patients with TSC2 mutations have significantly more hypomelanotic macules and learning disability compared with those with TSC1 mutations, suggesting that individuals with mutations in TSC2 have more severe symptoms. Tian et al. [66] analyzed the association between TSC mutation subtypes and the prevalence of LAM in women with TSC. The cohort consisted of 55 TSC women, including 30/55 (55%) with TSC2, 12/55 (22%) with TSC1, and 13/55 (23%) with no mutation identified (NMI). LAM and AMLs are more common in women with TSC harboring TSC2 mutations compared with women with TSC1 mutations. There was no association between TSC mutation subtype and the presence of MMPH, sclerotic bone lesions, and skin or brain involvement. Serum VEGF-D is a useful biomarker to suggest the presence of LAM in women with TSC.

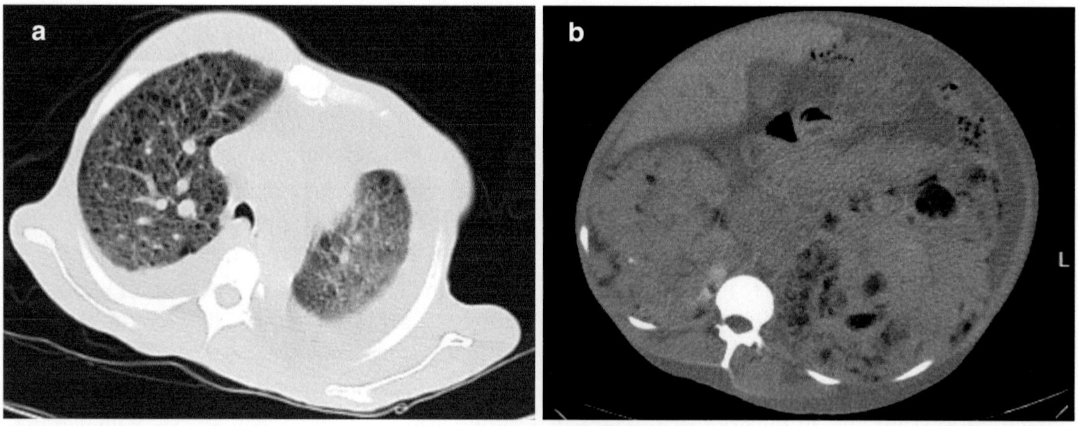

Fig. 17 (**a**) PLAM with pleural effusion. (**b**) Renal angiomyolipomas

References

1. Ferrans VJ, Yu ZX, Nelson WK, et al. Lymphangioleiomyomatosis (LAM). A review of clinical and morphological features. J Nippon Med Sch. 2000;67:311–29.
2. Flavin RJ, Cook J, Fiorentino M, et al. Beta-catenin is a useful adjunct immunohistochemical marker for the diagnosis of pulmonary lymphangioleiomyomatosis. Am J Clin Pathol. 2011;135:776–82.
3. Crooks DM, Pacheco-Rodriguez G, DeCastro RM, et al. Molecular and genetic analysis of disseminated neoplastic cells in lymphangioleiomyomatosis. Proc Natl Acad Sci U S A. 2004;101:17462–7.
4. Cai X, Pacheco-Rodriguez G, Fan QY, et al. Phenotypic characterization of disseminated cells with TSC2 loss of heterozygosity in patients with lymphangioleiomyomatosis. Am J Respir Crit Care Med. 2010;182:1410–8.
5. Kumasaka T, Seyama K, Mitani K, et al. Lymphangiogenesis in lymphangioleiomyomatosis: its implication in the progression of lymphangioleiomyomatosis. Am J Surg Pathol. 2004;28:1007–16.
6. Kumasaka T, Seyama K, Mitani K, et al. Lymphangiogenesis-mediated shedding of LAM cell clusters as a mechanism for dissemination in lymphangioleiomyomatosis. Am J Surg Pathol. 2005;29:1356–66.
7. Hayashi T, Fleming MV, Stetler-Stevenson WG, et al. Immunohistochemical study of matrix metalloproteinases (MMPs) and their tissue inhibitors (TIMPs) in pulmonary lymphangioleiomyomatosis (LAM). Hum Pathol. 1997;28:1071–8.
8. Zhe X, Yang Y, Jakkaraju S, et al. Tissue inhibitor of metalloproteinase-3 downregulation in lymphangioleiomyomatosis. Am J Respir Cell Mol Biol. 2003;28:504–11.
9. Odajima N, Betsuyaku T, Nasuhara Y, et al. Matrix metalloproteinases in blood from patients with LAM. Respir Med. 2009;103:124–9.
10. Lee PS, Tsang SW, Moses MA, et al. Rapamycin-insensitive up-regulation of MMP2 and other genes in tuberous sclerosis complex 2-deficient lymphangioleiomyomatosis-like cells. Am J Respir Cell Mol Biol. 2010;42:227–34.
11. Gupta N, Lee HS, Ryu JH, et al. The NHLBI LAM registry: prognostic physiologic and radiologic biomarkers emerge from a 15-year prospective longitudinal analysis. Chest. 2019;155:288–96.
12. Ryu JH, Moss J, Beck GJ, et al. The NHLBI lymphangioleiomyomatosis registry: characteristics of 230 patients at enrollment. Am J Respir Crit Care Med. 2006;173:105–11.
13. Schiavina M, Di Scioscio V, Contini P, et al. Pulmonary lymphangioleiomyomatosis in a karyotypically normal man without tuberous sclerosis complex. Am J Respir Crit Care Med. 2007;176:96–8.
14. Johnson SR, Tattersfield AE. Clinical experience of lymphangioleiomyomatosis in the UK. Thorax. 2000;55:1052–7.
15. Harknett EC, Chang WY, Byrnes S, et al. Use of variability in national and regional data to estimate the prevalence of lymphangioleiomyomatosis. QJM. 2011;104:971–9.
16. Cudzilo CJ, Szczesniak RD, Brody AS, et al. Lymphangioleiomyomatosis screening in women with tuberous sclerosis. Chest. 2013;144:578–85.
17. Steagall WK, Glasgow CG, Hathaway OM, et al. Genetic and morphologic determinants of pneumothorax in lymphangioleiomyomatosis. Am J Physiol Lung Cell Mol Physiol. 2007;293:L800–8.
18. Gonano C, Pasquier J, Daccord C, et al. Air travel and incidence of pneumothorax in lymphangioleiomyomatosis. Orphanet J Rare Dis. 2018;13:222.
19. Cohen MM, Pollock-BarZiv S, Johnson SR. Emerging clinical picture of lymphangioleiomyomatosis. Thorax. 2005;60:875–9.
20. Gupta R, Kitaichi M, Inoue Y, et al. Lymphatic manifestations of lymphangioleiomyomatosis. Lymphology. 2014;47:106–17.
21. Avila NA, Kelly JA, Chu SC, et al. Lymphangioleiomyomatosis: abdominopelvic CT and US findings. Radiology. 2000;216:147–53.
22. Theilig D, Doellinger F, Kuhnigk JM, et al. Pulmonary lymphangioleiomyomatosis: analysis of disease manifestation by region-based quantification of lung parenchyma. Eur J Radiol. 2015;84:732–7.
23. Adriaensen ME, Schaefer-Prokop CM, Duyndam DA, et al. Radiological evidence of lymphangioleiomyomatosis in female and male patients with tuberous sclerosis complex. Clin Radiol. 2011;66:625–8.
24. Kobylianskii J, Hutchinson-Jaffe A, Cabanero M, et al. Pathologically confirmed diffuse alveolar haemorrhage in lymphangioleiomyomatosis. BMJ Case Rep. 2021;14:e238713.
25. Avila NA, Dwyer AJ, Rabel A, et al. Sporadic lymphangioleiomyomatosis and tuberous sclerosis complex with lymphangioleiomyomatosis: comparison of CT features. Radiology. 2007;242:277–85.
26. Johnson SR, Cordier JF, Lazor R, et al. European respiratory society guidelines for the diagnosis and management of lymphangioleiomyomatosis. Eur Respir J. 2010;35:14–26.
27. McCormack FX, Gupta N, Finlay GR, et al. Official American Thoracic Society/Japanese Respiratory Society Clinical Practice Guidelines: lymphangioleiomyomatosis diagnosis and management. Am J Respir Crit Care Med. 2016;194:748–61.
28. Hirose M, Matsumuro A, Arai T, et al. Serum vascular endothelial growth factor-D as a diagnostic and therapeutic biomarker for lymphangioleiomyomatosis. PLoS One. 2019;14:e0212776.
29. Bissler JJ, McCormack FX, Young LR, et al. Sirolimus for angiomyolipoma in tuberous sclerosis complex or lymphangioleiomyomatosis. N Engl J Med. 2008;358:140–51.
30. McCormack FX, Inoue Y, Moss J, et al. Efficacy and safety of sirolimus in lymphangioleiomyomatosis. N Engl J Med. 2011;364:1595–606.
31. Sakurai T, Arai T, Hirose M, et al. Reduced risk of recurrent pneumothorax for sirolimus therapy

after surgical pleural covering of entire lung in lymphangioleiomyomatosis. Orphanet J Rare Dis. 2021;16:466.
32. Hu S, Wu X, Xu W, et al. Long-term efficacy and safety of sirolimus therapy in patients with lymphangioleiomyomatosis. Orphanet J Rare Dis. 2019;14:206.
33. Revilla-López E, Berastegui C, Méndez A, et al. Long-term results of sirolimus treatment in lymphangioleiomyomatosis: a single referral centre experience. Sci Rep. 2021;11:10171.
34. Wang Q, Luo M, Xiang B, et al. The efficacy and safety of pharmacological treatments for lymphangioleiomyomatosis. Respir Res. 2020;21:55.
35. Estenne M, de Francquen P, Wellens F, et al. Combined heart-and-lung transplantation for lymphangioleiomyomatosis. Lancet. 1984;1:275.
36. Khawar MU, Yazdani D, Zhu Z, et al. Clinical outcomes and survival following lung transplantation in patients with lymphangioleiomyomatosis. J Heart Lung Transplant. 2019;38:949–55.
37. Warrior K, Leard LE, Nair AR, et al. A survey of use of mTOR inhibitors in patients with lymphangioleiomyomatosis listed for lung transplant. Respir Med. 2022;195:106779.
38. Oprescu N, McCormack FX, Byrnes S, et al. Clinical predictors of mortality and cause of death in lymphangioleiomyomatosis: a population-based registry. Lung. 2013;191:35–42.
39. Yoon HY, Kim HJ, Song JW. Long-term clinical course and outcomes in patients with lymphangioleiomyomatosis. Respir Res. 2022;23:158.
40. Harari S, Torre O, Elia D, et al. Improving survival in lymphangioleio-myomatosis: a 16-year observational study in a large cohort of patients. Respiration. 2021;100:989–99.
41. Taveira-DaSilva AM, Johnson SR, Julien-Williams P, et al. Pregnancy in lymphangioleiomyomatosis: clinical and lung function outcomes in two national cohorts. Thorax. 2020;75:904–7.
42. Suzuki E, Kurihara M, Tsuboshima K, et al. The effects of total pleural covering on pneumothorax recurrence and pulmonary function in lymphangioleiomyomatosis patients without history of pleurodesis or thoracic surgeries for pneumothorax. J Thorac Dis. 2021;13:113–24.
43. Zhou L, Ouyang R, Luo H, et al. Efficacy of sirolimus for the prevention of recurrent pneumothorax in patients with lymphangioleiomyomatosis: a case series. Orphanet J Rare Dis. 2018;13:168.
44. Pollock-BarZiv S, Cohen MM, Downey GP, et al. Air travel in women with lymphangioleiomyomatosis. Thorax. 2007;62:176–80.
45. Taveira-DaSilva AM, Burstein D, Hathaway OM, et al. Pneumothorax after air travel in lymphangioleiomyomatosis, idiopathic pulmonary fibrosis, and sarcoidosis. Chest. 2009;136:665–70.
46. Carsillo T, Astrinidis A, Henske EP. Mutations in the tuberous sclerosis complex gene TSC2 are a cause of sporadic pulmonary lymphangioleiomyomatosis. Proc Natl Acad Sci U S A. 2000;97:6085–90.
47. Bissler JJ, Kingswood JC, Radzikowska E, et al. Everolimus for angiomyolipoma associated with tuberous sclerosis complex or sporadic lymphangioleiomyomatosis (EXIST-2): a multicentre, randomised, double-blind, placebo-controlled trial. Lancet. 2013;381:817–24.
48. Bissler JJ, Kingswood JC, Radzikowska E, et al. Everolimus long-term use in patients with tuberous sclerosis complex: four-year update of the EXIST-2 study. PLoS One. 2017;12:e0180939.
49. Taveira-DaSilva AM, Jones AM, Julien-Williams P, et al. Long-term effect of sirolimus on serum vascular endothelial growth factor D levels in patients with lymphangioleiomyomatosis. Chest. 2018;153:124–32.
50. Watanabe EH, Coelho FMA, Filho HL, et al. The effect of sirolimus on angiomyolipoma is determined by decrease of fat-poor compartments and includes striking reduction of vascular structures. Sci Rep. 2021;11:8493.
51. Avila NA, Bechtle J, Dwyer AJ, et al. Lymphangioleiomyomatosis: CT of diurnal variation of lymphangioleiomyomas. Radiology. 2001;221:415–21.
52. Taveira-DaSilva AM, Jones AM, Julien-Williams P, et al. Effect of fasting on the size of lymphangioleiomyomas in patients with lymphangioleiomyomatosis. Chest. 2015;148:1027–33.
53. WHO Classification of Tumours Editorial Board. WHO classification of tumours of the lung, pleura, thymus and heart. Lyon, France: International Agency for Research on Cancer; 2015.
54. Chu-Shore CJ, Major P, Camposano S, et al. The natural history of epilepsy in tuberous sclerosis complex. Epilepsia. 2010;51:1236–41.
55. Kobashi Y, Sugiu T, Mouri K, et al. Clinicopathological analysis of multifocal micronodular pneumocyte hyperplasia associated with tuberous sclerosis in Japan. Respirology. 2008;13:1076–81.
56. Muzykewicz DA, Black ME, Muse V, et al. Multifocal micronodular pneumocyte hyperplasia: computed tomographic appearance and follow-up in tuberous sclerosis complex. J Comput Assist Tomogr. 2012;36:518–22.
57. Tanaka M, Hirata H, Wataya-Kaneda M, et al. Lymphangioleiomyomatosis and multifocal micronodular pneumocyte hyperplasia in Japanese patients with tuberous sclerosis complex. Respir Investig. 2016;54:8–13.
58. Pannu BS, Apala DR, Kotecha A, et al. Multifocal micronodular pneumocyte hyperplasia (MMPH) in a patient with tuberous sclerosis-evidence for long term stability. Respir Med Case Rep. 2017;20:113–5.
59. Konno S, Shigemura M, Ogi T, et al. Clinical course of histologically proven multifocal micronodular pneumocyte hyperplasia in tuberous sclerosis complex: a case series and comparison with lymphangiomyomatosis. Respiration. 2018;95:310–6.

60. Daccord C, Nicolas A, Demicheli R, et al. Effect of everolimus on multifocal micronodular pneumocyte hyperplasia in tuberous sclerosis complex. Respir Med Case Rep. 2020;31:101310.
61. Shoji T, Niida Y, Osawa T, et al. Resolution of multifocal micronodular pneumocyte hyperplasia with everolimus in a patient with tuberous sclerosis complex. Respir Med Case Rep. 2021;34:101526.
62. O'Callaghan FJ, Shiell AW, Osborne JP, et al. Prevalence of tuberous sclerosis estimated by capture-recapture analysis. Lancet. 1998;351:1490.
63. Osborne JP, Fryer A, Webb D. Epidemiology of tuberous sclerosis. Ann N Y Acad Sci. 1991;615:125–7.
64. Jones AC, Shyamsundar MM, Thomas MW, et al. Comprehensive mutation analysis of TSC1 and TSC2-and phenotypic correlations in 150 families with tuberous sclerosis. Am J Hum Genet. 1999;64:1305–15.
65. Au KS, Williams AT, Roach ES, et al. Genotype/phenotype correlation in 325 individuals referred for a diagnosis of tuberous sclerosis complex in the United States. Genet Med. 2007;9:88–100.
66. Tian X, Glass JE, Kwiatkowski DJ, et al. Lymphangioleiomyomatosis association with underlying genotype in patients with tuberous sclerosis complex. Ann Am Thorac Soc. 2021;18:815–9.

Pulmonary Epithelioid Hemangioendothelioma

Xue-Peng Huang and Song Zhang

Pulmonary epithelioid hemangioendothelioma (PEH) is a rare low to intermediate malignant vascular tumor developing from vascular endothelial cells.

1 Classification

In 1975, PEH was initially described by Dail and Liebow and was named as intravascular bronchioloalveolar tumor (IVBAT) because they believed it to arise from type II alveolar cells which invaded adjacent blood vessels and small airways [1]. Corrin et al. [2] described three cases of Dial and Liebow's IVBAT. The electron microscopy did not support the alveolar cell origin and immunohistochemical techniques confirmed its endothelial lineage. Weldon-Linne et al. [3] confirmed that IVBAT consists of endothelial cells and is not related to the typical bronchioloalveolar tumor of lung using electron microscopy and showed a diffuse cytoplasmic staining of the malignant cells with a factor VIII-related antigen.

In 1982, Weiss and Ezinger [4] first introduced the term epithelioid hemangioendothelioma (EHE) to describe a vascular tumor showing pathological features between hemangioma and angiosarcoma. In the 2002 WHO classification, it was classified into the category of locally aggressive tumors with metastatic potential [5]. In the 2015 WHO classification, EHE was described as a low- to intermediate-grade malignant vascular tumor [6].

2 Pathology

Histologically, the tumor cells are epithelioid cells with abundant eosinophilic cytoplasm and arranged in nests and cords, and cytoplasmic vacuoles are commonly noted (Figs. 1 and 2). EHE typically shows a myxochondroid or hyaline stroma and often forms a primitive vascular lumen. The morphology of the majority of the tumor cells is moderate, including little necrosis or mitosis, and mild atypia. The presence of necrosis, increased mitotic activity, and increased atypia may differ intermediate-grade EHE from low-grade EHE [7]. Morphologic features such as intranuclear inclusions, intracytoplasmic vacuoles, and stromal changes (chondroid, myxoid, or hyalinized stroma) are more common in EHE, but blood lakes, proliferation of slit-like vessels, and prominent nucleoli favor high-grade epithelioid angiosarcoma (EAS) [7].

X.-P. Huang
Department of Respiratory and Critical Care Medicine, People's Hospital of Rizhao Lanshan, Rizhao, Shandong, China

S. Zhang (✉)
Department of Respiratory and Critical Care Medicine, Shandong Provincial Hospital Affiliated to Shandong First Medical University, Jinan, Shandong, China

S. Zhang (ed.), *Diagnostic Imaging of Lung Cancers*, https://doi.org/10.1007/978-981-99-6815-2_18

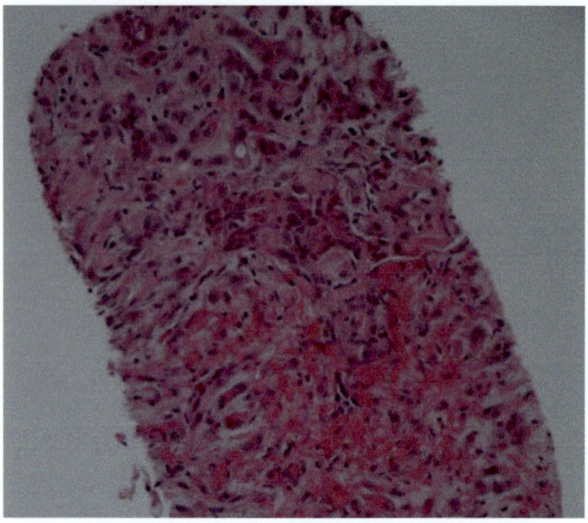

Fig. 1 Hematoxylin-eosin (×200)

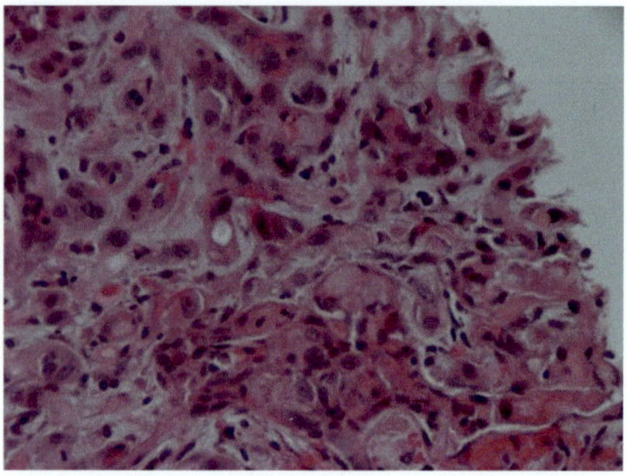

Fig. 2 Hematoxylin-eosin (×400)

Immunohistochemically, the endothelial markers may be useful to identify EHE. Tumor cells are positive for CD31 (Fig. 3a), CD34, and Fli-1. Fli-1 shows a better combined sensitivity and specificity than CD31 and CD34 and is most helpful in distinguishing EHE from metastatic carcinoma [8]. Other vascular markers include F8, ERG (Fig. 3b), EMA, and FKBNP12. Cytokeratin is focally positive in 25–30% of cases. Due to the absence of complete specificity of any of the endothelial markers for EHE, or of keratin cocktail for carcinoma, these markers are best used in combination. The combination of Fli-1 and CD31 may represent an ideal panel for the differential diagnosis [8].

3 Molecular Features

About 90% and 5% of EHE cases are associated with the WWTR1-CAMTA1 and YAP1-TFE3 fusion gene, respectively.

The translocation t(1;3) (p36.3;q25), resulting in WWTR1-CAMTA1 fusion, is the most commonly identified genetic abnormality with EHE. Errani et al. [9] demonstrated the presence of a WWTR1-CAMTA1 fusion in all EHE tested from soft tissue, bone, and visceral location (liver, lung) in keeping with a unique and specific pathological entity. A study by Anderson et al. [7] found thatWWTR1-CAMTA1 fusions in 4/7 low-grade and 23/23 intermediate-grade EHE by fluorescence in situ hybridization analysis. In EAS, CAMTA1 rearrangement was negative in all cases, whereas a WWTR1 complex abnormality was found in 1/5 cases. This provides an objective method to distinguish intermediate-grade EHE from EAS, especially on limited biopsies.

YAP1-TFE3 gene fusion has been identified in a small subset of WWTR1-CAMTA1 negative cases [10]. This subset has a distinct morphology with more obvious vasoformation, voluminous eosinophilic cytoplasm, and TFE3 expression on immunohistochemistry. Dermawan et al. [11] analyzed 24 cases of YAP1-TFE3-fused hemangioendothelioma: majority with YAP1 exon 1 fused to TFE3 exon 4 (88%), or less commonly, TFE3 exon 6 (12%). Tumors were most commonly located in soft tissue (50%), followed by bone (29%), lung (13%), and liver (8%). The 5-year progression-free survival probability was 88%, although approximately two-thirds presented with multifocal disease, including 7 cases with distant organ metastasis. Rosenbaum et al. [12] demonstrated that patients with WWTR1-CAMTA1 fusion had a poorer prognosis compared with the YAP1-TFE3 subset, the 5-year overall survival being 59% versus 86%, respectively.

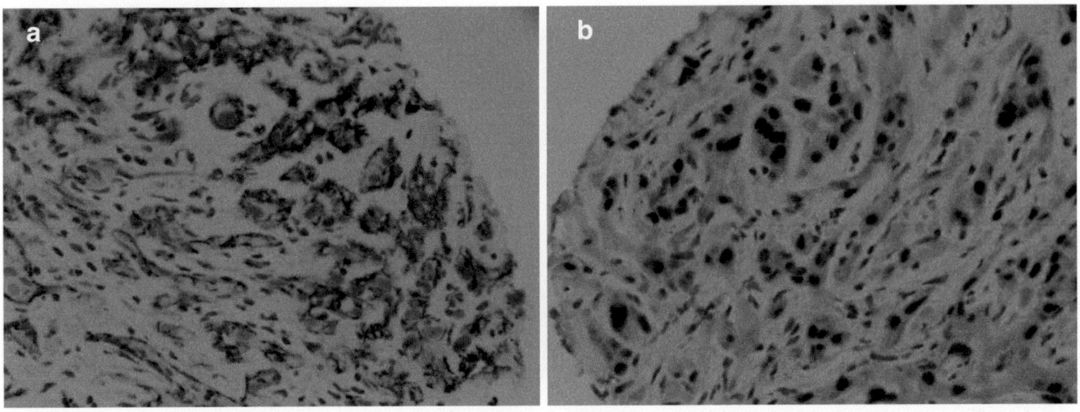

Fig. 3 (**a**) Immunohistochemistry for CD31 (×400). (**b**) Immunohistochemistry for ERG (×400)

4 Epidemiology

EHE represents less than 1% of all the vascular tumors. The prevalence of EHE is less than one in one million.

EHE occurs in various organs and tissues, predominantly the liver, lung, bone, and soft tissue, and has a tendency to be multifocal. Therefore, it is difficult to confirm whether the tumor is a primary, multicentric, or metastatic lesion. The International Hemangioendothelioma, Epithelioid Hemangioendothelioma and Related Vascular Disorders (HEARD) Registry showed that the most common EHE involvements are in the liver alone (21%), liver plus lung (18%), lung alone (12%), and bone alone (14%) [13].

PEH preferentially occurs in women at a rate fourfold greater than that in men, with a median age of 36 years, and a life expectancy of 15–30 years [14].

5 Clinical Features

Majority of the patients with PEH are asymptomatic on initial presentation. A few patients may present with dyspnea, chest pain, hemoptysis, and weight loss. Amin et al. [15] analyzed 93 PEH cases collected from the literature. The mean age of patients was 40.1 ± 17.3, and 73% were females. Nearly half of the patients were asymptomatic (49.5%). The common non-specific presentations were dyspnea (18.3%), cough (18.3%), chest pain (16%), hemoptysis (6.5%), and weight loss (6.5%). Other rare presentations include hypertrophic pulmonary osteodystrophy, pleural effusion, pulmonary thromboembolic disease with pulmonary hypertension, and scoliosis.

6 Radiographic Features

Thoracic EHE involves the lungs, pleurae, and mediastinum. There are three different imaging patterns identified in thoracic EHE [16]: multiple pulmonary nodules (Figs. 4 and 5), multiple pulmonary reticulonodular opacities, and diffuse infiltrative pleural thickening (Fig. 6). Individual cases may imitate lung cancer, presenting with a solitary pulmonary nodule or mass (Fig. 7).

The presentation of bilateral multiple nodules is the most common pattern of presentation and is easily mistaken for metastatic carcinoma. However, these nodules show little or no progression on serial chest CT examinations. Amin et al. [15] revealed that most of the nodules were multiple (84%) and of variable sizes (0.5–15 cm) but generally less than 2 cm (n = 36, 39%). Liu et al. [17] analyzed the CT findings of six patients with pathology-proven PHE. All cases showed multiple nodules/masses with irregular margin and 90% (160/178) of nodules were <1 cm in diameter. Nodules with pleural indentation (100%)

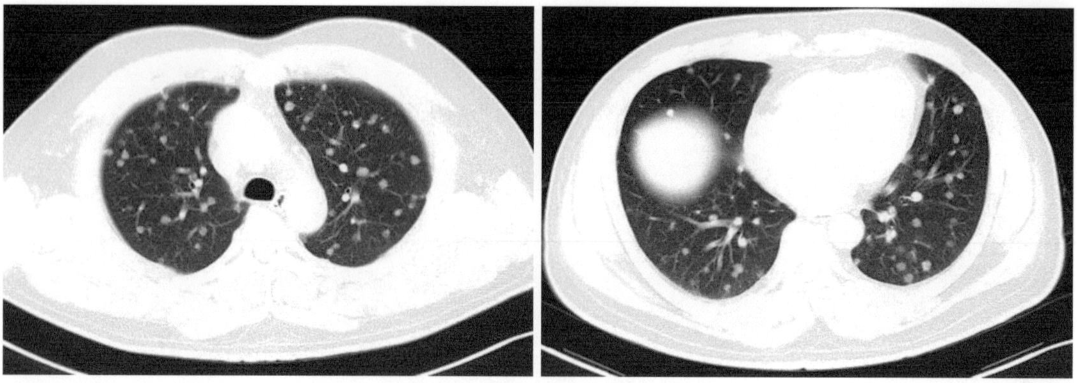

Fig. 4 A 28-year-old man with multiple pulmonary nodules in both lungs

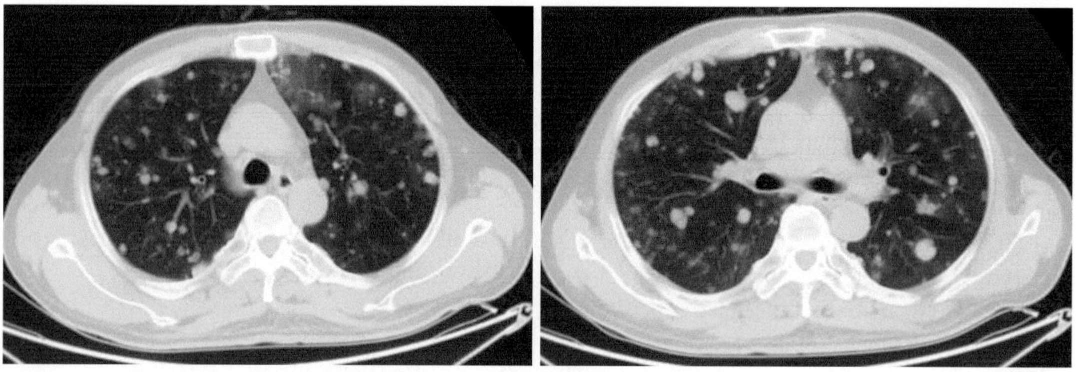

Fig. 5 A 55-year-old man with innumerable pulmonary nodules with halo sign

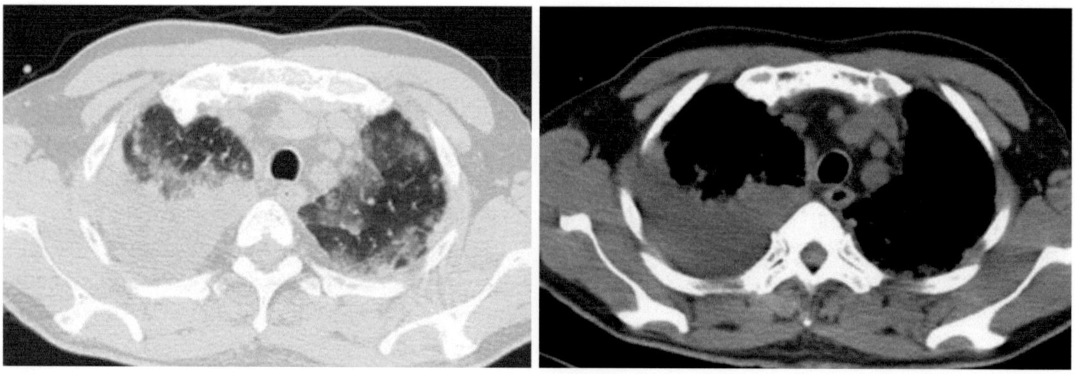

Fig. 6 A 60-year-old man with multiple pulmonary nodules, ground-glass opacities, and right pleural effusion

were common because of predilection for subpleural (93% within 2 cm from the pleura) and perivascular (100%) location. A total of 48% (86/178) of nodules/masses showed punctate calcification in four of six cases (Fig. 8).

Histopathologically, multiple reticulonodular lesions and interlobular septal thickening represent areas of multiple, small, infiltrating nodular proliferation of neoplastic cells within the lumina of small blood vessels and lymphatic vessels; the

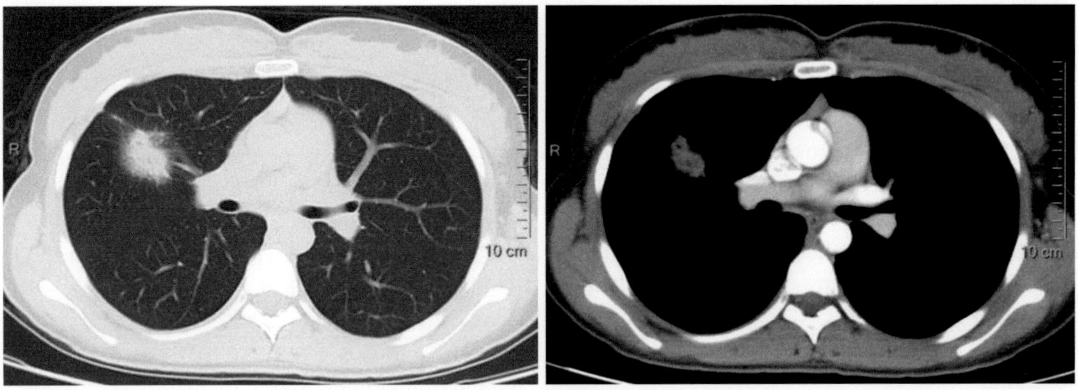

Fig. 7 A 18-year-old man with a mass in the right upper lobe

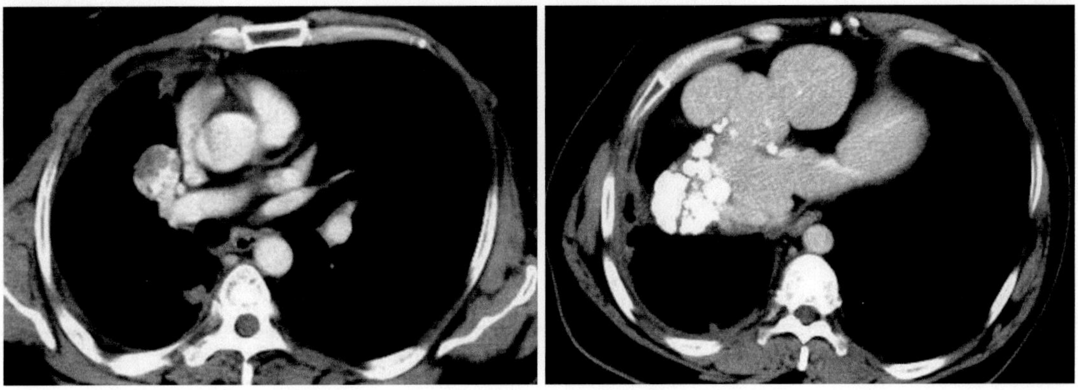

Fig. 8 A 48-year-old man with a right hilar and liver mass with calcifications

pleural lesions consist of diffuse irregular thickening of pleura and multifocal and variable-sized subpleural and intraparenchymal nodules of infiltrative growth [16]. Woo et al. [18] found that multiple pulmonary nodules were most common (n = 10), followed by parenchymal tumor with pleural invasion (n = 4), reticulonodular opacities (n = 3), and diffuse pleural thickening (n = 2). The lung multinodular pattern had longer median survival (8.5 months) than other patterns, whereas the nodule/mass with pleural involvement pattern had the shortest median survival (1 month).

7 Treatment

So far, there is no standard of treatment for PEH because of its low incidence worldwide. Surgery can be performed in cases of single nodule or unilateral multiple nodules with no evidence of metastasis [19]. Baba et al. [20] reported a 51-year-old woman with multifocal primary PEH (11 tumors) in the bilateral lungs. All of the tumors were surgically resected. The patient had no tumor recurred for 8 years after surgery until a single recurrent nodule appeared and was thoracoscopically resected.

Radiotherapy is considered ineffective for PHE because of its slow growth and radiobiological characteristics. Patients with unresectable bilateral multiple nodules or disseminated disease are usually treated with chemotherapy or immunotherapy. Paclitaxel or platinum-based chemotherapy regimens tend to be the most common options. Antiangiogenetic drugs such as thalidomide, lenalidomide, and bevacizumab can be considered because of its vascular origin. Kanemura et al. [21] reported a 31-year-old woman with EHE of the pleura underwent the fourth cycle of chemotherapy with carboplatin, pemetrexed, and bevacizumab, the disease was well controlled with a 90% reduction of the left pleural effusion. A retrospective study showed that patients with PEH demonstrated a good partial response to treatment with carboplatin, paclitaxel, bevacizumab, thalidomide, and α-interferon [22]. Combined therapy may be an effective option for PHE patients.

8 Prognosis

The prognosis of PHE is variable, ranging from spontaneous regression to rapid disease progression and death even with aggressive treatment. Kitaichi et al. [23] analyzed 21 PHE patients throughout Asia by a questionnaire. Three asymptomatic patients occurred partial spontaneous regression. Patients with fibrin fibrous pleuritis with extrapleural proliferation of tumor cells and spindle tumor cells had worse prognosis. Bagna et al. [19] reported a 5-year survival probability of 60% (range, 47–71%) in 80 PHE patients. Univariate analysis showed that anemia, loss of weight, pulmonary symptoms, and more particularly pleural hemorrhagic effusions were significant factors of poor prognosis, with a median survival of less than 1 year. Amin et al. [15] found that male, symptomatic patients, hemoptysis, presence of cough, chest pain, multiple unilateral nodules, pleural effusion, metastases to more than one site, and lymph node metastases were all significant risk factors for PEH. Symptomatic patients and presence of pleural effusion were the independent predictors of survival in PEH patients. Anderson et al. [7] analyzed 39 EHE patients with thoracic involvement (lung, pleura, mediastinum, heart, great vessels) and found that higher tumor grade and the presence of pleural involvement in lung and/or pleural tumors correlate with poor prognosis.

9 Case Analysis

9.1 Case 1

A 27-year-old man complained of cough and abdominal discomfort for 1 month. Blood routine showed pancytopenia.

Chest CT: Multiple ground-glass nodules in both lungs and liver (Fig. 9).

[Diagnosis] Epithelioid hemangioendothelioma.

[Diagnosis Basis] The lung biopsy of the patient was a vascular tumor, and immunohistochemistry showed positive for CD31, CD34, and Vimentin, and negative for CK20, CK7, EMA, and TTF-1. Histological and immunohistochemical findings support the diagnosis of EHE.

[Analysis] EHE most commonly occurs in liver and lungs, and bones, although it can present at multiple other sites such as soft tissue. Epelboym et al. [24] evaluated 29 EHE patients with median age of 16 years. 22 (70%) had multifocal disease. The common involved sites were lung (n = 25), liver (n = 16), bone (n = 12), soft tissue (n = 3), and lymph nodes (n = 1). In 18/25 with PHE, there were multiple nodules of varying sizes and characteristics. In 14/16 with hepatic disease, there were multiple nodules with predominantly peripheral distribution. Subcapsular retraction was observed in 10/16 and a "lollipop" sign (hepatic or portal vein tapering at the edge of a well-defined hypo-enhancing lesion) identified in 5/16. Of 12 osseous lesions, 11 were lytic, 8 involved vertebrae, and 9 involved the axial skeleton.

On imaging, hepatic epithelioid hemangioendothelioma (HEH) usually presents as an incidental finding of multifocal, heterogeneously enhancing nodules. Merriam et al. [25] examined 50 HEH patients, 80% were asymptomatic, 94% had multiple intrahepatic lesions, and 54% had

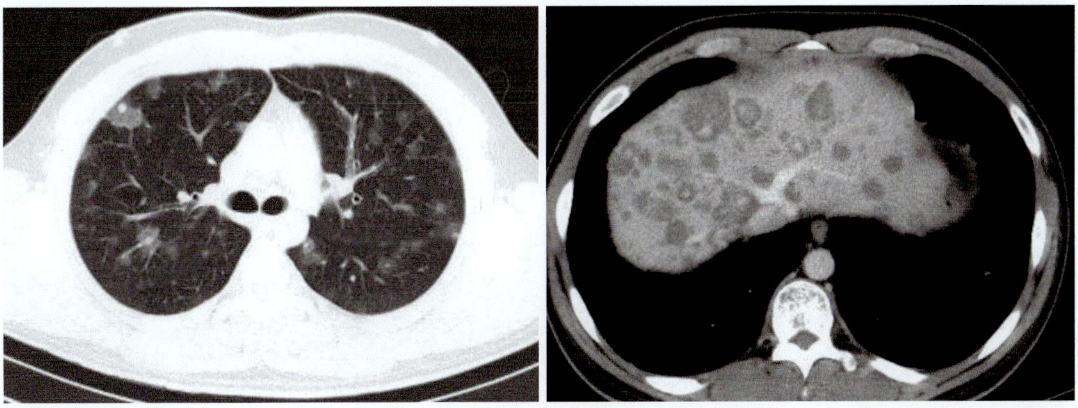

Fig. 9 Chest CT

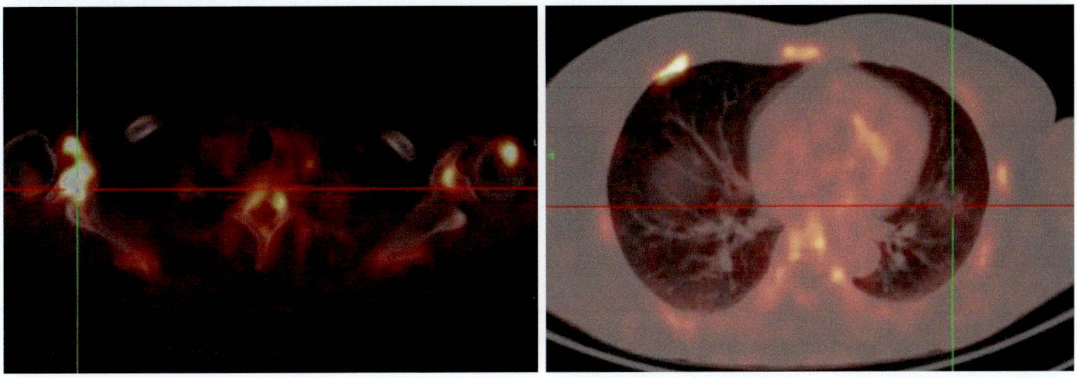

Fig. 10 PET/CT

extrahepatic metastases. Sixteen (88.9%) of 18 patients with initial observation had progressive disease (PD). Noh et al. [26] selected 79 patients diagnosed with HEH from 1973 to 2014 in the SEER database. The initial extent of disease was local in 22 (27.8%) patients, regional metastasis in 22 (27.8%), distant metastasis in 31 (39.2%), and unknown in 4 (5.1%). Surgical therapy was the only independent prognostic factor for survival based on multivariate analysis.

9.2 Case 2

A 47-year-old man complained of lumbodynia for 5 months. The pain was aggravated 20 days ago, accompanied by pain in the right ilium.

PET/CT: Increased uptake corresponding to lesions in the right ilium, multiple vertebral bodies of the spine, and multiple ribs (Fig. 10).

Chest CT: Multiple ground-glass nodules in both lungs (Fig. 11).

[Diagnosis] Epithelioid angiosarcoma.

[Diagnosis Basis] The patient underwent a needle biopsy of the right ilium, which revealed an epithelioid angiosarcoma (Fig. 12). Immunohistochemistry showed positive for CD31, CD34, FVIII, Fli-1, CKpan, and CK7, and negative for CK20, PSA, P504S, and TTF-1.

[Analysis] Angiosarcomas are rare, aggressive soft-tissue sarcomas of vascular endothelial cell

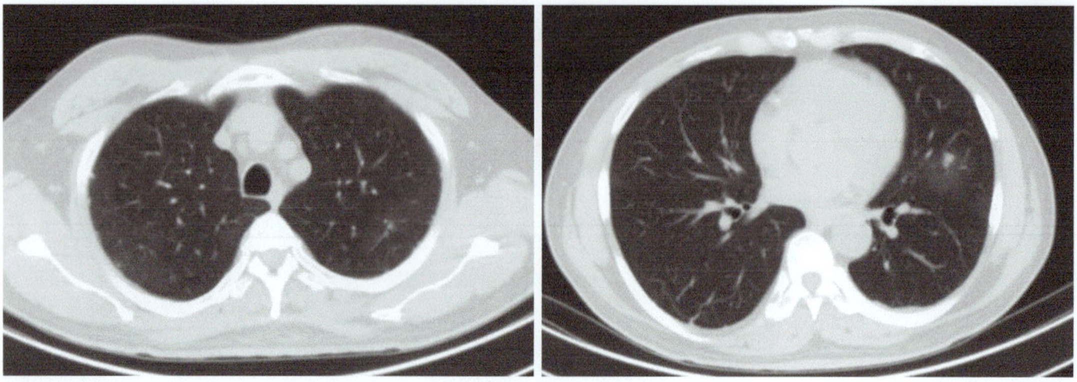

Fig. 11 Chest CT

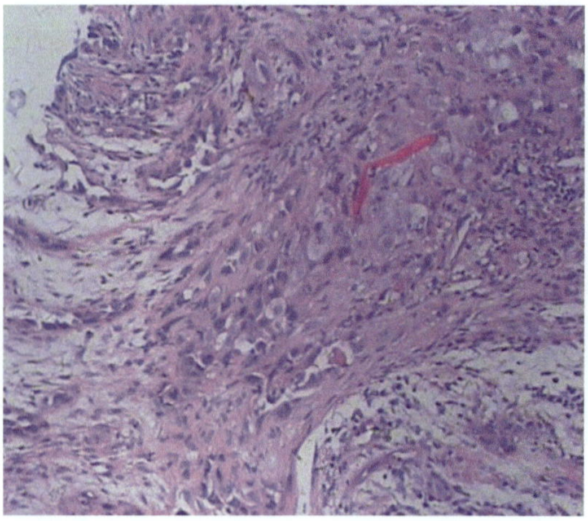

Fig. 12 Tumor cells are epithelioid with abundant eosinophilic cytoplasm, vesicular nuclei, and prominent nucleoli, and arranged in small nests or cords, showing immature vascular lumen

origin, accounting for 1–2% of all soft tissue sarcomas. It may affect any organ and often occurs in the deep soft tissues, skin, bone, adrenals, thyroid, liver, spleen, heart, and breast. 90% of angiosarcomas involving the lung are metastatic. Radiotherapy or chronic lymphoedema may induce angiosarcoma. Medical or occupational exposure to thorium dioxide, polyvinyl chloride, and arsenic has been also considered as risk factors [27]. Naka et al. [28] collected 99 cases of angiosarcoma through a nationwide Japanese study. The mean age at diagnosis was 62 years (3–92), with a 2:1 male to female ratio. The most common primary site was head and face (29 cases), followed by liver (17), trunk (13), heart (12), extremities (7), pleural cavity (6), chest wall (2), buttock (2), abdominal wall (2), and inguinal region (1). The majority of cases had metastases, including 72 cases of lung, 42 cases of bone, 36 cases of liver, 30 cases of regional lymph nodes, and 24 cases of adrenal gland. The 2-year survival rate was 17%. In Japan, chronic pyothorax, radiotherapy, and Thorotrast proved to be unique causative factors of angiosarcoma.

Histologically, angiosarcomas range from well-differentiated tumors with variable endothelial atypia to high-grade spindle cell malignancies, including classic and epithelioid variants. Epithelioid angiosarcoma (EAS) is a histologic subtype of angiosarcoma, with a structure characterized by epithelial cells and represents about 20–30% of angiosarcoma. Most EAS are soft-tissue angiosarcomas, and a few are located in the internal organs and skin. Primary pulmonary EAS is an extremely rare malignancy reported for the first time by Sheppard et al in a 65-year-old man in 1997 [29].

Classic angiosarcomas often show vasoformative features as anastomosing vascular channels lined by malignant endothelium. Compared with classical vasoformative angiosarcoma, epithelioid differentiation is considered to be a feature of higher malignant potential. EAS is characterized by solid-sheeted growth pattern with large, mildly to moderately pleomorphic epithelioid or spindled tumor cells with abundant eosinophilic cytoplasm, vesicular nuclei, and prominent nucleoli. Numerous intracytoplasmic lumina with extravasated red blood cells can usually be

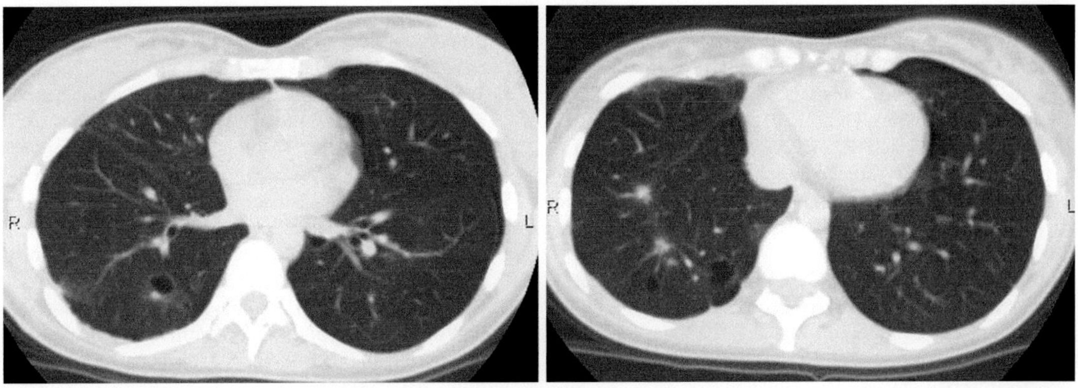

Fig. 13 Chest CT

observed, aiding in diagnosis. Obvious vasoformative foci is limited to a small proportion in EAS.

Immunohistochemically, EAS is positive for endothelial cell markers (CD31, CD34, FVIII, Fli-1, and Ulex europaeus agglutinin I), and vimentin. The expression of EMA or cytokeratin is variable.

9.3 Case 3

A 30-year-old woman complained of chest pain, cough, and hemoptysis for 1 week.

Chest CT: Multiple nodular and cystic lesions in both lungs (Fig. 13).

[Diagnosis] Epithelioid angiosarcoma.

[Diagnosis Basis] The pathology of the soft-tissue lesions in the right hand of the patient 2 months ago suggested epithelioid sarcoma, and the intrapulmonary lesions were considered for metastasis.

[Analysis] Primary pulmonary EAS mainly occurs in adults with an obvious predominance in males. Primary and metastatic pulmonary EAS have similar symptomatology and radiologic features. The common symptoms include chest pain, dyspnea, hemoptysis, cough, and weight loss. The CT findings include solitary pulmonary nodule or mass (particular as primary), multiple peripheral pulmonary nodules, diffuse and patchy consolidation, multiple thin-walled cysts, and ground-glass opacities (related to pulmonary hemorrhage) with or without pleural effusion. It is difficult to differentiate pulmonary EAS from other pulmonary malignant neoplasms by radiographic features.

Surgical resection and radiation therapy are the common options for pulmonary EAS. Chemotherapy is generally not effective due to aggressive, high-grade malignancy. Most patients die within 1 year of initial presentation.

References

1. Dail DH, Liebow AA. Intravascular bronchioalveolar tumor. Am J Pathol. 1975;78:6–7.
2. Corrin B, Manners B, Millard M, et al. Histogenesis of the so-called "intravascular bronchioloalveolar tumour". J Pathol. 1979;128:163–7.
3. Weldon-Linne CM, Victor TA, Fry WA, et al. Angiogenic nature of the intravascular bronchioloalveolar tumor of the lung: an electron microscopic study. Arch Pathol. 1981;105:174–9.
4. Weiss SW, Enzinger FM. Epithelioid hemangioendothelioma: a vascular tumor often mistaken for a carcinoma. Cancer. 1982;50:970–81.
5. Mertens F, Unni K, Fletcher CDM. World Health Organization classification of tumors. Pathology and genetics. Tumors of soft tissue and bone. Lyon: IRAC Press; 2002. p. 155.
6. Travis WD, Brambilla E, Nicholson AG, et al. The 2015 World Health Organization classification of lung tumors: impact of genetic, clinical and radiologic advances since the 2004 classification. J Thorac Oncol. 2015;10:1243–60.

7. Anderson T, Zhang L, Hameed M, et al. Thoracic epithelioid malignant vascular tumors: a clinicopathologic study of 52 cases with emphasis on pathologic grading and molecular studies of WWTR1-CAMTA1 fusions. Am J Surg Pathol. 2015;39:132–9.
8. Gill R, O'Donnell RJ, Horvai A. Utility of immunohistochemistry for endothelial markers in distinguishing epithelioid hemangioendothelioma from carcinoma metastatic to bone. Arch Pathol Lab Med. 2009;133:967–72.
9. Errani C, Zhang L, Sung YS, et al. A novel WWTR1-CAMTA1 gene fusion is a consistent abnormality in epithelioid hemangioendothelioma of different anatomic sites. Genes Chromosomes Cancer. 2011;50:644–53.
10. Antonescu CR, Le Loarer F, Mosquera JM, et al. Novel YAP1-TFE3 fusion defines a distinct subset of epithelioid hemangioendothelioma. Genes Chromosomes Cancer. 2013;52:775–84.
11. Dermawan JK, Azzato EM, Billings SD, et al. YAP1-TFE3-fused hemangioendothelioma: a multi-institutional clinicopathologic study of 24 genetically-confirmed cases. Mod Pathol. 2021;34:2211–21.
12. Rosenbaum E, Jadeja B, Xu B, et al. Prognostic stratification of clinical and molecular epithelioid hemangioendothelioma subsets. Mod Pathol. 2020;33:591–602.
13. Lau K, Massad M, Pollak C, et al. Clinical patterns and outcome in epithelioid hemangioendothelioma with or without pulmonary involvement: insights from an internet registry in the study of a rare cancer. Chest. 2011;140:1312–8.
14. Schattenberg T, Kam R, Klopp M, et al. Pulmonary epithelioid hemangioendothelioma: report of three cases. Surg Today. 2008;38:844–9.
15. Amin RM, Hiroshima K, Kokubo T, et al. Risk factors and independent predictors of survival in patients with pulmonary epithelioid haemangioendothelioma. Review of the literature and a case report. Respirology. 2006;11:818–25.
16. Kim EY, Kim TS, Han JH, et al. Thoracic epithelioid hemangioendothelioma: imaging and pathologic features. Acta Radiol. 2011;52:161–6.
17. Liu K, Xie P, Peng W, et al. The computed tomographic findings of pulmonary epithelioid hemangioendothelioma. Radiol Med. 2014;119:705–13.
18. Woo JH, Kim TJ, Lee KS, et al. Epithelioid hemangioendothelioma in the thorax: clinicopathologic, CT, PET, and prognostic features. Medicine (Baltimore). 2016;95:e4348.
19. Bagan P, Hassan M, Barthes FLP, et al. Prognostic factors and surgical indications of pulmonary epithelioid hemangioendothelioma: a review of the literature. Ann Thorac Surg. 2006;82:2010–3.
20. Baba H, Tomiyasu M, Makino H, et al. Surgical resection of a primary pulmonary epithelioid hemangioendothelioma in bilateral lungs. Gen Thorac Cardiovasc Surg. 2010;58:431–3.
21. Kanemura S, Kuribayashi K, Moriya Y, et al. Pemetrexed for epithelioid haemangioendothelioma of the pleura. Respirol Case Rep. 2016;4:e00191.
22. Ye B, Li W, Feng J, et al. Treatment of pulmonary epithelioid hemangioendothelioma with combination chemotherapy: report of three cases and review of the literature. Oncol Lett. 2013;5:1491–6.
23. Kitaichi M, Nagai S, Nishimura K, et al. Pulmonary epithelioid haemangioendothelioma in 21 patients, including three with partial spontaneous regression. Eur Respir J. 1998;12:89–96.
24. Epelboym Y, Engelkemier DR, Thomas-Chausse F, et al. Imaging findings in epithelioid hemangioendothelioma. Clin Imaging. 2019;58:59–65.
25. Merriam P, Nathenson MJ. Liver transplantation for hepatic epithelioid hemangioendothelioma. Cancer. 2021;127:3714–6.
26. Noh OK, Kim SS, Yang MJ, et al. Treatment and prognosis of hepatic epithelioid hemangioendothelioma based on SEER data analysis from 1973 to 2014. Hepatobiliary Pancreat Dis Int. 2020;19:29–35.
27. Young RJ, Brown NJ, Reed MW, et al. Angiosarcoma. Lancet Oncol. 2010;11:983–91.
28. Naka N, Ohsawa M, Tomita Y, et al. Angiosarcoma in Japan. A review of 99 cases. Cancer. 1995;75:989–96.
29. Sheppard MN, Hansell DM, Du Bois RM, et al. Primary epithelioid angiosarcoma of the lung presenting as pulmonary hemorrhage. Hum Pathol. 1997;28:383–5.

Pulmonary Sarcoma

Xue-Peng Huang and Song Zhang

Sarcomas are a heterogeneous group of malignant tumors and predominantly arise from the embryonic mesoderm. Sarcomas may be divided into two major categories, originating from the soft tissue such as muscle, tendons, and blood vessels and originating from the bone such as osteosarcoma and Ewing's sarcoma. Approximately 80% of sarcomas originate from soft tissue and 20% arise from the bone.

Primary pulmonary sarcomas (PPS) are very rare malignant tumors that arise from mesenchymal elements of the bronchial wall, vessels, or pulmonary stroma, representing 0.013%–1.1% of all lung malignancies.

1 Pathology

The classification of sarcomas and the recognition of new entities have evolved since the introduction of immunohistochemical and molecular diagnosis and the fifth edition of the WHO classification of soft tissue and bone tumors has been published in May 2020. These refinements may explain the incongruence in different histotype frequencies between different studies.

The common types of PPS are malignant fibrous histiocytoma, fibrosarcoma, synovial sarcoma, angiosarcoma, leiomyosarcoma, malignant peripheral nerve sheath tumor, undifferentiated pleomorphic sarcoma, liposarcoma, and rhabdomyosarcoma. Spraker et al. [1] found that the most frequently identified histologies were fibroblastic and myofibroblastic tumors (16.2%), accompanied by leiomyosarcoma (15%), synovial sarcoma (12%), fibrohistiocytic tumors (8%), blood vessel tumors (6%), and nerve sheath tumors (4%). Keel et al. [2] analyzed the pathologic features of 26 PPS. The histologic diagnoses were malignant fibrous histiocytoma (7), synovial sarcoma (6), malignant peripheral nerve sheath tumor (3), leiomyosarcoma (3), intimal sarcoma (2), angiosarcoma (2), fibrosarcoma (2), and one case of epithelioid hemangioendothelioma. A study by Duran-Moreno et al. [3] revealed histological subtypes including synovial sarcoma (40%), undifferentiated pleomorphic sarcoma (40%), epithelial sarcoma (4%), angiosarcoma (4%), fibrosarcoma (4%), inflammatory fibroblastic tumor (4%), and SMARCA4-deficient sarcoma (4%).

X.-P. Huang
Department of Respiratory and Critical Care Medicine, People's Hospital of Rizhao Lanshan, Rizhao, Shandong, China

S. Zhang (✉)
Department of Respiratory and Critical Care Medicine, Shandong Provincial Hospital Affiliated to Shandong First Medical University, Jinan, Shandong, China

S. Zhang (ed.), *Diagnostic Imaging of Lung Cancers*, https://doi.org/10.1007/978-981-99-6815-2_19

2 Epidemiology

PPS usually occur in middle-aged to elderly individuals with a mean age of 45 to 63 years according to different series. Gebauer et al. [4] reported no connection between PPS and smoking, environmental pollution, industrial toxins, or chronic bronchitis by a comparison of 41 primary sarcomas of the lungs with the 192 cases of carcinomas.

3 Radiographic Features

PPS usually infiltrates lung parenchyma, forming a large peripheral or hilar well-circumscribed, but not encapsulated mass, and may present as an endobronchial tumor in 10% of cases.

4 Treatment and Prognosis

Surgical resection is the first choice for resectable disease. Régnard et al. [5] performed 20 complete resections and three exploratory thoracotomies only for primary lung sarcomas in a 24-year period. One patient declined operation. All 4 patients who had no resection died within 15 months. The 5- and 10-year actuarial survival after complete resection was 48%. Complete resection and stage of disease were the sole significant prognostic factors, although almost half of the patients died of metastasis within 2 years of operation. Gołota et al. [6] estimated factors that may affect the overall survival (OS) and progression-free survival (PFS) of different types of radical operations for PPS. They concluded that there are no unambiguous factors affecting OS and PFS of patients who have undergone anatomical and non-anatomical resections. Yamada et al. [7] retrospectively reviewed the records of 24 PPS patients who underwent surgical resection. The 5-year OS rate of the patients was 50%. Incomplete resection, higher pathological grade, advanced pathological stage, and tumor size($\geq$7 cm) were unfavorable factors for long-term survival.

PPS patients may benefit from the appropriate combination of surgery, radiation, chemotherapy, and immunotherapy. Spraker et al. [1] analyzed the clinical characteristics and therapeutic strategies of PPS and their impact on OS by a large cohort of 365 PPS patients. OS of PPS patients were compared with a cohort of 10,909 extremity soft tissue sarcomas patients. 55% of PPS patients had large tumors (>5 cm), 76% were high-grade, and 16% had node-positive disease.75% of patients underwent surgery alone, 14% surgery and radiation therapy (RT), and 11% RT alone. Multivariate analysis showed reduced OS for patients with tumors more than 5 cm, high tumor grade, and unresectable disease. The 5-year OS for PPS patients versus sarcomas of the extremities was 35% versus 71%. Regarding therapy, the 5-year OS was 41% for those who underwent surgery alone, 25% for those who underwent surgery and RT, and 7% for those who underwent RT alone. Gołota et al. [8] analyzed 22 patients who underwent surgical treatment. The median OS of all patients was 22 months, 5- and 10-year OS was 27% and 18% respectively, whereas in patients who underwent non-anatomical lung resections, 5- and 10-year OS was 80% and 60% with median OS of 213 months. Primary radical surgical resection prolongs patient survival. Patients with tumors larger than 5 cm and men have worse prognoses. Hemoptysis was an adverse prognostic factor. Age, type of sarcoma, degree of histological malignancy, stage or adjuvant treatment did not affect on OS. Collaud et al. [9] retrospectively reviewed 13 patients who underwent resection for PPS. Eight (61.5%) patients received neoadjuvant treatment. Overall 5-year survival was 60%. Median disease-free survival was 17 months. Tumor size was a predictor for survival and recurrence. Sex and type of lung resection were predictors of survival. TNM stages for PPS were predictors for recurrence. Porte et al. [10] found that complete resection is the best therapeutic option for achieving an acceptable survival rate in PPS, pre-operative chemotherapy can serve as a useful adjunct in increasing the resectability of these tumors.

Tumor size has been considered as a prognostic factor with the greatest impact on survival.

However, Régnard et al. [5] and Porte et al. [10] did not find statistically significant differences in OS between patients with tumors greater or smaller than 5 cm.

Sarcoma spreads primarily via the bloodstream and only rarely through the lymphatic system [11]. The current study suggested that nodal status was not related to prognosis and histologic subtype. However, Régnard et al. [5] observed N2 development in 2 out of 20 patients who underwent surgical treatment and N1 development in another 3, which amounts to 22% of patients. A study by Spraker et al. [1] showed that the 5-year OS for patients with node-negative disease was 39%, whereas it was 14% for those with node-positive disease. Duran-Moreno et al. [3] presented a retrospective study of 26 PPS patients. Eight patients (33.33%) had mediastinal node invasion (MNI). Median disease-free interval was 15 months. The median OS of all patients were 10 months and 4 months for metastatic disease. Only surgery may affect survival. These studies suggest that nodal status may serve as an indication for surgical evaluation of mediastinum and locoregional PPS patients should be treated with a more aggressive approach.

5 Case Analysis

5.1 Case 1

A 47-year-old man complained of cough, expectoration, and hemoptysis for 2 weeks.

Chest CT: A heterogeneous mass in the right lower lobe with smooth border and intratumoral calcification and vessels (Fig. 1).

[Diagnosis] Primary pulmonary synovial sarcoma.

[Diagnosis Basis] The patient underwent right lower lobectomy. The tumor size was 8 × 7 × 3 cm and pathology showed peripheral synovial sarcoma. No nerve or intravascular invasion was seen. No regional lymph node metastasis was found. Immunohistochemistry showed positive for CK, EMA, vimentin, CK19, CD99, Calponin, Bcl-2, and negative for CD34, SMA, S-100, and desmin.

[Analysis] Synovial sarcoma (SS) is a malignant tumor and mainly arises in the deep soft tissues, especially near the large joints of the extremities (80%–95% of cases), therefore, it was mistakenly believed arising from synovium. It originates from pluripotent mesenchymal tissue located in various organs of the body rather than synovial tissue, so the term "synovial sarcoma" is a misnomer. SS represents 5%–10% of all soft tissue sarcomas.

Primary pulmonary SS (PPSS) is a very rare, highly aggressive tumor with less than 0.5% incidence among all pulmonary malignancies, arising most commonly from the lung parenchyma followed by the pleura and mediastinum. It was first reported by Zeren et al. in 1995 [12].

Most of PPSS are reported in non-smokers, and young and middle-aged adults with a median age of 31–50 years. Patients with mediastinal SS are younger with a male gender bias [13].

Clinical symptoms of PPSS are based on the histological type, tumor location, size, and degree of differentiation of the tumor. Peripheral tumors may be initially asymptomatic. The most common presenting symptoms are cough, dyspnea, and hemoptysis caused by obstructive pneumonia as the disease progresses. They can infiltrate the adjacent organs and result in chest pain, pleural or pericardial effusions, hemothorax, and recurrent pneumothorax.

Chest CT scan shows a well-circumscribed mass with round, lobulated borders, a pleural mass, partial or complete opacification of the hemithorax in large tumors, or endobronchial lesion (Fig. 2). Most tumors are larger than 5 cm, with heterogeneous enhancement because of the presence of a necrotic, cystic, or friable portion of the tumor interspersed with a solid enhancing component of the tumor (Fig. 3). Primary pulmonary and mediastinal SS has less intratumoral calcification (15%–17%) compared with soft tissue SS (≤30%) (Fig. 4). Cavitation or mediastinal adenopathy is rare. Kim et al. [14] retrospectively reviewed 14 patients with pathologically proven PPSS. The median tumor size was 10.2 cm. Half

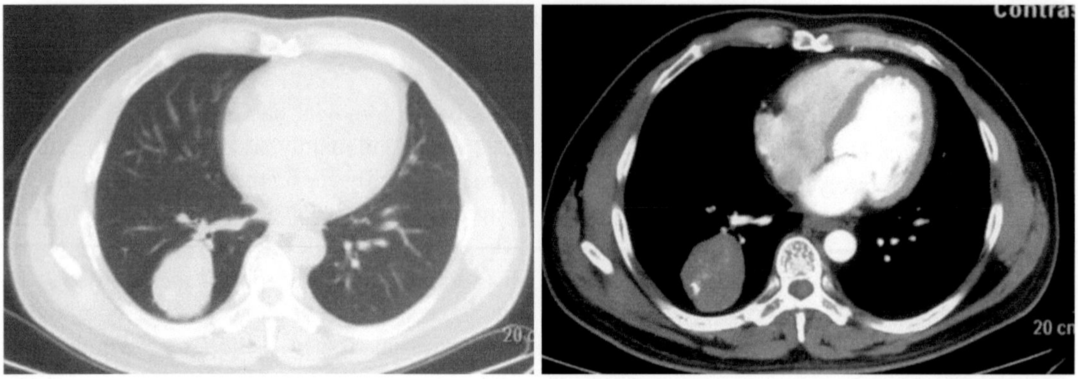

Fig. 1 Chest CT

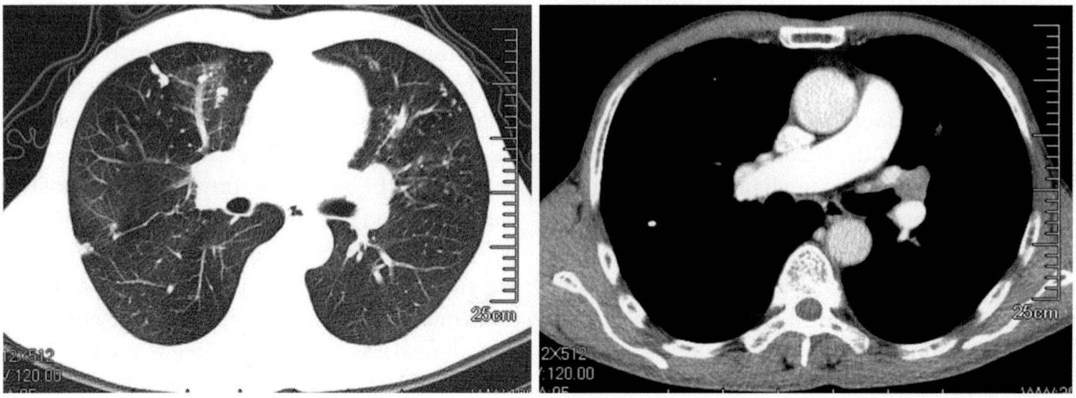

Fig. 2 A 58-year-old man with a lesion in the left upper lobe, growing along the lumen

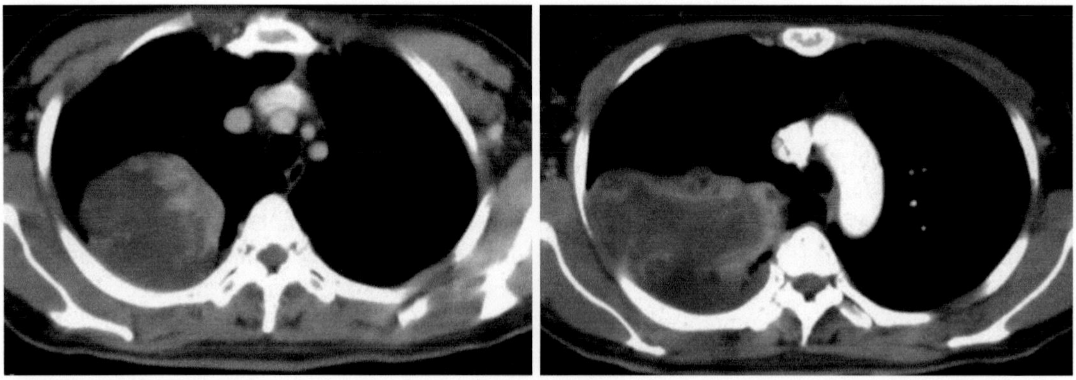

Fig. 3 A 48-year-old woman with a right pleura mass, showing obvious necrosis and cystic degeneration

of the tumors had intratumoral calcifications, and intratumoral vessels were frequently seen. Tumor rupture, pleural/chest wall extension, and pleural effusion occurred frequently. On MRI, PPSS shows triple signal areas of bright, dark, and gray attenuation representing the presence of tumor, hemorrhage, and necrosis, respectively.

Histologically, PPSS is mainly composed of two morphological types of epithelial cells or fibroblast-like spindle cells and is classified into

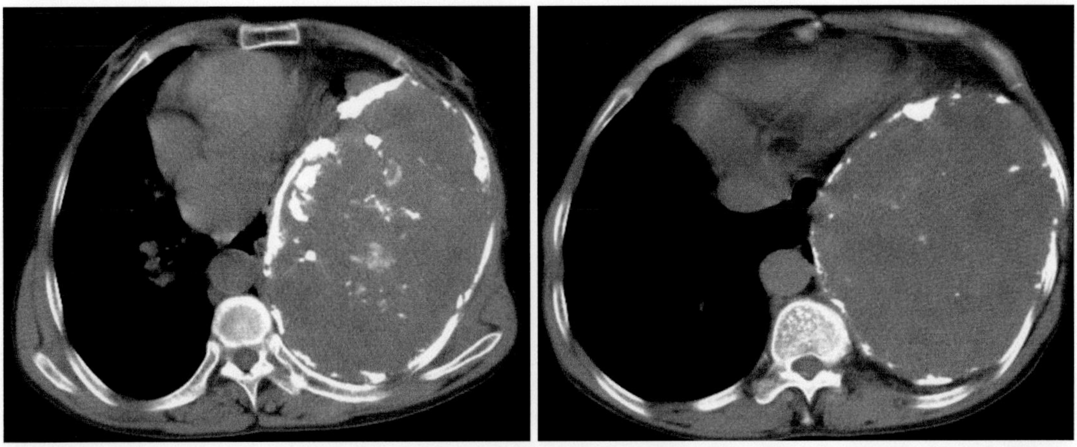

Fig.4 A 62-year-old woman with a huge mass in left thoracic cavity with obvious calcifications

four types: biphasic, poorly differentiated, monophasic fibrous (spindle cell), and monophasic epithelial type. The monophasic spindle cell type consists of relatively small and uniform spindle cells with ovoid, pale staining nuclei and inconspicuous nucleoli. The monophasic epithelial type has a uniformly glandular pattern and practically indistinguishable from adenocarcinoma in the absence of cytogenetic study. Biphasic SS is composed of both epithelial and spindle components. The epithelial cell component contains ovoid nuclei and has a cytoplasm that is organized in a glandular pattern. The poorly differentiated SS consists of spindle, polymorphic, and round cells, which is hard to be differentiated from the others through cell morphology. Immunohistochemically, SS is usually positive for cytokeratin, EMA, Bcl-2, CD99, vimentin and negative for S-100, desmin, smooth muscle actin, CD34, and vascular tumor markers.

Cytogenetically, the t(X:18) (p11.2;q11.2) translocation is exclusively observed in this tumor and remains the gold standard for the diagnosis. This translocation results in an SYT-SSX1, SYT-SSX2, or rarely SYT-SSX4 fusion transcript which is present in more than 95% of cases. Nilsson et al. [15] assessed the type of fusion transcript by reverse transcription-PCR and sequence analysis in 33 patients with primary SS. The 5-year metastasis-free survival for patients with SYT-SSX1 was 42% versus 89% for patients with SYT-SSX2.

Complete surgical resection is the first choice for patients with PPSS followed by chemotherapy and/or radiotherapy. SS has a relative chemosensitivity with about 50% response rates to ifosfamide and doxorubicin-based regimens [16].

Local recurrence of PPSS is common and frequently metastasizes to bone, liver, skin, brain, contralateral lung, spleen, abdomen, and subcutaneous tissue. PPSS has a poor prognosis, with an overall 5-year survival rate of 35%–50%. Tumor size, male gender, extensive tumor necrosis, higher histological grade, mitotic rate, the expression of SYT-SSX1 variants, and neurovascular invasion are negative prognostic factors.

5.2 Case 2

A 65-year-old man complained of cough for 1 month.

Chest CT: A heterogeneous mass in the left base of the lung involving the pleural surface and eroding of the adjacent rib (Fig. 5).

[Diagnosis] Primary pulmonary undifferentiated pleomorphic sarcoma.

[Diagnosis Basis] The patient underwent left thoracic tumor resection. The tumor was located in the posterior basal segment of the left lower

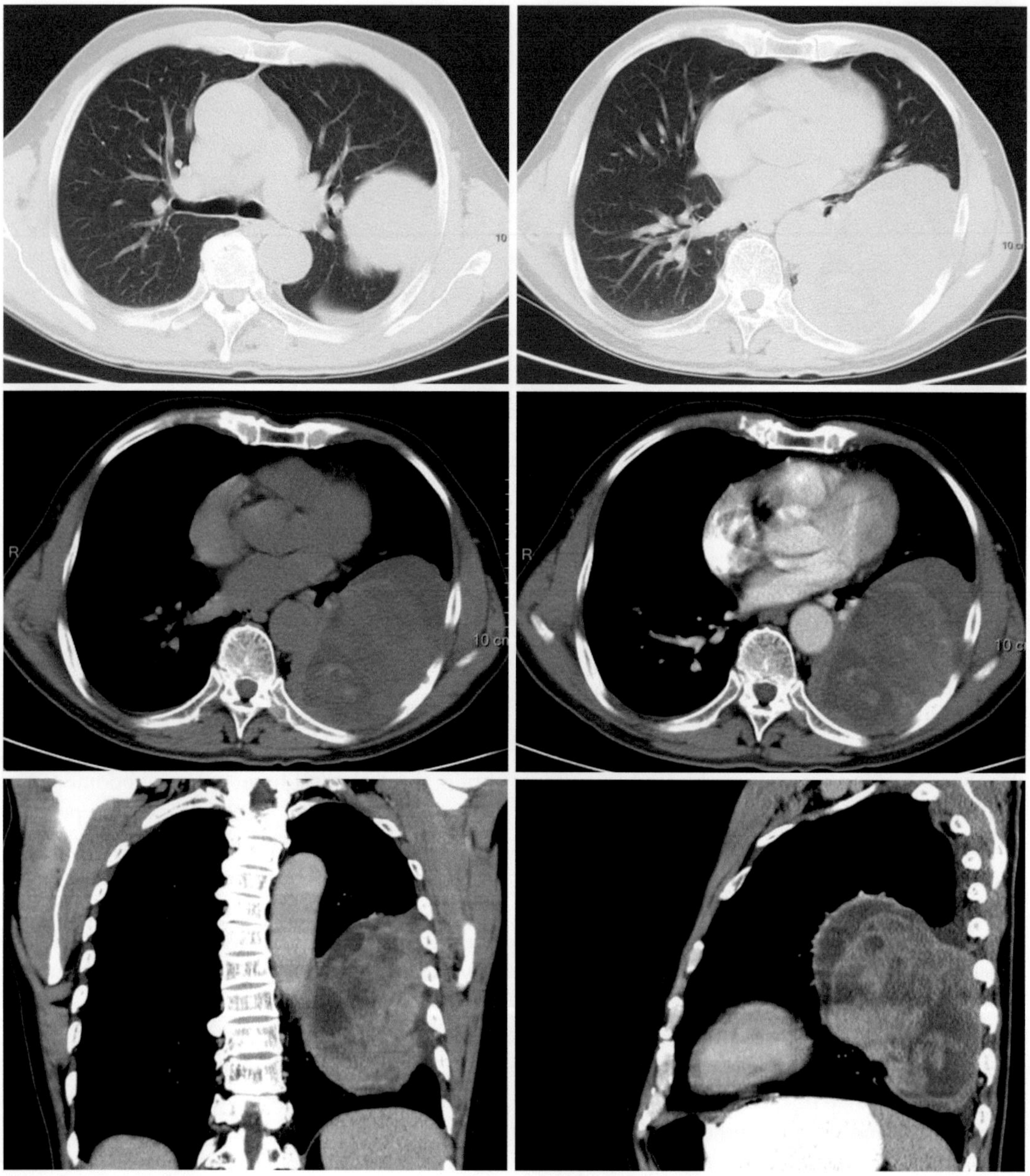

Fig. 5 Chest CT

lobe, with a size of about 15 × 10 × 10 cm, and invaded the left posterior chest wall and the seventh rib. The pathology was consistent with undifferentiated pleomorphic sarcoma. All surgical margins were free of malignancy, and no pleural nodule and lymph node metastasis were identified. Immunohistochemistry showed positive for bcl-2 (weak) and CD34(vascular), and negative for CK, CAM5.2, SMA, S-100, CR, CK5/6, desmin, HMB-45, Melan A, and EMA.

[Analysis] Undifferentiated pleomorphic sarcoma (UPS), formerly known as malignant fibrous histiocytoma (MFH), is a high-grade aggressive soft tissue sarcoma. It arises from mesenchymal stem cells rather than histiocytes as previously thought. MFH was first described in 1963 as a malignant soft tissue tumor with a fibrohistiocytic origin [17], however, further studies (electron microscopy, immunohistochemical techniques, or molecular studies) failed to find evidence of true fibrohistiocytic differentiation, and its morphologic pattern may be shared by a wide variety of poorly differentiated malignant neoplasms. Fletcher et al. [18] reassessed 159 tumors diagnosed as pleomorphic sarcomas. 97 cases (61% of total) proved to be specific sarcomas other than MFH, 20(12.6%) proved to be nonmesenchymal neoplasms, and 42(26.4%) were unclassifiable (of which 19 were small biopsies and 2 were subtotally necrotic). Only 13% ($n = 21$) of these cases were eligible for consideration as MFH. Therefore, MFH was removed from the 2013 WHO classification and renamed "undifferentiated pleomorphic sarcoma" [19].

UPS most commonly affects the extremities and the retroperitoneum of elderly patients (average 50–70 years) and metastasizes to several organs, especially the lungs. Primary pulmonary UPS(PPUPS) is extremely rare, which was first described by Bedrossian et al. in 1979 [20]. Yousem et al. [21] described 22 cases of primary pulmonary MFH. Chest wall invasion at diagnosis was found in four cases. Vascular invasion was observed in 50% of cases. Histologic features did not correlate with prognosis, and subsequent aggressive behavior was related primarily to symptomatic presentation, advanced stage at diagnosis, incomplete excision, invasion of the chest wall or mediastinum, and subsequent recurrence or metastasis.

Histologically, UPS consists of a storiform arrangement of highly pleomorphic and spindle-shaped cells and shows no discernible microscopic evidence of any specific form of differentiation such as lipoblasts, bone formation, and epithelial structures. Immunohistochemically, UPS is characteristically positive for histiocytic markers (CD68, α1-antichymotrypsin, vimentin), a reason why it was named as MFH in the past. UPS is a diagnosis of exclusion, which need wider immunohistochemical studies to rule out other neoplasms that can resemble UPS, including other types of sarcomas, sarcomatoid carcinoma, melanoma, or sarcomatoid mesothelioma. Desmin, actin, vimentin, keratin, TTF-1, S-100, myoglobin, D2-40, and neurogenic tumors are commonly used for the differential diagnosis.

Higuchi et al. [22] analyzed the data of PPUPS of 54 patients since 1979.This cohort included 33 men and 21 women. The mean age was 56.1 (range 12–86) years. The average tumor size was 7.3 cm.12 patients were positive for lymph node metastasis and 42 were negative. Of the 54 patients, 48 patients received surgical treatments including lobectomy in 35 patients, pneumonectomy in 8 patients, and other resection in 5 patients. The 2-, 5-, and 10-year overall survival rates were 46.4%, 40.2%, and 34.5%, respectively. The 5-year overall survival rate was 48.7% in no lymph node metastatic group and 16.7% in lymph node metastatic group. The effective treatment for UPS is complete resection, and appropriate surgical procedure is lobectomy.

5.3 Case 3

A 34-year-old man complained of intermittent hemoptysis for 4 months, aggravated by 1 day.

Chest CT: A heterogeneous mass in the left lower lobe (Fig. 6).

[Diagnosis] Primary pulmonary alveolar rhabdomyosarcoma.

[Diagnosis Basis] The patient underwent left lower lobectomy. The tumor was about 6.5 × 6.3 × 6.2 cm. Postoperative pathology showed sarcoma. All surgical margins were free of malignancy, and no pleural nodule and lymph node metastasis were identified. Immunohistochemistry showed positive for MYOD1 (sporadic cells), vimentin, bcl-2, desmin (sporadic cells), CD31 (weak), CD34 (weak), CD99, and STAT6, and negative for CK, Cam5.2, S-100, HMB-4, SOX10, and P63. The tumor was diagnosed as alveolar RMS based on the microscopic and immunohistochemical findings.

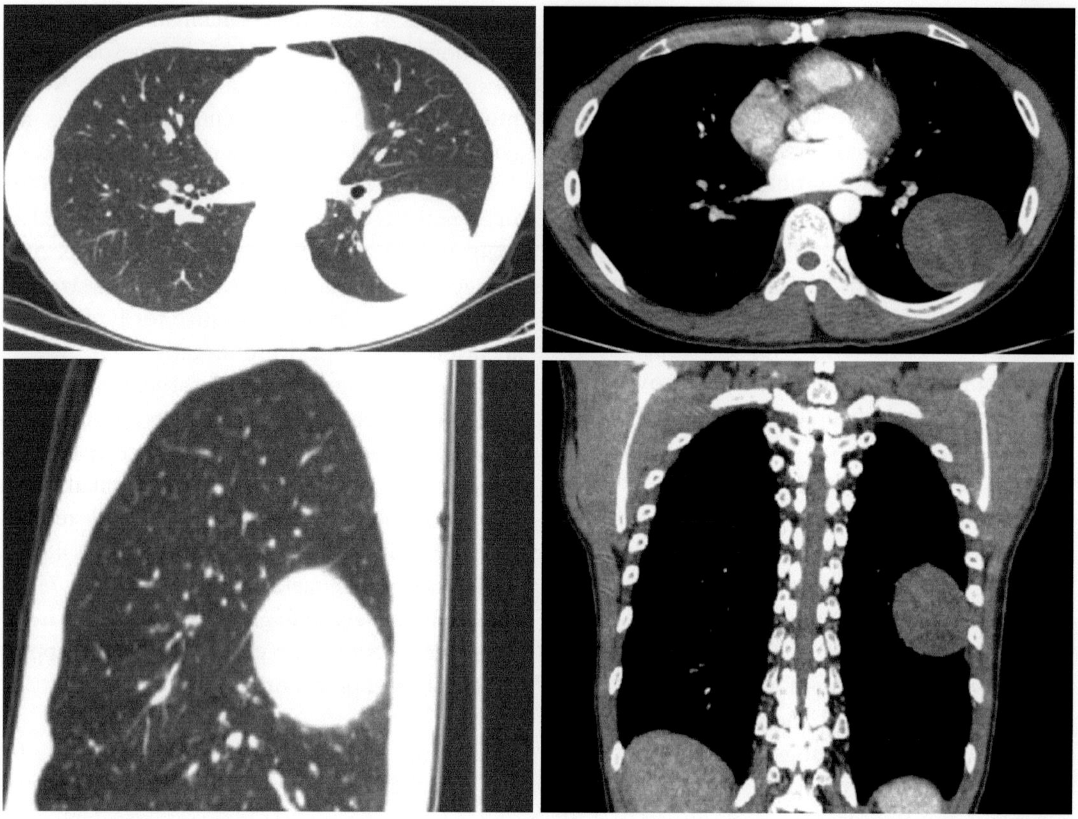

Fig. 6 Chest CT

[Analysis] Rhabdomyosarcoma (RMS) is a high-grade, malignant neoplasm with a propensity for myogenic differentiation and is the most common soft tissue sarcomas in children. Almost 90% of RMS present in individuals under 25 years of age, and about 70% are in children under 10 years of age. RMS represents less than 1% of adult malignancies and less than 5% of adult soft tissue sarcomas. Weber reported the first case of RMS in 1854, and McDonald et al. reported the first case of primary pulmonary RMS in 1939 [23]. RMS can arise in any site and occurs commonly in the head and neck region (35%–40%), followed by the urogenital system, extremities, and torso.

Primary pulmonary RMS occurring in adults is extremely rare and typically presents as a parenchymal mass. There are two possible reasons for the histogenesis of primary pulmonary RMS. The first states an origin from heterotopic islets of striated muscle, thus explaining the frequent association of RMS with pulmonary malformations such as bronchogenic cysts, cystic adenomatoid malformations, and extralobar sequestration, where these islets are usually present. The second hypothesis suggests a metaplasia of uncommitted mesenchymal cells in a normal lung like in other organs lacking intrinsic skeletal muscles such as bile ducts, eye, peripheral nerves, and cerebellum. Metaplasia seems more applicable for those cases in which no pre-existing lung malformation is present.

Environmental factors such as paternal tobacco smoking, advanced maternal age, maternal recreational drug use, and X-ray exposure in the uterus increase the risk for developing RMS. Genetic disorders such as neurofibromatosis type 1, hereditary retinoblastoma, Beckwith-Wiedemann syndrome, Li-Fraumeni syndrome, Rubinstein-Taybi syndrome, nevoid basal cell carcinoma syndrome, and Costello syndrome may play a role in the etiopathogenesis of RMS.

RMS was classified into four histological subtypes in the 2013 WHO classification of tumors of soft tissue and bone, including embryonal (60%), alveolar (20%), pleomorphic (10%), and spindle cell/sclerosing (10%). Pleomorphic RMS arises almost exclusively in adults. Three new subtypes have been proposed recently, namely RMS with MYOD1 mutations, RMS with TFCP2 fusions, and RMS with VGLL2/NCOA2 fusions. Two major RMS subtypes, alveolar RMS (ARMS) and embryonic RMS (ERMS), are driven by fundamentally different mechanisms. The diagnosis of RMS is based mainly on a combination of the histopathological, immunohistochemical, and molecular biological findings. Histopathologically, RMS cells are of heterogeneous shapes including undifferentiated and round cells, tadpole-like cells, ovoid cells, spindle-shaped cells and fully differentiated rhabdomyoblasts. ARMS comprises densely packed, small, round cells subdivided in nests by fibrous septa, whereas ERMS is typically composed of immature rhabdomyoblasts in a less dense, stroma-rich background without an alveolar pattern. Pleomorphic RMS comprises polymorphic, spindle, and multinucleated giant cells with abundant acidophilic cytoplasm. Highly differentiated striated rhabdomyoblasts are rarely found. Spindle cell/sclerosing RMS is characterized by extensive histologic heterogeneity. The presence of rhabdomyoblastic differentiation does not always equate to malignancy such as rhabdomyoma, nor to RMS, as some mesenchymal and epithelial malignancies may exhibit focal rhabdomyocytic differentiation such as mesenchymal chondrosarcoma and sarcomatoid carcinoma.

Immunohistochemically, RMS expresses skeletal muscle proteins, such as muscle-specific actin and myosin, desmin, myoglobin, Z-band protein, and MYOD1 or myogenin (Myf4). The expression of MYOD1 protein and myogenin is the easiest way to demonstrate rhabdomyoblastic differentiation of the sarcoma. Rekhi et al. [24] evaluated clinicopathologic and immunohistochemical features of 300 RMSs. Most cases, with the exception of polymorphic RMSs, occurred in the first two decades (228 cases) (76%), frequently in males, in the head and neck region (126) (42%). Immunohistochemically, desmin was positive in 292/299 (97.6%) tumors; myogenin in 238/267 (89.1%), and MYOD1 in 192/266 (72.2%) tumors. There was a significant association between high myogenin expression and ARMSs and high MYOD1 expression and spindle cell/sclerosing RMSs. Myogenin is a group of myogenic regulatory proteins whose expression determines commitment and differentiation of primitive mesenchymal cells into skeletal muscle. It is a useful marker in the differential diagnosis of RMS from other malignant small round cell tumors of childhood because its expression has been demonstrated to be highly specific for rhabdomyoblastic differentiation. In ARMS, the majority of tumor cells (75–100%) were positive for myogenin, in contrast to ERMS, in which the positivity ranged from rare + to 25% [25].

Molecularly, ARMS is characterized by t(2;13) (q35;q14) or t(1;13)(p36;q14) translocations encoding for PAX3- or PAX7-FOXO1 (FKHR) chimeric transcription factors, respectively, and is defined as fusion positive RMS (FP-RMS). The fusion gene alters the myogenic program and maintains the proliferative state while blocking terminal differentiation [26]. The fusion gene acts as a driver of malignancy in ARMS by disrupting tightly coupled but mutually exclusive pathways of proliferation and differentiation. FP-RMS has a worse prognosis compared to the more common fusion-negative RMS (FN-RMS). PAX3-FKHR and PAX7-FKHR fusion transcripts were detected in 55% and 22% of ARMS patients, respectively. PAX-FKHR fusion transcripts not only have specificity for ARMS, but the expression of PAX3-FKHR and PAX7-FKHR identifies a very high-risk subgroup and a favorable outcome subgroup, respectively, among patients presenting with metastatic ARMS [27]. Collins et al. [28] also confirmed that ARMS patients with PAX3-FKHR fusion have poorer prognosis owing to more marked cell cycle dysregulation compared to ARMS patients with the less common PAX7-FKHR fusion.

The genetic alteration in most of the ERMS patients is caused by the combination of copy number alterations (including loss of chromosomes 10 and 15, loss of heterozygosity at chromosome 11, polysomy of chromosome 8, and gains of 11q and 7q regions) and RAS pathway mutations such as Kirsten RAS oncogene homolog (KRAS), NRAS, fibroblast growth factor receptor 4 (FGFR4), neurofibromatosis 1 (NF1), and PIK3CA. Based on genetic features, spindle cell/sclerosing RMS is classified into three categories of MYOD1-mutated, gene fusion-driven, and a subset without a currently identified genetic driver event.

RMS has a higher propensity for lymph nodes metastasis compared with other types of soft tissue sarcoma. Nishida et al. [29] analyzed 44 RMS patients. The mean age of the patients at diagnosis was 26 (range 1–69) years, and 18(41%) were males. The histological subtypes included alveolar (17 patients), embryonal (10 patients), pleomorphic (7 patients), and unknown (10 patients). There were three cases of local relapse (two alveolar type and one unknown), ten cases of regional lymph node relapse, and three cases of in-transit metastasis (all alveolar type). Twenty-one patients (48%) developed distant metastases. Initial sites of metastases were bone (9 patients, 20%), lung (5 patients), and bone marrow dissemination (5 patients). Patients with alveolar type had a significantly high propensity for lymph node metastasis.

Adult RMS has poor prognosis as compared to childhood RMS. The treatment is usually multimodal with a combination of surgical resection, chemotherapy, and radiotherapy. The ARMS subtype is more aggressive and has a poorer prognosis. Metastatic ARMS is the most aggressive subtype with an 8% 5-year disease-free survival rate when PAX-FKHR fusion is present and a 29% 5-year disease-free survival rate when negative for a fusion event. ARMS patients without fusions are not different from those with ERMS in terms of prognosis and clinical course.

5.4 Case 4

A 52-year-old woman complained of chest tightness for 1 month.

Chest CT: A heterogeneous mass in the left lower lobe (Fig. 7).

[Diagnosis] Primary pulmonary leiomyosarcoma.

[Diagnosis Basis] The patient underwent lung biopsy. Pathology showed that the tumor was filled with dense spindle cells. Immunohistochemistry showed positive for vimentin, SMA, and H-caldesmon, and negative for S-100, HMB-4, CD34, and P63. The Ki-67 labeling index was 67.7%. The tumor was diagnosed as leiomyosarcoma based on the microscopic and immunohistochemical findings.

[Analysis] Leiomyosarcoma arises from any location but occurs most commonly in the uterus, retroperitoneum, or intraabdominal region. Primary pulmonary leiomyosarcoma (PPL) originates from the smooth muscle cells of the pulmonary parenchyma, blood vessels, or bronchial tree and accounts for less than 0.5% of all malignant lung tumors and 30% of primary pulmonary sarcomas. PPL was first described in 1903 by Davidsohn. Localized unilateral pulmonary mass with no detectable abnormality of the soft tissue, gastric intestinal tract, and genito-urinary system supports a primary pulmonary lesion.

Histologically, PPL shows malignant spindle cells with cigar-shaped nuclei arranged in interweaving fascicles. Calcification, cavitation, pneumothorax, and pleural effusions are rarely found. Immunohistochemistry showed positive for actin, smooth muscle actin, caldesmon, and vimentin, and negative for leukocyte common antigen, S-100, CD99, cytokeratins, neuroendocrine filaments, or carcinoembryonic antigen. Carvalho et al. [30] explored the differential expression of immunohistochemical markers in leiomyosarcoma. Smooth muscle actin was the

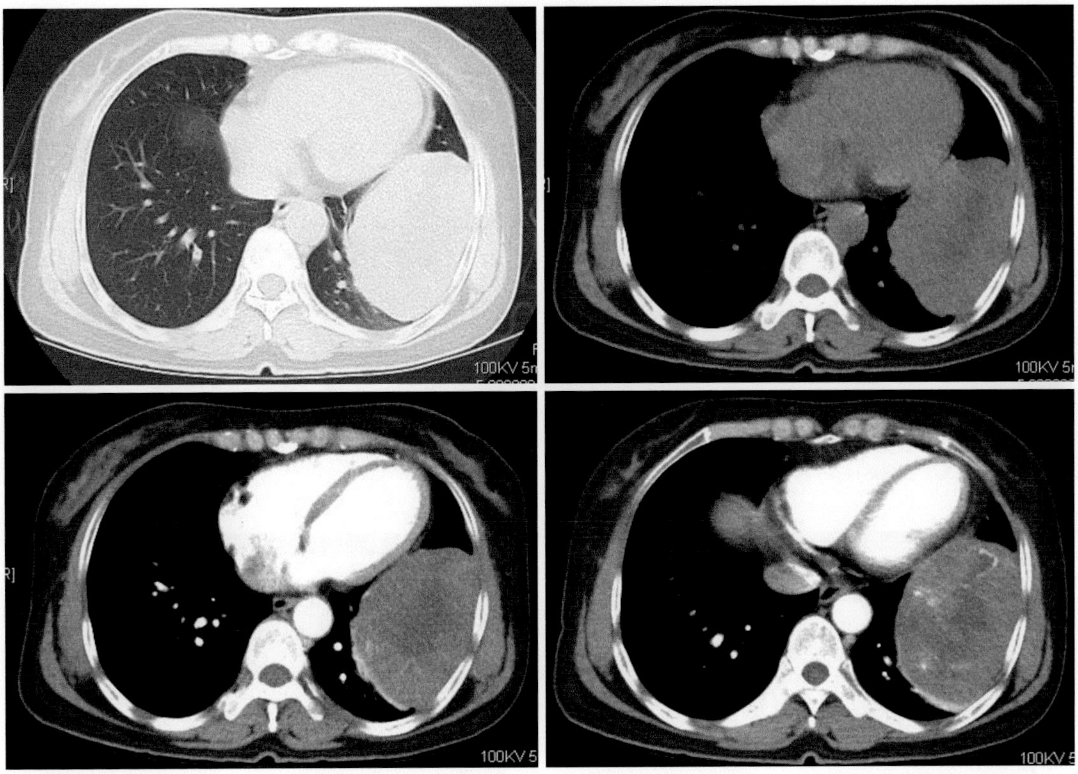

Fig. 7 Chest CT

most sensitive antibody (95%), followed by muscle-specific actin (91%), calponin (88%), desmin (73%), caldesmon (66%), and myosin (64%). Caldesmon and myosin were usually coexpressed and were highest in retroperitoneal tumors (94%). There was no discernable correlation noted between histologic differentiation and expression of smooth muscle marker. Estrogen receptor (ER) was much more common in women, with the highest incidence of retroperitoneal (86%) and uterine tumors (63%) in women. Nuclear Wilms tumor-1 protein (WT1) was expressed in 11% of all tumors and was limited to ER-positive uterine and female retroperitoneal tumors.

Complete surgical resection is the mainstay of therapy for pulmonary leiomyosarcoma. Adjuvant radiotherapy or chemotherapy treatment is used in cases with bilateral disease, extrathoracic dissemination, and refusal for surgery. Qin et al. [31] analyzed 231 PPL patients. Median overall survival (OS) of all patients was 14.0 months, and 1-, 3- and 5-year OS was 52.7%, 29.0%, and 22.2%, respectively. Cancer-directed surgery significantly improved median OS for PPL patients by almost 29.0 months (33.0 vs 4.0 months) and decreased risk of death by 57%.

5.5 Case 5

A 3-year-old boy was admitted to the hospital 2 years ago with intussusception. Physical examination revealed a right lower lobe cyst.

Chest CT (2008): A large cyst in the lower lobe of the right lung (Fig. 8).

Chest CT (2010):Cystic and solid mass in the right lower lobe (Fig. 9).

[Diagnosis] Pleuropulmonary blastoma.

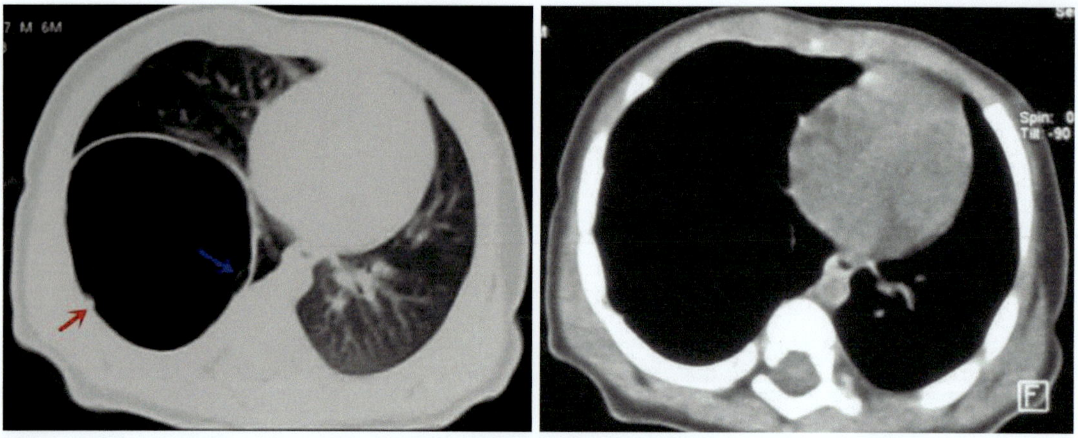

Fig. 8 Chest CT (2008)

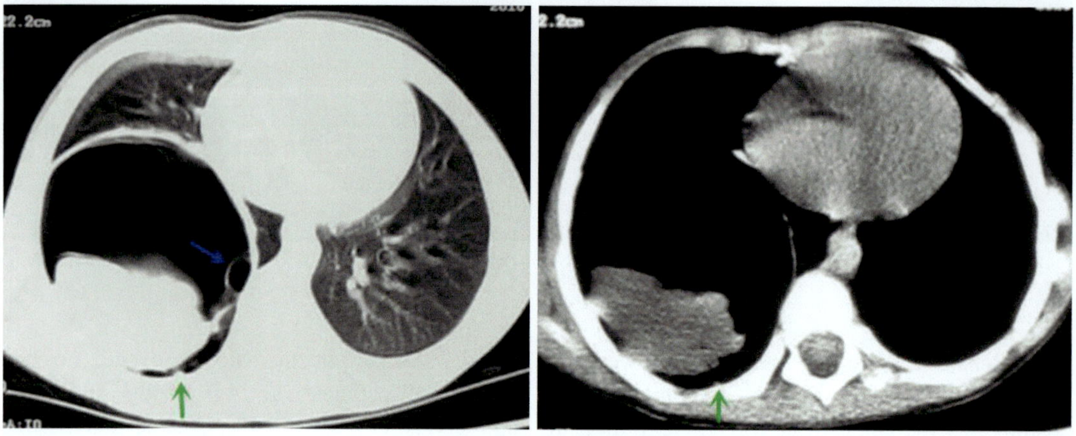

Fig. 9 Chest CT (2010)

[Diagnosis Basis] Physical examination of a 1-year-old child reveals a cystic lesion in the right lower lobe, with small nodule (red arrows) and small cyst (blue arrows) on the cyst wall. Two years later, a mass is seen at the bottom of the cyst, which is considered as nodular progression. New nodule (green arrows) is also found, and the small cyst is also larger than before. The above evolution supports the diagnosis of pleuropulmonary blastoma. The patient underwent surgical resection of the lesion. The resected lung tissue showed multiple cystic and solid masses, which were gray-yellow and gray-white in color. Microscopically, the epithelium was composed of small round, oval cells, and fascicular spindle cells without obvious differentiation. The tumor cells were deeply stained, nuclear atypia, and less cytoplasm, and chondrosarcoma components and stromal myxoid changes can be observed (Fig. 10). The diagnosis is type II pleuropulmonary blastoma because it contains both solid and cystic components. Immunohistochemistry showed positive for vimentin (Fig. 11a), Myo, CK (benign epithelial component) (Fig. 11b), and negative for HHF35, S-100, NSE, CD99, LCA, and Syn. The tumor was diagnosed as pleuropulmonary blastoma based on the microscopic and immunohistochemical findings.

[Analysis] Pleuropulmonary blastoma (PPB) is a rare, aggressive pediatric primary lung tumor, which originates from the lung parenchyma and/

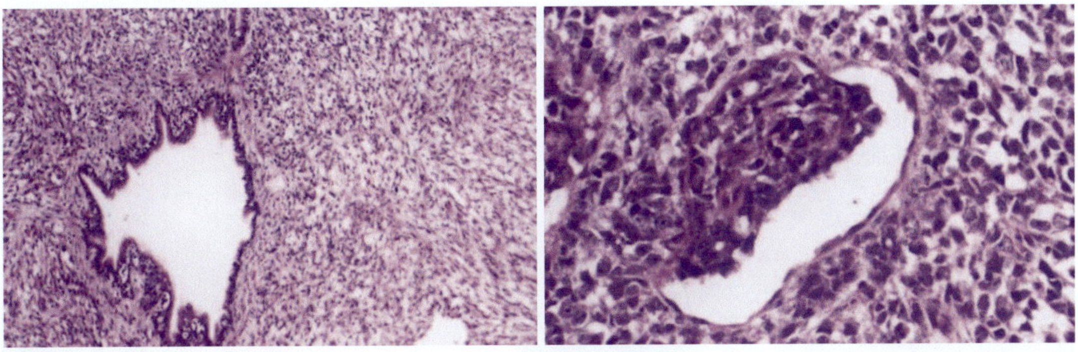

Fig. 10 (HE×100, HE×400) Tumor cells are mainly embryonal primordial sarcoma with a small amount of benign epithelial component

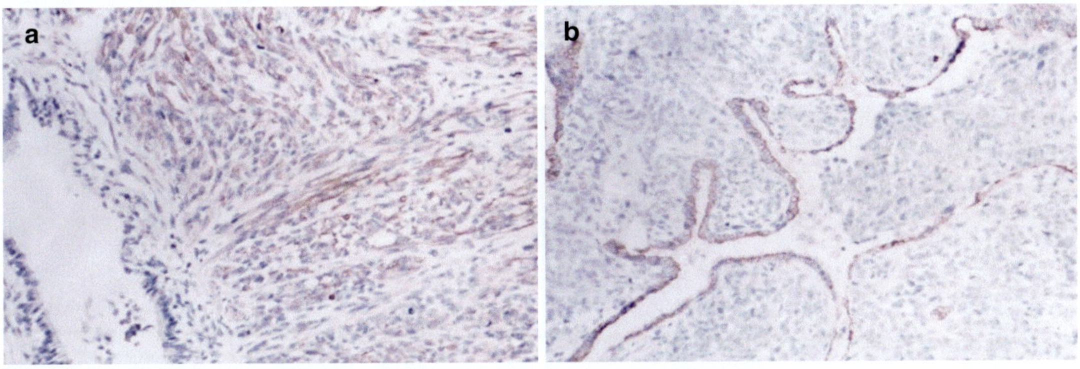

Fig. 11 (**a**) Diffuse strong cytoplasmic expression with vimentin stain. (**b**) CK expression in epithelial component

or pleura. It occurs primarily in children less than 6 years age and rarely happens beyond the first decade of life.

PPB is distinct from pulmonary blastoma and fetal adenocarcinoma. Microscopically, Spencer [32] first coined the term pulmonary blastoma in 1961 and suggested the tumor originating from mesodermal blastema. Pulmonary blastoma is composed of biphasic components including a mesenchymal and an epithelial malignant and immature component. Manivel et al. [33] first described PPB in children in 1988 as distinct tumor from pulmonary blastoma in adults because of its variable anatomic location, primitive embryonic-like blastema and stroma, lack of a carcinomatous component, and potential for sarcomatous differentiation (rhabdomyosarcoma, chondrosarcoma, liposarcoma). Fetal adenocarcinoma is characterized by an epithelial malignant and immature component. In the 2015 WHO classification, fetal adenocarcinoma is classified into the group of adenocarcinomas, pulmonary blastoma is classified into the group of sarcomatoid carcinoma, and PPB belongs to the group of mesenchymal tumors.

PPB is histopathologically classified into 3 types: cystic (type I), mixed cystic and solid (type II), and solid tumor (type III). The variant (type I-regressed, Ir) is added in 2006 and is histologically considered as a cystic lesion without malignant cells. These types represent a developmental continuum and can progress with time from type I to more aggressive type II and type III tumors. Moreover, type I PPB may also regress to type I-regressed, and no malignant cells are present.

On CT, type I PPB presents as a single or a multicystic lung lesions that have mass effect on adjacent structures, sometimes with contralateral mediastinal shift (Fig. 12). Type I PPB is often

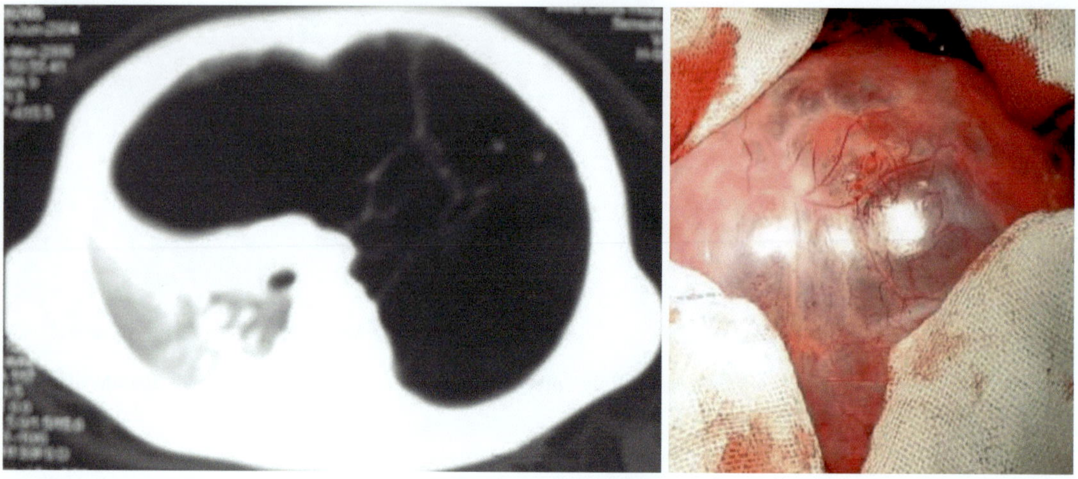

Fig. 12 A 2-year-old girl with type I PPB. There was a history of pneumothorax 1 year ago

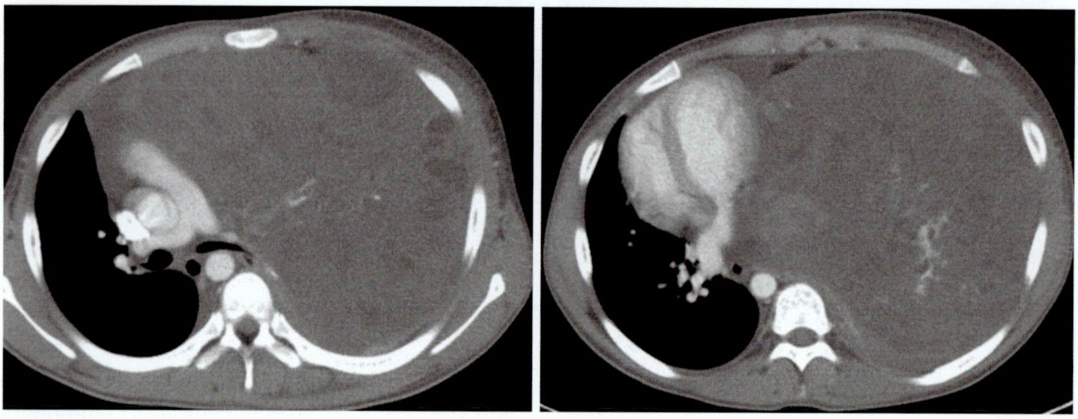

Fig. 13 A 13-year-old male with type III PPB

mistaken for unrelated entities such as congenital pulmonary airway malformation (CPAM), pulmonary sequestration, bronchogenic cysts, and congenital lobar emphysema. Type II PPB appears as solid components together air- or fluid-filled cavities with possible air-fluid levels. Type III PPB usually shows as large, well-circumscribed masse partly filling the hemithorax which invade mediastinum, vessels, and diaphragm (Fig. 13).

PPB has strong genetic association with the DICER1 mutation and recognized as a part of DICER syndrome comprising different type of tumor. DICER1-related tumors also include ovarian sex cord-stromal tumors, uterine cervical rhabdomyosarcoma, nodular hyperplasia of the thyroid gland and carcinoma, cystic nephroma, pineoblastoma, pituitary blastoma, nasal chondromesenchymal hamartoma, and ciliary-body medulloepithelioma. Messinger et al. [34] reviewed 350 PPB patients confirmed by central pathology and reported their clinical characteristics and outcomes. Germline DICER1 mutations were sought with Sanger sequencing. Type I PPB is defined as multilocular, air-filled cysts with thin septa. The cysts are lined with benign respiratory epithelium and mesenchyme, with an underlying component of malignant mesenchymal cells that may have rhabdomyoblastic differentiation. Type Ir PPB has the same multilocular cystic appearance as type I, but without the interspersed primitive malignant cells. Type II and type III PPB are similar in their histologic features within the solid areas, which consist of a collage of primitive sarcomatous patterns. Type II PPB contains residual cystic areas, whereas type III PPB is purely solid lesions without epithelial-lined cystic spaces. Thirty-three percent of all cases were type I or type I-regressed (type Ir), 35% were type II, and 32% were type III or type II/III. The median ages at diagnosis for type I, type II, and type III patients were 8, 35, and 41 months, respectively. The 5-year overall survival (OS) rate for type I/Ir patients was 91%; all deaths in this group were due to progression to type II or III. The 5-year OS rates (71% and 53%, respectively) and disease-free survival (DFS) (9% and 37%, respectively) of type II were significantly better than those of type III. The PPB type was the strongest prognostic factor. Metastatic disease at the diagnosis of types II and III was also an independent unfavorable prognostic factor. 66% of the 97 patients tested had a heterozygous germline DICER1 mutation. In this subset, the DICER1 germline mutation status was independent of the outcome. Surveillance of DICER1 carriers may allow the earlier detection of cystic PPB before its progression to type II or III PPB and thereby improve outcomes.

The mainstay of treatment for type I and type Ir PPB is radical surgery Adjuvant chemotherapy is often used in cases of intraoperative tumor spill, incomplete resection, or local invasion [35]. Surgical resection and adjuvant chemotherapy are the best choice for type II and type III PPB. The recommended chemotherapeutic agents are typically based on sarcoma regimens, including ifosfamide, vincristine, actinomycin D, and doxorubicin (IVADo regimen).

5.6 Case 6

A 58-year-old man complained of chest tightness and chest pain being for 1 month.

Chest CT: Complete occlusion of the right pulmonary artery, partial occlusion of the main pulmonary artery (Fig. 14).

[Diagnosis] Pulmonary artery intimal sarcoma.

[Diagnosis Basis] Enhanced CT scan shows intraluminal hypoattenuating lesions arising from main pulmonary artery and extending into the right pulmonary artery branches. The patient's symptoms are mild, and there is no obvious hemoptysis, dyspnea, hypotension, and shock symptoms. Imaging and clinical features do not support the diagnosis of pulmonary embolism and are more consistent with pulmonary intimal sarcoma. The postoperative pathology of the patient was a mesenchymal tumor located in the right pulmonary artery, consistent with intimal sarcoma, and no lymph node metastasis was found.

[Analysis] Primary pulmonary artery sarcoma (PAS) is rare malignant neoplasm that was first described in an autopsy by Mandelstamm in 1923 [36]. PAS is usually divided into intimal sarcoma and luminal sarcoma. The luminal type is rarely observed, and the most common pathological type is leiomyosarcoma developing along the medial smooth muscle of the large veins, mainly the vena cava. PAS mainly consists of intimal sarcoma arising from the intimal layer of the pulmonary artery. Pulmonary artery intimal sarcoma (PAIS) occurs in the pulmonary trunk, the left or right pulmonary artery and may rarely spread to the right ventricle and the pulmonary valve in a retrograde manner. It may also originate from the right ventricular outflow tract and the heart valves.

The incidence of PAIS is estimated to be 0.001%–0.03%. PAIS typically affects middle-aged adults with a mean age of 48–55 years old. The clinical presentation of PAIS may mimic acute and chronic pulmonary embolism, which leads to about 42.3% of PAIS patients misdiagnosed as pulmonary thromboembolism (PTE) and that had a significantly shorter overall survival than patients whose diagnosis was not misdiagnosed [37]. The symptoms of PAIS are more gradual in presentation compared with the acute nature of PTE. The most common clinical manifestation of PAIS is dyspnea, followed by chest pain, cough, hemoptysis and syncope, etc.

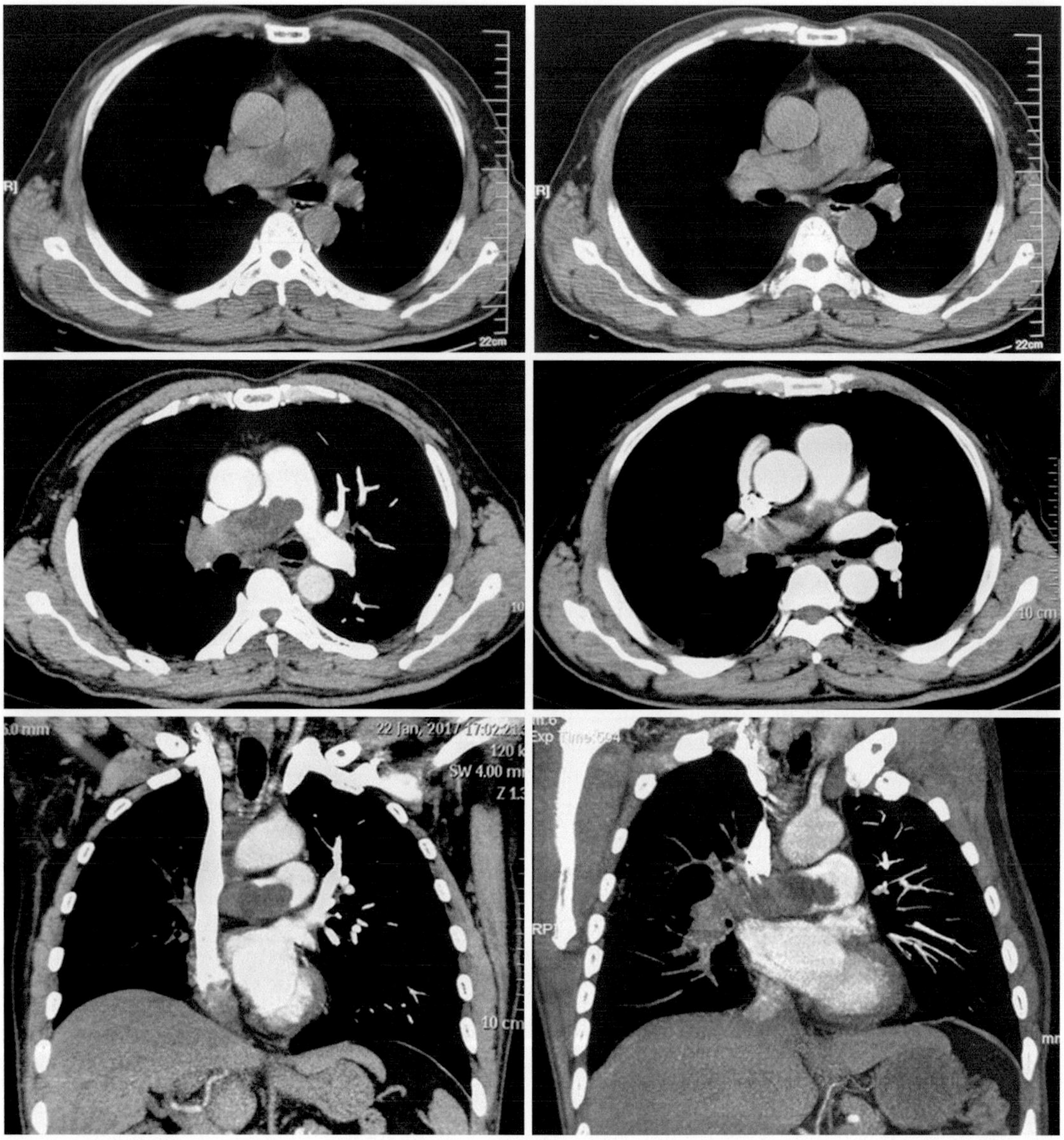

Fig. 14 Chest CT

some patients may be asymptomatic. Other findings include fever, cachexia, inflammatory anemia, and increased erythrocyte sedimentation rate also give a cue the diagnosis of PAIS, especially if the patient does not have any risk factors for deep venous thrombosis.

Histologically, PAIS is composed of spindle-shaped or epithelioid cells and shows various histological subtypes of differentiation, such as fibrosarcoma, leiomyosarcoma, anaplastic sarcoma, osteosarcoma, and chondrosarcoma. The 2013 WHO classification of soft tissue tumors defined intimal sarcoma as a soft tissue malignant tumor with uncertain differentiation, which may originate from multipotent mesenchymal cells in the intima, most of which are poorly differentiated spindle cell sarcomas with the feature of fibroblast and/or myofibroblast differentiation. Cell atypia, mitosis, and necrosis vary among cases. The 2015 WHO classification of the lung tumors defined PAIS as undifferentiated sarcoma with round cell features.

Immunohistochemically, MDM2, a proto-oncogene and negative regulator of p53 protein, is positive in at least 65%–100% of cases. The molecular hallmark of PAIS is MDM2 amplification. A majority of tumors show consistent genetic changes (gains and amplifications in the 12q13-14 region). Jimbo et al. [38] found that MDM2 and CDK4 were immunopositive in all 10 intimal sarcoma tumors, and high-level amplification of MDM2 was detected in eight tumors by both FISH and DISH. The other two tumors had polysomy of chromosome 12 and overexpression of p53 protein. As MDM2 amplification and p53 overexpression were mutually exclusive, disruption of the MDM2-p53 pathway may be an essential genetic event for this malignant tumor.

The diagnosis of PAIS relies mainly on echocardiography, computed tomography, magnetic resonance imaging (MRI), and positron emission tomography (PET). Biopsy is the gold standard for diagnosis. The CT features of PAIS are filling defect in the pulmonary artery lumen, extraluminal tumor invasion, and a nodular appearance. Kim et al. [37] described CT findings of PAIS compared with those of PTE. Tumoral impaction is the most common tumor pattern in PAIS. Heterogeneous attenuation, wall eclipse signs (WES), intratumoral vessels, acute interphase angles, single location, presence of lung ischemia, and central location were significantly more common in PAIS than in PTE. WES is defined as eclipsing of the pulmonary artery wall before the lesion infiltrated beyond the artery [39].

The mainstay of treatment is surgical resection. Multimodal treatment may provide better survival outcomes than monotherapy such as surgery alone. The prognosis of PAIS is extremely poor with a median survival of 1.5–3 months in non-operative patients. Blackmon et al. [40] analyzed survival data by an aggregate series derived from the published literature. The median survival was 36.5 ± 20.2 months for patients undergoing an attempt at curative resection compared with 11 ± 3 months for those undergoing incomplete resection. Median survival was 24.7 ± 8.5 months for patients undergoing multimodality treatment compared with 8.0 ± 1.7 months for patients having single-modality therapy. Lee et al. [41] evaluated potential prognostic factors in 20 PAS patients. The median age was 54 years (range, 33–75 years). The most common symptom was dyspnea (65%). The most common histologic type was spindle cell sarcoma (30%). Ten patients had a presumptive diagnosis of pulmonary embolism (PE) and received anticoagulation therapy. Seventeen patients underwent surgery, but only 5 patients had complete resection. Eleven patients received postoperative treatment (chemotherapy = 3, radiotherapy = 5, chemoradiotherapy = 3). Overall median survival was 24 months. Post-treatment pulmonary hypertension is associated with a poor prognosis.

References

1. Spraker MB, Bair E, Bair R, et al. An analysis of patient characteristics and clinical outcomes in primary pulmonary sarcoma. J Thorac Oncol. 2013;8:147–51.
2. Keel SB, Bacha E, Mark EJ, et al. Primary pulmonary sarcoma: a clinicopathologic study of 26 cases. Mod Pathol. 1999;12:1124–31.
3. Duran-Moreno J, Kokkali S, Ramfidis V, et al. Primary sarcoma of the lung-prognostic value of clinicopathological characteristics of 26 cases. Anticancer Res. 2020;40:1697–703.
4. Gebauer C. Primary pulmonary sarcomas: etiology, clinical assessment and prognosis with a comparison to pulmonary carcinomas—a review of 41 cases and 394 other cases of the literature. Jpn J Surg. 1982;12:148–59.
5. Régnard JF, Icard P, Guibert L, et al. Prognostic factors and results after surgical treatment of primary sarcomas of the lung. Ann Thorac Surg. 1999;68:227–31.
6. Gołota J, Osowiecka K, Orłowski T. Primary pulmonary sarcoma—treatment outcomes depending on the different types of radical operation. Kardiochir Torakochirurgia Pol. 2019;16:1–6.
7. Yamada Y, Kaplan T, Soltermann A, et al. Surgical outcomes and risk analysis of primary pulmonary sarcoma. Thorac Cardiovasc Surg. 2021;69:101–8.
8. Gołota J, Osowiecka K, Orłowski T. Primary pulmonary sarcoma - long-term treatment outcomes and prognostic factors. Kardiochir Torakochirurgia Pol. 2018;15:162–9.
9. Collaud S, Stork T, Schildhaus HU, et al. Multimodality treatment including surgery for primary pulmonary sarcoma: size does matter. J Surg Oncol. 2020;122:506–14.
10. Porte HL, Metois DG, Leroy X, et al. Surgical treatment of primary sarcoma of the lung. Eur J Cardiothorac Surg. 2000;18:136–42.

11. Pennacchioli E, Tosti G, Barberis M, et al. Sarcoma spreads primarily through the vascular system: are there biomarkers associated with vascular spread? Clin Exp Metastasis. 2012;29:757–73.
12. Zeren H, Moran CA, Suster S, et al. Primary pulmonary sarcomas with features of monophasic synovial sarcoma: a clinicopathological, immunohistochemical, and ultrastructure study of 25 cases. Hum Pathol. 1995;26:474–80.
13. Hartel PH, Fanburg-Smith JC, Frazier AA, et al. Primary pulmonary and mediastinal synovial sarcoma: a clinicopathologic study of 60 cases and comparison with five prior series. Mod Pathol. 2007;20:760–9.
14. Kim GH, Kim MY, Koo HJ, et al. Primary pulmonary synovial sarcoma in a tertiary referral center: Clinical characteristics, CT, and 18F-FDG PET findings, with pathologic correlations. Medicine (Baltimore). 2015;94:e1392.
15. Nilsson G, Skytting B, Xie Y, et al. The SYT-SSX1 variant of synovial sarcoma is associated with a high rate of tumor cell proliferation and poor clinical outcome. Cancer Res. 1999;59:3180–4.
16. Spurrell EL, Fisher C, Thomas JM, et al. Prognostic factors in advanced synovial sarcoma: an analysis of 104 patients treated at the Royal Marsden Hospital. Ann Oncol. 2005;16:437–44.
17. Ozzello L, Stout AP, Murray MR. Cultural characteristics of malignant histiocytomas and fibrous xanthomas. Cancer. 1963;16:331–5.
18. Fletcher CD. Pleomorphic malignant fibrous histiocytoma: fact or fiction? A critical reappraisal based on 159 tumors diagnosed as pleomorphic sarcoma. Am J Surg Pathol. 1992;16:213–28.
19. Jo VY, Fletcher CD. WHO classification of soft tissue tumours: an update based on the 2013 (4th) edition. Pathology. 2014;46:95–104.
20. Bedrossian CW, Verani R, Unger KM, et al. Pulmonary malignant fibrous histiocytoma: light and electron microscopic studies of one case. Chest. 1979;75:186–9.
21. Yousem SA, Hochholzer L. Malignant fibrous histiocytoma of the lung. Cancer. 1987;60:2532–41.
22. Higuchi M, Yamada H, Machino K, et al. Successful multidisciplinary treatment for aggressive primary pulmonary undifferentiated pleomorphic sarcoma. Case Rep Oncol. 2020;13:385–91.
23. McDonald SJ, Heather JC. Neoplastic invasion of the pulmonary veins and left auricle. J Pathol Bact. 1939;48:533–43.
24. Rekhi B, Gupta C, Chinnaswamy G, et al. Clinicopathologic features of 300 rhabdomyosarcomas with emphasis upon differential expression of skeletal muscle specific markers in the various subtypes: a single institutional experience. Ann Diagn Pathol. 2018;36:50–60.
25. Kumar S, Perlman E, Harris CA, et al. Myogenin is a specific marker for rhabdomyosarcoma: an immunohistochemical study in paraffin- embedded tissues. Mod Pathol. 2000;13:988–93.
26. Linardic CM. PAX3-FOXO1 fusion gene in rhabdomyosarcoma. Cancer Lett. 2008;270:10–8.
27. Sorensen PH, Lynch JC, Qualman SJ, et al. PAX3-FKHR and PAX7-FKHR gene fusions are prognostic indicators in alveolar rhabdomyosarcoma: a report from the children's oncology group. J Clin Oncol. 2002;20:2672–9.
28. Collins MH, Zhao H, Womer RB, et al. Proliferative and apoptotic differences between alveolar rhabdomyosarcoma subtypes: a comparative study of tumors containing PAX3-FKHR or PAX7-FKHR gene fusions. Med Pediatr Oncol. 2001;37:83–9.
29. Nishida Y, Tsukushi S, Urakawa H, et al. High incidence of regional and in-transit lymph node metastasis in patients with alveolar rhabdomyosarcoma. Int J Clin Oncol. 2014;19:53643.
30. Carvalho JC, Thomas DG, Lucas DR, et al. Cluster analysis of immunohistochemical markers in leiomyosarcoma delineates specific anatomic and gender subgroups. Cancer. 2009;115:4186–95.
31. Qin BD, Jiao XD, Zang YS. Primary pulmonary leiomyosarcoma: a population-based study. Lung Cancer. 2018;116:67–72.
32. Spencer H. Pulmonary blastoma. J Pathol Bacteriol. 1961;82:161–5.
33. Manivel JC, Priest JR, Watterson J, et al. Pleuropulmonary blastoma. The so-called pulmonary blastoma of childhood. Cancer. 1988;62:1516–26.
34. Messinger YH, Stewart DR, Priest JR, et al. Pleuropulmonary blastoma: a report on 350 central pathology-confirmed pleuropulmonary blastoma cases by the international Pleuropulmonary Blastoma registry: 350 centrally confirmed PPB cases. Cancer. 2015;121:276–85.
35. Knight S, Knight T, Khan A, et al. Current management of pleuropulmonary blastoma: a surgical perspective. Children (Basel). 2019;6:86.
36. Mandelstamm M. Uber primare Neubildungen des Herzens. Virchows Arch. 1923;245:43–54.
37. Kim C, Kim MY, Kang JW, et al. Pulmonary artery intimal sarcoma versus pulmonary artery thromboembolism: CT and clinical findings. Korean J Radiol. 2018;19:792–802.
38. Jimbo N, Komatsu M, Itoh T, et al. MDM2 dual-color in situ hybridization (DISH) aids the diagnosis of intimal sarcomas. Cardiovasc Pathol. 2019;43:107142.
39. Gan HL, Zhang JQ, Huang XY, et al. The wall eclipsing sign on pulmonary artery computed tomography angiography is pathognomonic for pulmonary artery sarcoma. PLoS One. 2013;8:e83200.
40. Blackmon SH, Rice DC, Correa AM, et al. Management of primary pulmonary artery sarcomas. Ann Thorac Surg. 2009;87:977–84.
41. Lee Y, Kim HJ, Yoon H, et al. Clinical characteristics and treatment outcomes of primary pulmonary artery sarcoma in Korea. J Korean Med Sci. 2016;31:1755–60.

Part III

Haematolymphoid Tumors

Pulmonary Lymphoma

Jing Liu and Song Zhang

Lymphoma is a heterogeneous group of malignancies arising from lymph nodes or other lymphoid tissues and can be classified as Hodgkin's lymphoma (HL) (10%) and non-Hodgkin's lymphoma (NHL) (90%). NHL is the most common hematologic malignancy and consists of more than 50 defined types with distinct genetic, morphologic, and clinical features. Most lymphomas (85–90%) originate from B lymphocytes, and others arise from T lymphocytes or natural killer (NK) lymphocytes.

1 Classification

Lymphoma accounts for approximately 5% of malignancies. The 2017 WHO classification tumors of hematopoietic and lymphoid tissues classified cancerous lymphomas into five classes: mature T/NK-cell lymphoma, precursor lymphoid hematopoietic system tumors, mature B-cell lymphoma, histocytes and dendritic cell neoplasms (HDCNs), and HL.

J. Liu
Department of Radiation Oncology, Shandong Cancer Hospital and Institute, Shandong First Medical University and Shandong Academy of Medical Sciences, Jinan, Shandong, China

S. Zhang (✉)
Department of Respiratory and Critical Care Medicine, Shandong Provincial Hospital Affiliated to Shandong First Medical University, Jinan, Shandong, China

Pulmonary lymphomas can be divided into primary pulmonary lymphoma (PPL) and secondary pulmonary lymphoma (SPL). PPL was first described as "peribronchial lymphosarcoma" by Emanuele Pekelis in 1931 [1]. PPL is a lymphocytic malignant clonal proliferative disease involving one or both lungs without any evidence of extrapulmonary involvement at the time of diagnosis or up to 3 months thereafter [2]. PPL is uncommon, accounting for 3–4% of extranodal lymphoma, fewer than 1% of malignant lymphomas, and approximately 0.3–1% of primary pulmonary malignancies. It most commonly occurs in adults and is particularly rare in children.

The most common pathological subtype of PPL is the low-grade marginal zone B-cell lymphoma of mucosa-associated lymphoid tissue (MALT) lymphoma, accounting for 60–80% of all cases, followed by diffuse large B-cell lymphoma (DLBCL), comprising 10–25% of all cases. Other rare types include plasmacytoma, lymphomatoid granulomatosis, small lymphocytic lymphoma (SLL), mantle B-cell lymphoma (MCL), follicular lymphoma (FL), and Burkitt lymphoma (BL). PPL of T-cell origin is extremely rare, with a main phenotype of anaplastic large-cell lymphoma (ALCL). The least common type of PPL is HL.

SPL is defined as secondary involvement of pulmonary by a systemic lymphoma and is more frequent, ranging from 25 to 40% in patients with a history of lymphoma. The most common sub-

S. Zhang (ed.), *Diagnostic Imaging of Lung Cancers*, https://doi.org/10.1007/978-981-99-6815-2_20

type of SPL is DLBCL, followed by MCL, MALT, FL, and BL.

2 Epidemiology

PPL often occurs in the sixth and seventh decades of life and rarely affects individuals under the age of 30 years. PPL has no obvious gender advantage or slight male predominance.

The incidence of lymphoma and the distribution of histologic subtypes not only show significant geographic differences and distinct time trends but also vary by sex, age, and race/ethnicity. The reason for these incidence patterns and time trends is poorly understood and can be attributed to immunodeficiency, various infections, familial aggregation, genetic predisposition, blood transfusion, diet, and chemical exposures to pesticides and solvents.

3 Clinical Features

PPL has nonspecific clinical symptoms, including cough, chest pain, dyspnea, hemoptysis, fever, apnea, fatigue, weight loss, night sweats, etc. B symptoms such as fever, night sweats, and weight loss occur in 15–27% of PPL patients [3]. Approximately 30–50% of PPL patients are asymptomatic at initial presentation.

The presence of B symptoms, more advanced disease stage, intermediate-high or high risks of international prognostic index (IPI) and NCCN-IPI, elevated inflammatory parameters (absolute lymphocyte count, CRP, β2-MG, and ferritin), and elevated cytokine levels (IL-2R, IL-6, and IL-10) were observed in SPL compared to PPL [4].

4 Radiographic Features

The radiological presentation of pulmonary lymphoma can be divided into five categories: nodular or mass-like, pneumonic or alveolar, bronchovascular or lymphangitic, miliary or hematogenous, and mixed. Consolidation is the most common radiological finding in PPL, while nodules or masses are the most frequent finding in SPL.

When lymphoma cells spread and infiltrate along the peribronchovascular lymph sinus, they present as nodules and masses with irregular morphology and uneven density. Nodule or mass can be single or multiple, and multiple nodules or masses are more common (Figs. 1 and 2). The lesions are well defined, lobulated, with or without burrs, and without pleural indentation. Air bronchogram sign and halo sign can be detected (Fig. 3). The halo sign is defined as ground glass attenuation surrounding a pulmonary nodule on CT scan (Fig. 4). In pulmonary lymphoma, it represents the surrounding interstitium invasiveness by less densely arranged tumor cells. Local necrosis can be detected in some larger mass, and

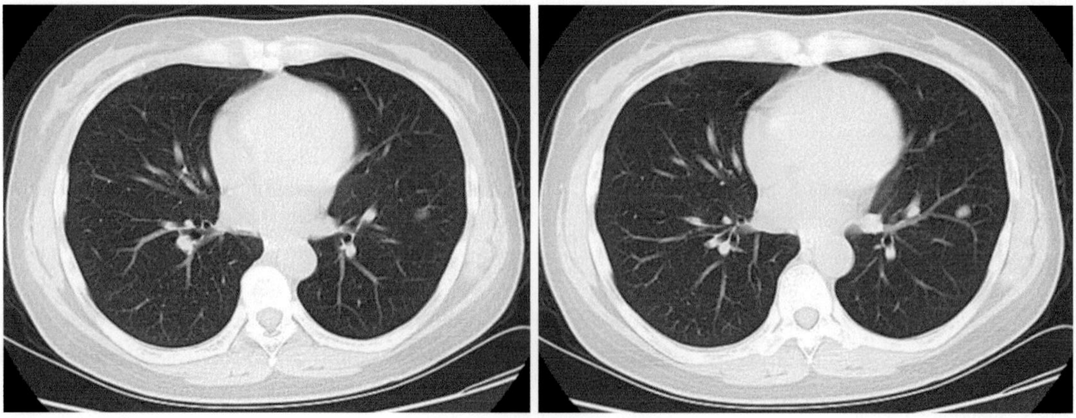

Fig. 1 A 43-year-old woman with MALT lymphoma. Chest CT shows single nodule in the left lower lung lobe

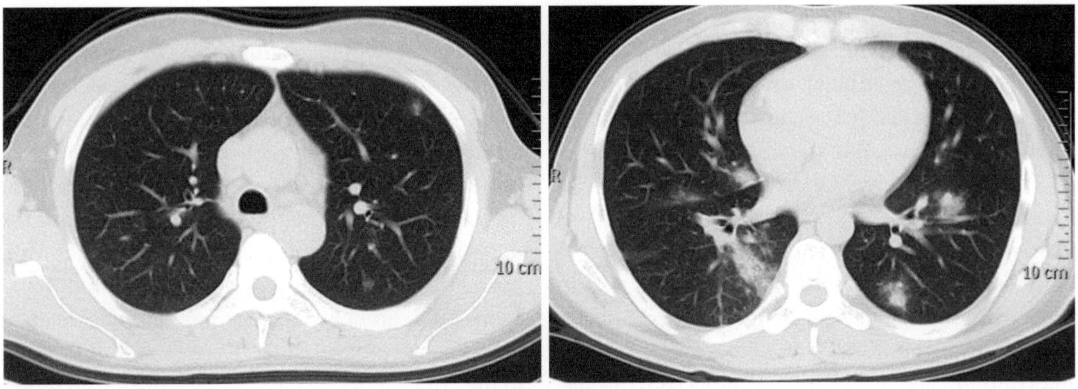

Fig. 2 A 23-year-old man with T-cell lymphoma. Chest CT shows multiple nodules

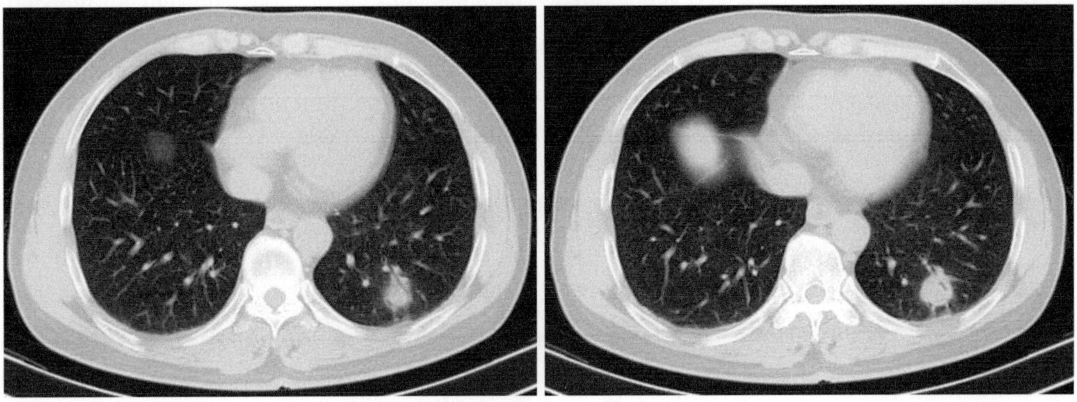

Fig. 3 A 58-year-old man with peripheral T-cell lymphoma, not otherwise specified (PTCL-NOS). Chest CT shows nodule with air bronchogram in the left lower lung lobe

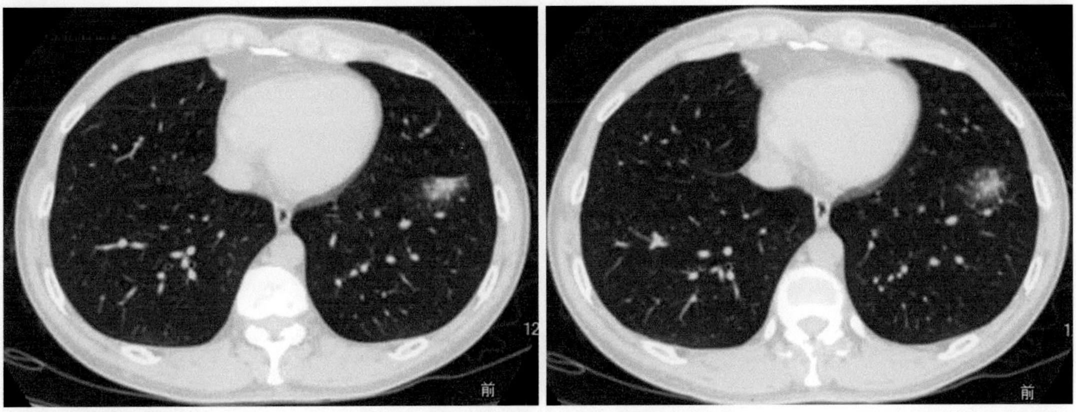

Fig. 4 A 47-year-old man with MALT lymphoma. Chest CT shows nodule with halo sign in the left lower lung lobe

small calcification lesions in the marginal zone are also observed (Fig. 5). The mass type is relatively easy to be related to enlargement of the hilar or mediastinal lymph, thickening or involvement of the pleura, and pleural effusion (Fig. 6).

Pneumonic or alveolar type manifests as patchy exudative lesions and/or consolidated masses involving lobe/segment (Fig. 7). Typical air bronchogram sign can be seen, similar to the performance of lobar pneumonia (Fig. 8). The reason is that tumor cells infiltrated and grew along the lung interstitium and bronchial submucosal tissue, while there is no tumor cell infiltration and destruction in the bronchial wall and bronchial lumen keeps smooth. Most of the pulmonary lymphomas are indolent tumors, and the tumor blood vessels are not abundant. The contrast-enhanced CT shows mild-to-moderate homogeneous enhancement of the lesions, and angiogram sign can be seen. The angiogram sign is an enhancing pulmonary vessel within pulmonary consolidation or masses and demonstrates an intact vascular network within consolidated lung of low attenuation after enhancement (Fig. 9). The mechanism is that tumor cells infiltrate along the peribronchovascular interstitium, leading to the consolidation of the lung tissue, but without invading the vascular wall. Tumor cells spread along pleura, interlobular septa, and bronchovascular bundles can lead to lung lesions crossing lobe fissures and infiltrating to the adjacent lobe (Fig. 10). Butterfly sign represents the distribution from the hilum to the periphery across lobe fissures. A consolidation with homogeneous attenuation, halo sign, air bronchogram sign, angiogram sign, cross-lobe sign, and butterfly sign contributes to differentiating pulmonary lymphoma from other pulmonary malignant tumors.

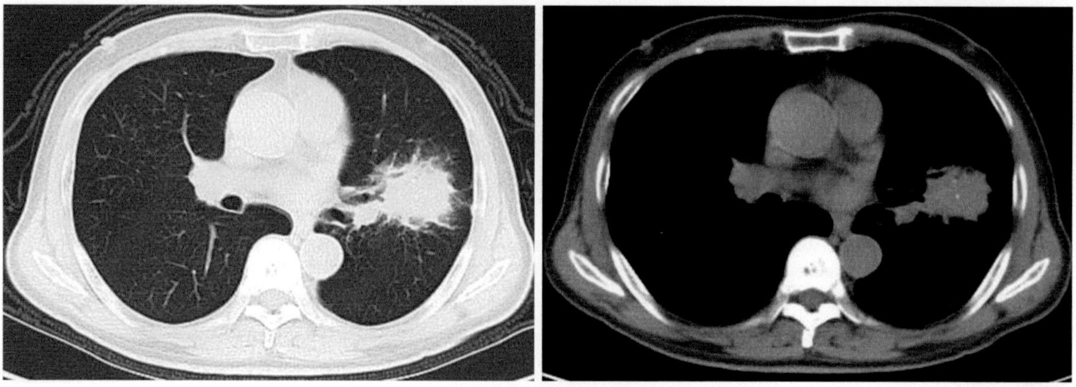

Fig. 5 An 80-year-old man with MALT lymphoma. Chest CT shows mass with punctate calcification in the left lingual lobe

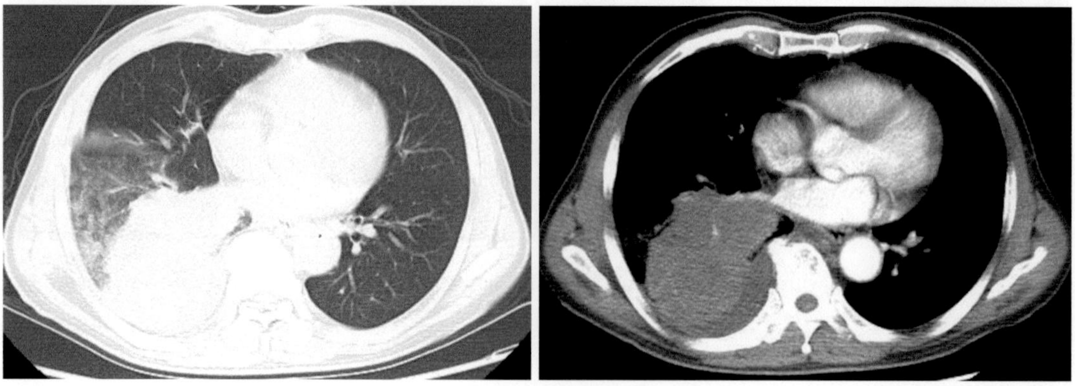

Fig. 6 A 68-year-old man with DLBCL. Chest CT shows mass with pleural effusion in the right lower lung lobe

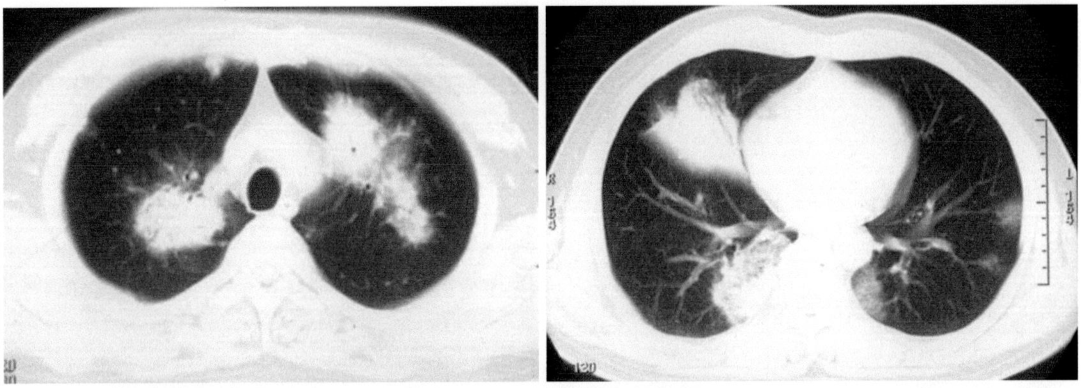

Fig. 7 A 56-year-old man with MALT lymphoma. Chest CT shows multiple consolidated lesions in bilateral lung

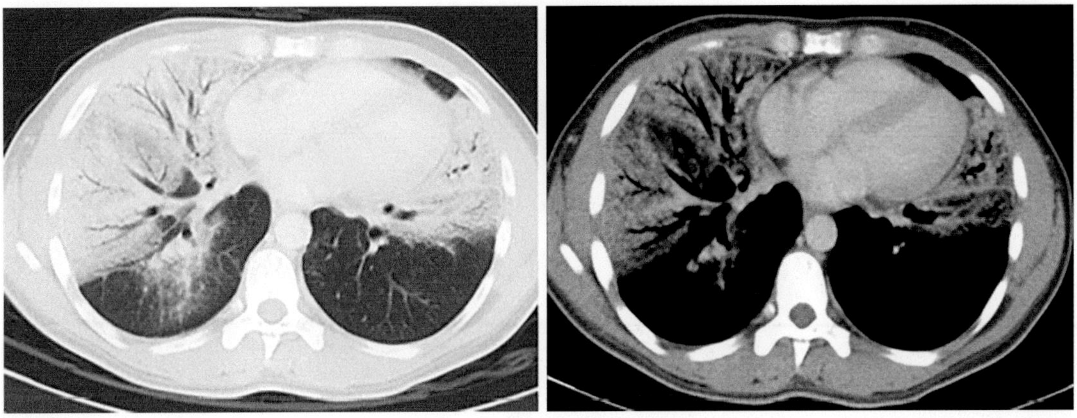

Fig. 8 A 40-year-old man with MALT lymphoma. Chest CT shows multiple consolidation with air bronchogram in bilateral lung

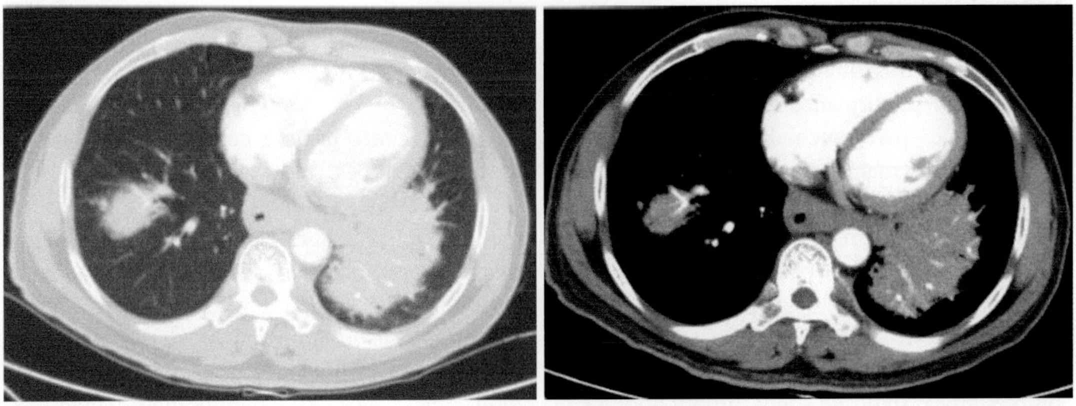

Fig. 9 A 42-year-old man with MALT lymphoma. Chest CT shows multiple consolidation with angiogram sign

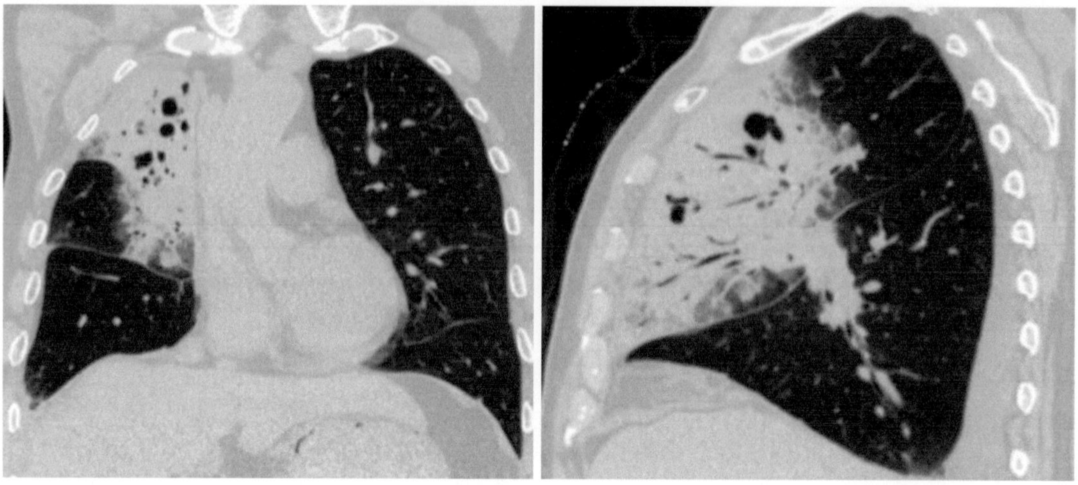

Fig. 10 A 50-year-old man with MALT lymphoma. Chest CT shows consolidation with cross-lobe sign

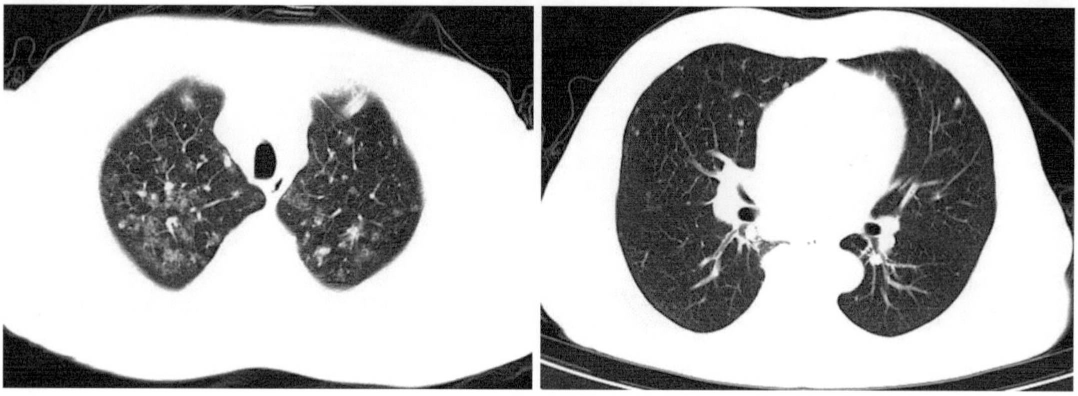

Fig. 11 A 60-year-old man with DLBCL. Chest CT shows diffuse ground glass opacity with interlobular septal thickening in bilateral parenchyma

The bronchovascular or lymphangitic type is a characteristic performance of SPL. Tumor cells infiltrate the peribronchial interstitium. The resultant lesions manifest as diffuse fine or coarse reticulate or small reticulonodular structures extending outward from the hilum or as ground glass opacity with interlobular septal thickening and distortion of the bronchovascular bundle (Fig. 11).

The miliary type invades the lung interstitium and presents as multiple small miliary nodules in a linear diffuse distribution along the bronchus. The nodules have rough boundaries and have little tendency to merge. No air bronchograms are found.

The mixed type is a combination of two or more above types.

Cozzi et al. [5] found that the most frequent features of PPLs were the presence of consolidations and ground glass opacities, accompanied by perilymphatic and/or bronchovascular spread. Nodules, consolidations with air bronchogram, and related lymphadenopathies were more common in MALT lymphomas than in DLBCL. Angiogram sign and pleural involvement were similar in both MALT and DLBCL.

5 Treatment

The therapeutic methods include surgery, chemotherapy, immunochemotherapy, immunotherapy, radiotherapy, or "wait and watch," but there is no established consensus on the optimal treatment strategy. Surgical resection for PPL is still debated. Limited PPL with no distant infiltration may consider surgery or local radiotherapy, and PPL with bilateral or extrapulmonary involvement, relapse, or progression may adopt chemotherapy. Cyclophosphamide, adriamycin, vincristine, and prednisolone (CHOP) regimen is the first treatment option for chemotherapy. The regimens of cyclophosphamide, vincristine, and prednisone (CVP); rituximab-CHOP (R-CHOP); and R-CVP also achieve good results.

6 Prognosis

The prognosis of PPL varies with different pathologic types and the stage of the disease. Most PPLs are indolent and progress slowly, with 50–85% of 5-year overall survival (OS) rates.

Low et al. [6] analyzed 2325 PPL patients diagnosed between 1983 and 2010 by the Surveillance, Epidemiology, and End Results (SEER) database. Multivariate analysis showed that older age at diagnosis, males, Hispanic race, non-marginal zone B-cell lymphoma of mucosa-associated lymphoid tissue histology, and Ann Arbor stage IV were significantly associated with worse OS. According to univariate analysis, all treatment modalities, including surgery, chemotherapy, and radiotherapy, were independent predictors of survival.

He et al. [7] analyzed 90 consecutive PPL cases. The estimated 5-year OS rates of MALT lymphoma and non-MALT lymphoma were 68.9% and 65.9%, respectively. Age over 60 years old, elevated LDH and β2-MG levels, clinical stage II2E disease or higher, and nonsurgical treatment were associated with poor prognosis in PPL patients. Age can be used as a potential independent prognostic factor for PPL.

Santopietro et al. [8] reviewed the medical records of 49 PPL patients. The complete response (CR) and overall response rate (ORR) were 83.7% and 95.9%. The estimated 5- and 10-year OS rates for all patients were 85% and 72.3%, for indolent PPL 89.2% and 80.3%, and for aggressive PPL 70.7% and 47.1%. Aggressive PPL often carried a high risk of progression in the first months. No advantages were found for indolent PPL who received immunochemotherapy non-anthracycline-containing regimens compared with other therapies, such as wait and watch, complete surgical resection, radiotherapy, or chemotherapy with chlorambucil. The multivariate Cox analysis confirmed that age was the only independent prognostic factor for OS.

7 Case Analysis

7.1 Case 1

A 28-year-old woman complained of cough, expectoration of sputum for 2 months, chest pain for half a month, and blood in sputum for 3 days. The patient's chest CT examination 2 months ago showed a mass in the left upper lung lobe and mediastinal lymphadenopathy. She was hospitalized 1 month ago, and bronchoscopy and two lung biopsies were performed. Bronchoscopy biopsy pathology showed a little lymphoid tissue and fibrous tissue. The lung biopsy pathology showed mature lymphocytes, plasma cells, alveolar epithelial hyperplasia, and fibrous tissue hyperplasia.

Chest CT: A left hilar mass with air bronchogram. The enhanced scan shows obvious homogeneous enhancement, and mediastinal lymph nodes are enlarged (Fig. 12).

[Diagnosis] Hodgkin's lymphoma.

[Diagnosis Basis] A young woman has a left hilar mass and mediastinal lymphadenopathy. Antibiotic therapy was ineffective. One bronchoscopy and two lung puncture biopsies are performed in other hospitals. No tumor cells are

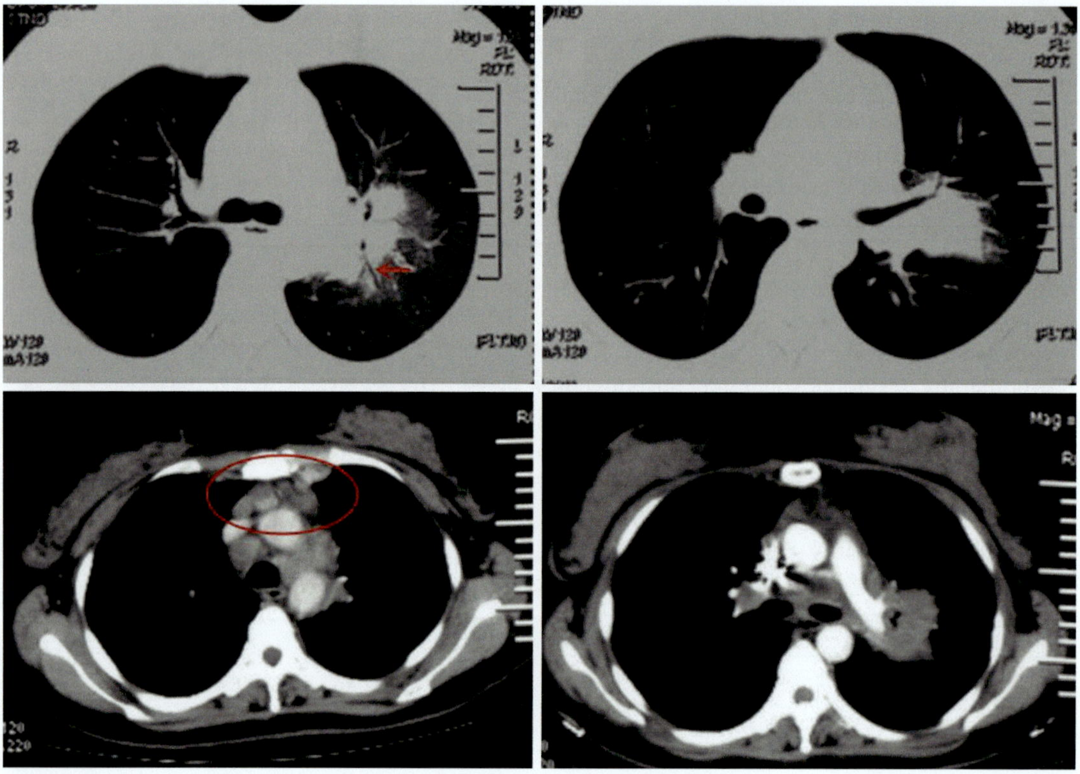

Fig. 12 Chest CT

found, but the image still indicated a high possibility of malignant tumor. In this case, multiple enlarged lymph nodes (red circles) are seen in the anterior mediastinum, and air bronchogram (red arrow) is seen at the edge of the mass. The possibility of Hodgkin's lymphoma is first considered. After admission, the patient refused to undergo bronchoscopy or lung biopsy again. Physical examination revealed a palpable enlarged right supraclavicular lymph node, about 1 × 1 cm in size. Lymph node biopsy showed lymphoid tissue hyperplasia, lymph node structure destruction, infiltration of a large number of neutrophils and eosinophils, scattered mononucleated and multinucleated large cells, and obvious nucleoli. Immunohistochemistry showed positive for CD20, PAX-5, CD30, MUM1, Bcl-6, and vimentin and negative for CD3, CD15, CD10, LCA, ALK, CK, and EMA. Histological and immunohistochemical findings support the diagnosis of mixed cellularity classical Hodgkin's lymphoma.

[Analysis] Hodgkin's lymphoma (HL), formerly called Hodgkin's disease, is a rare B-cell malignant neoplasm comprising two distinct entities: classical Hodgkin's lymphoma (CHL) and nodular lymphocyte-predominant Hodgkin's lymphoma (NLPHL).

CHL represents approximately 95% of all HL, and it is further classified into four subgroups on the basis of its morphological characteristics of the tumor cells and the composition of the reactive immune cell infiltrate of the tumor microenvironment (TME): nodular sclerosis (NSHL) (70%), mixed cellularity (MCHL) (20–25%), lymphocyte-rich (LRHL), and lymphocyte-depleted (LDHL). Epstein-Barr virus infection may be causally linked to 25–40% of CHL cases. Genome-wide association studies suggested that EBV status is an etiologically important classification of CHL [9].

NLPHL has distinct clinical and pathological features. Lymphocyte-predominant (LP) cells are the malignant cells in NLPHL. NLPHL is further subdivided into six patterns: classic nodular, serpiginous/interconnected nodular, nodular pattern with prominent extranodular LP cells, T-cell-rich nodular, diffuse pattern with a T-cell-rich microenvironment, and diffuse B-cell-rich pattern [10].

HL is characterized by Hodgkin and Reed-Sternberg (HRS) cells. The mononucleated and multinucleated cells are called Hodgkin cells and Reed-Sternberg cells, respectively. In 1832, Thomas Hodgkin reported six cases of primary lymph node tumors occurring in young adults presenting with enlarged cervical nodes, weight loss, and fever and leading to death in a few months in a paper titled "On some morbid appearances of the absorbent glands and spleen." In 1856, Samuel Wilkes first coined the term "Hodgkin's disease" in recognition of the first description of lymph system abnormalities by Thomas Hodgkin. In 1898, Carl Sternberg described the cells and believed that Hodgkin's disease was a form of tuberculosis. In 1902, Dorothy Reed Mendenhall described Reed-Sternberg cells and emphasized that Hodgkin's disease was unrelated to tuberculosis.

The classic Reed-Sternberg cell is a large cell and is binucleated with prominent eosinophilic nuclei that are surrounded by extensive inflammatory and immune effector cells. The HRS cells typically show a repressed B-cell program and defective immunoglobulin expression in CHL [11]. Immunohistochemical stains express CD30 (100% of cells), CD15 (75–80%), CD20 (30–40%), and PAX5 (95%) for confirming B-cell origin and usually lack expression of CD45 and molecules characteristic of the B- and T-cell lineages. Tzankov et al. [11] concluded that B-cell markers were expressed in 38% of CHL in the following rank order: CD20>CD79a>>CD138. In this case, although there are no typical Reed-Sternberg cells, there is a more obvious inflammatory background, and immunohistochemistry is positive for CD30, PAX-5, and CD20, which support the diagnosis of CHL.

HL is one of the most common neoplasms in adolescents and young adults, with an incidence in populations of European ancestry of 2–3 cases per 100,000 persons per year, although it can affect elderly individuals. HL has a bimodal peak at ages 15–34 years and over 60 years and shows a slight female preponderance (1.4:1).

Primary pulmonary Hodgkin's lymphoma (PPHL) is a rare entity and originates directly from lung tissue. Secondary pulmonary Hodgkin's lymphoma (SPHL) occurs in 12–40% of HL patients and usually arises from mediastinal or hilar lymph nodes. This case is SPHL. PHL patients often do not have the typical manifestations of lymphoma. The symptoms of this case were only cough, sputum, chest pain, and blood in the sputum. Although three biopsies were performed, the important sign of enlarged supraclavicular lymph nodes was ignored. When pulmonary lymphoma manifests as a central mass, it is similar to central lung cancer. Signs such as air bronchogram, angiogram, and cross lobe strongly suggest the diagnosis of pulmonary lymphoma.

7.2 Case 2

A 20-year-old man found lung lesions and enlarged cervical lymph nodes on physical examination.

Chest CT: Multiple nodules and consolidation in both lungs. Multiple enlarged lymph nodes in the hilum, mediastinum, and axilla (Fig. 13).

[Diagnosis] Hodgkin's lymphoma.

[Diagnosis Basis] A young woman has multiple nodules, consolidation, and ground glass opacities (green arrows) in both lungs. The interlobular septa are thickened (blue arrows). Lymphadenopathy can be seen in the neck, mediastinum, hilum, and axilla. The lesion is translobar fissure (white arrow), and air bronchogram (red arrow) is seen. These features support the diagnosis of lymphoma. A biopsy of cervical lymph node revealed lymphocyte-depleted Hodgkin's lymphoma.

[Analysis] The diagnostic criteria for PPHL include histological features of HL; restriction of the disease to the lung with or without minimal hilar lymph node involvement; and adequate

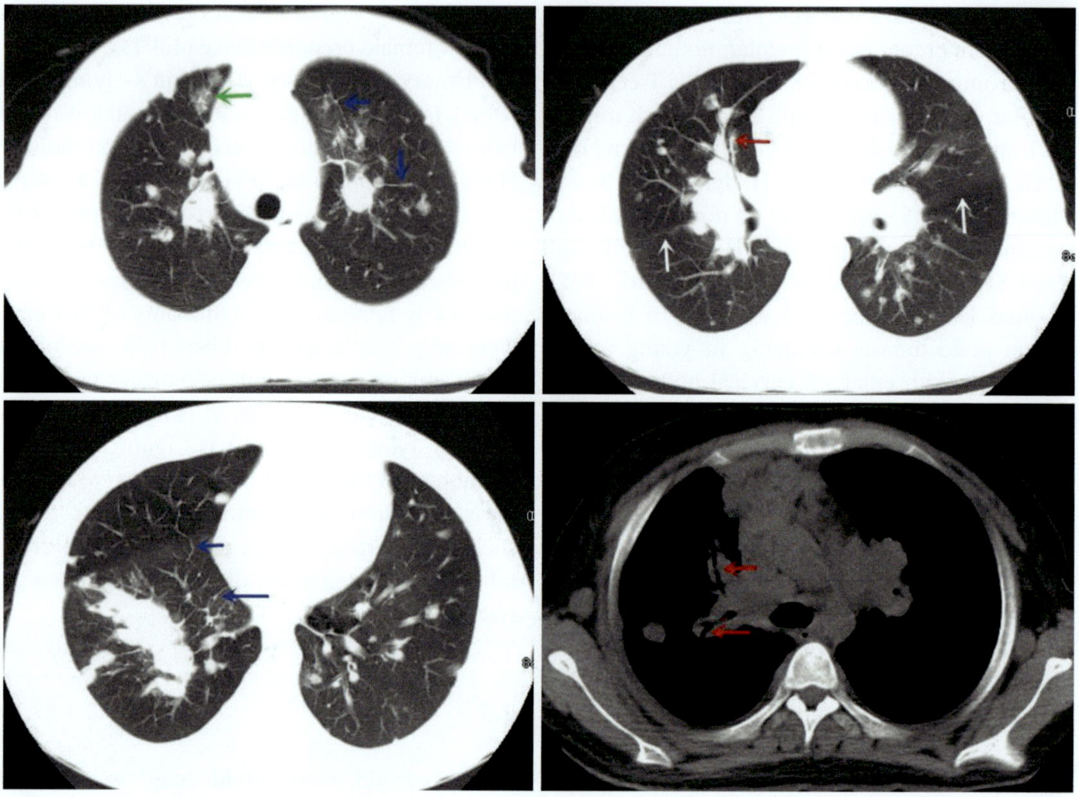

Fig. 13 Chest CT

clinical and/or pathological exclusion of the disease at distant sites. Our case does not meet the above diagnostic criteria and is considered SPHL.

Radiologically, PHL presents as a solitary nodule or mass, alveolar consolidation, multiple nodules, or cavitary pulmonary lesions. For patients with malignant tendencies in clinical symptoms and imaging findings, especially with mediastinal mass or enlarged superficial lymph nodes, the possibility of SPHL should be considered.

Combined modality treatment regimens including multiagent chemotherapy, radiation, and immunotherapy are effective in HL with about 80% cure rate. Bröckelmann et al. [12] evaluated 10 meta-analyses, 89 randomized and controlled trials, and 81 prospective or retrospective trials. In early stages, two cycles of ABVD (doxorubicin, bleomycin, vinblastine, and dacarbazine) and 20 Gy involved-site radiotherapy (IS-RT) are recommended. For the treatment of intermediate stages, two cycles of escalated BEACOPP (bleomycin, etoposide, doxorubicin, cyclophosphamide, vincristine, procarbazine, and prednisone) + two cycles of ABVD and 30 Gy IS-RT are administered. In advanced stages, two cycles of escalated BEACOPP are performed, followed by PET to guide further treatment: two further cycles of escalated BEACOPP are recommended if the PET is negative and four further cycles if it is positive, and then radiotherapy is performed on the PET-positive residual tumor tissue. The five-year survival rate of HL patients is 95%. In case of disease recurrence, high-dose chemotherapy followed by autologous stem cell transplantation is administered, and targeted drugs including brentuximab vedotin, nivolumab, and pembrolizumab are used.

7.3 Case 3

A 48-year-old woman complained of recurrent cough for more than 1 year.

Chest CT: Consolidation in the left upper lung lobe (Fig. 14).

[Diagnosis] Primary pulmonary MALT lymphoma.

[Diagnosis Basis] A middle-aged woman has a longer medical history. Chest CT shows segmental consolidation with air bronchogram (red arrow), adjacent pleural thickening (blue arrows), and clear, adducted margins (green arrows), which need to be considered for the diagnosis of lobar pneumonia, pneumonic lung adenocarcinoma, or pulmonary MALT lymphoma. Lobar pneumonia has obvious clinical symptoms, and anti-inflammatory treatment is effective. This case has a long history, regular lesion margins, and obvious stretch and dilation of the bronchus, which does not support the diagnosis. There are no signs of twisting or truncation of the bronchus

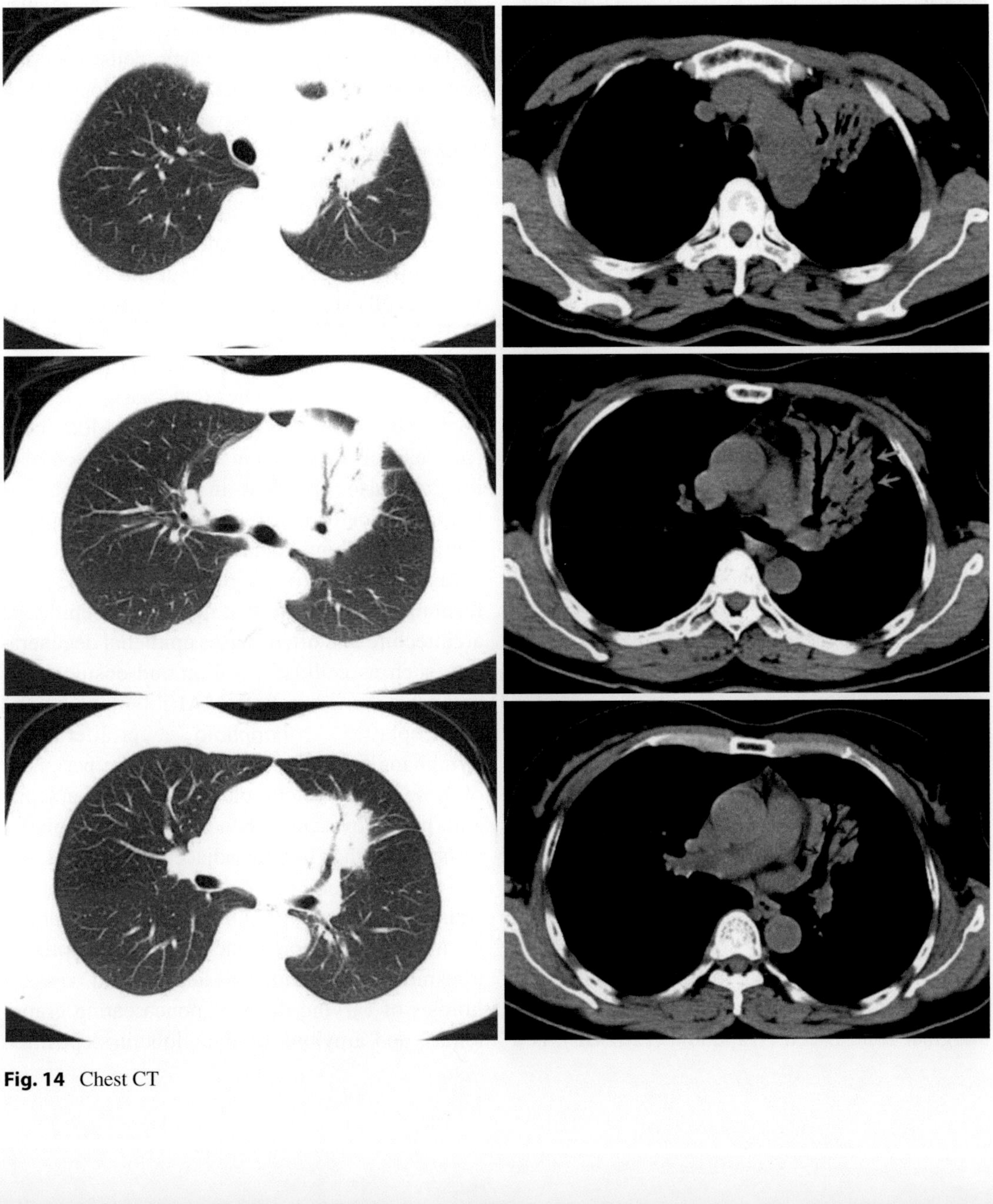

Fig. 14 Chest CT

in the lesion, no disseminated foci around the lesion, and no pleural depression and pleural effusion, which does not support the diagnosis of pneumonic lung adenocarcinoma. The above characteristics combined with the absence of obvious lymphadenopathy in the hilum and mediastinum are consistent with the diagnosis of pulmonary MALT lymphoma. The lesion was surgically removed, and the size of the mass was 9 × 7 × 5 cm. The cut surface was gray-white, and the boundary was clear. Pathology revealed diffuse proliferation of lymphocytes with slight atypia and several lymphoepithelial lesions, in keeping with a MALT lymphoma. Immunohistochemistry was positive for LCA, CD20, CD79a, CD3, CD45RO (scattered), and AE1/3 (weak) and negative for CD99 and EMA.

[Analysis] Mucosa-associated lymphoid tissue (MALT) is located along the surfaces of all mucosal tissues and is a disseminated collection of lymphoid tissues in multiple sites throughout the body. About half of immune system lymphocytes are in MALT. The primarily studied MALT sites include gut-associated lymphoid tissue (GALT), bronchus-associated lymphoid tissue (BALT), and nasopharynx-associated lymphoid tissue (NALT). Lacrimal duct-associated lymphoid tissue (LDALT), conjunctiva-associated lymphoid tissue (CALT), larynx-associated lymphoid tissue (LALT), and salivary duct-associated lymphoid tissue (DALT) have also been reported.

The pulmonary lymphoid system consists of BALT and pulmonary lymphatics. BALT is located beneath the areas of specialized bronchial epithelium throughout the airways, mostly at bifurcations of the bronchus, and is not present at birth, develops in children and adolescents, misses again in normal healthy adults, and can reappear in adults with antigenic stimulation, such as cigarette smoke, infection, chronic inflammation (asthma), collagen vascular disease, and AIDS.

Marginal zone lymphoma includes the nodal, extranodal, and splenic subtypes, which arise from post-germinal center marginal zone B cells. MALT lymphoma, also known as extranodal marginal zone B-cell lymphoma (EMZBL), is a monoclonal lymphoid proliferation classified as low-grade marginal zone B-cell lymphoma of mucosa-associated lymphoid tissue. MALT lymphoma was first described by Isaacson and Wright in 1983 [13] and develops in many different organs, such as gastrointestinal tract, orbit, salivary glands, thyroid gland, and lungs. MALT lymphomas most commonly occur at sites where MALT is not normally present, such as the stomach, orbit, salivary glands, lungs, and thyroid gland, rather than at sites that are physiologically rich in MALT, such as the Peyer's patches of the terminal ileum. Pulmonary MALT lymphoma originates from bronchial MALT and is also referred to as BALT lymphoma.

Histologically, the neoplastic cells are comprised of centrocyte-like cells, monocytoid B cells, small lymphocytes, and plasma cells and exhibit the presence of lymphoid infiltrate expanding the marginal zone of reactive lymphoid follicles. Scattered large transformed centroblast-like or immunoblast-like cells are frequently dispersed throughout the lymphoma. Plasma cells are often adjacent to the epithelium and contain intranuclear inclusions of immunoglobulins known as Dutcher bodies (intranuclear inclusions). Russell bodies (cytoplasmic vesicles containing immunoglobulin) and Mott cells (plasma cells that contain numerous Russell bodies) are also observed in MALT lymphoma. Lymphoid cells infiltrate the bronchial epithelium forming lymphoepithelial lesions, which are defined as three or more marginal zone cells forming an aggregate that disrupts the epithelial architecture and often causes epithelial degeneration such as cellular swelling and eosinophilia, and are common in both MALT lymphoma and nonneoplastic lymphoid proliferations. Lymphangitic spread can occur at the periphery of these lesions (along pleura, interlobular septa, and bronchovascular bundles), and neoplastic cells may invade into the adjacent pleura, vessels, and airways. Follicular colonization by the tumor cells can be observed. Other histologic features of MALT lymphoma include non-necrotizing transmural infiltration of large blood vessels, fibrosis of varying degrees, noncaseating granulomas, and amyloid/immunoglobulin deposition often associated with foreign-body giant cells and giant lamellar bodies formed at least in part from surfactant protein [14].

Immunohistochemically, MALT lymphoma cells are positive for B-cell-associated antigens, such as CD19, CD20, CD22, and CD79a, and negative for CD5, CD10, CD23, CD43, Bcl-6, and cyclin D1. Begueret et al. [15] found that 71.5% of MALT lymphomas showed the CD20+/CD43+ centrocyte-like cell phenotype. The determination of B-cell CD20+/CD43+ phenotype of the intraepithelial lymphocytes highly increased the specificity of lymphoepithelial lesions. The neoplastic cells express monotypic surface Ig and are more frequently IgM positive than IgG or IgA but are negative for IgD. Negative expression of lymphoma cells for IgD, CD5, CD10, Bcl-6, and cyclin D1 can help to rule out other small B-cell lymphomas. MALT lymphoma demonstrates light chain restriction defined as a cell population producing only one of the two types of light chain (either κ or λ) that occur in a monoclonal cell population.

Some studies have reported a potential relationship between IgG4-related disease and MALT lymphoma based on rare observations of ocular adnexal or cutaneous MALT lymphoma associated with heavy infiltrations of IgG4 plasma cells or arising from an underlying IgG4-related disease (IgG4-RD). Most cases derive from Asia. Bledsoe et al. [16] analyzed the spectrum of lymphomas among IgG4-RD patients in the Western world. They found that lymphomas in IgG4-RD are more varied in location and type than the experience reported from Asia to date. Persistence of lymphadenopathy or extranodal mass after appropriate treatment of IgG4-RD should be aware of the potential for lymphoma to develop in patients with IgG4-RD. The co-occurrence of IgG4-RD and lymphoma suggests a possible etiologic association. Tanahashi et al. [17] first reported a case of primary pulmonary MALT lymphoma with high IgG4 expression. The histological findings met the diagnostic criteria for MALT lymphoma and IgG4-related respiratory disease (IgG4-RRD). Polymerase chain reaction using paraffin sections revealed the clonality of the immunoglobulin heavy-chain variable region gene rearrangement, confirming the diagnosis of MALT lymphoma. This report reveals a potential association between IgG4 and primary pulmonary MALT lymphoma. Molecular based methods for B-cell clonality and interphase FISH are useful tools to differentiate reactive conditions from lymphoma.

MALT lymphoma is specifically associated with t(11;18)(q21;q21), t(14;18)(q32;q21), and t(1;14)(p22;q32). Translocation (11;18)(q21;q21) causes the inhibitor of apoptosis family member API2-MALT1 gene fusion, resulting in the expression of an API2/MALT1 fusion protein, while the t(1;14)(p22;q32) and t(14;18)(q32;q21) bring the BCL10 and MALT1 genes, respectively, to the IGH locus and deregulate their expression. The t(11;18)(q21;q21)/API2-MALT1 is most commonly detected in pulmonary(40%) and gastric tumors (25%) and is not found in other small B-cell lymphomas. The t(14;18)(q32;q21)/IgH-MALT1 is usually found in non-gastric sites, such as ocular adnexa/orbit, skin, and salivary glands. Approximately 4% of gastric and 8% of pulmonary MALT lymphomas carry a t(1;14)(p22;q32). Trisomies 3 and 18 each occurred most frequently in intestinal and salivary gland MALT lymphomas [18].

7.4 Case 4

A 66-year-old man presented with rheumatoid arthritis and found lung lesions during physical examination.

Chest CT: Multiple consolidations in the upper lobe of the right lung, the upper lobe and lower lobe of the left lung, with left hydropneumothorax (Fig. 15).

[Diagnosis] Primary pulmonary MALT lymphoma.

[Diagnosis Basis] The patient has no respiratory complaints, and the imaging findings are severe. The lesions invade multiple lung segments, all of which show consolidation, with air bronchogram and cystic changes in some areas. The enhanced scan shows mild homogeneous enhancement.

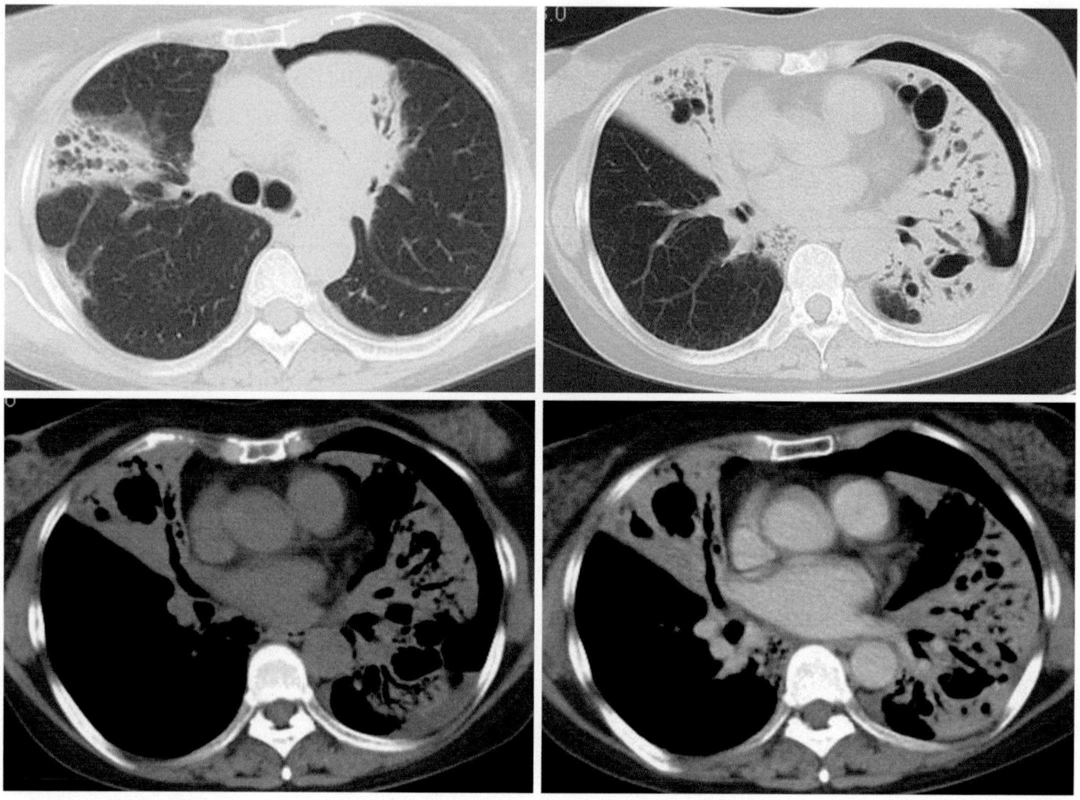

Fig. 15 Chest CT

Old age, mild clinical symptoms, bronchiectasis, and air bronchogram on chest CT images are useful to distinguish pulmonary MALT lymphoma from lobar pneumonia. The patient's percutaneous lung biopsy confirmed the diagnosis. Immunohistochemistry showed strong positive for CD20 and CD79a.

[Analysis] MALT lymphomas arise from antigenic stimulation or immunosuppression. The infectious agent does not directly infect and transform lymphoid cells, as do the lymphotropic oncogenic viruses Epstein-Barr virus (EBV), human T-lymphotropic virus 1 (HTLV-1), and human herpesvirus 8 (HHV8), but rather indirectly increases the probability of lymphoid transformation by chronically stimulating the immune system to maintain a protracted proliferative state [19]. MALT lymphomas have been proved to be associated with several distinct chronic inflammatory disorders, such as chronic infection by *Helicobacter pylori* in the stomach, *Chlamydia psittaci* in the ocular adnexa, *Borrelia burgdorferi* in the skin, *Campylobacter jejuni* in the small intestine, and hepatitis C virus in the spleen, as well as autoimmune disorders including Sjögren's syndrome, rheumatoid arthritis, dysgammaglobulinemia, collagen vascular diseases, amyloid deposits, lymphoepithelial sialadenitis, and Hashimoto thyroiditis. Most MALT lymphoma patients are former or active smokers.

The causative antigens associated with pulmonary MALT lymphoma have not been identified. Chanudet et al. [20] used PCR to detect DNA traces of *Chlamydophila pneumoniae*, *Chlamydia trachomatis*, *Chlamydia psittaci*, or *Mycoplasma pneumoniae* in tissues. Among 69 pulmonary MALT lymphomas, 30 other lymphoproliferative disorders (LPD) and 44 non-LPD *Chlamydia pneumoniae*, *Chlamydia trachomatis*, and *Chlamydia psittaci* were detected at low frequencies (<20%). The incidence of individual *Chlamydia* in MALT lymphoma was generally higher than that in non-LPD, although the difference was not statistically significant. *Mycoplasma pneumoniae* DNA was not detected. Adam et al. [21] used a specific nested PCR to examine the potential association of pulmonary MALT lymphoma with *Achromobacter xylosoxidans* (*A. xylosoxidans*). 57/124 (46%) pulmonary MALT lymphomas and 15/82 (18%) control tissues were positive for *A. xylosoxidans*. Borie et al. [22] investigated the presence of virus or any infectious agents in pulmonary MALT lymphoma by using metagenomic next-generation sequencing (mNGS). They identified *A. xylosoxidans* sequence in 4/13 pulmonary MALT lymphoma patients and in 4/10 controls. No clear evidence of a specific pathogen associated with pulmonary MALT lymphoma was identified. Aoyama et al. [23] also confirmed that *A. xylosoxidans* infection may not be related to pulmonary B-cell lymphoma in a Japanese case series. Large-scale international studies are needed to elucidate the role of *A. xylosoxidans* in pulmonary lymphoma.

Some autoimmune disorders greatly increase the risk of developing lymphoproliferative disorders in general, especially those of MALT type. Ekström et al. [24] performed a pooled analysis of self-reported autoimmune conditions and risk of NHL and its subtypes, encompassing 29,423 participants in 12 case-control studies. Sjögren syndrome was associated with a 6.6-fold increased risk of NHL, a 250-fold increased risk of parotid gland NHL, and a 1000-fold increased risk of parotid gland marginal zone lymphoma. Systemic lupus erythematosus was associated with a 2.7-fold increased risk of NHL overall and with increased risk of diffuse large B-cell and marginal zone lymphomas. Rheumatoid arthritis was not associated with the risk of NHL, but results were heterogeneous between studies.

The case has a history of rheumatoid arthritis, and chest CT shows multiple consolidations with air bronchogram, which is consistent with pulmonary MALT lymphoma. The association between pulmonary MALT lymphoma and pneumothorax is extremely rare, often related to therapeutic toxicity. Cyst formation and rupture due to lymphocytic interstitial pneumonia or other rare pulmonary lymphoid proliferative disorders may be associated with pneumothorax formation in pulmonary MALT lymphoma.

7.5 Case 5

A 42-year-old woman complained of cough, expectoration for 3 months, and shortness of breath for half a month.

Chest CT: Consolidation in the left lower lung lobe (Fig. 16).

[Diagnosis] Primary pulmonary MALT lymphoma.

[Diagnosis Basis] A middle-aged woman has a long course of disease and mild symptoms; chest CT shows consolidation in the left lower lung lobe with relatively clear borders (blue arrow), air bronchogram, distal bronchiectasis (green arrow), angiogram sign (red arrows), and a small patchy ground glass opacity in the right lung, supporting the diagnosis of pulmonary MALT lymphoma. The patient's left lower lung puncture confirmed the diagnosis, and immunohistochemistry was strongly positive for CD20 and CD79a, weakly positive for CD43 and CD21, and negative for CD3, CD5, and CD23.

[Analysis] MALT lymphoma accounts for about 6–8% of all NHLs in the Western hemisphere. The median age at diagnosis of pulmonary MALT lymphoma is 50–60 years, although rare cases in younger patients (<30 years) have been reported.

MALT lymphoma may occur in any lung lobe or large airway including the trachea and main bronchus. Variety of the location and extent of the lymphomatous infiltration results in different characteristics at CT. Consolidation and nodular/mass are the most frequent patterns. CT features include air bronchogram, well-marginated halo sign, angiogram sign, peribronchovascular thickening, septal lines, cystic bronchiectasis, and pulmonary cyst. Hilar or mediastinal lymphadenopathy and mild pleural effusion may also be observed.

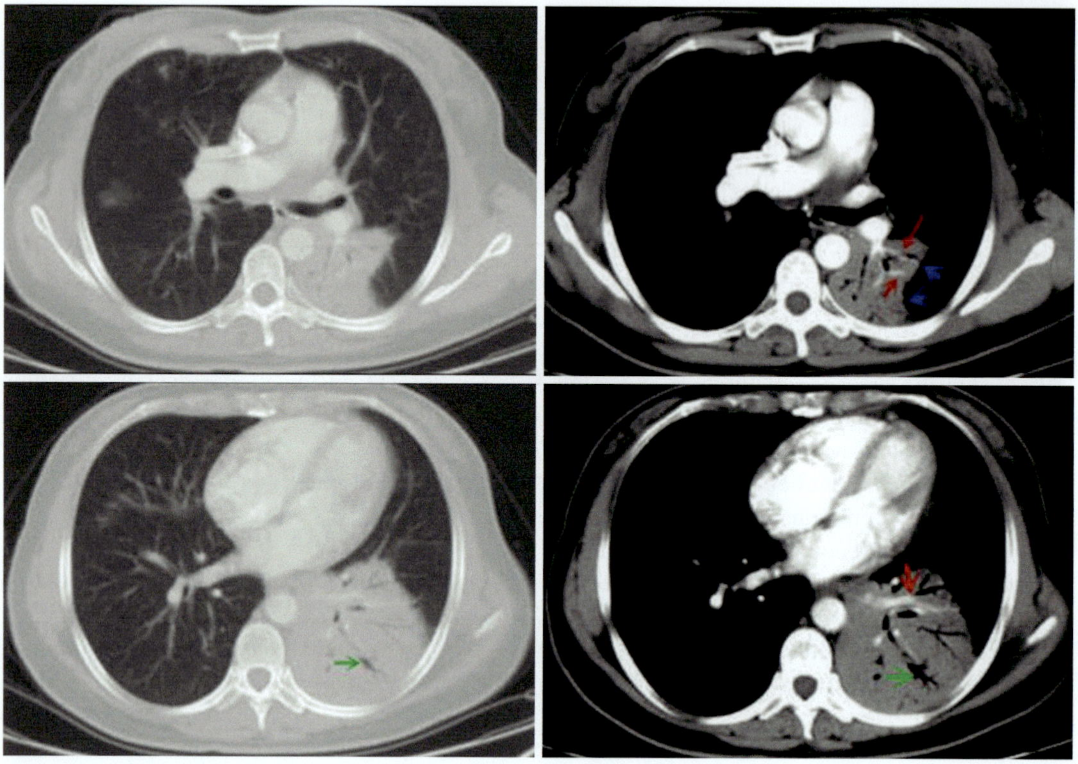

Fig. 16 Chest CT

The pathological changes corresponding to the diversity of imaging manifestations of pulmonary MALT lymphoma are the spread of tumor cells along the bronchovascular tree and interlobular septa, further infiltrating the alveolar and bronchiolar walls, thereby forming consolidations, masses, or nodules on imaging. The lesions are randomly infiltrating, showing the characteristics of multiple lobes and multifocal coexistence. The infiltration of the lymphoid cell along the bronchus and the vessel with almost intact underlying structure displays air bronchogram and angiogram sign. The infiltration of tumor cells forms a widening of the alveolar walls, collapses the residual alveolar lumens, and produces abundant fibrous tissue that can exert various traction on the bronchial wall, resulting in the appearance of bronchiectasis or cystic bronchiectasis. The tumor infiltrates the surrounding tissue, causing mild interstitial thickening or incomplete filling of the air cavity, resulting in ground glass opacity or halo sign at the edge of the lesion. Cystic lesions are frequently associated with amyloid or light-chain deposition.

Patients with MALT lymphoma have a good prognosis, with an overall 5-year survival rate of over 80% and a median survival of over 10 years. Thieblemont et al. [25] found that MALT lymphoma presents as a disseminated disease in one-third of the cases at diagnosis. The dissemination does not change the outcome of the patients.

There are no optimal frontline treatment strategies for pulmonary MALT lymphoma. Treatment options include surgery, radiotherapy, chemotherapy, immunotherapy, or "watch and wait" strategy in asymptomatic patients.

Early-stage primary pulmonary MALT lymphoma is indolent in nature. Troch et al. [26] found that pulmonary MALT lymphoma has the potential for spontaneous regression. Therefore, pulmonary MALT lymphoma might not require immediate treatment in the absence of symptoms, and a watch-and-wait policy could be adopted. Yan et al. [27] analyzed the clinical characters and effect on 28 patients with primary pulmonary MALT lymphoma (IE phase). The estimated median times of overall survival (OS) in the "watch-and-wait" cohort and immediate rituximab single-agent or combined chemotherapy cohort were 78 months and 76 months, which were also not statistically significant. Lin et al. [28] identified 953 patients with early-stage MALT-type PPL. Multivariate Cox regression analyses demonstrated that increasing age, tumors located in the lower lobe, and stage II were independent predictors of poorer OS, while increasing age and tumors located in the bilateral lungs resulted in lower cancer-specific survival (CSS). The treatment modalities were not correlated with OS and CSS in early-stage MALT-type PPL, suggesting that "watch and wait" may be a reasonable alternative.

Surgery or radiotherapy may be considered if the lesion is localized. Husnain et al. [29] analyzed 40 primary pulmonary MALT lymphoma patients with the aim of identifying clinical and radiological features associated with shorter survival and poorer treatment outcomes. Patients with elevated LDH at diagnosis, B symptoms, and advanced stage and who failed to achieve complete response (CR) after initial treatment had shorter progression-free survival (PFS). On CT scans, patients with multifocal lung disease, extrapulmonary MALT lymphoma, and cavitary lesions exhibited shorter PFS. However, no clinical or radiologic findings were related to shorter OS. All patients who underwent surgery ($n = 4$) and radiation therapy ($n = 3$) achieved and remained in CR. Primary pulmonary MALT lymphoma exhibited excellent outcomes with a 15-year OS of 94.9%. Radiotherapy and surgery are potentially curative strategies for local primary pulmonary MALT lymphoma.

Chemotherapy and/or immunotherapy is permitted in cases of bilateral or extrapulmonary disease, or in cases of disease recurrence or progression. Borie et al. [30] identified 63 cases of primary pulmonary MALT lymphoma. The median age was 60 years. 23 patients (36%) had no symptoms at diagnosis. 29 (46%) patients had at least one extrapulmonary location of lymphoma. The estimated 5- and 10-year overall survival rates were 90% and 72%, respectively. Age (>60 years) and performance status were the only two adverse prognostic factors for shorter overall survival. Extrapulmonary location of lymphoma was not a prognostic factor for progression-free survival or overall survival. Treatment with chlorambucil had better progression-free survival, when compared with cyclophosphamide or anthracycline. Other studies showed that multiagent chemotherapy, such as cyclophosphamide, hydroxydaunorubicin, vancomycin, and prednisone (CHOP), is not superior to single-agent chemotherapy with chlorambucil or fludarabine. The IELSG-19 study (Randomized Trial of Chlorambucil Versus Chlorambucil Plus Rituximab Versus Rituximab in MALT Lymphoma) showed significantly better 5-year event-free survival rates (68% versus 50%) and complete response rate (78% versus 65%) observed in the double-therapy group compared with the monotherapy group, but not significantly [31].

7.6 Case 6

A 74-year-old man complained of chest tightness and shortness of breath for more than 10 days.

Chest CT: Multifocal nodules in both lungs (Fig. 17).

[Diagnosis] Primary pulmonary diffuse large B-cell lymphoma.

[Diagnosis Basis] The patient underwent a lung biopsy, and the pathology revealed diffuse large B-cell lymphoma (Fig. 18). Immunohistochemistry was positive for LCA, CD20, CD79a, CD30, and EBER and negative for CD3, CD15, and CD34. The Ki-67 index was 30–40%.

[Analysis] Diffuse large B-cell lymphoma (DLBCL) consists of a heterogeneous group of tumors and is the most common type of non-Hodgkin's lymphoma worldwide, accounting for almost 30–40% of all cases in different geographic regions. In the 2016 revision of the WHO classification of lymphoid neoplasms, DLBCL is defined as a neoplasm of large B cells arranged in a diffuse pattern with a nuclear size at least equal

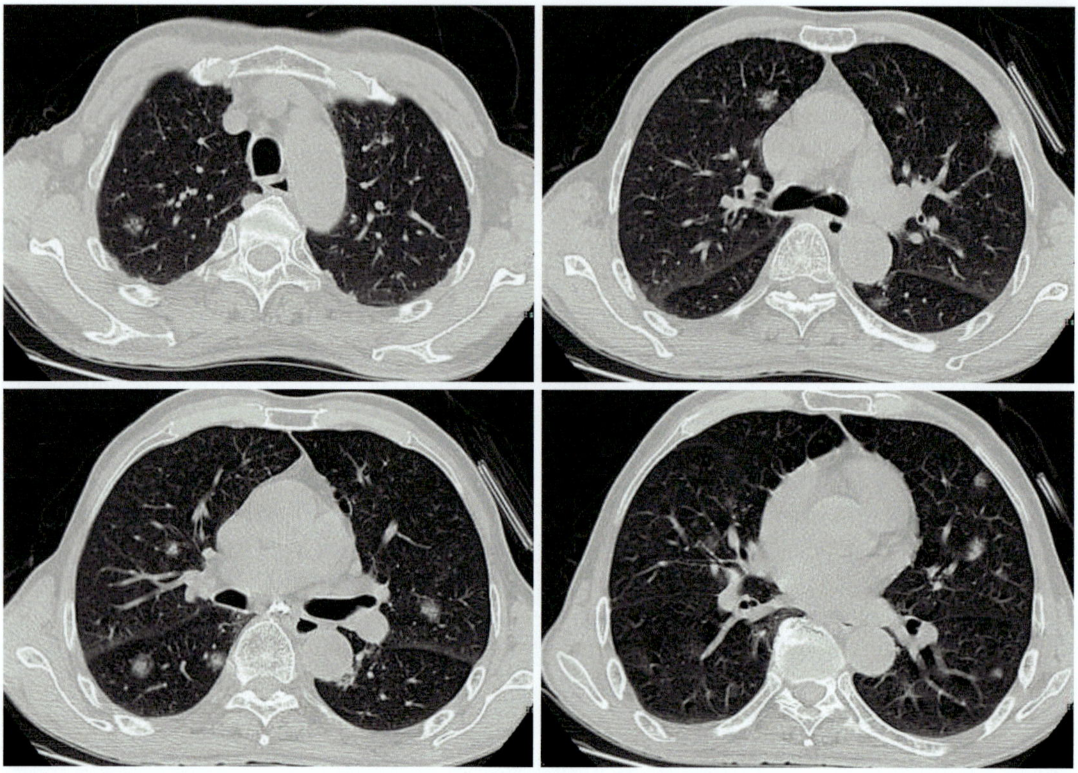

Fig. 17 Chest CT

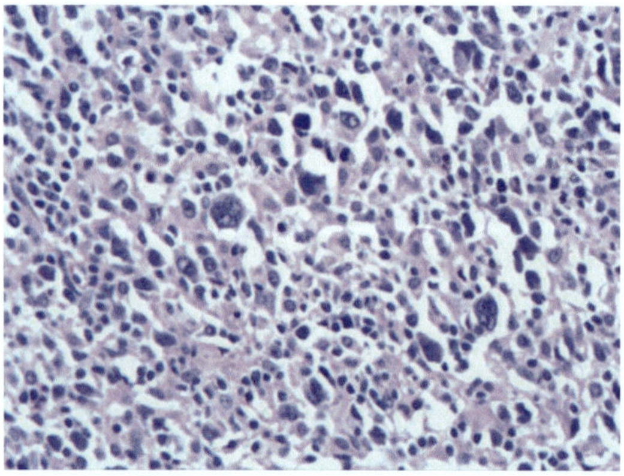

Fig. 18 Hematoxylin-eosin staining shows diffuse proliferation of large cells with scattered large, oddly shaped nuclei resembling Reed-Sternberg cells

to that of the normal macrophage nucleus or more than twice the size of the small lymphocyte. Several subtypes of DLBCL have been designated distinct entities, including primary mediastinal (thymic) large B-cell lymphoma (LBCL), primary DLBCL of the central nervous system, primary cutaneous DLBCL leg type, intravascular LBCL, plasmablastic lymphoma, ALK-positive DLBCL, T-cell/histiocyte-rich LBCL, Epstein-Barr virus (EBV)-positive DLBCL, DLBCL associated with chronic inflammation, LBCL with IRF4 rearrangement, lymphomatoid granulomatosis, primary effusion lymphoma, and HHV8-positive DLBCL. 80–85% of cases cannot be assigned to any specific subgroup/subtype and are named DLBCL, not otherwise specified (NOS).

DLBCL-NOS is divided into two distinct molecular subtypes based on gene expression profiling, germinal center B-cell-like (GCB), and activated B-cell-like (ABC) subtypes, with about 10–15% of cases being unclassifiable. These subtypes arise from different stages of lymphoid differentiation (cell of origin), relying on separate oncogenic mechanisms. Patients with the GCB subtype usually have better outcome than patients with the ABC subtype (3-year progression-free survival, approximately 75% vs. 40–50%) [32].

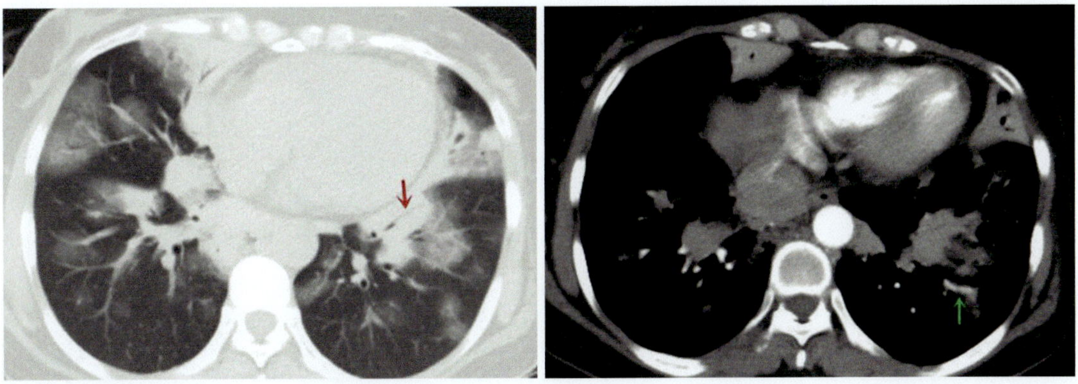

Fig. 19 A 53-year-old woman with DLBCL. Chest CT shows multiple consolidations and ground glass opacities in both lungs. Air bronchogram (red arrow) and angiogram sign (green arrow) are observed

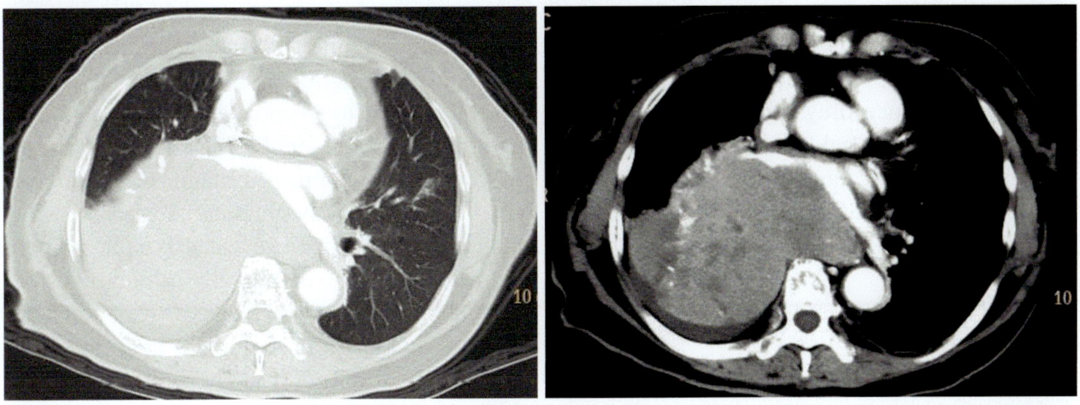

Fig. 20 A 74-year-old woman with DLBCL. Chest CT shows a huge mass in the right thoracic cavity with right pleural effusion

The GCB subtype expresses genes commonly detected in germinal center B cells, including BCL6 and EZH2, whereas the ABC subtype of DLBCL is characterized by chronic B-cell receptor signaling and activation of nuclear factor κB.

Histologically, the lymphoma cells are large and grow diffusely, totally, or partially effacing normal nodal or extranodal architecture. A variable number of background reactive small T cells and histiocytes are present. Three main variants of DLBCL have been described: centroblastic, immunoblastic, and anaplastic. The neoplastic cells express pan B-cell antigens such as CD19, CD20, and CD79a as well as B-cell transcription factors such as PAX5, BOB.1, and OCT2. About 50–70% of cases express surface or cytoplasmic immunoglobulin, most common IgM followed by IgG and IgA. All of the cases are negative for pan T-cell antigens.

On CT scans, pulmonary DLBCL has patchy or irregular consolidations (Fig. 19), single or multiple nodules or huge lumps (Fig. 20), and thick-walled cavities of occasional manifestation (Fig. 21). Interstitial involvement can also occur in pulmonary DLBCL cases. When pulmonary DLBCL infiltrates walls of the chest, thickening pleural nodule with pleural effusion may be observed. Mediastinal lymph node enlargement is occasionally merged.

The standard therapy for patients with DLBCL is rituximab plus cyclophosphamide, doxorubicin, vincristine, and prednisone (R-CHOP) and may cure two-thirds of DLBCL patients. About 30–40% of DLBCL patients are refractory or

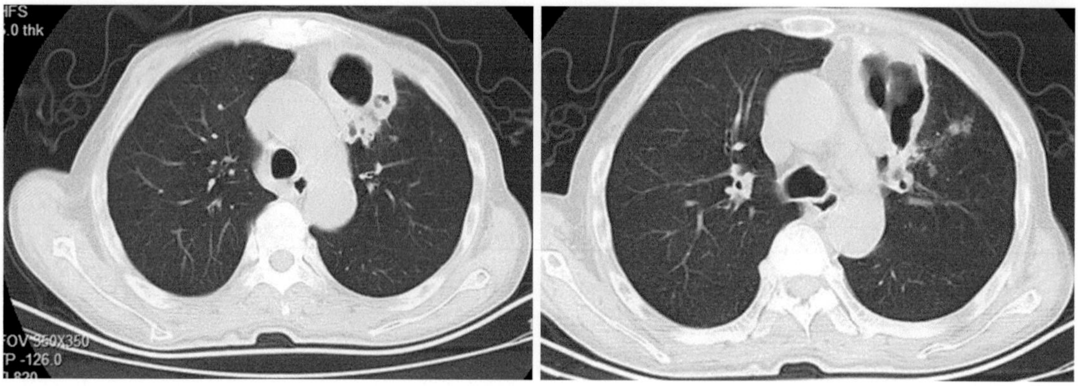

Fig. 21 A 63-year-old man with DLBCL. Chest CT shows an irregular thick-walled cavity next to the aortic arch

resistant to standard therapy. The current treatment options for these patients include autologous stem cell transplantation, chimeric antigen receptor T cells, bispecific T-cell engagers, immunomodulatory drugs, immune checkpoint inhibitors, monoclonal antibodies, molecular pathway inhibitors, antibody-drug conjugates, and epigenetic-modifying drugs. The current 5-year overall survival rate is 60–70%.

7.7 Case 7

A 53-year-old man complained of cough, chest tightness, intermittent fevers to 39 °C, and weight loss for 4 months. He was treated with antibiotics without improvement. Laboratory tests revealed the following results: total leukocyte count, 4650 cells/mm^3; hemoglobin concentration, 11.1 g/dL; platelet count, 172,000/μL; albumin, 30.2 g/L; serum lactate dehydrogenase, 1093 U/L; and arterial oxygen tension, 53.2 Torr. Abdominal B-ultrasound showed splenomegaly. Echocardiography showed moderate pulmonary hypertension (PASP 60 mmHg). No obvious abnormality was found in bone marrow biopsy.

Chest CT: Diffusely spreading ground glass opacities (GGOs) in bilateral lungs (Fig. 22).

PET/CT: A high uptake in the bilateral lungs (Fig. 23).

[Diagnosis] Primary pulmonary intravascular large B-cell lymphoma.

[Diagnosis Basis] A middle-aged man has B symptoms, anemia, hypoalbuminemia, splenomegaly, and significantly elevated lactate dehydrogenase, suggesting a diagnosis of lymphoma. The patient has hypoxemia and moderate pulmonary hypertension, and PET/CT reveal increased FDG uptake, supporting a diagnosis of intravascular large B-cell lymphoma. A transbronchial lung biopsy specimen revealed lymphoma cells in the lumen of small blood vessels. Immunohistochemistry was positive for CD20, CD34 (vascular+), CD31, and TTF-1 and negative for CD3 and CD10. The Ki-67 index was 40%. Combined with immunohistochemistry, it is consistent with intravascular large B-cell lymphoma. He received four courses of R-CHOP, and the status and laboratory findings were dramatically improved.

[Analysis] Intravascular large B-cell lymphoma (IVLBCL) is a rare type of extranodal large B-cell lymphoma characterized by selective growth of tumor cells in the lumina of small to medium-sized blood vessels in systemic organs, especially capillaries. It was first described as a cutaneous small-vessel neoplasm of presumed endothelial origin under the name angioendotheliomatosis proliferans systemisata by Pfleger and Tappeiner [33] in 1959 and was also known as malignant angioendotheliomatosis and angiotropic large-cell lymphoma [34]. Some studies confirmed the lymphoid origin of the tumor cells with B-cell phenotype, supporting that IVLBCL

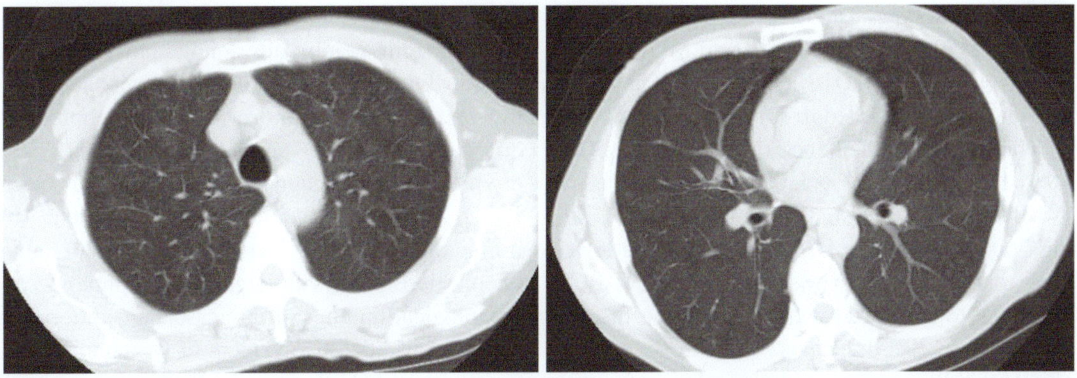

Fig. 22 Chest CT

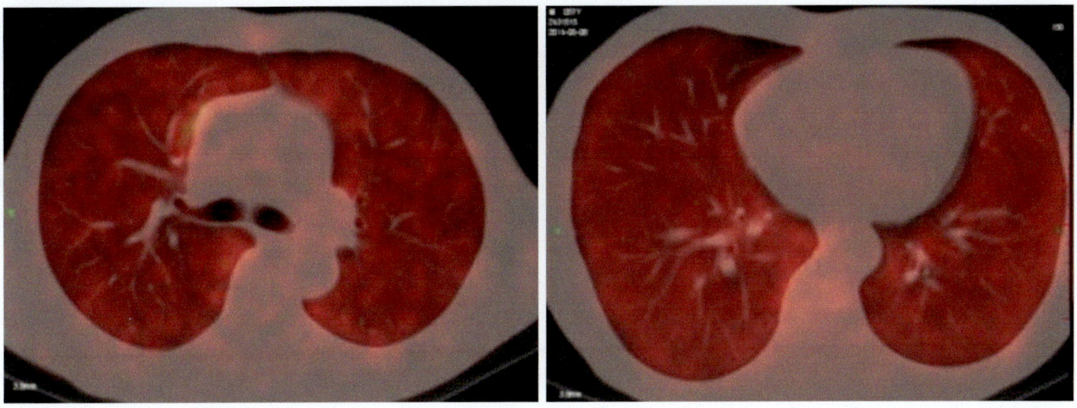

Fig. 23 PET/CT

is more appropriate than malignant angioendotheliomatosis as a name for this disease [34, 35]. In 2008, the WHO classification of hematopoietic tumors classified it as a distinct disease entity and a subtype of diffuse large B-cell lymphoma.

The mechanisms for the selective intravascular growth of tumor cells remain unknown. Ponzoni et al. [36] hypothesized that the intravascular growth pattern could be secondary to a defect of lymphoma cell homing receptors, such as lack of adhesion molecules CD29 (B1 integrin) and CD54 (ICAM-1). However, subsequent studies have not confirmed these findings. Shimada et al. [37] found that the expression of specific adhesion molecules was no loss using patient-derived xenograft (PDX) models. Inhibition of cell migration might be involved in IVLBCL pathogenesis. Some studies have reported the PD-L1 expression of tumor cells in IVLBCL cells, which implies an association between PD-L1 expression and IVLBCL pathogenesis. Suzuki et al. [38] examined neoplastic PD-L1 expression in 34 IVLBCL cases and compared clinicopathological characteristics between patients with PD-L1+ and PD-L1− IVLBCL. 35% (12/34) of cases showed positivity for PD-L1. The PD-L1+ group had significantly lower survival rates compared with the PD-L1− group. The worse prognosis of the PD-L1+ group might be caused by immune evasion mechanisms, which are linked to PD-L1 expression.

Histologically, large, atypical lymphocytes grow within the lumen of small blood vessels and alveolar wall capillaries. The tumor cells are large in size with one or more nucleoli, scant cytoplasm, and frequent mitotic figures. Various degrees of cellulose thrombosis are observed. IVLBCL cells show mature peripheral B-cell immunophenotype. Tumor cells are positive for CD20, CD79a, PAX5, BCL-6, and MUM-1, but negative for CD3, CD10, and CD56. The T-cell marker CD5 is detected in some cases.

The estimated incidence of IVLBCL is 300–400 patients annually in Japan. The incidence of IVLBCL was 0.095 per 1,000,000 per year during 2000–2013 in the USA [39], which is lower than that in Japan. The increase of IVLBCL attributes to improved awareness of the disease and more precise diagnosis. The disease mainly affects middle-aged and elderly individuals, with an average age at diagnosis of 70 years, with no sex differences.

IVLBCL is difficult to diagnose early because of the absence of lymphadenopathy, a common feature of malignant lymphoma, and extracellular tumor mass. IVLBCL lesions are found in almost all organs; the most commonly involved organs are the skin, central nervous system (CNS), bone marrow, and lung. It presents with nonspecific symptoms, such as unexplained fever, night sweat, weight loss, and impaired consciousness. The common respiratory symptoms include cough, sputum production, dyspnea, hypoxemia, pulmonary embolism, and pulmonary hypertension. The laboratory abnormalities include anemia, thrombocytopenia, low levels of serum albumin, and high levels of serum LDH, ESR, CRP, sIL2R, and ferritin.

The clinical manifestations are classified as the classic type and the hemophagocytic syndrome-associated variant (also known as the Asian variant) based on published 2017 WHO criteria. IVLBCL patients in Western countries usually present symptoms of CNS and skin involvement. In contrast, patients with IVLBCL in Asian countries usually show medullary involvement and hemophagocytic syndrome, mainly including pancytopenia and hepatosplenomegaly. Murase et al. [40] proposed diagnostic criteria for Asian variant: (1) Clinical and laboratory criteria (at least two out of three are required): (a) cytopenia (not caused by hypoplastic or dysplastic marrow), affecting at least one of the two lineages, i.e., erythrocytes and platelets. Leukocytes are not included. It is prescribed by hemoglobin (<11 g/dL) or RBC ($<3.5 \times 10^{12}$/L) and/or platelet count ($<100 \times 10^9$/L); (b) hepatomegaly and/or splenomegaly, identified by computerized tomography, ultrasonography, or physical examination; (c) absence of overt lymphadenopathy and tumor formation. (2) Histopathological criteria (all three terms are required): (a) erythrocyte-hemophagocytosis; usually seen mildly or moderately in hemopoietic system; (b) immunophenotypical evidence of proliferating neoplastic B cells with large-cell morphology; (c) pathological findings of intravascular proliferation and/or sinusoidal involvement of lymphoma cells. Ferreri et al. [41] described a “cutaneous variant” with disease limited to the skin, tending to occur in young female patients with a normal platelet count and exhibiting a significantly better outcome. In our case, the patient exhibits findings typical of an Asian variant.

The most common chest CT abnormality is bilateral diffuse ground glass opacities, which are histopathologically correlated with the expanded alveolar septal vasculatures and perivascular spaces filled with neoplastic lymphoid cells [42]. The other CT findings include peribronchovascular and interlobular septal thickening, nodules, and consolidation, suggesting lymphatic and hematological spread. FDG-PET/CT is a useful tool for the early diagnosis of IVLBCL. Intense and diffuse fluorodeoxyglucose uptake in the lungs without corresponding abnormal performance on CT should consider the diagnosis of IVLBCL [43].

Systemic chemotherapy with an anthracycline-based regimen is the recommended treatment for IVLBCL. The use of rituximab (R-CHOP) has resulted in significantly better outcomes compared with CHOP. In Western patients with IVLBCL, the addition of rituximab can improve complete remission rate (90% vs. 50%), event-free survival (3 years: 89% vs. 35%), and overall survival (3 years: 89% vs. 38%) [44]. In Japan, progression-free survival (PFS) and overall survival (OS) rates of patients in the R-chemotherapy group at 2 years after diagnosis were significantly higher than those in the chemotherapy group (PFS, 56%; OS, 66% vs. PFS, 27%; OS, 46%) [45]. Matsue et al. [46] found that about 60% of IVLBCL patients were possible to survive more than 5 years with combination chemotherapy. R-CHOP regimen can improve the outcomes of

IVLBCL patients, but the prognosis remains unsatisfactory. Autologous hematopoietic stem cell transplantation has shown additional promise in small retrospective studies [47].

IVLBCL often results in a delayed diagnosis and poor prognosis. Rajyaguru et al. [39] analyzed 344 IVLBCL patients. The median age at diagnosis was 70 years with most patients (84.9%) being of white race. After propensity matching, the median OS for VLBCL patients was 45.3 months, while for DLBCL patients, it was 44 months. The 1-, 3-, and 5-year survival rates of the IVLBCL (67.6%, 52.5%, and 46.4%, respectively) were comparable to those of the DLBCL-NOS (63.3%, 51.2%, and 46.5%, respectively). On multivariate analysis, advanced age, advanced stage, and having Medicaid or Medicare insurance predicted worse OS, whereas female gender, treatment at academic facility, and use of radiation therapy predicted better OS. Boonsakan et al. [48] found that C-MYC/BCL2 double expression may be a useful prognostic indicator, with significantly higher incidence rate to mortality compared with nondouble expressors. Bonnet et al. [49] conducted a retrospective study on 65 IVLBCL patients treated from 2000 to 2016 in LYSA cooperative group centers. Median age at diagnosis was 69 years. The most frequent extranodal locations were bone marrow (n = 34; 52%), central nervous system (n = 25; 39%), and skin (n = 21; 33%). 0.41% of patients (n = 26) had macrophage activation syndrome. Tumor cells were frequently CD5 positive (52%) with a non-germinal center origin (86%). Eighty-seven percent of all samples analyzed (n = 20) expressed BCL2, and 43% of patients had a MYC/BCL2 double expression. Fifty-six patients received chemotherapy regimen containing rituximab, among whom 73% reached complete remission. The median progression-free survival (PFS) and median overall survival (OS) were 29.4 months and 63.8 months, respectively. History of autoimmune disorder, lack of anthracycline, nodal involvement, or no intensification at first-line regimen was associated with worse PFS. The use of high-dose methotrexate was not associated with better PFS or OS.

7.8 Case 8

A 60-year-old man complained of intermittent cough and weight loss for 3 months. Multiple lung nodules were found for more than 1 month.

Chest CT: Multiple nodules and consolidations in both lungs (Fig. 24).

[Diagnosis] Pulmonary lymphomatoid granulomatosis.

[Diagnosis Basis] Patient has mild clinical symptoms and weight loss. Chest CT shows multiple nodules and consolidations with lobulation, burrs, pleural indentation (green arrows), adjacent pleura thickening (blue arrows), air bronchogram (red arrows), angiogram sign (yellow arrows), and a peribronchovascular distribution. All of the above are in line with the diagnosis of pulmonary lymphoma, especially MALT lymphoma and lymphomatoid granulomatosis. Central necrosis within the nodule is more consistent with the diagnosis of lymphomatoid granulomatosis. The patient underwent thoracoscopic resection of the left upper lung nodule. Histopathological examination showed marked infiltration of lymphocytes around the blood vessels. The alveoli cavities were obliterated by large atypical lymphoid cells intermixed with mature lymphocytes, plasma cells, and histiocytes. Necroses were also seen. Immunohistochemistry was positive for CD3, CD20, CD34 (vascular+), and TTF-1. The tumor was diagnosed as lymphomatoid granulomatosis.

[Analysis] Lymphomatoid granulomatosis (LYG), also known as angiocentric lymphoma and angiocentric immunoproliferative lesion, is a rare angiocentric and angiodestructive B-cell lymphoproliferative disease associated with Epstein-Barr viral infection. It was first described in 1972 by Liebow et al. [50] and was initially thought to be a T-cell disorder because of the predominance of T cells on pathologic examination [51, 52]. Veltri et al. [53] first reported an LYG patient presenting initially a reactivated Epstein-Barr virus (EBV) infection. In 1990, Katzenstein and Peiper [54] identified EBV DNA in 21 of 29 cases (72%) by means of the polymerase chain

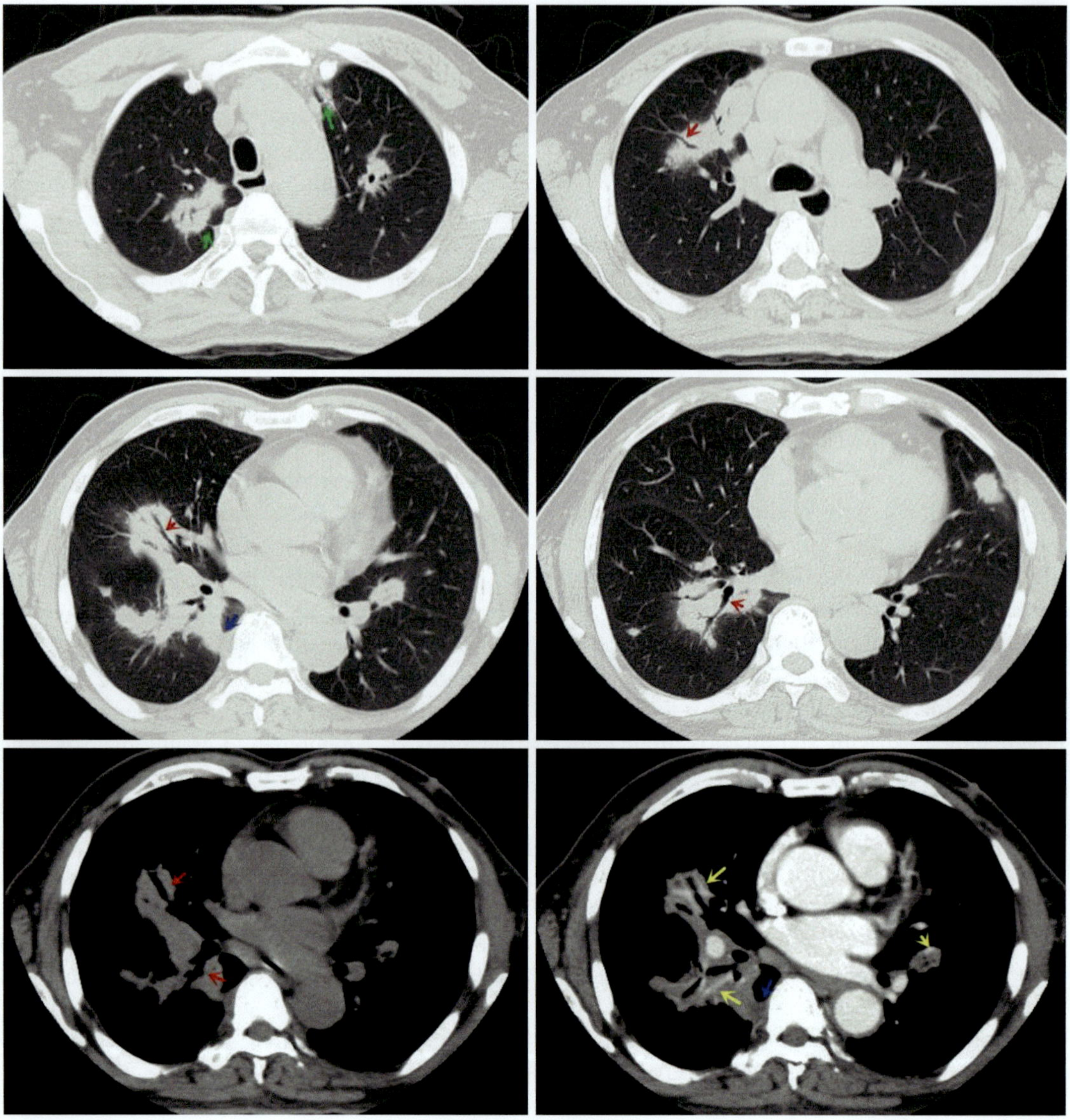

Fig. 24 Chest CT

reaction (PCR) technique on paraffin-embedded formalin-fixed tissue and revealed the role of EBV in the pathogenesis of LYG. In 1994, Guinee et al. [55] confirmed the presence of EBV sequences within B (CD20+) cells and the absence of Epstein-Barr within T cells (CD45RO+) by immunohistochemistry and in situ hybridization in LYG and suggested that most cases of pulmonary LYG represent a proliferation of EBV-infected B cells with a prominent T-cell reaction and vasculitis. In 1995, Myers et al. [56] also confirmed that some cases of LYG are B-cell lymphoma associated with EBV infection.

EBV is a ubiquitous human herpesvirus and primarily infects the B cells, resulting in protective immunity mediated by EBV-specific cytotoxic T cells and natural killer cells. Immunocompromised individuals with EBV infection can severely retard EBV eradication and cannot inhibit the proliferation of EBV-infected B cells, which are predisposed to develop LYG. LYG may be idiopathic or occur in the setting of congenital or acquired immunosuppression, including viral infections, immunosuppressive therapies, autoimmune diseases, organ transplantation, and lymphoproliferative disorders.

According to 2001 WHO classification of tumors of hematopoietic and lymphoid tissues, LYG was a lymphoproliferative disorder of indeterminate potential. The 2008 WHO classification placed it under the category of large B-cell lymphomas and described it as an extranodal, angiocentric, T-cell-rich B-cell lymphoma. It was categorized as a distinct mature B-cell neoplasm in the 2016 revision.

LYG often presents between the fourth and sixth decades of life and occurs more often in men, with a male-to-female ratio of 2:1 to 3:1. It presents sometimes in children with immunodeficiency disorders and is more diagnosed in Western countries than in Asia. Lung is the most commonly affected site (>90%). Other organ systems involved concomitantly or separately include the skin (20–50%), kidneys (15–32%), and central nervous system (20–38%). Upper respiratory tract, gastrointestinal tract, liver, spleen, bone marrow, and lymph nodes are rarely involved.

The clinical feature of LYG can mimic infectious diseases, vasculitis, or malignancies. Patients may present with systemic symptoms or be associated with organ involvement. The common chest symptoms include cough, chest pain, and dyspnea. Skin manifestations include nodules, erythematous papules, and ulcerations. Neurological involvement can present as peripheral neuropathy or focal deficits.

Histologically, LYG is characterized by a triad of polymorphic lymphoid infiltrate, transmural infiltration of vasculature by the lymphoid cells (angiitis), and granulomatosis. Varying numbers of large, atypical, CD20-positive B lymphocytes are present within a background containing numerous small, reactive, CD3-positive T lymphocytes and scattered admixed histiocytes and plasma cells. EBV-encoded RNA (EBER) positivity in situ hybridization is often revealed within these atypical B cells. The infiltrate is angiodestructive, with fibrinoid necrosis of involved vessel walls. The term of granulomatosis is used to describe the focal areas of necrosis within the lymphoid infiltrates, but typical well-formed granulomas may not be observed. The large atypical B cells are also positive for CD79a; positive or negative for CD30; and negative for CD15.

LYG is graded based on the proportion of EBV-positive large B lymphocytes by in situ hybridization of EBER and necrosis: grade 1 lesion is composed of scattered EBV-positive large B cells (<5/high-power field) without necrosis; grade 2 lesions reveal an increased number of EBV-positive large B cells (>5–20/high-power field) and some necrosis; and grade 3 lesions consist mainly of many EBV-positive cells (>50 per high-power field) with extensive necrosis. This B-cell proliferation is polyclonal in grade 1, oligoclonal or monoclonal in grade 2, and monoclonal in grade 3. Immunoglobulin gene rearrangement studies showed a higher percentage of clonal rearrangements in grade 2 (50%) and grade 3 (69%) as compared with grade 1 (8%) [57].

On chest CT, pulmonary LYG shows multiple nodules, masses, or consolidation with lymphatic (predominantly peribronchovascular) distribution representing the lymphoproliferative nature. Single nodule (Fig. 25) and mediastinal lymph node enlargement is rare. Lesions may contain cavitation, air bronchograms, and a peripheral ground glass halo (Fig. 26). Central low attenuation, ground glass halo, and peripheral enhancement of the nodules/masses are likely related to the angioinvasive nature of LYG [58].

At present, there is no validated treatment for LYG. Therapeutic options include systemic corticosteroids, interferon-alpha, rituximab, chemotherapy, and autologous hematopoietic stem cell transplantation. The treatment strategy depends on the presence and severity of symptoms, spread of extrapulmonary involvement, histopathologic grade of the lesion, and underlying diseases. Treatment for low-grade (grades 1–2) LYG is watch and wait, with serial examinations or given immunostimulatory therapy with interferon-alpha to augment host anti-EBV responses. High-grade (grade 3) or symptomatic and advanced patients require combination immunochemother-

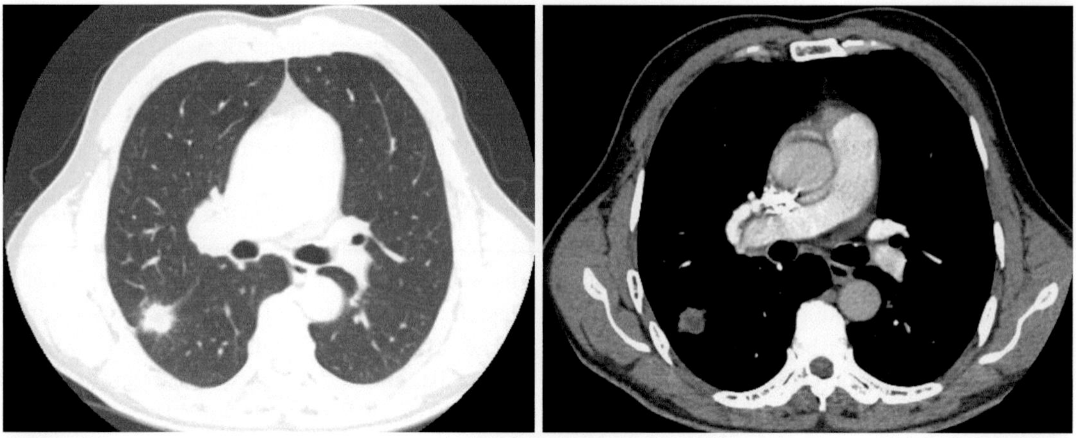

Fig. 25 Chest CT shows single nodule in the right lower lobe, with uneven enhancement and a large area of necrosis

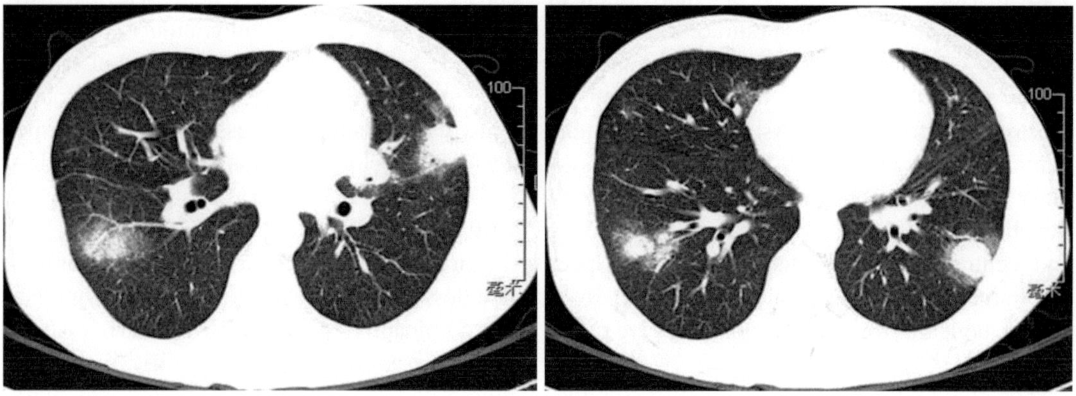

Fig. 26 Chest CT shows multiple nodules with halo sign

apy analogous to treatment for diffuse large B-cell lymphoma. Chavez et al. [59] analyzed 9 pulmonary LYG patients treated with rituximab-based chemotherapy. The overall response rate and complete response rate were 63.6% and 36.44%, respectively. The median overall survival and progression-free survival were 23 and 12.2 months, respectively.

The clinical course of LYG is variable. About 20% of patients may witness spontaneous remission, but most cases are generally progressive. Grade 1–2 patients receiving immunomodulation may progress to grade 3, while immunochemotherapy for grade 3 patients can impair the antiviral response, resulting in relapse with grades 1–2. The prognosis is poor with a mean survival of 2 years and 5-year mortality rate of 60–90%.

References

1. Pekelis E. Linfosarcoma peribronchiale con sviluppo prevalentemente intrapolmonare rapido [Peribronchial lymphosarcoma with rapid intrapulmonary development].Pathologica. 1931;23:66–71.
2. Cordier JF, Chailleux E, Lauque D, et al. Primary pulmonary lymphomas. A clinical study of 70 cases in nonimmunocompromised patients. Chest. 1993;103:201–8.
3. Ferraro P, Trastek VF, Adlakha H, et al. Primary non-Hodgkin's lymphoma of the lung. Ann Thorac Surg. 2000;69:993–7.
4. Zhang MC, Zhou M, Song Q, et al. Clinical features and outcomes of pulmonary lymphoma: a single center experience of 180 cases. Lung Cancer. 2019;132:39–44.
5. Cozzi D, Dini C, Mungai F, et al. Primary pulmonary lymphoma: imaging findings in 30 cases. Radiol Med. 2019;124:1262–9.

6. Low SK, Zayan AH, Istanbuly O, et al. Prognostic factors and nomogram for survival prediction in patients with primary pulmonary lymphoma: a SEER population-based study. Leuk Lymphoma. 2019;60:3406–16.
7. He H, Tan F, Xue Q, et al. Clinicopathological characteristics and prognostic factors of primary pulmonary lymphoma. J Thorac Dis. 2021;13:1106–17.
8. Santopietro M, Kovalchuk S, Battistini R, et al. Treatment and prognosis of primary pulmonary lymphoma: a long-term follow-up study. Eur J Haematol. 2021;106:49–57.
9. Urayama KY, Jarrett RF, Hjalgrim H, et al. Genome-wide association study of classical Hodgkin lymphoma and Epstein-Barr virus status-defined subgroups. J Natl Cancer Inst. 2012;104:240–53.
10. Fan Z, Natkunam Y, Bair E, et al. Characterization of variant patterns of nodular lymphocyte predominant Hodgkin lymphoma with immunohistologic and clinical correlation. Am J Surg Pathol. 2003;27:1346–56.
11. Tzankov A, Zimpfer A, Pehrs AC, et al. Expression of B-cell markers in classical Hodgkin lymphoma: a tissue microarray analysis of 330 cases. Mod Pathol. 2003;16:1141–7.
12. Bröckelmann PJ, Eichenauer DA, Jakob T, et al. Hodgkin lymphoma in adults. Dtsch Arztebl Int. 2018;115:535–40.
13. Isaacson P, Wright DH. Malignant lymphoma of mucosa-associated lymphoid tissue. A distinctive type of B-cell lymphoma. Cancer. 1983;52:1410–6.
14. Kurtin PJ, Myers JL, Adlakha H, et al. Pathologic and clinical features of primary pulmonary extranodal marginal zone B-cell lymphoma of MALT type. Am J Surg Pathol. 2001;25:997–1008.
15. Begueret H, Vergier B, Parrens M, et al. Primary lung small B-cell lymphoma versus lymphoid hyperplasia: evaluation of diagnostic criteria in 26 cases. Am J Surg Pathol. 2002;26:76–81.
16. Bledsoe JR, Wallace ZS, Stone JH, et al. Lymphomas in IgG4-related disease: clinicopathologic features in a western population. Virchows Arch. 2018;472:839–52.
17. Tanahashi H, Yamaguchi K, Koura T, et al. Primary pulmonary mucosa-associated lymphoid tissue lymphoma with the high expression of IgG4. Intern Med. 2022;61:1043–8.
18. Streubel B, Simonitsch-Klupp I, Müllauer L, et al. Variable frequencies of MALT lymphoma-associated genetic aberrations in MALT lymphomas of different sites. Leukemia. 2004;18:1722–6.
19. Suarez F, Lortholary O, Hermine O, et al. Infection-associated lymphomas derived from marginal zone B cells: a model of antigen-driven lymphoproliferation. Blood. 2006;107:3034–44.
20. Chanudet E, Adam P, Nicholson AG, et al. Chlamydiae and Mycoplasma infections in pulmonary MALT lymphoma. Br J Cancer. 2007;97:949–51.
21. Adam P, Czapiewski P, Colak S, et al. Prevalence of Achromobacter xylosoxidans in pulmonary mucosa-associated lymphoid tissue lymphoma in different regions of Europe. Br J Haematol. 2014;164:804–10.
22. Borie R, Caro V, Nunes H, et al. No evidence for a pathogen associated with pulmonary MALT lymphoma: a metagenomics investigation. Infect Agent Cancer. 2021;16:10.
23. Aoyama S, Masaki A, Sakamoto Y, et al. Achromobacter infection is rare in Japanese patients with pulmonary B-cell lymphoma. Intern Med. 2018;57:789–94.
24. Ekström Smedby K, Vajdic CM, Falster M, et al. Autoimmune disorders and risk of non-Hodgkin lymphoma subtypes: a pooled analysis within the InterLymph Consortium. Blood. 2008;111:4029–38.
25. Thieblemont C, Berger F, Dumontet C, et al. Mucosa-associated lymphoid tissue lymphoma is a disseminated disease in one third of 158 patients analyzed. Blood. 2000;95:802–6.
26. Troch M, Streubel B, Petkov V, et al. Does MALT lymphoma of the lung require immediate treatment? An analysis of 11 untreated cases with long-term follow-up. Anticancer Res. 2007;27:3633–7.
27. Yan W, Wu B, Liao AJ, et al. Watch-and-wait or immediate immunotherapy/immunochemotherapy in patients with phase IE primary pulmonary MALT lymphoma? A multicenter retrospective study. Ann Hematol. 2021;100:709–14.
28. Lin H, Zhou K, Peng Z, et al. Surgery and chemotherapy cannot improve the survival of patients with early-stage mucosa-associated lymphoid tissue derived primary pulmonary lymphoma. Front Oncol. 2022;12:965727.
29. Husnain M, Kuker R, Reis IM, et al. Clinical and radiological characteristics of patients with pulmonary marginal zone lymphoma: a single center analysis. Cancer Med. 2020;9:5051–64.
30. Borie R, Wislez M, Thabut G, et al. Clinical characteristics and prognostic factors of pulmonary MALT lymphoma. Eur Respir J. 2009;34:1408–16.
31. Zucca E, Conconi A, Laszlo D, et al. Addition of rituximab to chlorambucil produces superior event-free survival in the treatment of patients with extranodal marginal-zone B-cell lymphoma: 5-year analysis of the IELSG-19 randomized study. J Clin Oncol. 2013;31:565–72.
32. Scott DW, Mottok A, Ennishi D, et al. Prognostic significance of diffuse large B-cell lymphoma cell of origin determined by digital gene expression in formalin-fixed paraffin-embedded tissue biopsies. J Clin Oncol. 2015;33:2848–56.
33. Pfleger L, Tappeiner J. On the recognition of systematized endotheliomatosis of the cutaneous blood vessels reticuloendotheliosis? Hautarzt. 1959;10:359–63.
34. Domizio P, Hall PA, Cotter F, et al. Angiotropic large cell lymphoma (ALCL): morphological, immunohistochemical and genotypic studies with analysis of previous reports. Hematol Oncol. 1989;7:195–206.
35. Sheibani K, Battifora H, Winberg CD, et al. Further evidence that "malignant angioendotheliomatosis" is

an angiotropic large-cell lymphoma. N Engl J Med. 1986;314:943–8.
36. Ponzoni M, Arrigoni G, Gould VE, et al. Lack of CD 29 (beta1 integrin) and CD 54 (ICAM-1) adhesion molecules in intravascular lymphomatosis. Hum Pathol. 2000;31:220–6.
37. Shimada K, Shimada S, Sugimoto K, et al. Development and analysis of patient-derived xenograft mouse models in intravascular large B-cell lymphoma. Leukemia. 2016;30:1568–79.
38. Suzuki Y, Kohno K, Matsue K, et al. PD-L1 (SP142) expression in neoplastic cells predicts a poor prognosis for patients with intravascular large B-cell lymphoma treated with rituximab-based multiagent chemotherapy. Cancer Med. 2020;9:4768–76.
39. Rajyaguru DJ, Bhaskar C, Borgert AJ, et al. Intravascular large B-cell lymphoma in the United States (US): a population-based study using surveillance, epidemiology, and end results program and National Cancer Database. Leuk Lymphoma. 2017;58(9):1–9.
40. Murase T, Nakamura S, Kawauchi K, et al. An Asian variant of intravascular large B-cell lymphoma: clinical, pathological and cytogenetic approaches to diffuse large B-cell lymphoma associated with haemophagocytic syndrome. Br J Haematol. 2000;111:826–34.
41. Ferreri AJ, Campo E, Seymour JF, et al. Intravascular lymphoma: clinical presentation, natural history, management and prognostic factors in a series of 38 cases, with special emphasis on the 'cutaneous variant'. Br J Haematol. 2004;127:173–83.
42. Cha MJ, Lee KS, Hwang HS, et al. Pulmonary intravascular lymphomatosis: clinical, CT, and PET findings, correlation of CT and pathologic results, and survival outcome. Radiology. 2016;280:602–10.
43. Wagner T, Brechemier D, Dugert E, et al. Diffuse pulmonary uptake on FDG-PET with normal CT diagnosed as intravascular large B-cell lymphoma: a case report and a discussion of the causes of diffuse FDG uptake in the lungs. Cancer Imaging. 2012;12:7–12.
44. Ferreri AJM, Dognini GP, Bairey O, et al. The addition of rituximab to anthracycline-based chemotherapy significantly improves outcome in 'Western' patients with intravascular large B-cell lymphoma. Br J Haematol. 2008;143:253–7.
45. Shimada K, Matsue K, Yamamoto K, et al. Retrospective analysis of intravascular large B-cell lymphoma treated with rituximab-containing chemotherapy as reported by the IVL study group in Japan. Clin Oncol. 2008;26:3189–95.
46. Matsue K, Abe Y, Narita K, et al. Diagnosis of intravascular large B cell lymphoma: novel insights into clinicopathological features from 42 patients at a single institution over 20 years. Br J Haematol. 2019;187:328–36.
47. Meissner J, Finel H, Dietrich S, et al. Autologous hematopoietic stem cell transplantation for intravascular large B-cell lymphoma: the European Society for Blood and Marrow Transplantation experience. Bone Marrow Transplant. 2017;52:650–2.
48. Boonsakan P, Iamsumang W, Chantrathammachart P, et al. Prognostic value of concurrent expression of C-MYC and BCL2 in intravascular large B-cell lymphoma: a 10-year retrospective study. Biomed Res Int. 2020;2020:1350820.
49. Bonnet A, Bossard C, Gabellier L, et al. Clinical presentation, outcome, and prognostic markers in patients with intravascular large B-cell lymphoma, a lymphoma study association (LYSA) retrospective study. Cancer Med. 2022;11(19):3602–11. https://doi.org/10.1002/cam4.4742.
50. Liebow AA, Carrington CR, Friedman PJ. Lymphomatoid granulomatosis. Hum Pathol. 1972;3:457–558.
51. Nichols PW, Koss M, Levine AM, et al. Lymphomatoid granulomatosis: a T-cell disorder? Am J Med. 1982;72:467–71.
52. Lipford EH, Margolick JB, Longo DL, et al. Angiocentric immunoproliferative lesions: a clinicopathologic spectrum of post-thymic T-cell proliferations. Blood. 1988;72:1674–81.
53. Veltri RW, Raich PC, McClung JE, et al. Lymphomatoid granulomatosis and Epstein-Barr virus. Cancer. 1982;50:1513–7.
54. Katzenstein AL, Peiper SC. Detection of Epstein-Barr virus genomes in lymphomatoid granulomatosis: analysis of 29 cases by the polymerase chain reaction technique. Mod Pathol. 1990;3:435–41.
55. Guinee D Jr, Jaffe E, Kingma D, et al. Pulmonary lymphomatoid granulomatosis. Evidence for a proliferation of Epstein-Barr virus infected B-lymphocytes with a prominent T-cell component and vasculitis. Am J Surg Pathol. 1994;18:753–64.
56. Myers JL, Kurtin PJ, Katzenstein AL, et al. Lymphomatoid granulomatosis. Evidence of immunophenotypic diversity and relationship to Epstein-Barr virus infection. Am J Surg Pathol. 1995;19:1300–12.
57. Song JY, Pittaluga S, Dunleavy K, et al. Lymphomatoid granulomatosis—a single institute experience: pathologic findings and clinical correlations. Am J Surg Pathol. 2015;39:141–56.
58. Chung JH, Wu CC, Gilman MD, et al. Lymphomatoid granulomatosis: CT and FDG-PET findings. Korean J Radiol. 2011;12:671–8.
59. Chavez JC, Sandoval-Sus J, Horna P, et al. Lymphomatoid granulomatosis: a single institution experience and review of the literature. Clin Lymphoma Myeloma Leuk. 2016;16(Suppl):S170–4.

Pulmonary Langerhans Cell Histiocytosis

Jing Liu and Song Zhang

Langerhans cell histiocytosis (LCH) is a rare histiocytic disorder characterized by proliferation of abnormal Langerhans cells. Histiocyte is an archaic term (meaning tissue cell or tissue macrophages) and derives from hematopoietic myeloid progenitors, which further differentiate into antigen-processing cells (monocytes and macrophages) and antigen-presenting cells (dendritic cells and Langerhans cells). The histiocytoses are rare disorders characterized by infiltration of myeloid cells with diverse macrophage or dendritic cell phenotypes in various tissues and organs. In 1987, histiocytoses were classified by the Working Group of the Histiocyte Society into three categories: Langerhans cell related, non-Langerhans cell related, or malignant [1]. In 2016, the revised classification system consists of five groups of diseases: Langerhans, cutaneous and mucocutaneous, malignant, Rosai-Dorfman disease, and hemophagocytic lymphohistiocytosis and macrophage activation syndrome [2].

J. Liu
Department of Radiation Oncology, Shandong Cancer Hospital and Institute, Shandong First Medical University and Shandong Academy of Medical Sciences, Jinan, Shandong, China

S. Zhang (✉)
Department of Respiratory and Critical Care Medicine, Shandong Provincial Hospital Affiliated to Shandong First Medical University, Jinan, Shandong, China

1 Origin of LCH

In 1868, Paul Langerhans [3] first described the presence of gold-positive dendritic cells in the epidermis and considered as intraepidermal nerve endings because gold chloride was thought to be specific for neurons, later named Langerhans cells. Between 1893 and 1920, Alfred Hand, Artur Schüller, and Dr. Henry A. Christian elaborated the classical triad of skull defects, exophthalmos, and diabetes insipidus [4–6]. This complex syndrome is now known as Hand-Schüller-Christian disease. Erich Letterer reported an acute fulminant, non-leukemic disorder of the reticuloendothelial system in a 6-month-old child in 1924 [7]. Sture Siwe described a similar case of a very young child with splenomegaly, hepatomegaly, lymphadenopathy, bone tumors, hemorrhaging, and generalized histiocytic hyperplasia in 1933 [8]. In 1936, Arthur Abt and Edward Denenholz reported another patient with similar findings and named it Letterer-Siwe disease after reviewing the prior literature [9]. Sadao Otani and Joseph Ehrlich [10] and Louis Lichtenstein and Henry L. Jaffe [11] almost simultaneously reported solitary granulomatous histiocytic lesions of bone and named the disease eosinophilic granuloma. The three entities of eosinophilic granuloma, Hand-Schüller-Christian disease, and Letterer-Siwe disease were linked on the basis of similar radiologic and histologic findings by Farber in 1941

S. Zhang (ed.), *Diagnostic Imaging of Lung Cancers*, https://doi.org/10.1007/978-981-99-6815-2_21

[12] and William T. Green and Sidney Farber in 1942 [13]. In 1953, Lichtenstein first recognized that the three entities have common clinical and pathological characteristics and named them as histiocytosis X, with the X indicating an uncertain cell of origin [14]. In 1961, Birbeck et al. [15] found characteristic ultrastructural cytoplasmic inclusions called Birbeck granules in Langerhans cells. Using the Birbeck granule as a marker, Friedman and Hanaoka in 1969 [16] and Nezelof et al. [17] in 1973 concluded that the lesions of histiocytosis X were the result of the proliferation and dissemination of abnormal histiocytic cells of the Langerhans cell system. In 1983, Risdall et al. [18] renamed histiocytosis X as LCH based on the understanding that the Langerhans cell was the common key player, and all the different clinical presentations were just different forms of the disease spectrum.

2 Etiology

The pathogenesis of LCH remains speculative. Previous studies suggested that LCH arises from malignant transformation and metastasis of epidermal Langerhans cells. Allen et al. [19] found that Langerhans cells are transcriptionally more similar to bone marrow-derived immature myeloid dendritic cells than to epidermal Langerhans cells.

Dendritic cell (DC) is a member of the mononuclear phagocyte system and consists of a heterogenous population of cells whose primary function is to serve as antigen-presenting cells to T cells. Langerhans cell (LC) is a subset of DC found in the epidermis and under the epithelium of the bronchial tree and other mucosae and is characterized by the presence of cell surface markers CD1a and CD207 (langerin).

Pulmonary Langerhans cell histiocytosis (PLCH) was initially considered as an inflammatory/reactive granulomatous process because of the near-universal association with smoking and instances of remission upon smoking cessation. Tobacco smoke induces the accumulation of DCs and monocytes in the lungs, which release cytokines such as TNF-α, interleukin 1 beta, GM-CSF, TGF-β, and chemokine of dendritic cells (CCL20) and express excessive osteopontin, resulting in PLCH lesion [20].

BRAF V600E mutation or other mitogen-activated protein kinase (MAPK) mutations have been identified in some PLCH patients, suggesting that at least a subset of PLCH represents a myeloid neoplasm with inflammatory properties. BRAF V600E mutation induces a constitutive activation of the MAPK signaling pathway, which is involved in several physiological cellular processes, including proliferation, differentiation, transformation, migration, and survival. Badalian-Very et al. [21] identified the oncogenic BRAF V600E mutation in 35 of 61 archived specimens (57%). TP53 and MET mutations were also observed in one sample each. High-prevalence, recurrent BRAF mutations in LCH indicate that it is a neoplastic disease that may respond to RAF pathway inhibitors. Jouenne et al. [22] genotyped a large number of adult LCH biopsies. Out of 69 cases, 59 (86%) detected MAPK pathway alterations (BRAF V600E mutation: 36%, BRAF N486-P490 deletion: 28%, MAP2K1 mutations: 15%, isolated NRAS Q61 mutations: 4%), while KRAS mutations were almost nonexistent in PLCH lesions. BRAF V600E status did not influence the risk of LCH progression over time. Animal models have also shown that MAPK pathway is involved in myeloid differentiation, apoptosis resistance, dysfunctional migration, and senescence-associated secretory phenotype, leading to the formation of LCH lesions [23].

Liu et al. [24] established a cigarette smoke-exposed (CS-exposed) BRAF-V600E-mutant mouse model to further analyze the role of smoking in PLCH in the context of MAPK pathway activation. They found that CD11c-targeted expression of BRAF-V600E increases DC responsiveness to stimuli, including the chemokine CCL20, and the accumulation of mutated cell in the lungs of CS-exposed mice is due to both increased cellular viability and enhanced recruitment. Moreover, they reported that the chemokine CCL7 is secreted from DCs and human peripheral blood monocytes in a BRAF-V600E-dependent manner, suggesting that smoking most likely plays a triggering role for the development of PLCH.

3 Pathology

The characteristic lesions of PLCH are associated with destructive granulomas, which contain numerous LCs and cysts. PLCH begins with an infiltration and destruction of distal bronchiolar walls and epithelium by LCs. These cells develop into stellate nodules containing the LCs, lymphocytes, fibroblasts, eosinophils, neutrophils, plasma cells, and pigmented macrophages. PLCH lesions progressively envelope the terminal bronchioles and obstruct the small airways, leading to the distal perilesional airspace enlargement and cyst formation. As the disease progresses, nodules are gradually replaced by fibroblastic proliferation and develop into stellate fibrotic scars surrounded by cystic areas and honeycombing.

LCs are relatively large with moderate amount of eosinophilic cytoplasm and pale, elongated nuclei with delicate folds and clefts (Fig. 1a). Immunohistochemical staining is positive for CD1a (Fig. 1b) and CD207 (langerin). The expression of S-100 protein may be present but is not specific. Birbeck granules (pentalaminar rod-shaped intracellular structures) are characteristic of LCs on electron microscope. Inflammatory eosinophilic granulomas may be observed based on the stage of disease progression. Owing to the fact that most PLCH patients are smokers, the background lung parenchyma might show signs of other smoking-related diseases including respiratory bronchiolitis, desquamative interstitial pneumonia, and emphysema [25].

4 Epidemiology

The incidence of adult LCH is estimated at 1–2 cases per million/year. PLCH is most commonly diagnosed in 20–40 years of age, without gender predominance. In Japan, the estimated crude prevalence was 0.27 and 0.07 per 100,000 population in males and females, respectively [26]. This may be related to the fact that the number of female smokers in Asia is much smaller. About 90–95% of PLCH patients are tobacco smokers. The intensity and/or duration of smoking do not influence the development of PLCH.

The estimated incidence of LCH in children is 2.6–8.9 cases per million/year. Isolated PLCH is extremely rare in children, and most of them are associated with passive exposure to tobacco smoke. Multisystemic LCH in children is more prevalent than in the adult population, and approximately 10–30% of children with multisystem LCH exhibit pulmonary lesions. Familial cases of LCH occur occasionally, but no genetic predisposition toward LCH was found.

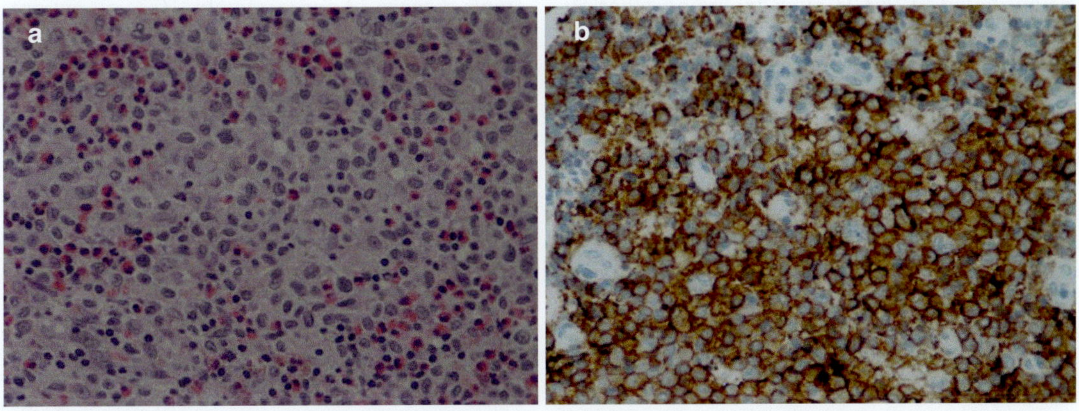

Fig. 1 (**a**) Langerhans cells are relatively large with reactive inflammatory cell background including eosinophils, small lymphocytes, and macrophages. (**b**) Langerhans cells marked with CD1a (membranous staining)

Some studies have described the association between LCH and other malignancies, especially other myeloproliferative neoplasms. The incidence ranges from 2.6% in children to 32% in adults [27, 28]. Of 132 adult LCH patients, the incidence of solid tumors (especially lung and thyroid cancer), lymphoma, and other hematological malignancies was 39 (74%), 9 (17%), and 5 (9%), respectively [28].

5 Clinical Features

PLCH may occur as part of multisystem LCH, or more commonly as isolated LCH (single-system PLCH). Patients with PLCH have a variable clinical presentation, including asymptomatic disease detected incidentally, spontaneous regression (more often in young smokers), or progressive multi-organ failure and death. Approximately 5–25% of patients are asymptomatic, and two-thirds of patients present with nonproductive cough and exertional dyspnea as the initial complaint. About 10–20% of patients present with constitutional symptoms such as fever, fatigue, and weight loss. Pneumothorax is the initial symptom of PLCH in 10–30% of patients and occurs in 30–45% of cases during the course of the disease. PLCH patients with spontaneous pneumothorax as the initial sign are younger, more frequently men, and had greater respiratory impairment than those who had no pneumothorax [29]. Hemoptysis is uncommon and can only be attributed to PLCH after excluding other etiologies and alternative diagnoses. Pulmonary hypertension, dyspnea at rest, and right ventricular circulatory failure occur in the late stages of PLCH. Extrathoracic lesions of PLCH in adults are rare, usually involving bones (lytic lesions), pituitary stalks (diabetes insipidus), and more rarely skin.

Singla et al. [30] analyzed 94 PLCH patients. Median age at diagnosis was 40 years. Average interval between symptom onset and diagnosis was 2.9 years. The most common manifestation was dyspnea on exertion (89%), followed by fatigue (74%), cough (72%), chest pain (65%), constitutional symptoms such as fever, sweats, and/or chills (42%), and weight loss (32%). Other manifestations included diabetes insipidus (29%), pulmonary hypertension (29%), bone lesions or bone pain (26%), lymphadenopathy (23%), spontaneous pneumothorax (23%), and hemoptysis (8%).

6 Radiographic Features

Early imaging findings of PLCH show bilateral, upper-middle lobe predominant, irregular, small (<1 cm), centrilobular or peribronchovascular nodules with sparing of the costophrenic angles (>90%) (Fig. 2). As disease progresses, nodules increasingly evolve to cavities and thick-walled cysts (Fig. 3). The cysts initially appear to be round and small (<1 cm) and become gradually larger, irregular, thin-walled, bizarre, bilobed, cloverleafed, or branched (Fig. 4). The irregularity of the cysts derives from further cystic dilatation and adjacent cyst fusion (Fig. 5a, b). Fibrosis may appear at the affected areas in end-stage disease. Approximately 10% of patients may have enlarged lymph nodes. The coexistence of upper-middle nodules, cavities, and bizarre cysts in a smoker allows a confident diagnosis of PLCH.

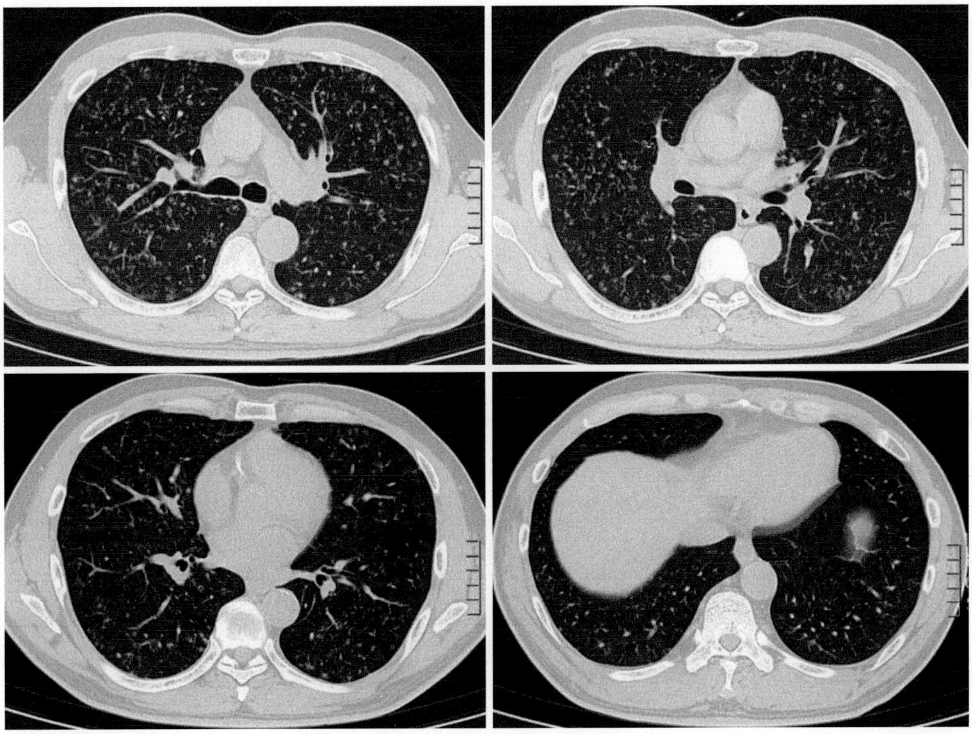

Fig. 2 A 52-year-old man with smoking history of 30 years. Chest CT shows small intralobular nodules, tree in bud, and cavitated nodules

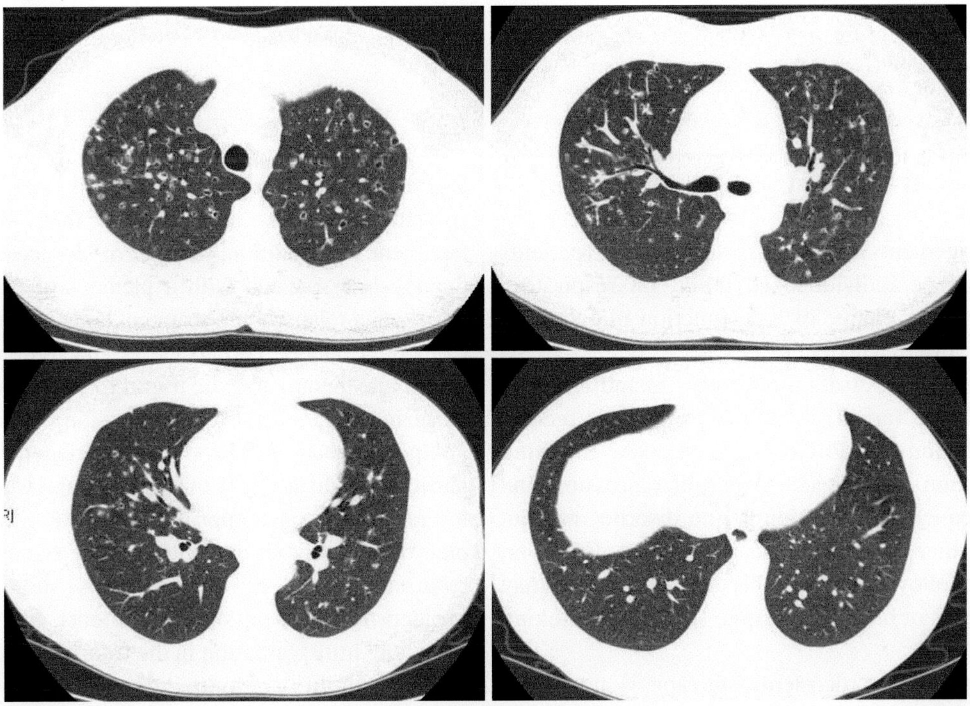

Fig. 3 A 33-year-old man with PLCH. Chest CT shows upper-middle lobe predominant, small nodules, and cavities

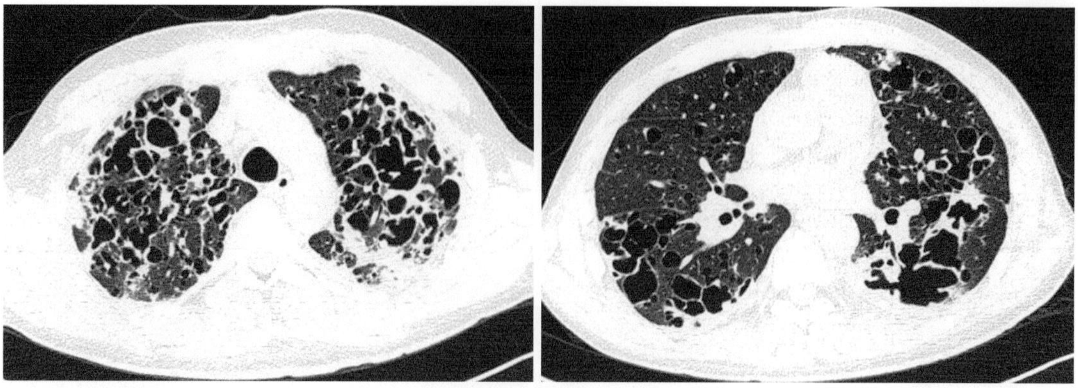

Fig. 4 A 32-year-old man with PLCH. Chest CT shows large, bizarre cysts

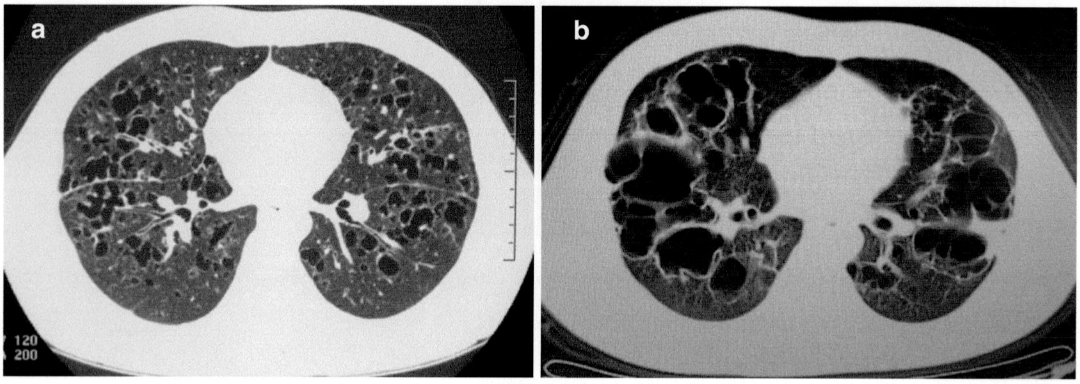

Fig. 5 (**a**) A 23-year-old man with smoking history. Chest CT shows small round, partially fused cysts. (**b**) After 3 years, the cysts are larger, with obvious fusion

7 Treatment

Management of single-system PLCH patients should be individualized based on respiratory symptoms, degree of lung function impairment, and radiologic extent of disease.

Smoking cessation (all forms including marijuana and vaping) is the most important recommendation in PLCH management. Smoking cessation alone leads to partial regression and subsequent stabilization of the disorder without any other pharmacological treatment. However, close follow-up is vital, because the disease may progress or reactivate despite successful smoking cessation.

Systemic corticosteroid therapy is no longer recommended because some symptomatic, radiological, and functional improvements are due to smoking cessation alone rather than steroid treatment. In addition, long-term corticosteroid therapy is associated with a plethora of adverse effects, and relapse after treatment is also common. Combined inhaled corticosteroid and long-acting β2-agonist therapy may be useful for patients with wheezing and moderate obstructive lung disease.

Spontaneous pneumothorax management is particularly difficult. If managed conservatively, the recurrence rates approach 50–60%. Surgical pleurodesis may significantly reduce the risk of recurrence to 0–20%. Pleurodesis should be avoided as far as possible in patients who may need lung transplantation in the future, but it does not constitute a contraindication for lung transplantation.

Systemic therapy is recommended for patients who do not respond to smoking cessation or are unable to quit smoking with persistent or worsening symptoms. Vinblastine or methotrexate has limited efficacy in isolated PLCH. Some studies have shown that cladribine (2-chlorodeoxyadenosine), a synthetic cytotoxic purine analogue, can improve lung function in isolated PLCH and is the preferred systemic therapy. Its long-term effects and tolerance are being evaluated in a phase II clinical trial (NCT01473797).

Targeted therapies directed at MAPK mutations may be a clinically useful future strategy in PLCH. Lorillon et al. [31] reported a case of an 18-year-old young smoking patient with multisystem LCH whose lung involvement progressed despite treatment with cladribine and who improved following therapy with the MEK inhibitor trametinib.

Patients with advanced PLCH or severe pulmonary hypertension may be candidates for lung transplantation (LT), although disease recurrence has been described in the transplanted lungs, which highlights the neoplastic nature of PLCH. Wajda et al. [32] analyzed 87 patients with PLCH who underwent LT in the United States. The mean age at LT for PLCH patients was 49 years, with a near-equal gender distribution. Median post-LT survival for PLCH patients was similar to post-LT survival in other lung diseases (5.1 vs. 5.5 years). The actuarial Kaplan-Meier post-LT survival rates for PLCH patients were 85%, 65%, 49%, and 22% at 1, 3, 5, and 10 years, respectively. Females had a significantly increased median survival compared to male PLCH LT recipients (9.3 vs. 3.9 years). The exact reasons for this gender-based contrast in outcomes are not entirely clear.

8 Prognosis

The prognosis of PLCH is highly variable, ranging from spontaneous resolution to chronic respiratory failure (CRF) and pulmonary hypertension (PH), ultimately resulting in lung transplantation or death. Adverse prognostic factors include age, smoking, severe obstruction, decreased PaO_2, higher SGRQ score, pulmonary hypertension, and multiple organ involvement, particularly risk organs.

Previous reports have shown that the median survival after diagnosis of the disease was 12–13 years. However, the long-term prognosis of PLCH is significantly more favorable than has previously been reported because a significant proportion of patients with mild disease are lost to follow-up.

Benattia et al. [33] analyzed 206 PLCH patients. The estimated rate of survival at 10 years was 93%. The cumulative incidences of CRF and/or PH were <5% at both 5 and 10 years, and 58% of these patients died. Eight (5.1%) of the 157 patients with isolated PLCH developed extrapulmonary involvement.

Patients must be closely monitored after diagnosis in order to detect severe complications early.

9 Case Analysis

9.1 Case 1

A 32-year-old man complained of left paroxysmal headache and numbness of the right limb for 2 months. He had convulsions and syncope four times. Brain MRI showed swelling and enhancement of the left frontal parietal gyrus and enhancement of the pia mater. The quantity of cerebrospinal fluid protein was slightly higher. After treatment with antiepileptic drugs, headache was relieved and limb convulsions did not occur again. Multiple pulmonary nodules were found on physical examination 1 day ago.

Chest CT: Multiple nodules, nodules with cavities, and cysts in bilateral lungs (Fig. 6).

[Diagnosis] Langerhans cell histiocytosis.

[Diagnosis Basis] Chest CT scan shows the coexistence of nodules, cystic nodules, and cysts in both lungs, fully reflecting the evolution of PLCH. In combination with the patient's age and history of brain lesions, the diagnosis of LCH should be considered. This image should be dif-

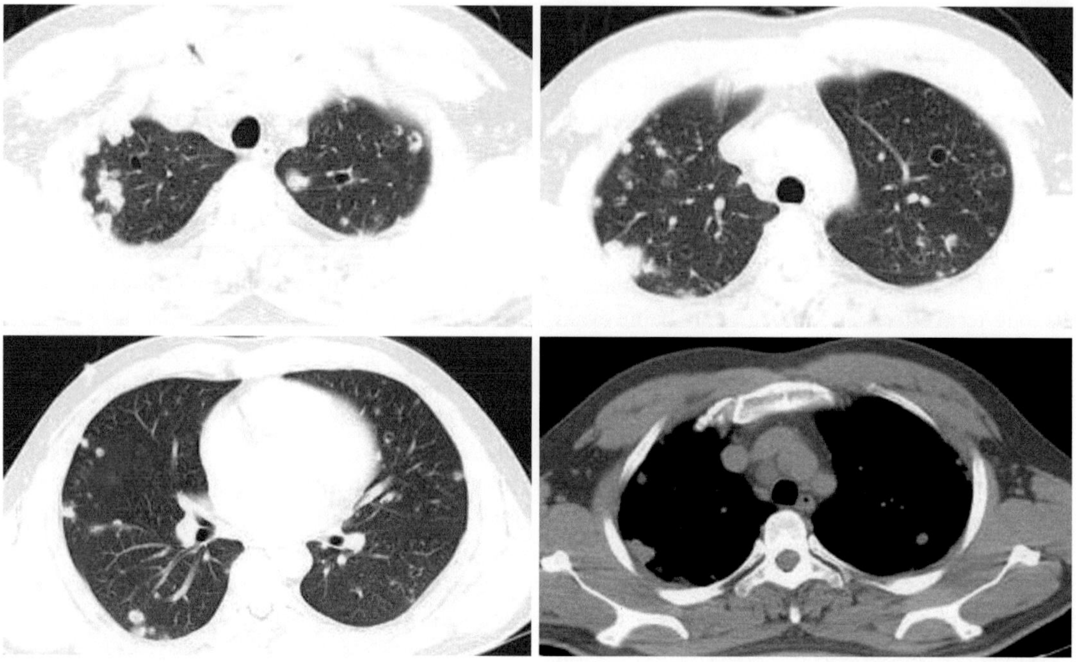

Fig. 6 Chest CT

ferentiated from cryptococcosis and metastatic tumor. Cryptococcosis can also affect the lungs and brain. The chest CT findings of cryptococcosis may show multiple nodules, halo sign around the nodules, and cavities, but cysts are rare. Most of the metastatic tumors have a history of primary tumors, and nodules are more common in lower lobes than in upper lobes because they usually develop via a hematogenous route and the bloodstream is more abundant in lower lobes. Nodules of PLCH are usually distributed in the centers of secondary lobules around small airways. Cystic changes in lung metastatic nodules are more common in larger nodules than in smaller ones. The patient underwent percutaneous lung biopsy, and the pathology was Langerhans cell histiocytosis. Immunohistochemistry was positive for CD1a, S-100, CD68, and vimentin. The Ki-67 index was 10%.

[Analysis] LCH presents with various degrees of systemic involvement, ranging from a solitary eosinophilic granuloma to widespread disseminated disease. Based on the site of lesions, and number of involved sites (single or multisystem/local or multifocal), it is divided into two types: single-system LCH (SS-LSH) and multisystem LCH (MS-LCH). MS-LCH is less common than SS-LSH, accounting for about 20% of cases. SS-LSH affects single or multiple involvement of the single organs or systems: bone, with involvement of a single or multiple bones and many foci in many bones; skin; isolated pulmonary involvement; lymph nodes, excluding lymph nodes that drain the area of histiocyte infiltration or multiple lymph nodes (i.e., more than one lymph node group); hypothalamus-hypophysis/CNS; other, with involvement of oral mucosa, thyroid, thymus, or intestine. MS-LCH affects two or more organs or systems and may further be classified into low-risk multisystem and multisystem with risk organ involvement. Risk organs include hematopoietic system, spleen, and liver. Involvement of central nervous system (CNS) "risk" bones (temporal, sphenoid, ethmoid, zygomatic, mastoid, maxilla, and orbit) or pituitary is associated with higher risk of diabetes insipidus, endocrinopathies, and/or CNS involvement, including late neurodegenerative sequelae [34, 35].

Ronceray et al. [36] retrospectively analyzed 420 consecutive patients with MS-LCH. 102

(24%) presented pulmonary involvement at diagnosis. In multivariate analysis, lung involvement was not an independent prognostic variable and is excluded from the definition of risk organ involvement in MS-LCH.

Lung involvement in childhood LCH is rare. Le Louet et al. [37] found that 111 (7.4%) had lung involvement among 1482 children (<15 years). Seventeen (1.1%) were admitted to ICU due to respiratory failure. Of the 17 patients, 14 presented with lung involvement at the LCH diagnosis, and 7 patients (41%) had concomitant involvement of risk organ (hematologic, spleen, or liver). Lung involvement is associated with high mortality. They suggested that treatment guidelines should be improved for this group of patients, including viral infection prophylaxis and early administration of a new LCH therapy such as targeted therapy.

The prognosis of LCH depends on the number and location of affected organs. In adults, LCH most commonly involves the lungs, bones, skin, and pituitary gland. Hazim et al. [38] analyzed 240 LCH patients. 112 (47%) had pulmonary signs or symptoms at presentation. 108 (45%) were SS-LSH. The 5-year survival rates of SS-LCH, MS-LCH, and multisystem without lung involvement (MSNL-LCH) were 94%, 78%, and 75%, respectively.

9.2 Case 2

A 33-year-old woman complained of cough and shortness of breath for 1 year. She has a history of smoking.

Chest CT: Multiple cysts with varying sizes in both lungs (Fig. 7).

[Diagnosis] Pulmonary Langerhans cell histiocytosis.

[Diagnosis Basis] Chest CT scan shows diffuse cysts in both lungs, and the diagnosis of PLCH or pulmonary lymphangioleiomyomatosis (PLAM) should be considered. The patient has a definite history of smoking; the cysts are of varying sizes and irregular morphology, with nodules of varying sizes in some areas, which is more consistent with PLCH. The patient underwent lung biopsy to confirm the diagnosis of PLCH.

[Analysis] With the increase in smoking or second-hand smoke exposure among Asian women, the incidence of PLCH among women is on the rise. Wang et al. [39] retrospectively analyzed a cohort of Asian patients with PLCHs. Patients were subdivided into isolated pulmonary group and extrapulmonary recidivism group. The characteristics of the isolated group included predominantly young males under 40 years, a history of smoking, respiratory symptoms, more cystic lesions in CT scanning, more cellular Langerhans granulomas under the microscope, overexpression of P16 (66.7%), high PD-1 (100%) and low PD-L1 (33.3%) expressions, and no BRAF V600E mutation. In contrast, the extrapulmonary recidivism group showed significantly older age (>40 years old), recurrent spontaneous pneumothorax, more nodular changes in CT scanning, more interstitial fibrosis histologically, expression rates of 100% of P16,

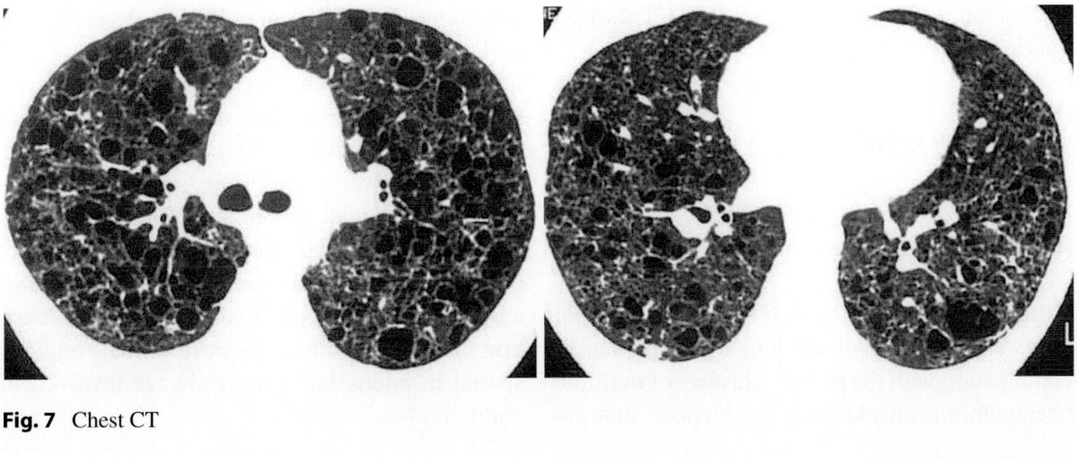

Fig. 7 Chest CT

66.7% of PD-1, and 33.3% of PD-L1, and importantly, BRAF V600E mutation was detected in 33.3% of this subdivision. The extremely low BRAF gene mutation in adult PLCH suggested that there might be other pathogeneses for this disease among Asian patients.

Gatalica et al. [40] analyzed 24 cases of neoplastic histiocytic diseases using immunohistochemical and mutational analysis in search of biomarkers for targeted therapy. BRAF V600E mutations were detected in 4/11 LCH and 4/4 Erdheim-Chester disease (ECD) cases. A pathogenic PTEN gene mutation and loss of PTEN protein expression were identified in the case of histiocytic sarcoma (HS). Increased expression of PD-L1 was seen in 3/4 ECD, 7/8 LCH, 3/3 follicular dendritic cell sarcoma (FDCS), and 1/1 HS. These results first found significant expression of the PD-L1 immune checkpoint protein in these disorders, which may provide theoretical basis for addition of immune checkpoint inhibitors to treat disseminated and/or refractory histiocytoses.

9.3 Case 3

A 3-year-old boy found a neck mass for 5 months, coughing and panting intermittently for 5 days. The child had multiple pneumothorax attacks in the past. Chest radiograph showed left-lung pneumothorax. Closed thoracic drainage was performed. Physical examination showed that the skin eczema was obvious on the scalp and trunk, and the left chest had a clear sense of holding snow. Scattered subcutaneous nodules can be found on the abdomen. Nails have protrusions, congestion, and breakage. Abdominal CT showed multiple liver cysts and right renal cyst.

Chest CT: Multiple cysts in both lungs (Fig. 8).

Brain CT: Skull defect and lytic lesions (red arrow) (Fig. 9).

[Diagnosis] Langerhans cell histiocytosis.

[Diagnosis Basis] Chest CT shows multiple thin-walled cysts, with obvious cystic fusion. In combination with the patient's history of multiple pneumothorax attacks, neck lymph node enlargement, rash, skull lesions, multiple liver cysts, and right kidney cyst, the diagnosis of LCH should be considered. The biopsy pathology of skin and left frontal skull was Langerhans cell histiocytosis.

[Analysis] LCH affects people of all ages, but occurs more commonly in children, with a peak incidence of 1–3 years of age. All of the organs or systems can be involved; the most commonly affected organ is the skeleton (80%), followed by skin (33%), pituitary (25%), liver (15%), spleen (15%), hematopoietic system (15%), lungs (15%), lymph nodes (5–10%), and central nervous system excluding the pituitary (2–4%) [41].

Skeletal involvement may present as single osteolytic lesion, multi-ostotic single system disease, or part of multisystem disease. The craniofacial bones are the most common site of involvement; no lesions are found in the hand or foot. Skeletal lesions in child rarely cause functional impairment [42]. Radiographically, osseous involvement in children with LCH is very similar to that seen in multiple myeloma, presenting as single or multiple lytic lesions. Compared with multiple myeloma, LCH lesions may be accompanied by periosteal reaction.

Skin involvement may be the most common manifestation in patients <2 years of age. Seborrheic dermatitis or eczematous eruption on the scalp and trunk is most common. Dhar et al. [43] retrospectively analyzed a total of 126 children less than 18 years diagnosed with LCH. Sixty-eight percent of cases affected only skin, and 32% of cases presented multisystem involvement at the initial presentation. Scaly papules were the most common morphologic finding in skin. 27.9% of cases showed progression of skin to systemic involvement. 76.7% of skin lesions cleared over a period of 2–4 years. Complete remission was seen in 56.9% of children over a period of 3–7 years, while 8.1% children died of complications and 31.8% were lost to follow-up.

Lung involvement is exceedingly rare in children. Only a small percentage of PLCH patients have respiratory symptoms and generally affect other organs. CT features of PLCH are similar in adult and pediatric populations with the exception that lung base near the costophrenic angle is spared in adults but almost always involved in children [44].

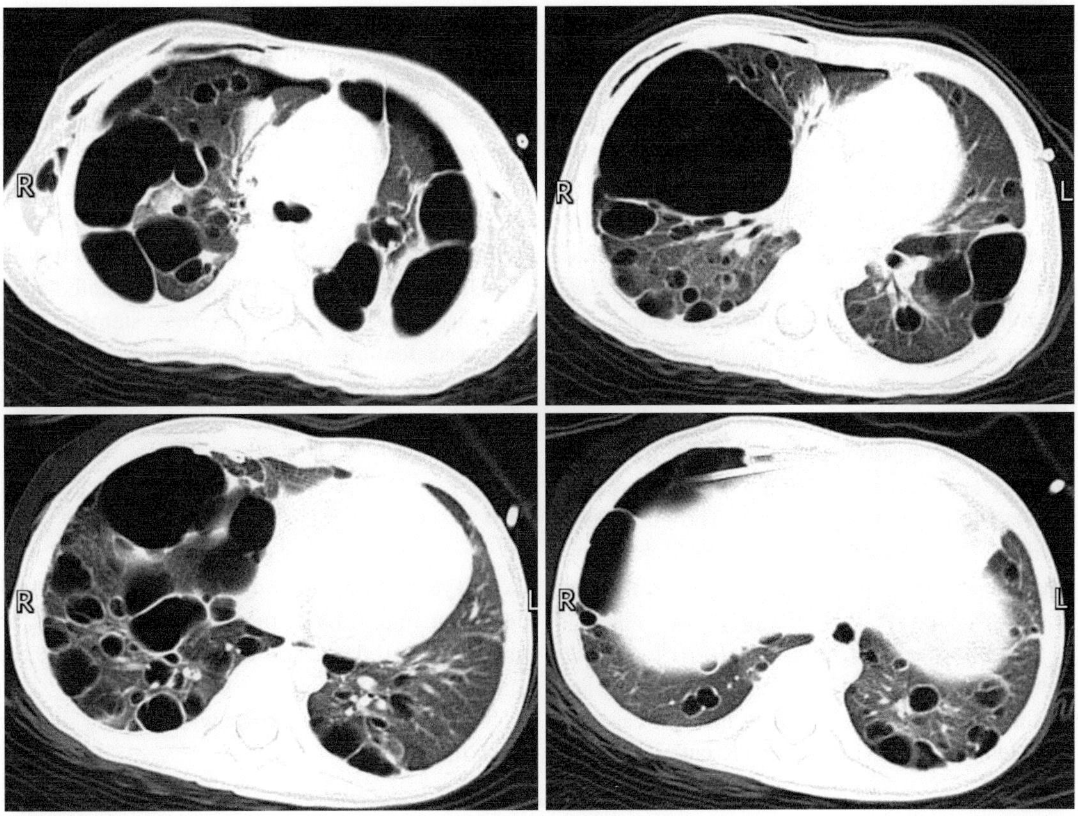

Fig. 8 Chest CT

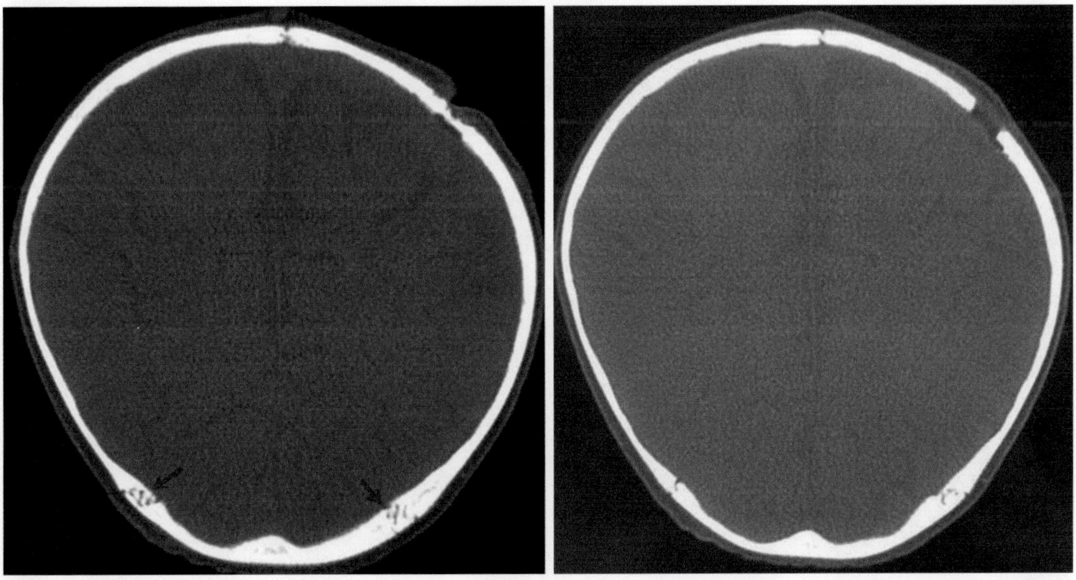

Fig. 9 Brain CT

Sequelae are common after LCH, although some are mild. Chow et al. [45] retrospectively reviewed 70 patients with a mean observation time of 12 years. The incidence of LCH-related sequelae was 56% (n = 39), which was more common in patients with multisystem diseases and reactivation. Prevalence of sequelae is as follows: orthopedic related 27%, diabetes insipidus 19%, growth retardation 13%, cosmetic 10%, neurological 7%, anterior pituitary hormone deficiency 7%, hearing 7%, hepatobiliary 4%, and ophthalmological 3%. Neurological sequelae could occur even 10 years after initial diagnosis of LCH. Reactivations, presence of CNS risk lesions, and radiation therapy were associated with a higher rate of sequelae. The cumulative incidence of reactivation was 34%. Most reactivations occurred in the first 2.5 years after diagnosis.

In multisystem LCH, up to 50–70% of cases recur after initial remission. In view of the fact that LCH is a neoplasm driven in most cases by oncogenic RAS/RAF/MEK/ERK pathway mutations, when LCH recurs, it is more reasonable to replace the concept of reactivation with the concept of disease recurrence or progression, and reactivation suggests a primary immunoregulatory etiology [46].

Some studies have evaluated the relationship between MAPK mutations and clinical manifestations and prognosis of PLCH. In children with LCH, BRAF V600E mutation is associated with increased risk of recurrence in systemic LCH, high-risk features (with risk organs), permanent injury, and poor short-term response to chemotherapy [47].

9.4 Case 4

A 34-year-old man complained of cough and fever for more than 2 months, expectoration for more than 10 days, and weight loss of 5 kg. He has a history of smoking.

Chest CT: Multiple cysts with varying sizes in both lungs (Fig. 10).

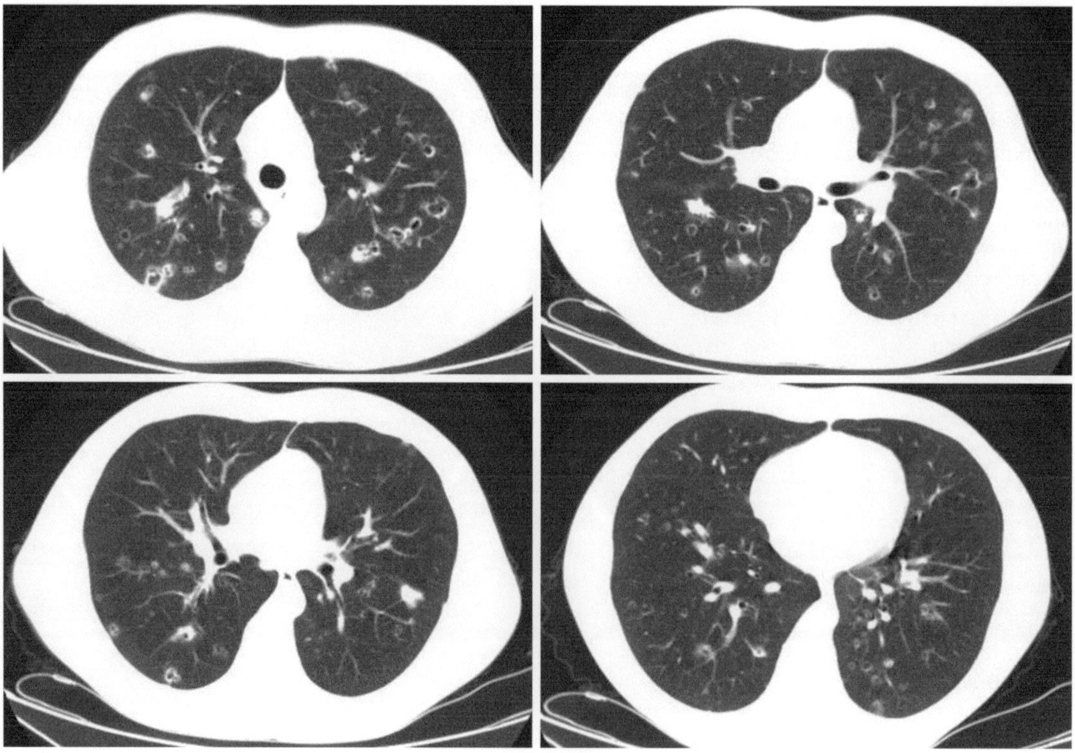

Fig. 10 Chest CT showed multiple cysts with varying sizes in both lungs

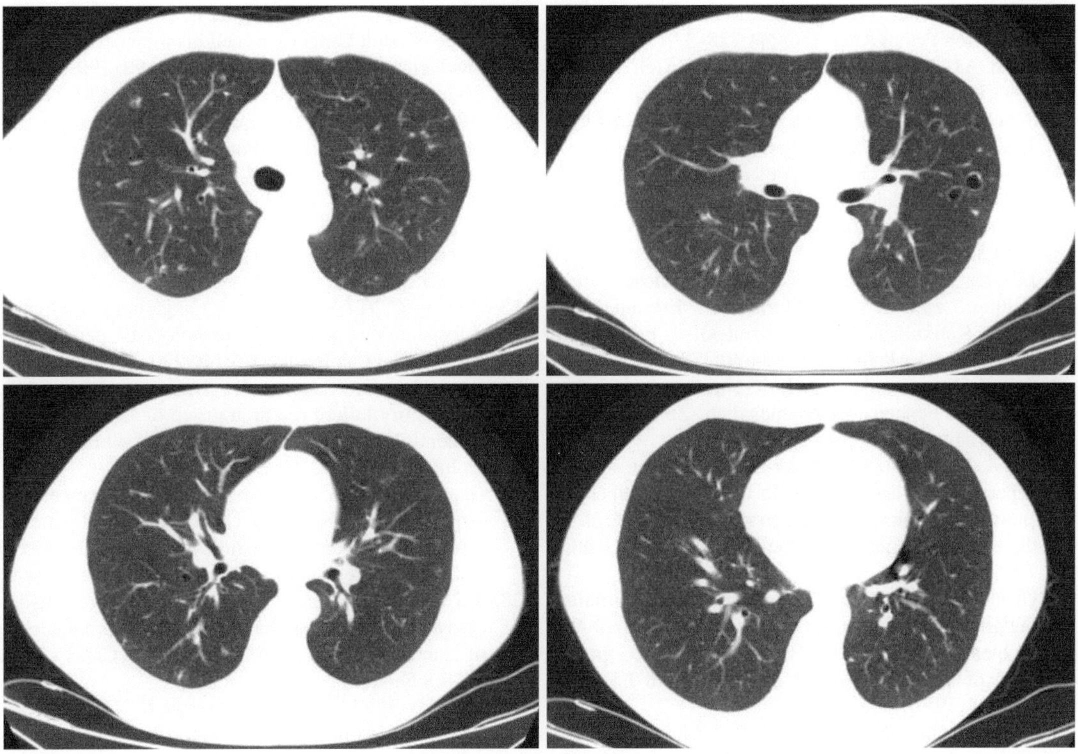

Fig. 11 Chest CT showed that the lesions were obviously absorbed

[Diagnosis] Pulmonary Langerhans cell histiocytosis.

[Diagnosis Basis] A young male has a history of smoking. Chest CT shows multiple nodules, cavities, and cysts with variable wall thickness and shape, which is consistent with PLCH imaging diagnosis. Lung biopsy confirmed the diagnosis of PLCH. The patient has smoking cessation for half a year, and chest CT showed that the lesions were obviously absorbed (Fig. 11).

[Analysis] The prognosis in PLCH is variable. Patients may experience clinical and radiological remission (25%), stabilization (50%), or disease progression (15–25%) after smoking cessation. In this case, CT scans demonstrate variable evolution of pulmonary nodules and cysts, including changes in size, thinning of walls, and a pattern of collapse into irregular small nodules and regression.

According to the appearance and distribution of the cysts, PLCH can be differentiated from lymphangiomyomatosis (LAM), lymphocytic interstitial pneumonia (LIP), and Birt-Hogg-Dubé syndrome (BHD). In PLCH, cysts are irregular in shape and size, have the middle and lung predominance, and are accompanied by nodules. In LAM, there are no nodules, the cysts are uniform and thin walled with homogeneous distribution, and the diameter is about 2–10 mm. As the disease progresses, cysts may coalesce and acquire larger size, and even progress to fibrosis. The cysts of LIP are variable shaped and larger (<3 cm) and have a random distribution, with basal, perivascular, or subpleural predominance, accompanied by subpleural nodules and septal thickening. In BHD, cysts show thin walls and multiple shapes and are mainly located at the basal and paramediastinal regions.

References

1. Histiocytosis syndromes in children. Writing Group of the Histiocyte Society. Lancet. 1987;1:208–209.
2. Emile JF, Abla O, Fraitag S, et al. Revised classification of histiocytoses and neoplasms of the macrophage-dendritic cell lineages. Blood. 2016;127:2672–81.

3. Langerhans P. Uber die nerven der menschlichen haut. Arch Pathol Anat. 1868;44:325–37.
4. Hand AJ. Polyuria and tuberculosis. Arch Pediatr. 1893;10:673–5.
5. Schüller A. Über eigenartige Schädeldefekte im Jugendalter. Fortschr Roentgenstr. 1915;23:12–8.
6. Christian HA. Defects in membranous bones, exophthalmos and diabetes insipidus: an unusual syndrome of dyspituitarism. Med Clin North Am. 1919;3:849–71.
7. Letterer E. Aleukamische retikulose (ein Beitrag zu den proliferativen Erkrankungen des Retikuloendothelialapparates). Frankfurter Zeitschritte der Pathology. 1924;30:377–94.
8. Siwe S. Die reticuloendotheliose-ein neues krankheitsbild unter denhepatosplenomegalien. Zeitschrift Fur Kinderheilkunde. 1933;55:212–47.
9. Abt A, Denenholz E. Letterer-Siwe's disease: splenohepatomegaly, associated with widespread hyperplasia of non-lipoid-storing macrophages; discussion of the so-called reticulo-endotheliosis. Am J Dis Child. 1936;51:499–22.
10. Otani S, Ehrlich J. Solitary granuloma of bone simulating primary neoplasm. Am J Pathol. 1940;16:479–90.
11. Lichtenstein L, Jaffe HL. Eosinophilic granuloma of bone. With report of a case. Am J Pathol. 1940;16:595–604.
12. Farber S. The nature of "solitary or eosinophilic granuloma" of bone. Am J Pathol. 1941;17:625.
13. Green WT, Farber S. Eosinophilic or solitary granuloma of bone. J Bone Joint Surg. 1942;24:499–526.
14. Lichtenstein L. Histiocytosis X; integration of eosinophilic granuloma of bone, Letterer-Siwe disease, and Schuller-Christian disease as related manifestations of a single nosologic entity. AMA Arch Pathol. 1953;56:84–102.
15. Birbeck MS, Breathnach AS, Everall JD. An electron microscope study of basal melanocytes and high-level clear cells (Langerhans cells) in vitiligo. J Invest Dermatol. 1961;37:51–63.
16. Friedman B, Hanaoka H. Langerhans cell granules in eosinophilic granuloma of bone. J Bone Joint Surg Am. 1969;51:367–74.
17. Nezelof C, Basset F, Rousseau MF. Histiocytosis X histogenetic arguments for a Langerhans cell origin. Biomedicine. 1973;18:365–71.
18. Risdall RJ, Dehner LP, Duray P, et al. Histiocytosis X (Langerhans' cell histiocytosis). Prognostic role of histopathology. Arch Pathol Lab Med. 1983;107:59–63.
19. Allen CE, Li L, Peters TL, et al. Cell-specific gene expression in Langerhans cell histiocytosis lesions reveals a distinct profile compared with epidermal Langerhans cells. J Immunol. 2010;184:4557–67.
20. Vassallo R, Harari S, Tazi A. Current understanding and management of pulmonary Langerhans cell histiocytosis. Thorax. 2017;72:937–45.
21. Badalian-Very G, Vergilio JA, Degar BA, et al. Recurrent BRAF mutations in Langerhans cell histiocytosis. Blood. 2010;116:1919–23.
22. Jouenne F, Chevret S, Bugnet E, et al. Genetic landscape of adult Langerhans cell histiocytosis with lung involvement. Eur Respir J. 2020;55:1901190.
23. Bigenwald C, Le Berichel J, Wilk CM, et al. $BRAF^{V600E}$-induced senescence drives Langerhans cell histiocytosis pathophysiology. Nat Med. 2021;27:851–61.
24. Liu H, Osterburg AR, Flury J, et al. MAPK mutations and cigarette smoke promote the pathogenesis of pulmonary Langerhans cell histiocytosis. JCI Insight. 2020;5:e132048.
25. Roden AC, Yi ES. Pulmonary Langerhans cell histiocytosis: an update from the pathologists' perspective. Arch Pathol Lab Med. 2016;140:230–40.
26. Watanabe R, Tatsumi K, Hashimoto S, et al. Respiratory failure research group of Japan. Clinicoepidemiological features of pulmonary histiocytosis X. Intern Med. 2001;40:998–1003.
27. Haupt R, Nanduri V, Calevo MG, et al. Permanent consequences in Langerhans cell histiocytosis patients: a pilot study from the histiocyte society-late effects study group. Pediatr Blood Cancer. 2004;42:438–44.
28. Ma J, Laird J, Chau K, et al. Langerhans cell histiocytosis in adults is associated with a high prevalence of hematologic and solid malignancies. Cancer Med. 2019;8:58–66.
29. Radzikowska E, Błasińska-Przerwa K, Wiatr E, et al. Pneumothorax in patients with pulmonary Langerhans cell histiocytosis. Lung. 2018;196:715–20.
30. Singla A, Kopras EJ, Gupta N. Spontaneous pneumothorax and air travel in pulmonary Langerhans cell histiocytosis: a patient survey. Respir Investig. 2019;57:582–9.
31. Lorillon G, Jouenne F, Baroudjian B, et al. Response to Trametinib of a pulmonary Langerhans cell histiocytosis harboring a MAP2K1 deletion. Am J Respir Crit Care Med. 2018;198:675–8.
32. Wajda N, Zhu Z, Jandarov R, et al. Clinical outcomes and survival following lung transplantation in patients with pulmonary Langerhans cell histiocytosis. Respirology. 2020;25:644–50.
33. Benattia A, Bugnet E, Walter-Petrich A, et al. Long-term outcomes of adult pulmonary Langerhans cell histiocytosis: a prospective cohort. Eur Respir J. 2022;59:2101017.
34. Girschikofsky M, Arico M, Castillo D, et al. Management of adult patients with Langerhans cell histiocytosis: recommendations from an expert panel on behalf of Euro-Histio-Net. Orphanet J Rare Dis. 2013;8:72.
35. Picarsic J, Jaffe R. Nosology and pathology of Langerhans cell histiocytosis. Hematol Oncol Clin North Am. 2015;29:799–82.
36. Ronceray L, Potschger U, Janka G, et al. Pulmonary involvement in pediatric-onset multisystem Langerhans cell histiocytosis: effect on course and outcome. J Pediatr. 2012;161:129–33.e1–3.
37. Le Louet S, Barkaoui MA, Miron J, et al. Childhood Langerhans cell histiocytosis with severe lung

involvement: a nationwide cohort study. Orphanet J Rare Dis. 2020;15:241.
38. Hazim AZ, Ruan GJ, Hu M, et al. Langerhans cell histiocytosis with lung involvement in isolation and multisystem disease: staging, natural history, and comparative survival. Am J Hematol. 2021;96:1604–10.
39. Wang J, Xie L, Miao Y, et al. Adult pulmonary Langerhans cell histiocytosis might consist of two distinct groups: isolated form and extrapulmonary recidivism type. Ann Transl Med. 2021;9:357.
40. Gatalica Z, Bilalovic N, Palazzo JP, et al. Disseminated histiocytoses biomarkers beyond BRAFV600E: frequent expression of PD-L1. Oncotarget. 2015;6:19819–25.
41. Haupt R, Minkov M, Astigarraga I, et al. Langerhans cell histiocytosis (LCH): guidelines for diagnosis, clinical work-up, and treatment for patients till the age of 18 years. Pediatr Blood Cancer. 2013;60:175–84.
42. Abdelaal AHK, Sedky M, Gohar S, et al. Skeletal involvement in children with Langerhans cell histiocytosis: healing, complications, and functional outcome. SICOT J. 2020;6:28.
43. Dhar S, Srinivas SM, Dhar S, et al. Langerhans cell histiocytosis in children: a retrospective case series of 126 cases. Pediatr Dermatol. 2020;37:1085–9.
44. Bano S, Chaudhary V, Narula MK, et al. Pulmonary Langerhans cell histiocytosis in children: a spectrum of radiologic findings. Eur J Radiol. 2014;83:47–56.
45. Chow TW, Leung WK, Cheng FWT, et al. Late outcomes in children with Langerhans cell histiocytosis. Arch Dis Child. 2017;102:830–5.
46. Egeler RM, Katewa S, Leenen PJ, et al. Langerhans cell histiocytosis is a neoplasm and consequently its recurrence is a relapse: in memory of Bob Arceci. Pediatr Blood Cancer. 2016;63:1704–12.
47. Héritier S, Emile JF, Barkaoui MA, et al. BRAF mutation correlates with high-risk Langerhans cell histiocytosis and increased resistance to first-line therapy. J Clin Oncol. 2016;34:3023–30.

GPSR Compliance

The European Union's (EU) General Product Safety Regulation (GPSR) is a set of rules that requires consumer products to be safe and our obligations to ensure this.

If you have any concerns about our products, you can contact us on ProductSafety@springernature.com

In case Publisher is established outside the EU, the EU authorized representative is:

Springer Nature Customer Service Center GmbH
Europaplatz 3
69115 Heidelberg, Germany

Batch number: 08049554

Printed by Printforce, the Netherlands